Core Curriculum for

Ambulatory Care Nursing

Second Edition
Candia Baker Laughlin, MS, RN, C

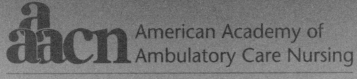

American Academy of
Ambulatory Care Nursing

Real Nurses. Real Issues. Real Solutions.

ISBN: 0-9768125-5-X

Published for AAACN by
Anthony J. Jannetti, Inc., East Holly Avenue, Box 56, Pitman, NJ 08071-0056
856-256-2300; FAX 856-589-7463; www.ajj.com

DISCLAIMER

The authors, reviewers, editors, and publishers of this book have made serious efforts to ensure that treatments, practices, and procedures are accurate and conform to standards accepted at the time of publication. Due to constant changes in information resulting from continuing research and clinical experience, reasonable differences in opinions among authorities, unique aspects of individual clinical situations, and the possibility of human error in preparing such a publication require that the reader exercise individual judgment when making a clinical decision, and if necessary, consult and compare information from other authorities, professionals, or sources.

Contributors

Nancy M. Albert, PhD, CCNS, CCRN, CNA
Director, Nursing Research and Innovation
Clinical Nurse Specialist
The Cleveland Clinic
Cleveland, Ohio

Ida M. Androwich, PhD, RN, BC, FAAN
Professor and Director, Health Systems
Management
Loyola University
Chicago, Illinois

Cindy Angiulo, MSN, RN, C
Assistant Administrator, Patient Care Services
University of Washington Medical Center
Seattle, Washington
Past President
American Academy of Ambulatory Care Nursing

Jo Ann Appleyard, PhD, RN
Clinical Assistant Professor
University of Wisconsin
Milwaukee College of Nursing
Milwaukee, Wisconson
Past President
American Academy of Ambulatory Care Nursing

Carole A. Becker, MS, RN
Director, Clinical Development
McKesson Provider Technologies
Medical Management Systems
Scottsdale, Arizona

Mary Anne Bord-Hoffman, MN, RN, C
Nurse Manager
VA Palo Alto HealthCare System, San Jose Clinic
San Jose, California

Linda Brixey, RN
Program Manager, Clinical Education
Kelsey-Seybold Clinic
Houston, Texas

Rebecca Elliot Bryan, MS, RN, C
Executive Director
Hospice of Redmond, Sisters
Redmond, Oregon

Michelle M. Budzinski-Braunscheidel, BSN, RN
Ambulatory Clinical Instructor
The Cleveland Clinic
Cleveland, Ohio

Renée Y. Cecil, BSN, RN
Nurse Coordinator, Sickle Cell Clinical Program
Children's Hospital of Philadelphia
Philadelphia, Pennsylvania

Linda D'Angelo, MSN, RN, MBA, CMPE
Independent Consultant
Champaign, Illinois
Past President
American Academy of Ambulatory Care Nursing

Pamela Del Monte, MS, RN, C
Field Communications Program Manager
Department of Veterans Affairs
Durham, North Carolina

Gail De Luca, MS, RN, CS, FNP
Instructor
Loyola University
Chicago, Illinois

Elizabeth Dickey, MPH, RN, FNP
Practice Management Consultant
Tucson, Arizona
Past President
American Academy of Ambulatory Care Nursing

Linda L. Edwards, RN, MHS, CDE
Diabetes Education Coordinator
Kaiser Permanente
Denver, Colorado

Eileen M. Esposito, RN, C, MPA, CPHQ
Assistant Executive Director
Ambulatory Patient Care Services and Quality
North Shore – LIJ Health System
Great Neck, New York

Contributors

Linda L. Gehring, PhD, APNP, RN, BC
Assistant Professor
Alverno College
Milwaukee, Wisconsin

Carrol Gold, PhD, RN
Distinguished Professor Emerita
Loyola University
Chicago, Illinois

Sheila A. Haas, PhD, RN, FAAN
Dean; Professor
Niehoff School of Nursing, Loyola University
Chicago, Illinois
Past President
American Academy of Ambulatory Care Nursing

Clare E. Hastings, PhD, RN, FAAN
Chief, Nursing and Patient Care Services
National Institutes of Health Clinical Center
Bethesda, Maryland
Past President
American Academy of Ambulatory Care Nursing

Traci S. Haynes, MSN, RN, CEN
Nurse Manager, Clinical Services
McKesson Corporation
Scottsdale, Arizona

Lois J. Iiams, MSHCA, RN, HEM
Director, Nursing Practice
Kaiser Permanente
Rockville, Maryland

E. Mary Johnson, BSN, RN, CNA
Consultant
The Cleveland Clinic
Cleveland, Ohio
Past President
American Academy of Ambulatory Care Nursing

Margaret Ross Kraft, PhD, RN
Assistant Professor
Loyola University
Chicago, Illinois

Sharon L. Lanzetta, MSN, RN, C
Ambulatory Care Nurse Manager
University of Michigan Health System
Ann Arbor, Michigan

Candia Baker Laughlin, MS, RN, C
Director of Nursing, Ambulatory Care Services
University of Michigan Health System
Ann Arbor, Michigan
Past President
American Academy of Ambulatory Care Nursing

Anita Markovich, MSN, BSN, MPA, CPHQ
Director, Quality Services Division
Our Lady of Lourdes Memorial Hospital
Binghamton, New York

Margaret Fisk Mastal, PhD, RN
Director, Special Projects
Delmarva Foundation for Medical Care
Washington, DC
Past President
American Academy of Ambulatory Care Nursing

Stephanie G. Metzger, MS, RN, CPNP
Pediatric Nurse Practitioner
Virginia Treatment Center for Children
Richmond, Virginia

Rachel Nosowsky, JD
Assistant General Counsel
University of Michigan
Ann Arbor, Michigan

Susan M. Paschke, MSN, RN, BC, CNA
Associate Chief Nursing Officer, Operations
The Cleveland Clinic
Cleveland, Ohio

Carolyn Pritchyk, MSN, RN, CNOR
Perioperative Clinical Specialist
Kaiser Permanente
Falls Church, Virginia

Contributors

Rebecca Linn Pyle, MS, RN
Regional Nursing Practice Leader
Kaiser Permanente
Aurora, Colorado
Past President
American Academy of Ambulatory Care Nursing

Christine Schaefer, MSN, RN, CDE, BC-ADM
Diabetes Care Manager
Kaiser Permanente
Denver, Colorado

Beth Ann Swan, PhD, FAAN, CRNP
Associate Professor
Jefferson College of Health Professions
Department of Nursing, Thomas Jefferson
University
Philadelphia, Pennsylvania
President, 2006-2007
American Academy of Ambulatory Care Nursing

Jane Westmoreland Swanson, PhD, RN, CNAA, BC
Director, Institute for Professional Development
Cedars-Sinai Medical Center
Los Angeles, California
Past President
American Academy of Ambulatory Care Nursing

Barbara G. White, MS, RN
Clinical Associate Professor
Arizona State University College of Nursing
Tempe, Arizona
Past President
American Academy of Ambulatory Care Nursing

Carol Jo Wilson, PhD, RN, CS, FNP
Associate Dean
University of St. Francis
Joliet, Illinois

Statements of Disclosure

Clare E. Hastings: This is to certify that Chapter 2, "The Ambulatory Care Practice Arena," fits the description in the U.S. Copyright Act of a "United States government work." It was written as part of the author's official duties as a government employee. While it cannot be copyrighted, this chapter is freely available to the American Academy of Ambulatory Care Nursing (AAACN) for publication without a copyright notice. There are no restrictions on its use, now or subsequently, and the author retains no rights in the article.

JoAnn Appleyard: The author is a member of the Speakers' Bureau for GlaxoSmithKline, Medtronic, Nitromed, and Scios. She is also a consultant for GlaxoSmithKlinke and Medtronic.

Ida M. Androwich: The author is an unpaid member of the Advisory Board of CINAHL, a past consultant to Zynx, an unpaid member of the Zynx Advisory Board, and an unpaid Fellow in the Centers for Classification Studies (NIC and NOC).

All other authors have no statements to disclose.

Reviewers

Mary Anne Bord-Hoffman, MN, RN, C
Nurse Manager
VA Palo Alto HealthCare System, San Jose Clinic
San Jose, California

Traci L. Brooks, BSN, RN, C
Duty Under Instruction
University of San Diego, United States Navy
San Diego, California

Nancy Burns, MSN, RN
Clinical Nurse Manager
Baystate Medical Center
Springfield, Massachusetts

Catherine Cahill, MS, RN, C
Associate Director, Pediatric Subspecialty Service
Children's Hospital of Montefiore
Bronx, New York

Jaclynn Cunningham, MS, RN, C
Administrative Director, Outpatient Clinic
William Beaumont Hospital
Royal Oak, Michigan

Ellen M. Curran, RN, CEN, RN, C
Staff Nurse
Intellicare Inc.
Portland, Maine

Judy Dawson-Jones, RN, MPH
Director, Ambulatory Nursing
Children's Hospital of Philadelphia
Philadelphia, Pennsylvania

Grace L. Doherty, MS, BSN, RN
Director, Satellite Services
Children's Memorial Hospital
Chicago, Illinois

Marilyn K. Douglas, DNSc, RN, FAAN
Editor, *Journal of Transcultural Nursing*
Associate Chief of Nursing Service for Research
VA Palo Alto Health Care System
Palo Alto, California

Karen Griffin, MSN, RN, CNAA
Associate Chief, Nursing Service, Ambulatory Care
South Texas Veterans Healthcare System
San Antonio, Texas

Kathleen P. Krone, MS, RN
Past President
American Academy of Ambulatory Care Nursing
Ann Arbor, Michigan

Lenora J. Matthews-Flint, MS, MSN, RN, CNS, PHN
Director, Population Care Management
Kaiser Permanente
Baldwin Park, California

Debbie McCash, BSN, RN
Clinical Education Program Administrator
University of Texas Southwestern Medical Center,
Ambulatory Services
Dallas, Texas

Patricia A. Menendez, BSN, RN, C
Assistant Director, Department of Accreditation
The Cleveland Clinic
Cleveland, Ohio

MaryAlice Morro, MSN, BSN
NC, USN/Director, Patient Services
United States Naval Hospital
Yokosuka, Japan

Regina C. Phillips, MSN, RN
Process Manager, Delegation Compliance
Humana, Inc.
Chicago, Illinois
Past President
American Academy of Ambulatory Care Nursing

Sandra W. Reifsteck, MS, RN, FACMPE
Regional Consultant
Institute for Healthcare Communications
Champaign, Illinois
Past President
American Academy of Ambulatory Care Nursing

Reviewers

Joan Robinson, MS, RN
Consultant
J. Robinson Consulting
Charlevoix, Michigan
Editor
*Core Curriculum for Ambulatory Care Nursing,
First Edition*

Carol C. Saxman, MSN, RN, C
Patient Care Specialist
Lehigh Valley Hospital
Allentown, Pennsylvania

Kitty Shulman, MSN, RN, C
Director, Children's Specialty Center
St. Luke's Regional Medical Center
Boise, Idaho

Maridel Candy Soutar, MSN, RN
Lieutenant, Nurse Corps, United States Navy Reserve
Department Administrator, OB/GYN Services
Kaiser Permanente South Bay Medical Center
Harbor City, California

Rowena Pat Stevens-Ross, MSN, BSN, RN
CDR, NC, USN/Deputy Director, Branch Clinics
Naval Hospital Camp Pendleton
Oceanside, California

Vivene E. Walters, MSN, RN, C
Health Care Integrator
United States Air Force, Andrews Air Force Base
Clinton, Maryland

Charlene Williams, BSN, RN, C, BC, MBA
Manager, Nurse on Call
The Cleveland Clinic
Cleveland, Ohio
President-Elect, 2006-2007
American Academy of Ambulatory Care Nursing

Marcia Winston, MSN, CPNP, AE, C
Certified Pediatric Nurse Practitioner
Certified Asthma Educator
Children's Hospital of Philadelphia
Philadelphia, Pennsylvania

Cassandra Fox Wood, BSN, RN, C
Staff Nurse, Infectious Diseases
Kaiser Permanente
Lafayette, Colorado

Cheryl A. Zeise-Schmidt, BSN, RN, C
Staff Nurse
Group Health Cooperative, HMO
Madison, Wisconsin

David C. Zimmerman, RN, MHA, C
Captain, United States Air Force
Chief, Healthcare Integration
United States Air Force
Yokota, Japan

Preface

The mission of the American Academy of Ambulatory Care Nursing (AAACN) is to "Advance the art and science of ambulatory care nursing." This second edition of the *Core Curriculum for Ambulatory Care Nursing* represents a major effort toward that goal. The original text served its purpose well as a state-of-the-art document on ambulatory care nursing, and this text is intended to continue in that vein. Nursing in ambulatory care is growing in volume, magnitude, and complexity as demands for health care continue to shift to ambulatory care settings. Additionally, ambulatory care nursing is growing in its body of knowledge and its required competencies. Ambulatory care nurses are challenged daily to find cost-effective ways to assist patients and families in promoting wellness, preventing illness, and managing acute, chronic and terminal conditions to achieve the most positive health status attainable. Ambulatory care nurses accomplish this through episodic interactions with patients in a variety of settings and through a variety of methods. This second edition is offered as a resource to support that specialty practice in all its complexity and breadth.

The *Core Curriculum for Ambulatory Care Nursing, Second Edition,* is intended as a reference for nurses in the ambulatory care practice arena to advance their knowledge and understanding of patient care issues, as well as their role and the context of nursing in ambulatory care settings in the current health care environment. In recognition of the value of this continuing education activity, contact hours are offered following the study of each chapter. Additionally, the text was organized and written for the purpose of providing a comprehensive review for those nurses who work in ambulatory care and wish to prepare for certification as an expert ambulatory care nurse through the American Nurses Credentialing Center's certification examination. Nurses who practice in other settings and are considering transitioning to ambulatory care will find it valuable in understanding this specialty area. Furthermore, those nurses who have decided to make such a transition will find the text a valuable resource in orienting to their new role in ambulatory care. Managers and others who support the practice and development of ambulatory care nurses, such as staff development personnel and preceptors, will find the text valuable as a resource both for themselves and also for use in assisting staff to advance their knowledge and skills. Faculty and students in schools of nursing may use this text to understand the unique attributes of the ambulatory care nursing role in preparing future nurses who should understand the role in the continuum of nursing care, as well as consider it in building a career in nursing.

The *Ambulatory Care Nursing Conceptual Framework*, developed by a "think tank" of AAACN expert members in 1998, is the basis for the text's organization. The sections of the book reflect the framework's three roles identified for the ambulatory care nurse: organization/systems role, professional role, and clinical role. The core areas of knowledge and skills within each of those three roles are reflected in those sections of the text. The core knowledge and skill dimensions that are part of the clinical role are applied to patient populations served by ambulatory care nurses, and are defined as well, acutely ill, chronically ill, or terminally ill.

Section One addresses the core knowledge and skills of the **organizational/systems role**. It includes updated content on the Conceptual Framework, standards of practice, the practice arena and context of delivering ambulatory nursing care, financial considerations, legal aspects, advocacy, informatics, telehealth, and other conceptual and operational dimensions of care. Section Two speaks to the **professional nursing role** of the ambulatory care nurse, including updated as well as new content on leadership, ethics, regulatory compliance, patient safety, professional development, and application of evidence and performance improvement in practice. Section Three starts with two new chapters about the core concepts and skill dimensions of the **clinical nursing role**, including application of the nursing process, technical skills, and multicultural nursing care. The new Chapter 19 addresses the concepts and skills of patient education and counseling, and clinical knowledge content related to preventive health counseling. Section Three is completed with four chapters of content on the care of the four ambulatory care patient populations described in the Conceptual Framework: the well patient, the acutely ill patient, the chronically ill patient, and the terminally ill patient. The clinical conditions and preventive care issues selected for inclusion are those most common to patients seen across the wide variety of ambulatory patient care settings.

The content is presented in outline format for easy review and reference. Key terms that are defined in the text are also captured in the Glossary. Many Web resources, community agencies and published references are identified throughout the text and at the end of chapters for further information. It is important to realize that this content captured the best information available at a point in time, and the reader is encouraged to seek current sources of information on rapidly changing areas, such as immunization science and recommendations.

The American Academy of Ambulatory Care Nursing and the association management firm of Anthony J. Jannetti, Inc. are commended for their vision and leadership in supporting the publication of the *Core Curriculum for Ambulatory Care Nursing, Second Edition*. It is fortunate that so many authors and reviewers provided a wealth of expertise from their diverse settings, backgrounds, and geographic locations across the United States. One of the greatest member benefits of AAACN is the rich network that the organization offers, and this text is another method through which it is enjoyed. All these individuals and groups have demonstrated tremendous commitment to advancing the art and science of ambulatory care nursing that is evident in the pages that follow.

Candia Baker Laughlin, MS, RN, C

Acknowledgments

The authors who researched and wrote the 23 chapters in this publication are all experts in ambulatory care nursing, and it has been my privilege to work with all of them. Many of them had contributed similar content in the first edition, and they carefully researched, updated, and revised it to support best practices in today's health care environment. I was also pleased to recruit some new authors, all of whom proved to be excellent and rose to the challenges of the scope and nature of this text. Additionally, I thank the content experts who reviewed every page, most of whom reviewed several chapters. Writing and reviewing content for a textbook requires hard work and perseverance. Only those passionate about ambulatory care nursing as a specialty would do such a thing. I owe a debt of gratitude to each and every one of them for their responsiveness and commitment.

I would also like to thank those individuals who supported the development of this second edition. I thank Sheila Haas, who lead the AAACN expert "think tank" that originated the *Ambulatory Care Nursing Conceptual Framework*, which is the organizing framework of this core curriculum. I am immensely grateful to Lori Ann Tornatore, who provided her support and expertise in managing deadlines, tracking chapters, communicating with authors and reviewers, and reassuring me when I became anxious. I thank Carol Ford for her guidance, encouragement, support, and superb editorial skill. I thank the AAACN Board of Directors for offering me this opportunity and particularly Charlene Williams, who served as Board Liaison.

Finally, I want to thank those who provided me personal and professional mentorship, counsel, encouragement, and support. My parents, Frederick and Patricia Baker, taught me that hard work is the most important factor in reaching high goals. My wonderful husband, Harry, was the person who ultimately told me that I "had to" take on this project and has provided every bit of the support that he promised in order to make it possible. My sons, Tom and Patrick, provided me with support with their love and tolerance of my time constraints. My friend and AAACN partner, Cynthia Nowicki Hnatiuk, who has recognized and encouraged my passion for AAACN for many years, persuaded me that I was ready to do this, and that she was "counting on me." Most of all, I thank Joan Robinson, who not only edited the outstanding first edition of this text, but has been my mentor as a nurse and leader in ambulatory care nursing at the University of Michigan and in AAACN. Her faith in me has always exceeded my own, and I am grateful.

Candia Baker Laughlin, MS, RN, C

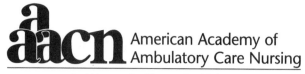

American Academy of
Ambulatory Care Nursing

Real Nurses. Real Issues. Real Solutions.

IDENTITY STATEMENT: The American Academy of Ambulatory Care Nursing (AAACN) is the association of professional nurses and associates who identify ambulatory care practice as essential to the continuum of accessible, high quality, and cost-effective health care.

MISSION AND CORE PURPOSE: Advance the art and science of ambulatory care nursing.

CORE VALUES: The following values guide member and the organization vision, actions and relationships:
1) Responsible health care delivery for individuals and communities.
2) Visionary and accountable leadership.
3) Productive partnerships and alliances.
4) Diversity.
5) Continual advancement of professional ambulatory care nursing practice.
6) Collaborative professional community.

GOALS:

○ **KNOWLEDGE –** AAACN will be the recognized source for knowledge in ambulatory care nursing.

○ **EDUCATION –** Nurses will have the leadership skills and capabilities to articulate, promote, and practice nursing successfully in an ambulatory care setting.

○ **ADVOCACY –** Nurses, employers, and third party payers will recognize and value ambulatory care nursing.

○ **COMMUNITY –** Ambulatory care nurses will have a supportive and collaborative community in which to share professional interests, experience, and practice.

ABOUT AAACN: AAACN (formerly the American Academy of Ambulatory Nursing Administration) was founded in 1978 as a not for profit, educational forum. In 1993, the organization's name was changed to the American Academy of Ambulatory Care Nursing (AAACN). Membership was broadened to include nurses in direct practice, education, and research roles as well as those in management and administration. Today, membership is open to nurses and other professionals interested in ambulatory care nursing. Corporations and individual corporate representatives are also welcomed as members.

Ambulatory practice settings include universities, medical centers, HMOs, group practices, urgent care centers, physician office settings, hospital based ambulatory care settings, military, community health, and others. The Academy serves as a voice for ambulatory care nurses across the continuum of health care delivery and has membership in the Nursing Organizations Alliance (NOA). The Alliance provides a forum for nursing organizations to dialogue, collaborate, and facilitate policy formulation on professional practice and national health.

MEMBERSHIP BENEFITS: Academy membership benefits include discounted rates to the AAACN National Preconference and Conference, distance learning programs, publications, and the ANCC ambulatory care nursing certification exam; the annual conference includes multiple practice innovations, industry exhibits, and numerous networking opportunities; the bimonthly newsletter - Viewpoint; subscription to **one** of four journals — *Nursing Economic$, MEDSURG Nursing, Dermatology Nursing, or Pediatric Nursing;* opportunity to join a special interest group in the area of: Leadership; Patient Education; Pediatrics; Staff Education; Telehealth Nursing Practice; Veterans Affairs; and Tri-Service Military; awards and scholarship programs; access to national experts and colleagues through AAACN's online membership directory, monthly E-newsletter, list serves and web site **aaacn.org**; and online Career Center.

AAACN PUBLICATIONS/EDUCATION RESOURCES:

- ○ Ambulatory Care Nurse Staffing: An Annotated Bibliography
- ○ Ambulatory Care Nursing Administration and Practice Standards
- ○ Ambulatory Care Nursing Certification Review Course Syllabus
- ○ Ambulatory Care Nursing Certification Review Course CD-ROM
- ○ Guide to Ambulatory Care Nursing Orientation and Competency Assessment
- ○ Ambulatory Care Nursing Self-Assessment
- ○ Telehealth Nursing Practice (TNP) Administration and Practice Standards
- ○ Telehealth Nursing Practice Core Course (TNPCC) Manual
- ○ Telehealth Nursing Practice Core Course (TNPCC) CD-ROM
- ○ Telehealth Nursing Practice Resource Directory

AAACN COURSES:

- • Ambulatory Care Nursing Certification Review Course*
- • Telehealth Nursing Practice Core Course (TNPCC)*

  *Both courses can be presented at your location.

ANNUAL CONFERENCE:

AAACN provides cutting edge information and education at its annual conference, usually held in the month of March or April. Nurses from across the country as well as international colleagues come together to network, learn from each other, and share knowledge and skills. Renowned speakers in the field of ambulatory care present topics of current interest offering over 30 contact hours. An Exhibit Hall featuring the products and services of vendors serving the ambulatory care community provides information and resources to attendees.

LIVE AUDIO SEMINARS:

Monthly continuing education on timely topics is convenient for nurses and cost effective.

CERTIFICATION:

AAACN values the importance of certification and promotes achieving this level of competency through its educational products to prepare nurses to take the ambulatory care nursing and telephone nursing practice certification examinations.

CORPORATE COLLABORATIONS:

Together, working with corporate colleagues, AAACN continues to advance the delivery of ambulatory care to patients. AAACN is open to alliances or collaborations with corporate industry to achieve mutual goals. Corporations are encouraged to contact the national office to suggest ways AAACN can work with corporations to advance the practice of ambulatory care nursing.

American Academy of Ambulatory Care Nursing
P.O. Box 56, Pitman, NJ 08071-0056
Phone: 800-262-6877   Fax: 856-589-7463
E-mail: aaacn@ajj.com   Web site: www.aaacn.org

Contents

The Organizational/ Systems Role of the Ambulatory Care Nurse

Chapter 1

Ambulatory Care Nursing Specialty Practice

Sheila A. Haas, PhD, RN, FAAN

Objectives

Study of the information presented in this chapter will enable the learner to:
1. Discuss the characteristics of ambulatory care nursing practice.
2. Differentiate ambulatory care nursing practice from other forms of specialty nursing practice.
3. Discuss the ambulatory care nursing conceptual framework.
4. Enumerate opportunities for nurses in ambulatory care nursing.
5. Discuss ambulatory care standards.

Key Points

1. The definition of ambulatory care nursing must delineate the scope and unique dimensions of ambulatory care nursing practice and differentiate ambulatory care nursing from other areas of specialty nursing practice.
2. A simple, concise blueprint of ambulatory care nursing practice is essential.
3. Change creates opportunities for nurses in ambulatory care.
4. Standards promote effective management of increasingly complex ambulatory care nursing roles and responsibilities in a changing health care environment.

mbulatory care nursing is a unique realm of nursing practice. It is characterized by rapid, focused assessments of patients, long-term nurse/patient/family relationships, and teaching and translating prescriptions for care into doable activities for patients and their caregivers. Ambulatory care nursing is a specialty practice area that is characterized by nurses responding rapidly to high volumes of patients in a short span of time while dealing with issues that are not always predictable. Because ambulatory care nursing spans all populations of patients, and care ranges from wellness/prevention to illness and support of the dying, there is a need for an ambulatory care nursing conceptual framework that specifies (1) the concepts unique to ambulatory care nursing, and (2) how these core concepts are linked in ambulatory care nursing practice. Ambulatory care nursing provides multiple opportunities as well as challenges for nurses. It offers great interdisciplinary as well as autonomous practice opportunities. It demands that ambulatory care nurses develop processes and procedures that meet the needs of ambulatory care patients. Ambulatory care standards define the structure and process of ambulatory care nursing.

Characteristics of Ambulatory Care Nursing Practice

Characteristics are unique features of ambulatory care nursing practice.
A. Differences between ambulatory care nursing and inpatient nursing practice are often overlooked.
B. Assumptions are made that practice styles, policies, and approaches used in inpatient care apply equally in ambulatory care, when in fact they often do not.
C. Ambulatory care focuses on the individual patient, with some population-based care protocols versus population-focused public health practice.
D. Focus groups (Haas, 1998) of experienced ambulatory care nurses identified the following characteristics of nursing practice in ambulatory care:
1. Nursing autonomy.
2. Patient advocacy.
3. Skillful, rapid assessment.
4. Holistic nursing care.
5. Client teaching.
6. Wellness and health promotion.

7. Coordination and continuity of care.
8. Long-term relationships with patients and families.
9. Telephone triage, consultation, follow up, and surveillance.
10. Patient and family control as major care-givers, users of the health care systems, and decision-makers regarding compliance with care regimen.
11. Collaboration with other health care providers.
12. Case management.

E. Challenges and characteristics of ambulatory care nursing evolve from each of the following:
1. Control of care by patient and family.
2. Timing pressure where visits are short and assessment time is compressed.
3. The need to make nursing care visible through documentation and use of nursing standardized languages.
4. The need for collaboration where roles are less clear.
5. Multitude of mechanisms for reimbursement for care.
6. Use of communication devices as alternatives to face-to-face encounters for clinical practice.
7. The need to protect patient privacy and comply with the Health Insurance Portability and Accountability Act (HIPAA) regulations.
8. Desire to standardize care delivered.

Definition of Ambulatory Care Nursing

The definition of ambulatory care nursing must delineate the scope and unique dimensions of ambulatory care nursing practice and differentiate ambulatory care nursing from other areas of specialty nursing practice.

A. Traditional definitions of ambulatory care nursing.
1. Ambulatory care nursing is defined by individual practice settings such as HMO, physician group practice, and hospital/clinic.
2. Ambulatory care nurses would see patients who were generally nonacute and able to walk in for appointments.
3. Ambulatory care nursing is defined by length of care episodes (less than 24 hours).

B. Today, ambulatory care nursing is defined in terms of:

1. Wellness or functional goals.
2. Patient expectations.
3. Patient population served.
4. Setting and encounter.

C. Definition of ambulatory care nursing (American Academy of Ambulatory Care Nursing/American Nurses' Association [AAACN/ANA], 1997).
1. Ambulatory care nursing includes clinical, management, educational, and research activities.
2. Ambulatory care nurses work with patients who seek care for health promotion, health maintenance, or health-related problems.
3. Ambulatory care patients provide their own care or have family or significant others as caregivers.
4. Ambulatory care nursing encounters are episodic and are less than 24 hours in duration. Encounters may occur singly or in a series lasting days/weeks/months/years.
5. Ambulatory care nursing sites are community-based including, but not limited to, hospitals, schools, workplaces, or homes.
6. Ambulatory care nursing encounters may occur face-to-face or via telephone or other communication device.
7. Ambulatory care nursing services focus on cost-effective ways to maximize wellness, prevent illness, and manage acute and chronic diseases to effect the most attainable positive health status over the patient's life span up to and including a peaceful death (AAACN/ANA, 1997).

Development of an Ambulatory Care Nursing Conceptual Framework

To guide the education/orientation of nurses who wish to work in ambulatory care and to assist nurses wishing to demonstrate their expertise in ambulatory care, a simple, concise blueprint of ambulatory care nursing practice is essential.

A. A conceptual framework is a diagram or map that specifies:
1. Essential major concepts, skills, and competencies in an area of practice.
2. Relationships between major content and skill areas.

B. An ambulatory care nursing conceptual framework

can assist in:
1. The design of ambulatory care delivery models.
2. Development of educational materials for ambulatory care nursing.
3. Development of testing materials for competencies and certification.
4. Development of orientation programs for ambulatory care nursing.
5. Development of performance appraisal instruments for ambulatory care nurses.
C. The AAACN Ambulatory Care Conceptual Framework was developed by an AAACN expert member "think tank" in 1998.
  1. The AAACN Think Tank Group used a nominal group approach to delineate major areas of practice, knowledge, and skills.
  2. The Group identified 61 core areas of knowledge and skills.
  3. Group members specified how these 61 areas were related to each other and the ambulatory care nurse role.
  4. The 61 areas were categorized under three roles that are a part of every ambulatory care nurse's practice. Ambulatory care nurses practice within the organization/system's role when they manage and coordinate resources and workflow in their setting; they practice within the professional role as they continuously practice according to standards, evaluate the outcomes of practice, develop themselves and other staff; and finally, they practice in the clinical role as they provide care within each of the clinical dimensions (Haas, 1998).
    a. Organizational/systems role.
      (1) Practice/office support.
      (2) Health care fiscal management (reimbursement and coding).
      (3) Collaboration/conflict management.
      (4) Informatics (for example, management of information and data that become information).
      (5) Context of care delivery/models.
      (6) Care of the caregiver.
      (7) Priority management/delegation /supervision.
      (8) Ambulatory culture/cross-cultural competencies.
      (9) Ongoing political/entrepreneurial skills.

(10) Structuring customer-focused systems.
(11) Workplace regulatory compliance (such as the Equal Employment Opportunity Commission [EEOC] and the Occupational Safety and Health Administration [OSHA]).
(12) Advocacy interorganizational and in community.
(13) Legal issues.
(14) Workload
    b. Professional role.
      (1) Evidence-based practice.
      (2) Leadership inquiry and research utilization.
      (3) Clinical quality improvement.
      (4) Staff development.
      (5) Regulatory compliance (for example, risk management).
      (6) Provider self-care.
      (7) Ethics.
    c. Clinical nursing role.
      (1) Patient education.
      (2) Advocacy.
      (3) Care management.
      (4) Assess, screen, triage.
      (5) Telehealth nursing practice.
      (6) Collaboration/resource identification and referral.
      (7) Clinical procedures, independent/interdependent/dependent.
      (8) Primary, secondary, and tertiary prevention.
      (9) Communication/documentation.
      (10) Outcome management.
      (11) Protocol development/usage.
  5. Core knowledge and skill dimensions that are a part of the clinical role are also related to the patient populations served.
    a. Think Tank Group members defined ambulatory patient populations in categories of well, acute, chronic, and terminally ill.
    b. Think Tank Group members defined characteristics of ambulatory patient populations:
      (1) Patient/family/significant other initiates encounter/visit.
      (2) Patient/family/significant other lives in the community.

Figure 1-1

Ambulatory Care Nursing Conceptual Framework

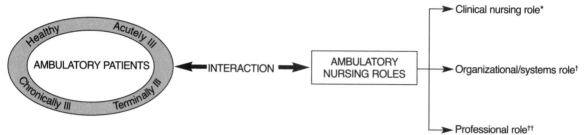

*CLINICAL NURSING ROLE
Patient education
Advocacy (compassion, caring,
    emotional support)
Care management
Assess, screen, triage
Telephone practice
Collaboration/resource
Identification and referral
Primary, secondary, and tertiary prevention
Clinical procedures, independent/
    interdependent/dependent
Communication/documentation
Outcome management
Protocol development/usage

†ORGANIZATIONAL/SYSTEMS ROLE
Practice/office support
Healthcare fiscal management (reimburse-
    ment and coding)
Collaboration/conflict management
Informatics
Context of care delivery/models
Care of the caregiver
Priority Management/delegation/supervi-
    sion
Ambulatory culture/cross cultural
Competencies
Ongoing political/entrepreneurial skills
Structuring customer-focused systems
Workplace regulatory compliance (EEOC,
    OSHA)
Advocacy inter-organizational and in
    community
Legal issues
Workload

††PROFESSIONAL ROLE
Evidence-based practice
Leadership inquiry and research
Utilization
Clinical quality improvement
Staff development
Regulatory compliance (risk management)
Provider self-care
Ethics

Source: Adapted from Haas, 1998.

(3) Patient/family/significant other collaborates with ambulatory interdisciplinary team regarding treatment regime.

(4) Patient/family/significant other manages and provides health care between visits.

(5) Patient/family/significant other controls health care decisions and has choices.

(6) Patient/family/significant other can have long-term relationships with ambulatory care providers.

c. Think Tank Group members recognized that ambulatory care patient populations may also be defined in terms of:

(1) Age (such as pediatrics, gerontology).

(2) Health states or illness categories (such as primary care, cardiac clinic, diabetes clinic, oncology clinic).

(3) Type of reimbursement (such as capitation versus fee-for-service).

(4) Source of reimbursement (such as Medicare, Medicaid, private insurance, federal employee, TriService).

d. Ambulatory Care Nursing Conceptual Framework (ACNCF) (AAACN, 2004a; Haas, 1998) (see Figure 1-1).

(1) Within the roles (clinical, organizational, and professional) specified in the ACNCF depicted in Figure 1-1, the nurse modifies the nursing process to meet the needs of patient populations (Haas, 1998).

(2) Ambulatory patient population health status:
(a) Well or essentially healthy.
(b) Acutely ill but otherwise healthy

(such as patients with ear infections or appendicitis).

(c) Chronically ill (such as patients with diabetes or heart disease); chronically ill persons can have acute illness and/or exacerbations of chronic disease (for example, the diabetic with the flu who also has hypoglycemia).

(d) Terminally ill (such as the patient with end-stage liver failure).

(e) Ambulatory patients can exhibit more than one of these states simultaneously.

(f) Ambulatory care nurses must be cognizant of all operative health states for patients encountered.

(3) The ACNCF (Haas, 1998) in Figure 1-1 assumes the patient's health status to be dynamic and to change between encounters such that persons with an acute illness at one encounter may be well at the next, and that a chronically ill patient may have an acute exacerbation at intervals.

(4) The ACNCF (Haas, 1998) in Figure 1-1 represents characteristics of a patient's health status at the encounter and for the duration of care initiated at the encounter.

(5) The ACNCF (Haas, 1998) in Figure 1-1 assumes that the overall goals of ambulatory care nurses are:
(a) To foster and maintain health.
(b) To prevent illness.
(c) To diagnose illness early and treat effectively.
(d) To manage chronic illness.
(e) To prevent complications and initiate rehabilitation early to regain optimal functioning.

(6) The ACNCF (Haas, 1998) in Figure 1-1 assumes that persons at all stages of health-illness in this continuum could benefit from nursing interventions at all three levels of prevention (Leavell & Clark, 1965): Primary prevention, secondary prevention, and tertiary prevention.

(a) The three levels of prevention are the classic framework for organizing health promotion and disease prevention used by nurses and physicians.

(b) Primary prevention includes health promotion (HP) interventions and specific protections (SP); it may be directed at individuals, groups, or populations; targeted at well populations or those already ill (for example, HP = nutrition education or sex education; SP = use of seat belts, avoidance of allergens, or inoculations).

(c) Secondary prevention involves early diagnosis and prompt treatment to avoid disability (for example, screening, biopsies, medication, surgery).

(d) Tertiary prevention involves rehabilitation to return maximum use of remaining capacities (such as maximizing functional status of the COPD patient with pulmonary toilet and oxygen administration).

(7) Ambulatory care nurses are required to simultaneously address the concurrent needs of patients across the health-illness continuum. For example:
(a) In the clinical role.
(i) Patient education dimension: The nurse understands that although chronically ill, patients still require wellness education.
(ii) Case management dimension: The nurse recognizes that cost effectiveness is maximized if case management protocols are implemented for chronically or terminally ill, and that case management protocols can also enhance recovery, pre-

vent complications, and decrease costs in acute illnesses.

(b) In the organizational role.

   (i) Management dimension: The nurse understands that reimbursement for some interventions may differ if the patient is acutely ill versus well at the time of the encounter.

   (ii) Care of the caregiver dimension: Although ambulatory nurses are attuned to caregivers of chronically or terminally ill patients, they also work with caregivers of acutely ill patients who need counseling or advice to see them through an exhausting acute illness.

(c) In the professional role.

   (i) Evidence-based practice dimension: The nurse understands that protocols can be applied to health promotion for well populations as well as treatment interventions for the chronically or terminally ill.

   (ii) Staff development dimension: Ambulatory care nurses are responsive to needs of staff for development in areas of new therapies and pharmacologic agents for acute or chronically ill patients, but they are also aware of needs for staff development in use of therapies and drugs for palliative care of the terminally ill.

6. All AAACN members had the opportunity to review the ACNCF and provide feedback on how well it represented the reality of ambulatory care nursing practice.

7. The ACNCF was used to organize the content for this *Core Curriculum* text.

8. Benefits of use of the ACNCF include:

   a. Provides clarity of the nursing role dimensions versus role dimensions of other health care providers.

   b. Reflects the uniqueness of the ambulatory care nursing role.

   c. Provides a resource for developers of performance standards and competency measures.

   d. Acts as a catalyst for further refinement of the role.

Change Creates Opportunities for Nurses in Ambulatory Care

A. Movement of U.S. health care system from specialty-based acute care to primary care-oriented ambulatory care offers diverse opportunities for ambulatory care nurses.

   1. Primary care clinic nurses.

   2. Nurse practitioners and nurse midwives.

   3. Nurse educators for wellness, health promotion, and disease prevention.

B. Movement from fee-for-service to capitated payment systems offers opportunities.

   1. Nurse case managers.

   2. Telephone nursing practice.

      a. Cost-effective: Decreases number of patient visits.

      b. Increases patient satisfaction.

      c. Enhances rapidity of response to patient problems.

   3. Nurse specialist (such as breast care, gastroenterology, wound care, skin care).

C. Movement of acute-care into ambulatory settings offers opportunities.

   1. Ambulatory infusion services, both cancer and non-cancer related.

   2. Ambulatory surgery and procedure-related care, nurse anesthetists, and post-anesthesia recovery.

   3. Ambulatory pediatric care for children with asthma and other chronic illnesses where therapies help prevent hospitalization.

   4. Day hospitals for psychiatric patients.

   5. Nurse-managed clinics (anticoagulation clinics, wound care clinics, incontinence clinics).

   6. Support of technologies used in homes, such as home ventilation programs.

D. There is potential for regulations to require use of

RNs in ambulatory care (for example, need for RNs to monitor/evaluate conscious sedation patients).

E. Increasing demand for nurse managers in ambulatory settings.
   1. Demand for nurse managers in areas where strict adherence to quality standards is paramount.
   2. Physician group practice management.
   3. Supervision of assistive personnel.
   4. Supervision of telehealth practice centers.
   5. Supervision of high-risk, high-volume procedure areas.
   6. Management of clinical effectiveness or outcomes performance management.
F. Preparation for these emerging opportunities includes:
   1. Patient teaching methods and strategies for health promotion, as well as disease prevention and disease treatment.
   2. Understanding of community resources.
   3. Expertise with specific patient populations.
   4. Care management skills.
   5. Telehealth nursing practice knowledge skills and competencies.
   6. Experience with acute care nursing modalities (critical care, OR, PACU).
   7. Understanding of health care payment methods.
G. Resources to assist in preparation for opportunities:
   1. Formal course work in undergraduate and graduate nursing programs. Aiken, Clarke, Cheung, Sloane, and Silber (2003) have found better patient outcomes when care is delivered by baccalaureate prepared nurses.
   2. Continuing education programming offered through professional organizations such as AAACN, the Oncology Nursing Society (ONS), and the Association of Operating Room Nurses (AORN).
   3. Readings in professional journals.
   4. Programming available via phone conference and on Internet/cable TV.
H. Nurses currently working in ambulatory care will also provide opportunities through:
   1. Design changes in nursing practice systems in ambulatory care.
   2. Alterations in role and job descriptions for ambulatory care nurses.
   3. Enhanced ambulatory care nursing experiences for nursing students.

Ambulatory Care Nursing Administration and Practice Standards

A. Standards promote effective management of increasingly complex ambulatory care nursing roles and responsibilities in a changing health care environment.
   1. The *AAACN Ambulatory Care Nursing Administration and Practice Standards* (2004b) are revised and updated every 3 years.
   2. The first edition of the *AAACN Telehealth Nursing Practice Administration and Practice Standards* was published in 1997. These standards are revised every 3 years and now use the title *Telehealth Nursing Practice Administration and Practice Standards* (AAACN, 2004c).
   3. The AAACN standards are the result of a collaborative effort of nurses from an array of ambulatory settings in a variety of geographic locations.
   4. Ambulatory care nursing values are reflected in the AAACN standards. The values of AAACN as an organization (AAACN, 2004b) are:
      a. Responsible health care delivery for individuals and communities.
      b. Visionary and accountable leadership.
      c. Productive partnerships and alliances.
      d. Innovative and responsible risk taking.
      e. Responsive member services.
      f. Diverse and committed membership.
      g. Continual advancement of professional ambulatory care nursing practice.
B. Definitions: Used as the common foundation in the development of standards (AAACN, 2004b).
   1. *Standard* – An authoritative statement developed and disseminated by a professional organization or governmental or regulatory agency by which the quality of practice, services, research, or education can be judged.
   2. *Patient* – An individual who requests or receives nursing services. Also called client, consumer, member, or customer in many settings.
   3. *Family* – Family members are defined by the patient in his or her own terms and may include individuals related by blood or marriage, or in self-defined relationships. (This

Table 1-1

Ambulatory Care Nursing Administration and Practice Standards

Standard I. Structure and Organization of Ambulatory Care Nursing
Ambulatory care nursing is provided within an environment that supports the nurse to provide quality patient care that is caring, efficient, effective, and evidence-based.

Standard II. Staffing
An adequate number of ambulatory care nurses are available to meet the patient care needs for the practice setting and maintain a safe and caring work environment.

Standard III. Competency
Professional ambulatory care nurses demonstrate technical, critical thinking, and interpersonal skills necessary to complete their expected job responsibilities.

Standard IV. Ambulatory Nursing Practice
The nursing process is the foundation used by professional ambulatory care nurses in making clinical decisions as they assess and identify patient and family health status, establish outcomes, plan, implement, and evaluate the care they provide.

Standard V. Continuity of Care
Professional ambulatory care nurses facilitate continuity of care utilizing the nursing process, interdisciplinary collaboration, and coordination of all appropriate health care services, including available community resources.

Standard VI. Ethics and Patient Rights
Professional ambulatory care nurses recognize the dignity, diversity, and worth of individuals and families; respect individual cultural, spiritual, and psychosocial differences; and apply philosophical and ethical concepts that promote access to care, equality, and continuity of care.

Standard VII. Environment
Professional ambulatory care nurses participate in a coordinated system-wide process that creates and maintains a safe, ergonomically correct, comfortable, and hazard-free environment for patients, visitors, and staff.

Standard VIII. Research
Professional ambulatory care nurses conduct and participate in clinical and health care systems research. Research findings are disseminated. Evidence-based information is used to improve health care and organizational effectiveness.

Standard IX. Performance Improvement
The performance improvement process is coordinated and integrated with that of the organization and includes the continuous data collection, evaluation, and improvement of the safety, quality, and appropriateness of ambulatory care nursing. Ambulatory care nursing leaders set expectations, provide resources and education, foster communication and coordination, and participate in improvement activities. Ambulatory care nursing leaders create an environment in which patients, their families, and organizational staff can identify and manage opportunities for improvement.

Source: AAACN, 2004b.

Table 1-2

Telehealth Nursing Practice Administration and Practice Standards

Standard I. Structure and Organization
Professional telehealth nursing practice is provided within an environment provided that supports the provision of quality patient care that is caring, efficient, effective, and evidence-based. It is practiced within the context of shared responsibility between patients, families, support systems, and health care providers.

Standard II. Staffing
An adequate number of competent telehealth nursing staff is available to meet the patient care needs for the telehealth practice setting. Staffing models address the complexity of the telehealth encounter care needs while maintaining a safe and caring work environment.

Standard III. Competency
Telehealth nurses demonstrate competency in clinical knowledge, critical thinking, and interpersonal and technical skills to provide efficient, effective, and evidence-based care.

Standard IV. Telehealth Nursing Practice
The nursing process is used with each telehealth encounter by registered nurses when making clinical decisions during the provision of health care interventions.

Standard V. Continuity of Care
Nurses manage telehealth encounters to facilitate continuity of care by utilizing the nursing process, interdisciplinary collaboration, and coordination of all appropriate health care services, including available community resources.

Standard VI. Ethics and Patient Rights
Professional telehealth nurses recognize the dignity and worth of individuals and families; respect cultural, spiritual, and psychosocial differences; and apply philosophical and ethical concepts that promote access to care, equality, and continuity of care.

Standard VII. Environment
A safe, hazard-free, ergonomically correct and efficient environment is provided for telehealth nursing staff.

Standard VIII. Research
Telehealth nurses participate in research that is consistent with their level of education, position, and practice environment. Telehealth nurses are able to critically evaluate, share findings, and apply research to practice.

Standard IX. Performance Improvement
The performance improvement process for telehealth care is coordinated and integrated with the organization and includes continuous data collection, evaluation, and improvement of the safety, quality, and appropriateness of care.

Source: AAACN, 2004c.

definition is intended to include the family in nursing care as appropriate. It is not intended as a legal definition of family.)

4. *Nursing staff* – Staff members who participate in delivering nursing care. These staff members are either registered nurses or are supervised by a registered nurse.

5. *Health care team* – Includes the patient, fam-

ily, and other members of the health care system who are involved in the development, and implementation and evaluation of the care plan.

6. *Nursing services* – Organized services delivered to groups of patients by nursing staff. Includes nursing care as well as services to support or facilitate direct care (such as

referral and coordination of care).

7. *Competency* – Refers to the knowledge, skills, and behaviors identified as performance standards constituting the acceptable demonstration of ability in a role.

8. *Evidence-based nursing practice* – Process by which nurses make clinical decisions using the best available research evidence, their clinical expertise, and patient preferences in the context of available resources.

C. Components of each standard.
   1. Standard statement.
   2. Rationale: A concise statement of the underlying reason for the standard.
   3. Measurement criteria: Specific, measurable indicators that demonstrate compliance with the standard.

D. Assumptions.
   1. Ambulatory care nurses use AAACN standards and nursing practice standards developed by professional nursing organizations such as ANA, ONS, AORN, and the Emergency Nurses Association (ENA) for care specific to patient populations.
   2. Ambulatory care nurses also use Clinical Practice Guidelines developed by federal agencies such as the Agency for Research and Quality (AHRQ) to guide care for specific patient populations. AHRQ guidelines can be obtained via the Internet at www.ahrq.gov

E. Purposes for use of *Ambulatory Care Nursing and Administration Practice Standards*:
   1. Provide guidance for the structure and processes in delivery of ambulatory care nursing.
   2. Serves as a guide for provision of quality patient care.
   3. Facilitates professional nursing development.
   4. Facilitates evaluation of professional nursing performance.

5. Stimulates participation in research and use of research findings.
6. Serves as a guide for quality management.
7. Serves as a guide for ethics and patient advocacy.

F. Content addressed in standards:
   1. Structure and organization of ambulatory care nursing.
   2. Staffing.
   3. Competency.
   4. Ambulatory nursing practice/telehealth nursing practice.
   5. Continuity of care.
   6. Ethics and patient rights.
   7. Environment.
   8. Research.
   9. Performance improvement.

G. Nine *AAACN Ambulatory Care Nursing Administration and Practice Standards* (see Table 1-1).

H. Nine *AAACN Telehealth Nursing Practice and Administration Standards* (see Table 1-2).

References

Aiken, L.H., Clarke, S.P., Cheung, R.B., Sloane, D.M., & Silber, J.H. (2003). Educational levels of hospital nurses and surgical patient mortality. *Journal of the American Medical Association, 290*(12), 1617-1623.

American Academy of Ambulatory Care Nursing (AAACN). (2004a). Ambulatory care nursing conceptual framework. In *Ambulatory care nursing administration and practice standards* (p. 5). Pitman, NJ: Author.

American Academy of Ambulatory Care Nursing (AAACN). (2004b). *Ambulatory care nursing administration and practice standards.* Pitman, NJ: Author.

American Academy of Ambulatory Care Nursing (AAACN). (2004c). *Telehealth nursing practice administration and practice standards.* Pitman, NJ: Author.

American Academy of Ambulatory Care Nursing/American Nurses' Association (AAACN/ANA). (1997). *Nursing in ambulatory care: The future is here.* Washington, DC: American Nurses Publishing.

Haas, S. (1998). Ambulatory care conceptual framework. *AAACN Viewpoint, 20*(3), 16-17.

Leavell, H., & Clark, E. (1965). *Preventive medicine for the doctor in his community: An epidemiologic approach.* New York: McGraw-Hill.

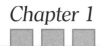

Ambulatory Care Nursing Specialty Practice

This test may be copied for use by others.

COMPLETE THE FOLLOWING:

Name: _____

Address: _____

City: _____ State: _____ Zip:_____

Preferred telephone: (Home)_____ (Work)_____

E-mail_____

AAACN Member Expiration Date: _____

Registration fee: AAACN Member: $12.00
                     Nonmember: $20.00

Objectives

This educational activity is designed for nurses and other health care professionals who practice in ambulatory care. For those wishing to obtain CE credit, an evaluation follows. After studying the information presented in this offering, you will be able to:

1. Discuss the characteristics of ambulatory care nursing practice.
2. Differentiate ambulatory care nursing practice from other forms of specialty nursing practice.
3. Discuss the ambulatory care nursing conceptual framework.
4. Enumerate opportunities for nurses in ambulatory care nursing.
5. Discuss ambulatory care standards.

Answer Form:

1. If you applied what you have learned from this activity into your practice, what would be different?

_____

_____

_____

Evaluation	Strongly disagree				Strongly agree
2. By completing this activity, I was able to meet the following objectives:					
a. Discuss the characteristics of ambulatory care nursing practice.	1	2	3	4	5
b. Differentiate ambulatory care nursing practice from other forms of specialty nursing practice.	1	2	3	4	5
c. Discuss the ambulatory care nursing conceptual framework.	1	2	3	4	5
d. Enumerate opportunities for nurses in ambulatory care nursing.	1	2	3	4	5
e. Discuss ambulatory care standards.	1	2	3	4	5
3. The content was current and relevant.	1	2	3	4	5
4. The objectives could be achieved using the content provided.	1	2	3	4	5
5. This was an effective method to learn this content.	1	2	3	4	5
6. I am more confident in my abilities since completing this material.	1	2	3	4	5

7. The material was (check one) ___new ___review for me.

8. Time required to read this chapter: _____minutes

I verify that I have completed this activity: _____
                                                    Signature

Comments: _____

_____

_____

Posttest Instructions

1. To receive continuing education credit for individual study after reading the article, complete the answer/evaluation form to the left.

2. Detach and send the answer/evaluation form along with a check or money order payable to the *American Academy of Ambulatory Care Nursing (AAACN)*, East Holly Avenue Box 56, Pitman, NJ 08071–0056.

3. Test returns must be postmarked by August 1, 2011. Upon completion of the answer/evaluation form, a certificate for **1.4** contact hour(s) will be awarded and sent to you. Should the material contained in this chapter become outdated prior to the above expiration date, AAACN reserves the right to withdraw this CE test.

This activity is co-provided by the *American Academy of Ambulatory Care Nursing (AAACN)* and Anthony J. Jannetti, Inc. (AJJ). AJJ is accredited as a provider of continuing nursing education by the American Nurses' Credentialing Center's Commission on Accreditation (ANCC-COA). AAACN is a provider approved by the California Board of Registered Nurses, provider number CEP 05336.

This article was reviewed and formatted for contact hour credit by Sally S. Russell, MN, CMSRN, AAACN Education Director; and Candia Baker Laughlin MS, RN, C, Editor.

Chapter 2

The Ambulatory Care Practice Arena

Clare E. Hastings, PhD, RN, FAAN

Objectives

Study of the information presented in this chapter will enable the learner to:
1. Describe the domain of ambulatory care nursing practice.
2. Discuss the characteristics of patients seen in ambulatory care and the implications of nursing practice.
3. Compare nursing practice in ambulatory and acute inpatient settings.
4. Identify and describe current practice settings for ambulatory care nursing.
5. Discuss challenges faced by nurses moving from inpatient to ambulatory care settings and describe strategies to facilitate the transition.

Key Points

1. The domain of ambulatory care nursing practice is defined as the overall scope of nursing practice in the ambulatory arena.
2. Ambulatory care is defined as outpatient care in which patients stay less than 24 hours and are discharged to their normal residential situation after care.
3. Practice setting is defined as the type of organizational delivery system in which the nurse practices.

Nurses in ambulatory care practice are in a diverse and changing environment. As health care increasingly moves out of the acute care hospital and into the community and home settings, nurses looking to ambulatory care as a practice setting find a broad array of possible settings, roles, and opportunities. It is important for nurses practicing in ambulatory care to be aware both of the diversity in roles and practice settings, as well as the common themes that are present across ambulatory practice settings. This chapter will provide nurses in ambulatory care with an overview of the broad domain of ambulatory practice and clarify the common factors that occur in all ambulatory care settings. The differences between ambulatory and inpatient practice and the often unexpected challenges faced by nurses transitioning from traditional inpatient roles to ambulatory care will also be discussed. An understanding of the effect of the practice setting on nursing practice is important to enable nurses to effectively contribute to the health care team. Significant content in this chapter is abstracted with permission from the monograph *Nursing in Ambulatory Care: The Future is Here* (American Academy of Ambulatory Care Nursing/American Nurses' Association [AAACN/ANA], 1997).

The Domain of Ambulatory Nursing Practice

The domain of ambulatory care nursing practice is defined as the overall scope of nursing practice in the ambulatory arena. It includes attributes of the environment in which practice occurs, patient requirements for care, and specific nursing role dimensions.
A. The movement of health care out of the hospital.
   1. Fueled by changes in reimbursement.
      a. Prospective payment for inpatient services has compressed hospital length of stay and pushed care into the ambulatory setting.
      b. Growth of HMOs and managed care has created incentives for keeping patients out of the hospital.
      c. Growth of population-based and capitated care has placed increased emphasis on preventive services, which are often provided in the ambulatory care setting.
      d. Growth of 23-hour short stay units has increased the use of outpatient observation or short-stay status as alternatives to an inpatient admission.
   2. Further speeded by changes in technology.
      a. Minimally invasive surgical techniques

that shorten recovery time.

   b. Improved methods for short-term anesthesia that shorten recovery time that allow more procedures to be performed on an outpatient basis.

   c. Innovations in vascular access and intravenous pump technologies that allow patients to remain out of the hospital during long-term intravenous therapy.

3. Early discharge creates the requirement for ambulatory followup, often in combination with home health visits.

   a. Enhanced surgical techniques have shortened stays, but recovery still must be monitored, drains removed, and wound healing assessed.

   b. Shortened hospital stays mean that pre- and post-intervention patient education and support must be done on an ambulatory basis.

4. Advances in the care of chronically ill patients.

   a. A growing elderly population requires ongoing ambulatory treatment, monitoring, and followup for chronic illness.

   b. Ambulatory infusion centers are used as alternatives to inpatient care.

   c. Outpatient invasive testing and treatment centers allow much of the ongoing care for severe chronic illness (heart disease, cancer, renal failure) to be provided in an ambulatory care setting.

   d. Nurses are becoming involved in multidisciplinary disease management teams for the chronically ill.

B. Descriptions of the domain of ambulatory care nursing.

1. Early literature on the ambulatory care nursing role changes in the 1970s (Johnston, 1980; Marzalek, 1980).

   a. Appearance of anecdotal descriptions noting the differences between inpatient and ambulatory nursing.

   b. Descriptions of underutilization and downward substitution of nurses.

   c. New efforts to understand ambulatory care nursing as a distinct specialty practice area in nursing.

2. Verran's Taxonomy of Ambulatory Care Nursing Practice (Verran, 1981).

   a. First attempt to systematically describe the role of professional nurses in ambulatory care.

   b. First time that a distinct domain of practice for ambulatory care nursing was proposed.

   c. Taxonomy formed the basis for several studies of the role dimensions of nurses in ambulatory care (Bunting, 1994; Hastings & Muir-Nash, 1989; Tighe, Fisher, Hastings, & Heller, 1985).

   d. Taxonomy also became the basis for attempts to classify nursing care requirements in ambulatory care and measure nursing intensity (Hastings, 1987; Parrinello, Brenner, & Vallone, 1988; Verran, 1986; Verran & Reid, 1987).

3. American Academy of Ambulatory Care Nursing.

   a. Only professional nursing organization with a focus on nursing practice in ambulatory care.

   b. Clearinghouse for information and consensus on the role of nursing in ambulatory care.

   c. Publishes and regularly updates *Ambulatory Care Nursing Administration and Practice Standards* (AAACN, 2004a), *Telehealth Nursing Practice Administration and Practice Standards* (AAACN, 2004b), and the monograph *Ambulatory Care Nursing: The Future is Here* (AAACN/ANA, 1997).

4. Research and conceptual development regarding nursing role in ambulatory care.

   a. Complexity and role confusion (Schim, Thornburg, & Kravutske, 2001)

   b. Ambulatory nursing role dimensions (Hackbarth, Haas, Kavanaugh, & Vlasses, 1995; Schroeder, Trehearne, & Ward, 2000a).

   c. Ambulatory nursing in the context of the interdisciplinary team (Dickey, 1998; Gesell & Gregory, 2004; Hastings, 1997; Hendershot et al., 2005).

   d. Impact of ambulatory nurses on outcomes in specific settings (Abercrombie,

2001; Adams, 1997; Burnett, Chapman, Wishart, & Purushotham, 2003; Eck, Picagali, & Boyle, 1997; Janikowski & Rockefeller, 1998; Loftus & Weston, 2001; Mayer, 1996; Scott, 2000; Schroeder, Trehearne, & Ward, 2000b).

C. Current consensus on role dimensions in ambulatory nursing (Haas, 1998). Components include:
  1. Assessment and triage.
  2. Prevention.
  3. Clinical procedures.
  4. Collaboration.
  5. Care management.
  6. Patient education.
  7. Advocacy.
  8. Telephone practice.
  9. Communication and documentation.
  10. Outcome management.
  11. Protocol development and use.

Ambulatory Patient Characteristics

A. Ambulatory patients are not ambulatory any more.
  1. Patients may not walk in and walk out.
  2. Increasing numbers of patients have chronic illnesses managed at home with complex treatment regimens and medical equipment.
  3. Movement of elective surgeries to the ambulatory setting means patients have to be recovered after invasive procedures and anesthesia.
  4. Ambulatory sites may also provide service to patients who are actually inpatients at another facility.
  5. Ambulatory services are often delivered over the telephone or via the Internet.
B. Ambulatory patients are as diverse as inpatients in their clinical presentation. They may be:
  1. Acutely ill requiring triage and possible emergency care.
  2. Acutely ill requiring support, diagnosis, and treatment.
  3. Chronically ill with an acute exacerbation.
  4. Chronically ill requiring ongoing monitoring and assistance with self-management.
  5. In need of a clearly defined treatment or procedure, including recovery, monitoring, and discharge instructions.

  6. In need of education, reassurance, and support.
  7. In need of preventive services and self-care education.
C. Ambulatory patients are informed consumers.
  1. Media coverage and the availability of comparative quality of care data have created a skeptical and informed consumer group.
  2. Many people have access to the Internet; they come already knowing much about their condition, its prognosis, and current treatment.
  3. As health care begins to adopt systematic assessment of patient satisfaction, patients themselves have become more willing to come forward with complaints and provide feedback.
  4. Because of the growth in consumerism, nurses in ambulatory care are very likely to encounter situations in which patients question the rationale or quality of care.
D. Each patient has a constituency of family members and/or concerned others who may become involved with care and care decisions.
  1. Ambulatory care is community-based, often involving care that must be continued in the home between ambulatory visits.
  2. With the increase in early hospital discharge and self-managed chronic disease, it is necessary to involve others as caregivers in the home.
  3. Involving family members or other significant individuals can enhance the effectiveness of patient education and increase the likelihood of adherence to the plan of care.

Comparison of Nursing Practice in Inpatient Acute Care and Ambulatory Care

Inpatient acute care is defined as hospital-based care in which patients are admitted overnight for diagnosis, treatment of an acute problem, or treatment of an acute exacerbation of a chronic problem. Ambulatory care is defined as outpatient care in which patients stay less than 24 hours and are discharged to their normal residential situation after care.
A. Summary of differences between the nursing role in ambulatory and inpatient settings (see Table 2-1).

Table 2-1.

Differences Between Nursing Role in Ambulatory and Inpatient Settings

Aspect of Role	Inpatient Practice	Ambulatory Practice
Treatment episode	Inpatient admission	Visit or phone encounter
Observation mode	Direct and continuous	Episodic, often using patient as informant
Management of treatment plan	By nurse, with input from patient and family	By patient and family, with input from nurse
Primary intervention mode	Direct	Consultative
Organizational presence of nursing	Nurse-managed department	May or may not be formal structure for nursing
Workload variability and intensity	Determined by bed capacity and admission criteria	Theoretically determined by scheduling system; may also be affected by telephone volume

Source: Adapted from Hastings, 1987.

1. The key to the difference between nursing care in inpatient and ambulatory settings lies in differences in the underlying assumptions about the relationship (or "contract") between the patient and the nurse (Hastings, 1987).
2. Distinct differences exist in the level of accountability for care and control over the treatment plan assumed by both the patient and the nurse in the two settings.
3. Although it is a requirement that RNs be present at all times in the inpatient setting to provide or coordinate patient care, this requirement does not universally exist in ambulatory care.
4. Differences in the focus of nursing practice in the two types of settings have led to different evolutions in the structure of care delivery and understanding of staffing requirements (see Chapter 10, *Staffing and Workload*).

B. Patient contacts in the hospital setting.
   1. Patients are admitted to the hospital because they require nursing care. This fact is the basis for the requirement that all hospitalized patients be under the care of a registered nurse while they are admitted.
   2. Accountability for managing care is trans-ferred to the nurse when the patient is admitted.
      a. This includes even those activities in which the patient was competent, such as medication administration.
      b. The nurse assumes total accountability for care and observation during admission.

C. Patient contacts in the ambulatory setting.
   1. Ambulatory visits usually initiated by the patient for the purpose of seeking medical care.
   2. Most prevalent site for ambulatory care is still the physician's office.
   3. Between provider visits, patients are expected to manage their own self-care and treatments prescribed by the provider, and seek additional help if needed.
   4. Need for nursing in ambulatory care is not universal as it is in the hospital setting.
      a. Must define patients or groups of patients requiring nursing care.
      b. Must define level of care to be provided.
      c. No universal professional or regulatory standards exist on this issue.

D. Differences in the definition of treatment episode.
   1. Episode of care in acute care nursing is the hospital admission.

a. Episode has defined beginning and end points (admission and discharge).

b. Treatment period is continuous with an admission.

2. Episode of care in ambulatory care is a visit or phone encounter.

a. Treatment is episodic rather than continuous.

b. Treatment period may include multiple episodes.

c. Treatment period often has poorly defined beginning and end point.

E. Differences in observation mode.

1. In acute care, the nurse has the opportunity to continuously observe the patient and collect assessment data.

a. Variations in disease process and treatment effectiveness can be directly observed.

b. Physical assessment can be used to corroborate patient-reported findings on an ongoing basis.

2. In ambulatory care, opportunity for direct observation and physical assessment is minimal.

a. The nurse must rely on the patient's report and description of symptoms, self-care, and results.

b. The nurse must have a comprehensive understanding of the patient's condition and treatment to effectively probe for additional data.

c. The nurse must often rely on the report of family members if the patient is unable to describe the situation.

d. The assessment is compressed into a much shorter time frame.

e. There are often gaps in critical information needed to make judgments about diagnosis and care.

F. Differences in management of the treatment plan.

1. In acute care, control over implementation of the treatment plan resides primarily with the nurse, with the patient playing the role of active participant.

a. Determining the approach.

b. Timing of care.

c. Modifications and adaptations to improve effectiveness or tolerance of treatment.

2. In ambulatory care, control over implementation of the treatment plan resides primarily with the patient (and family), with the nurse serving in a consultative role.

a. Approach is described and recommended during the visit, with possible demonstration by patient or family members.

b. Timing is prescribed.

c. Actual implementation occurs under the control of the patient when the nurse is not present.

d. Adaptations and modification are made by the patient, often not in consultation with health care providers.

e. Changes in implementation may be made without a detailed understanding of the rationale for treatment and implications of making changes.

G. Differences in nursing interventions.

1. Until recently, there was a clearly discernable difference in the types of interventions and locus of control over interventions between the hospital and ambulatory care nursing.

a. Historically, hospital-based care was initiated by the nurse, and related to either monitoring, treatment, or self-care activities that the patient would be unable to perform.

b. Hospital-based interventions are often technologically complex and involve hands-on care.

c. In contrast, interventions by ambulatory care nurses historically tended to be patient-initiated, focused on health care advice or instructing patients how to manage care at home or prepare for tests and procedures.

2. Recent changes in the health care system have blurred the boundaries of inpatient and outpatient care.

a. Patients with complex conditions and treatment regimens are being cared for in outpatient and day hospital settings.

b. There has been a dramatic growth in 23-hour short-stay units.

c. Complexity of ambulatory surgery has

increased.

    d.   Increasingly, outpatients are being seen on inpatient units for evaluation and triage (for example, oncology and labor and delivery).

H. Differences in the organizational position of nursing.

    1.   Traditionally, inpatient nursing staff are part of an organized department of nursing and have a defined nurse executive with a voice at the governing body level.

    2.   Traditionally, ambulatory care nurses work within a variety of structures.

        a.   Often report to a non-nursing administrator.

        b.   May be hired directly by physicians in a group practice.

        c.   Except for large hospital-based or group practices, may not have a defined nursing administrative structure.

        d.   Even in the same organization, nurses in different ambulatory roles may have different reporting and supervisory relationships.

I. Differences in workload variability and intensity.

    1.   In acute care, the inpatient unit has a defined capacity that is based on bed size.

        a.   Although acuity and census may fluctuate, there is at least a theoretical limit to the number of patients for whom care is provided.

        b.   Unit admission and discharge criteria set a level of care, which predicts what types of patients may be seen.

    2.   In ambulatory care, workload is theoretically predicted by the appointment system.

        a.   Ambulatory care nurses know that the appointment system is easily bypassed by walk-ins and urgent visits.

        b.   No-show patients and resulting overbooking practices also add to problems predicting workload.

        c.   Workload is also projected based on telephone volumes, which may or may not be proportionate to appointments scheduled.

Current Practice Settings for Ambulatory Care Nurses

Practice setting is defined as the type of organizational delivery system in which the nurse practices.

A. The context for ambulatory nursing practice.

    1.   Nurses practice within a broad continuum of ambulatory care settings (see Figure 2-1).

    2.   The ambulatory health care system spans primary care, when the patient first seeks care, through acute care, chronic follow-up and palliative care.

    3.   Nurses care for patients in every phase of preventive care, health maintenance, diagnosis, treatment, and follow-up as patients move in and out of acute care settings.

B. Ambulatory care nurses practice within several distinct organizational settings.

    1.   Characteristics of the setting are determined by its organizational structure, its patient population, its financial and reimbursement structure, and the organization of its primary providers (usually physicians).

    2.   Within each type of setting, there are also differences based on size, regional location, affiliation with a network or health system, and regional differences in health finance administration.

    3.   Dimensions of clinical nursing practice are similar across settings; however, the frequency of performance of certain dimensions varies a great deal by setting (Haas, Hackbarth, Kavanaugh, & Vlasses, 1995).

    4.   Major categories of practice setting include:

        a.   University hospital outpatient departments.

        b.   Community hospital outpatient departments.

        c.   Solo and group medical practices.

        d.   Health maintenance organization (HMO) clinics and services.

        e.   Government health systems (federal, state, and local).

        f.   Community and freestanding centers such as:

            (1) Occupational health centers.

            (2) School health clinics.

Figure 2-1.

Context for Ambulatory Care Nursing Practice

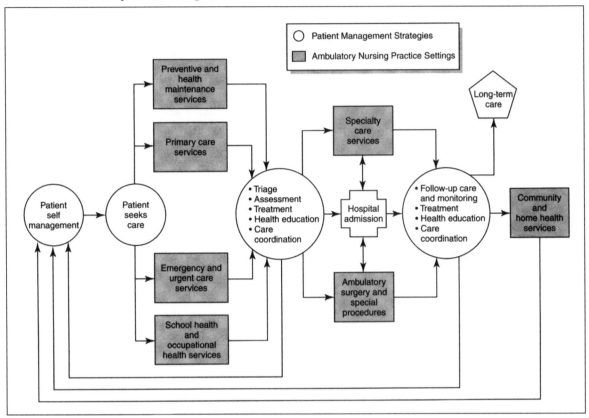

Source: Developed by Clare Hastings. Adapted from AAACN/ANA, 1997.

(3) Shelters for the homeless.
(4) Surgery/special procedure centers.
(5) Urgent care centers.
C. University hospital outpatient departments.
   1. History and development.
      a. Teaching hospital outpatient clinics have been used since the early 1900s to provide teaching opportunities for medical students, residents, and other health care providers.
      b. Traditionally, care was provided free or at minimal charge to those primarily in the local community.
      c. Have also included specialty clinics based on the expertise of medical faculty members that pull referrals from a greater distance.
   2. Ambulatory nursing role.
      a. Nurses have been active collaborators in the development of teaching hospital clinics and programs.
      b. Nurses are often the only constant for patients receiving chronic illness care through cycles of rotating residents.
      c. Nurses in academic medical centers were among the first to begin to describe the role of the nurse in ambulatory care.
      d. Teaching hospital clinics are often the site for innovations in nursing care, including nurse-run clinics and other forms of collaborative practice.

e. Because of the teaching focus, many teaching clinics have been plagued by long waits, poor access to urgent care, and difficulties obtaining medical records.

f. Recently, financial pressures and changing reimbursement have forced many academic medical centers to reorganize their teaching clinics, streamline operations and improve patient support services (Billi, Wise, Bills, & Mitchell, 1995), or consider closing in the face of increasing costs and decreasing revenues (Ervin, Chang, & White, 1998; Hunter, Ventura, & Kervus, 1998).

D. Community hospital outpatient centers.
1. History and development.
   a. Began as an outgrowth of the dispensary movement in the 1800s to serve the urban poor.
   b. As financial incentives and pressures changed, community hospital outpatient centers became more focused on adjunctive services, such as ambulatory surgery and short-stay units.
   c. Not financially or operationally competitive as a large source of primary care services.
2. Ambulatory nursing role.
   a. Usually small programs with limited numbers of nursing staff.
   b. Focus on the use of ancillary staff and use of RNs as working managers.
   c. As more high-tech programs were implemented, use of RNs increased.

E. Medical group practices.
1. History and development.
   a. Medical group practices are an outgrowth of the economic pressures on solo physician private practices.
   b. Movement of patients out of the hospital, and rapid growth of large multi-specialty practices have increased the intensity of services provided in the medical group practice setting (Curran, 1995).
2. Ambulatory care nursing role.
   a. The nursing role is focused on facilitating the care of patients and the work of physicians.

b. The physician is usually the employer and often the supervisor of nurses.
c. Role components include triage and access management, managing and coordinating care, providing technical support for complex clinical procedures, and patient education.

F. Health maintenance organizations (HMOs).
1. History and development.
   a. Since the 1970s, the number of prepaid comprehensive health plans that provide all services to members based on a fixed fee per month has grown.
   b. This organizational structure created a whole new set of incentives and needs for care management.
   c. Emphasis on reducing use of hospital days and utilization in general stimulated development of processes to triage patients and directed them to a different level of care.
   d. Incentives to reduce hospital utilization also led to a new focus on prevention and health maintenance.
2. Ambulatory care nursing role.
   a. Extensive involvement in assessment and triage.
   b. First sites to identify telephone triage as a specific nursing function.
   c. Nurses are also involved in health maintenance activities, technical procedures (such as outpatient chemotherapy), and care management.

G. Federal health systems.
1. History and development.
   a. Include federally mandated programs to serve specific populations.
      (1) Department of Defense programs for active duty and retired military personnel.
      (2) Department of Veterans Affairs programs.
      (3) U.S. Public Health Service programs, including Native American Health Service hospitals, clinics, and community health centers.
   b. Systems represent large networks of organizations operating on a fixed budget.

    c. Until recently, most services were provided free of charge to members of enrolled populations.

  2. Ambulatory care nursing role.

    a. Nursing practice supported by a long-standing tradition of well-trained unlicensed assistive personnel (Navy corpsmen and Army medics).

    b. The nursing role has developed rapidly in recent years, involving nurses in health assessment and promotion/disease prevention, patient education, and the provision of complex procedures in the outpatient setting.

    c. Federal health systems have been sites for development of innovative models and approaches to nurses providing primary ambulatory care services.

H. Community and freestanding centers.

  1. Program types include:

    a. Surgery centers.

    b. Diagnostic centers.

    c. Local health departments.

    d. Free and grant-supported experimental clinics.

    e. College health centers.

    f. Occupational health offices in large employers.

  2. Ambulatory care nursing role.

    a. Many centers small in size and scope.

    b. Nurses assume multiple roles.

    c. Many such sites have been experimental sites for piloting nurse-run clinics.

Transitioning into Ambulatory Care Nursing

A. Reasons nurses are making the transition to ambulatory care.

  1. Increased emphasis on ambulatory care as a care delivery site.

  2. Expansion of complex services offered in ambulatory care, with resulting needs for nursing support.

  3. Nurses seeking alternative practice settings to the hospital.

    a. Opportunities for greater professional autonomy.

    b. Opportunities for increased collaboration with physicians.

    c. Scheduling and lifestyle advantages.

    d. Expectations that ambulatory care will provide a low-stress work environment.

B. Transition challenges.

  1. Change in locus of control.

    a. Experience of diminished control.

      (1) Over the general treatment regimen.

      (2) Over the timing and method of implementation.

      (3) Especially noticed by nurses transitioning from critical care.

    b. Combined with general sensory overload.

      (1) Large numbers of patients arriving for care.

      (2) Large numbers of providers.

    c. Lack of a shift start and end, with resulting requirement that the nurse stays to see to the needs of all patients in the setting.

    d. Changes in expected workload.

    e. Difficulty planning time and controlling pace of work.

  2. Changes in data available.

    a. Requirement that clinical decisions be made with less than usual amount of data.

    b. Unavailability of continuous observation that allows the nurse to pick up subtle changes in the patient's condition.

    c. Reliance on new methods of assessment and integration of information.

      (1) Nuances of patient self-reporting.

      (2) Rapid observation and synthesis, combined with probing and assessment skills.

  3. Changes in scope of services provided.

    a. Scope dictated by both needs of the patient and the purpose of the visit.

      (1) May not be able or required to meet all assessed needs at a given visit.

      (2) May use referral or recommendation as opposed to direct intervention.

      (3) May create conflict in a newly transitioned nurse used to meeting the total needs of each patient.

    b. May apply health assessment standards

based on inpatient experience.
  (1) Not appropriate for ambulatory visits.
  (2) This practice creates an unnecessary burden on both the nurse and the patient.
  (3) Critical transition task is to learn how to assess only the essential data for purpose of the visit and the patient's need.
  c. Scope of services may vary substantially from visit to visit.
  (1) For one visit, the nurse may briefly review the patient record and assign the patient to an unlicensed staff member.
  (2) For another visit, the nurse may do a complete assessment and provide education and counseling or direct care.
  d. Important that population assessment be done.
  (1) Establish overall needs for nursing care within the population.
  (2) Identify major visit types and level of nursing care required for each.
  (3) Establish a process by which patients may gain access to the nurse as needed.
4. Changes in collaborative relationships.
  a. Relationships among health team members change.
  b. Focus of nursing care shifts.
  (1) Away from the medical plan of care and implementing that plan.
  (2) Toward a more consultative role with patients, families, and physicians.
  c. The nurse is seen more as the coordinator and manager of care and less as direct implementer.
  (1) Creates opportunities for collaborative practice with physicians.
  (2) Identified by nurses practicing in ambulatory care as a valued aspect of the role.
  d. The nurse becomes a conduit between the physician directing care and the patient/family managing care at home.
  e. Requires demonstration of key compe-

tencies to be accepted as a colleague in patient management by physicians.
  (1) Clinical competence.
  (2) Confidence in decision-making.
  (3) Ability to communicate effectively.
5. Diversity in practice assignments.
  a. Often a shock for nurses transitioning from single specialty inpatient units.
  b. Due to the episodic nature of care, some specialty programs may meet only once or twice per week.
  c. The nurse may be assigned in multiple locations to fill out the week.
  d. Requires broad competency to manage care for diverse groups of patients.
  e. For experienced ambulatory nurses, this variability is the "spice" in their roles.
  f. For the new nurse, it may seem like chaos.
C. Strategies to support a successful transition.
  1. Nurses transitioning to ambulatory care need full orientation to the setting and the practice styles for each area assigned.
  2. Although clinical competency is not usually the major issue, the new nurse will need assistance adapting practice approaches to the new setting.
  3. Attention should be paid to signs that the new staff member is becoming overwhelmed with multiple demands.

References

Abercrombie, P.D. (2001). Improving adherence to abnormal Pap smear follow-up. *Journal of Obstetric, Gynecologic, and Neonatal Nursing, 30*(10), 80-88.

Adams, J.H. (1997). Using RN care managers in community health centers. *Nursing Economic$, 14*(3), 153-156.

American Academy of Ambulatory Care Nursing and American Nurses' Association (AAACN/ANA). (1997). *Nursing in ambulatory care: The future is here.* Washington, DC: American Nurses Publishing.

American Academy of Ambulatory Care Nursing (AAACN). (2004a). *Ambulatory care nursing administration and practice standards.* Pitman, NJ: Author.

American Academy of Ambulatory Care Nursing (AAACN). (2004b). *Telehealth nursing practice administration and practice standards.* Pitman, NJ: Author.

Billi, J.E., Wise, C.G., Bills, E.A., & Mitchell, R.L. (1995). Potential effects of managed care on specialty practice at a university medical center. *Journal of the American Medical Association, 333*(13), 979-984.

Bunting, L.K. (1994). *Role of the ambulatory care nurse in the Indian Health Service.* Unpublished master's thesis, Johns

Hopkins School of Nursing, Baltimore, MD.

Burnett, K., Chapman, D., Wishart, G., & Purushotham, A (2004). Nurse specialists in breast care: A developing role. *Nursing Standard, 18*(45), 38-42.

Curran, C. (1995). An interview with Linda D'Angelo. *Nursing Economic$, 13*(4), 193-196.

Dickey, E. (1998). Outpatient visit planning: Turning episodic care into comprehensive care. *Nursing Economic$, 16*(2), 88-90.

Eck, S.A., Picagali, D., & Boyle, S. (1997). Improving health outcomes in under-served women. *AAACN Viewpoint, 19*(4), 1, 4-5, 9.

Ervin, N.E., Chang, W-Y., & White, J. (1998). A cost analysis of a nursing center's services. *Nursing Economic$, 16*(6), 307-312.

Gesell, S.B., & Gregory, N. (2004). Identifying priority actions for improving patient satisfaction with outpatient cancer care. *Journal of Nursing Care Quality, 19*(3), 226-233.

Haas, S. (1998). Ambulatory care nursing conceptual framework. *AAACN Viewpoint, 20*(3), 16-17.

Haas, S.A., Hackbarth, D.P., Kavanaugh, J.A., & Vlasses, E. (1995). Dimensions of the staff nurse role in ambulatory care. Part II: Comparison of role dimensions in four ambulatory settings. *Nursing Economic$, 13*(3), 152-165.

Hackbarth, D.S., Haas, S., Kavanaugh, J.A., & Vlasses, E. (1995). Dimensions of the staff nurse role in ambulatory care. Part I: Methodology and analysis of data on current staff nurse practice. *Nursing Economic$, 13*(2), 89-98.

Hastings, C. (1987). Classification issues in ambulatory care nursing. *Journal of Ambulatory Care Management, 10*(3), 50-64.

Hastings, C. (1997). The changing multidisciplinary team. *Nursing Economic$, 15*(2), 106-108, 105.

Hastings, C., & Muir-Nash, J. (1989). Validation of a taxonomy of ambulatory nursing practice. *Nursing Economic$, 7*(3), 142-149.

Hendershot, E., Murphy, C., Doyle, S., Van-Clief, J., Lowry, J., & Honeyford, L. (2005). Outpatient chemotherapy administration: Decreasing wait times for patients and their families. *Journal of Pediatric Oncology Nursing, 22*(1), 31-37.

Hunter, J.K., Ventura, M.R., & Kearns, P.A. (1999). Cost analysis of a nursing center for the homeless. *Nursing Economic$, 17*(1), 20-28.

Janikowski, D.L., & Rockefeller, C.A. (1998). Awake and talking: Ambulatory surgery and conscious sedation. *Nursing Economic$, 16*(1), 37-43.

Johnston, M. (1980). Ambulatory care into the 80's – Looking ahead to a decade of dilemmas. *American Journal of Nursing, 80*, 70-79.

Loftus, L.A., & Weston, V. (2001). The development of nurse-led clinics in cancer care. *Journal of Clinical Nursing, 10*, 215-220.

Marzalek, E. (1980). Ambulatory nursing: At the crossroads? *Nursing & Health Care, 1*, 245-255.

Mayer, G.G. (1996). Case management as a mindset. *Quality Management in Health Care, 5*(1), 7-16.

Parrinello, K.M., Brennan, P.S., & Vallone, B. (1988). Refining and testing a nursing patient classification instrument in ambulatory care. *Nursing Administration Quarterly, 13*(1), 54-65.

Schim, S.M., Thornburg, P., & Kravutske, M.E. (2001). Time, task and talents in ambulatory care nursing. *Journal of Nursing Administration, 31*(6), 311-315.

Scott, J. (2000). A nursing leadership challenge: Managing the chronically ill in rural settings. *Nursing Administration Quarterly, 24*(3), 21-32.

Schroeder, C.A., Trehearne, B., & Ward, D. (2000a). Expanded role of nursing in ambulatory managed care part I: Literature, role development, and justification. *Nursing Economic$, 18*(1) 14-19.

Schroeder, C.A., Trehearne, B., & Ward, D. (2000b). Expanded role of nursing in ambulatory managed care part II: Impact on outcomes of costs, quality, provider, and patient satisfaction. *Nursing Economic$, 18*(2), 71-78.

Tighe, M.G., Fisher, S.G., Hastings, C., & Heller, B.A. (1985). Study of the oncology nurse role in ambulatory care. *Oncology Nursing Forum, 12*(6), 23-27.

Verran, J. (1981). Delineation of ambulatory care nursing practice. *Journal of Ambulatory Care Management, 4*(2),1-13.

Verran, J.A. (1986). Patient classification in ambulatory care. *Nursing Economic$, 4*(5), 247-251.

Verran, J.A., & Reid, P.J. (1987). Replicated testing of the nursing technology model. *Nursing Research, 36*(3), 190-194.

The Ambulatory Care Practice Arena

This test may be copied for use by others.

COMPLETE THE FOLLOWING:

Name: _____

Address: _____

City: _____ State: _____ Zip: _____

Preferred telephone: (Home)_____ (Work)_____

E-mail_____

AAACN Member Expiration Date: _____

Registration fee: AAACN Member: $12.00
                     Nonmember: $20.00

Answer Form:

1. If you applied what you have learned from this activity into your practice, what would be different?

_____

_____

_____

Objectives

This educational activity is designed for nurses and other health care professionals who practice in ambulatory care. For those wishing to obtain CE credit, an evaluation follows. After studying the information presented in this offering, you will be able to:

1. Describe the domain of ambulatory care nursing practice.
2. Discuss the characteristics of patients seen in ambulatory care and the implications of nursing practice.
3. Compare nursing practice in ambulatory and acute inpatient settings.
4. Identify and describe current practice settings for ambulatory care nursing.
5. Discuss challenges faced by nurses moving from inpatient to ambulatory care settings and describe strategies to facilitate the transition.

Evaluation

	Strongly disagree				Strongly agree
2. By completing this activity, I was able to meet the following objectives:					
a. Describe the domain of ambulatory care nursing practice.	1	2	3	4	5
b. Discuss the characteristics of patients seen in ambulatory care and the implications of nursing practice.	1	2	3	4	5
c. Compare nursing practice in ambulatory and acute inpatient settings.	1	2	3	4	5
d. Identify and describe current practice settings for ambulatory care nursing.	1	2	3	4	5
e. Discuss challenges faced by nurses moving from inpatient to ambulatory care settings and describe strategies to facilitate the transition.	1	2	3	4	5
3. The content was current and relevant.	1	2	3	4	5
4. The objectives could be achieved using the content provided.	1	2	3	4	5
5. This was an effective method to learn this content.	1	2	3	4	5
6. I am more confident in my abilities since completing this material.	1	2	3	4	5

7. The material was (check one) ___new   ___review for me.
8. Time required to read this chapter: _____minutes

I verify that I have completed this activity: _____
                                                        Signature

Comments: _____

_____

_____

Posttest Instructions

1. To receive continuing education credit for individual study after reading the article, complete the answer/evaluation form to the left.

2. Detach and send the answer/evaluation form along with a check or money order payable to the *American Academy of Ambulatory Care Nursing (AAACN)*, East Holly Avenue Box 56, Pitman, NJ 08071–0056.

3. Test returns must be postmarked by August 1, 2011. Upon completion of the answer/evaluation form, a certificate for **1.2** contact hour(s) will be awarded and sent to you. Should the material contained in this chapter become outdated prior to the above expiration date, AAACN reserves the right to withdraw this CE test.

This activity is co-provided by the *American Academy of Ambulatory Care Nursing (AAACN)* and Anthony J. Jannetti, Inc. (AJJ). AJJ is accredited as a provider of continuing nursing education by the American Nurses' Credentialing Center's Commission on Accreditation (ANCC-COA). AAACN is a provider approved by the California Board of Registered Nurses, provider number CEP 05336.

This article was reviewed and formatted for contact hour credit by Sally S. Russell, MN, CMSRN, AAACN Education Director; and Candia Baker Laughlin MS, RN, C, Editor.

Chapter 3

The Context of Ambulatory Care Nursing

Margaret Fisk Mastal, PhD, RN

Objectives

Study of the information presented in this chapter will enable the learner to:

1. Trace the evolutionary changes of the concept of health from the early 1900s to the present time.
2. Discuss the application of health concepts in the ambulatory care environment.
3. Discuss the effects of consumerism on health care providers and organizations.
4. Identify major societal and health care industry trends and their impact on the ambulatory care environment.
5. Describe diverse nursing care delivery models in ambulatory settings.

Key Points

1. Health as a concept expanded over the 20th century to include disease prevention and health promotion as well as the treatment and/or cure of disease and illness, reshaping the focus of ambulatory care practice to a greater emphasis on disease prevention and wellness.
2. New concepts of health coupled with the responses of ambulatory care systems to societal and health industry trends brought about an emphasis on primary care, the rise of managed care, and the development of new practices in complex ambulatory care organizations.
3. Professional ambulatory care nursing practice has diverse delivery models that promote access to care and delivery of nursing services using clinical and administrative expertise.

A number of evolutionary societal, regulatory, and health industry trends form the context of the ambulatory care environment, effecting changes in ambulatory delivery systems and professional nursing practice. Delivery systems have evolved into sophisticated, highly complex organizations. Professional nursing roles have shifted from an emphasis on technological skills to a broader focus, one that requires diverse professional knowledge and competencies.

This chapter initially provides an overview of how the concept of health evolved over the 20th century to the present, discusses the application of health care concepts in ambulatory settings, and identifies the impact of societal and health industry trends on ambulatory care organizational practices. Additionally, it describes the professional nursing models currently operating in ambulatory settings, models categorized as those that (1) facilitate access, (2) provide direct health care services, or (3) manage or coordinate care across the continuum.

Concept

Over the past two centuries, health as a concept has expanded from a focus on preventing illness, treating disease, and minimizing symptoms to one that includes health promotion and targets achieving optimal health states for both individuals and populations. In the late 20th century, as health care industry activities shifted from hospital-centered to outpatient settings, evolving notions of health have been integrated into the ambulatory environment.

A. Health: Historical perspectives.
  1. *Medieval era* – Defined by isolation and quarantine of those with communicable diseases.
  2. *19th century* – Defined by emerging control and management of environmental factors, such as waste disposal, sanitation and hygiene, and adequate housing.
    a. Hand-washing practices emphasized (initiated by Isaac Semmelweis).
    b. Vector control practices initiated – Eradication of rats, fleas, mosquitoes, etc.

c. Influence of Florence Nightingale adopted – Emphasis on clean environments, nutrition, etc.

d. Lillian Wald spotlighted health care for women and children at the Henry Street Settlement.

3. *Early-mid 20th century* – Focused upon prevention of disease and treatment of mental illness.

a. New emphasis on the individual as responsible for his or her own health care emerged.

b. Immunizations and antibiotics were developed.

c. Tranquilizers and antidepressants became available for the treatment of mental health problems.

4. *Latter part of the 20th century* – Perspectives begin to expand.

a. Lalonde Report: Marc Lalonde, Canadian Health Minister, 1974.

(1) Lalonde hypothesized that health is affected by multiple factors (human biology, lifestyle choices, the organization of health care, and the social and physical environments).

(2) The report initiated a shift from the focus of treating disease to one of disease prevention and health promotion (McDonald & Bunton, 1992).

b. World Health Organization (WHO) (1978) publicized the Alma Ata Declaration, committing the WHO organization to work for the health of all world citizens by the year 2000.

(1) The Declaration expanded the conceptualization of primary scare to primary health care.

(2) Primary health care was defined as "essential health care . . made universally accessible to individuals and families in the community . . . through their full participation and at a cost that the community and country can afford" (WHO, 1978, p. 3).

c. Institute of Medicine (IOM) (1978) issued the first definition of primary care.

(1) Primary care was conceptualized in terms of personal health services rather than public health services.

(2) Primary care should be "accessible, comprehensive, coordinated, and continual by accountable providers of personnel [sic] health services" (IOM, 1978, p. 16).

(3) Increased emphasis was placed on prevention, removing barriers to care, coordination, continuity, and the inclusion of patients and families in the decision-making process (Hackbarth, 1995).

d. U.S. Surgeon General's 1979 report, *Healthy People: The Surgeon General's Report on Health Promotion and Disease Prevention*, declared that disease prevention and health promotion were separate but equal concepts.

(1) Disease prevention was defined as protection from environmental threats.

(2) Health promotion was considered in terms of positive lifestyle changes (U.S. Department of Health and Human Services [DHHS], 1991).

e. U.S. Surgeon General's report, *Promoting Health/Preventing Disease: Objectives for a Nation*, was issued in 1980.

(1) This report identified specific, quantifiable objectives for promoting health and preventing disease.

(2) Objectives were organized around 15 priority areas (for example, blood pressure and cancer screening, timely immunizations, smoking cessation, reduction of alcohol use, etc.) (DHHS, 1991).

f. The Ottawa Charter (1987) evolved from a meeting of the WHO, Health and Welfare Canada, and the Canadian Public Health Association.

(1) Health was broadly defined as individuals' ability to achieve physical, mental, and social well-being by their abilities to identify and realize aspirations, satisfy their needs, and change or cope with the environment.

(2) Health promotion was broadly defined as a process enabling people to increase their control over abilities to improve health.

(3) Health was perceived as a resource for daily life, not the objective of living.

(4) Health was described as a positive concept emphasizing social and personal resources as well as physical capacities, going beyond healthy lifestyles to well-being.

(5) Five major health promotion actions were outlined:

    (a) Build health public policy.

    (b) Create supportive environments.

    (c) Develop personal skills.

    (d) Strengthen community action.

    (e) Re-orient health services (WHO, 1987).

g. *Healthy People 2000* – Created a platform for action to help Americans fulfill their health potential (Morgan & Marsh, 1998).

(1) Three broad goals were outlined:

    (a) Increase the span of healthy life.

    (b) Reduce health disparities.

    (c) Achieve access to preventive services.

(2) Three hundred measurable objectives were established.

(3) Health promotion strategies were described in terms of:

    (a) Actions are related to individual lifestyle.

    (b) Personal choices are made in a social context (for example, physical activity, use of substances, family planning, mental health, and abusive or violent behaviors) (DHHS, 1991).

h. *Healthy People 2010* was initiated at a meeting of the *Healthy People 2000* Consortium in New York City, November 1996 (DHHS, 1999).

(1) Builds on prior health initiatives, the Surgeon General's Reports of 1979 and 1980, and the Healthy People 2000 movement as an instrument to improve health for the first decade of the 21st century.

(2) Overarching purpose – "Promoting health and preventing illness, disability, and premature death" (DHHS, 2000, p. 1).

(3) Assumption – The context of change and innovation will reshape the practice of medicine and health care (DHHS, 1999):

    (a) Advances will occur in preventive therapies, vaccines, pharmaceuticals, assistive technologies, and computer technologies.

    (b) New relationships between public health departments and health care organizations will be defined.

    (c) U.S. demographic changes (such as older and more racially diverse) will create new demands on the health care system.

    (d) Global forces (fluctuating food supplies, emerging infectious diseases, environmental interdependence) will present new public health challenges.

(4) Goals of *Healthy People 2000* (DHHS, 2000, pp. 8-16).

    (a) *Goal 1 – Increase the quality and years of healthy life.* Evaluation includes measuring changes in the following indicators:

        (i) *Life expectancy* – Average number of years people born in a given year are expected to live based on a set of age-specific death rates.

        (ii) *Health-related quality of life* – Subjective, personal sense of physical and mental health, and the ability to react to factors in the physical and social environments.

(iii) *Global assessments* – Personal ratings of one's own health status.

(iv) *Years of healthy life* – Average amount of time spent in less than optimal health as a result of chronic or acute limitations.

(b) *Goal 2 – Eliminate health disparities among different segments of the population.* Evaluation will occur by measuring the decrease in health status gaps that exist because of:

(i) Gender.

(ii) Race and ethnicity.

(iii) Income and education.

(iv) Disability.

(v) Rural or urban location.

(vi) Sexual orientation.

(5) 2010 objectives (467 objectives in 28 focus areas) will be distinguished from *Healthy People 2000* by having:

(a) Broadened preventive, scientific base.

(b) Improved surveillance and data systems.

(c) Heightened awareness and demand for preventive health services and quality health care.

(d) Integrated the changes in demographics, science, technology, and disease spread that will affect health in the 21st century.

(6) *Healthy People 2000* will be the United States' contribution to the WHO "Health for All" strategy.

(7) The U.S. effort will be characterized by key partnerships – that is, collaboration between and among federal, state, local, and private sectors as well as community participation (DHHS, 2000).

5. The shift in perspectives about health over the latter part of the 20th century and the possibilities that present for the 21st century have significant implications for ambulatory care settings.

B. Ambulatory environment: Crucible for the integration of health concepts.

1. Ambulatory settings are the sites in the community where care is usually initiated.

2. Optimal milieu for providers to initiate and integrate practices that reflect the current concepts of holistic health into the delivery of health care services.

Health Care Concepts in the Ambulatory Environment

The outpatient setting is uniquely poised to integrate current health care concepts into the delivery of care. Ambulatory services, the traditional site of primary care in America, focus on health promotion and disease prevention, as well as the treatment of acute and minor illness and chronic disease. Over the latter quarter of the 20th century, the scope of ambulatory care services has expanded significantly. Care has emerged from an emphasis on the single physician dispensing health care for an individual patient to a group of providers facilitating access to a broad array of diverse, comprehensive, and integrated services designed to meet community needs.

A. Primary care is regarded as *essential* health care and is the cornerstone for ambulatory health services (Shi & Singh, 1998).

1. Not all settings where patients walk in are considered primary care (for example, a hospital Emergency Department is not considered primary care).

2. Definitions vary slightly depending on differing viewpoints, but the one generally accepted definition comes from the IOM.

a. "Primary care is the provision of integrated, accessible health care services by clinicians who are accountable for addressing a large majority of *personal* health care needs, developing a sustained partnership with patients, and practicing in the context of family and community" (IOM, 1996, p. 5).

b. IOM definitional concepts – The definition of primary care embodies a number of concepts including:

(1) *Comprehensiveness* – Means that care addresses any health concern at any stage across the individual's life span.

(2) *Coordinating* – Refers to the function that ensures that the care (any combination of therapies and services) occurs to holistically meet the individual's needs.

(3) *Continuity* – Refers to the care that is received over time and that is being delivered or coordinated by a single provider or team of health care professionals.

(4) *Accessible* – Refers to the ease with which consumers can initiate interaction with a clinician about health problem(s). It includes activities to eliminate barriers raised by geography, financing, culture, race, language, etc.

(5) *Accountability* – Embodies both the provider and the consumer.

   (a) The clinical system is accountable for providing quality care, effecting consumer satisfaction, using resources efficiently, and acting in an ethical, culturally competent manner.

   (b) Consumers are accountable for their health and for using health care resources judiciously.

c. A second definition of primary care focuses on community-oriented primary care (COPC). It is a model that incorporates the elements of the IOM model but adds a population-based approach that identifies and addresses community health needs (Shi & Singh, 1998).

(1) The traditional definition of primary care centered on a biopsychosocial paradigm with medical care rendered to the individual in an encounter-based system.

(2) The evolving COPC model has a broader biopsychosocial paradigm, one that emphasizes the health of populations as well as the individual.

3. In primary care, the relationship of provider and consumer is one of partnership.

a. Roles played by each will vary over time and circumstances.

b. The hallmarks of the partnership are mutual trust, respect, and responsibility (Shi & Singh, 1998).

4. Primary care "specialties" are capable of addressing a wide variety of health care needs. They are most commonly designated as:

a. Adult medicine.

b. Pediatrics.

c. Family medicine.

d. Obstetrics and gynecology (OB/GYN) – Some practice settings consider OB/GYN a specialty rather than primary care.

5. Primary care, the conceptual foundation for ambulatory health services, is expected to coordinate access to and use of *secondary care* levels, such as routine hospitalization and surgery, specialty referrals, advanced diagnostic/therapeutic care, and *tertiary care,* (for example, highly specialized and highly technological care) (Shi & Singh, 1998).

A. Ambulatory health care occurs in a wide variety of settings that are generally defined by a community's demographics, health needs, and the resources available (refer to Chapter 2, *The Ambulatory Care Practice Arena,* for a listing of ambulatory care settings).

B. The nature of the modern ambulatory care environment is dynamic. Hallmarks of ambulatory care settings include:

1. Encounters are high-volume, time-sensitive, and generally based on an appointment schedule.

2. Patients ordinarily initiate their encounters through the appointment procedure; however, it is also common for patients to present themselves for care (walk in) without appointments.

3. The true nature of an individual's presenting problem(s) is frequently unknown until he or she accesses the system. Problems have a broad scope, ranging from emergency or urgent situations, through acute illness and

minor problems, chronic illness, and preventive health services, to a patient's desire for health care at his or her convenience.

C. In contrast to care systems throughout most of the 20th century, the single physician as provider is uncommon in today's ambulatory environment; rather, the physician now serves as a fulcrum to a diverse managed care system.

   1. From the historical perspective, ambulatory services are as old as the healing arts themselves (Williams, 1993).

      a. The physician was traditionally the central point of care. He or she treated patients in offices and/or during home visits.

      b. Rapidly advancing technology dating from the mid-20th century initiated a shift in the locus of ambulatory treatment, from offices and homes to the community hospital setting.

      c. Physicians gravitated toward hospital-based offices that offered easier access to diagnostic services, pharmacy, etc.

      d. Today, physicians commonly serve as leverage for individual consumers to access comprehensive arrays of health services in what is now a managed care environment.

D. *The managed care environment* – The concept and realities of managed care have evolved over the past quarter-century in response to societal concerns about rising health care costs and efforts to contain them.

   1. Definition of *managed care* – Incorporation of controls over the health care utilization behaviors of both providers and consumers (Shi & Singh, 1998).

      a. Managed care can be considered in two different contexts:

         (1) As a *mechanism or process* of providing health care services that integrates the key functions of insurance, care delivery, and payment in one organizational setting that exercises control over utilization.

         (2) As a *type of organizational form* (Shi & Singh, 1998).

      b. Ambulatory care organizational forms include diverse types of managed care organizations (refer to Chapter 6, *Health Care Fiscal Management*).

   2. Factors contributing to the emergence of today's managed care include events that resulted from cost containment efforts.

      a. The emergence of hospital insurance before World War II and advances in technology after World War II spurred the fiscal growth and care capabilities of the health care industry.

      b. The amendments to the *Social Security Act* in 1965 created Medicare and Medicaid, making subsidized hospital care available to the aged and poor. This landmark legislation created equal opportunity for health care for the older adult and poverty level populations, but it also spurred the rise of health care costs.

      c. During the 1970s, rising costs initiated the first serious cost control efforts including the *Health Maintenance Act* of 1973 that:

         (1) Allocated federal funds to establish and expand new HMOs.

         (2) Represented the government's first attempt to establish alternatives to fee-for-service reimbursement.

         (3) Required employers with 25-plus employees to offer an HMO option as an employee benefit.

      d. During the 1980s, an explosive growth of prepaid, capitated health plans occurred.

      e. During the 1990s, managed care arrangements dominated health care delivery services and utilization (Shi & Singh, 1998).

The Rise of Consumerism: Customer-Focused Health Care in Ambulatory Settings

During the 1990s, marketing approaches evolved in ambulatory care settings in a manner similar to the hospital industry that had adopted marketing approaches in 1980s. Increasingly, organizations were encouraging service industry strategies in provider-patient encounters. Employees were also encouraged to use these strategies in their work relationships. The "customer" was defined differently from various perspectives, but in all cases, it was the person, group, or population that became the central focus of the action or interaction.

A. The consumer as customer: In ambulatory care settings, the consumer generally initiates the encounter, expecting high levels of care and service from each member of the health care team.

1. Ambulatory health care is largely *self-administered by the individual* in the context of family and the social, economic, and cultural environments.

2. The focus of care is on the dignity and worth of the individual and his or her right to participate in:
   a. Making decisions about his or her health care.
   b. Setting goals about his or her health care.
   c. Being informed about and participating in the choice of therapy from among alternative therapies.

3. There are 3 categories of consumer concerns:
   a. Access to health care – Conceptually defined as "the fit among personal, socio-cultural, economic, and system-related factors that enable individuals, families, and communities to have timely, needed, necessary, continuous, and satisfactory health services" (Gulzar, 1999, p. 17).
      (1) Access addresses the availability of both primary care and specialty providers to consumers when they need or want an appointment.
      (2) Consumer expectations about waiting for access (or an appointment) to the primary care provider or specialist vary, depending on the individual's perception of the urgency of the need or want.
      (3) Different providers on the health care team ensure access according to their unique professional expertise.
         (a) Physicians (primary care providers and specialists) gen-

erally care for patients with medical emergencies, severe illness, and those with complex medical problems.
         (b) Advanced practice nurses (APNs) have a variety of roles, depending on the practice setting and the practice styles of others on the team. In general, they care for patients with acute minor illness, those who need oversight for the management of chronic disease and/or health education, and those with health and/or wellness concerns.
         (c) In many settings, clinical nurses triage unexpected demands for care, administer appropriate nursing interventions in acute situations, provide health education about disease prevention and health promotion, and serve as the conduit for information between the patient, the physician, and the organization.
         (d) Technicians and unlicensed personnel furnish technical support (for example, apply casts, screen vital signs, prepare patients for physical examinations, make follow-up appointments, etc.).
   b. Reasonable costs – American consumers generally desire quality health care services with minimal out-of-pocket costs. Costs of care should be fully disclosed and the payment plan(s) appropriately addressed.
   c. Quality health care – Consumers expect high-quality care, usually defined from their perspective in terms of:
      (1) Rapid, accurate diagnosis of their health care problem(s).
      (2) Appropriate therapies and pharmaceuticals that relieve their symptoms and restore them to their normal lifestyle.

    (3) Reasonable reassurance that their health concern(s) can be cured, minimized, or managed.

    (4) Complete, accurate, and understandable information about their condition.

    (5) Courteous and caring health care team members who treat their family members and them with dignity and respect.

    (6) Individualized care that is focused on their individual differences and uniqueness.

B. Provider team members as customer: Regardless of any particular setting, ambulatory health care delivery usually occurs within the context of a multidisciplinary team of providers in partnership with the patient, his or her family, and significant others.

  1. Service industry methods include providers approaching each other as customers.

  2. Ambulatory care staff practice as members of teams of health care providers that include a range of professional and allied staff.

  3. Modern team members are expected to relate among themselves and with other institutional staff using customer-oriented approaches, that is, placing the other person at the center of the interaction.

    a. Interact with each other with consideration, respect, and dignity.

    b. Interact so as to meet or exceed the other person's expectations.

C. Nursing roles on the ambulatory health care team.

  1. Historically, nursing roles focused on technical care (for example, injections, intravenous therapy, assisting with procedures, etc.).

  2. Increasingly, today's nursing role is a collaborative professional practice and includes:

    a. Assisting patients and families to coordinate their health care.

    b. Performing professional nursing interventions.

    c. Communicating nursing interventions and outcomes among team members (Haas & Hackbarth, 1995).

    d. Evaluating nursing performance and out-comes of care.

3. The sponsoring organization influences the structure and operating style of the multidisciplinary team.

  a. Historical origins of the organization (for example, hospital-based, private practice, HMOs) affect beliefs, strategies, and the way the individual practice environment serves its consumer population.

  b. Roles and functions of team members, including nurses, vary within different organizations and even within different units of the same organization.

    (1) Traditional: Physician is leader and chief decision-maker; team members function according to the physician's directions (commonly seen in, but not exclusive to, private physician offices).

    (2) Care partners: Physician and nurse team together to assume responsibility for the health care of a designated population (for example, oncology patients).

      (a) Follow patients across the continuum of care (hospital, clinic, and home).

      (b) The nurse is also sometimes referred to as the primary nurse (Bedlek, 1996).

    (3) Participatory, multidisciplinary teams: Physicians, advanced practitioners, managers, nurses, staff, etc. work collaboratively according to mutually developed and clearly defined roles and functions.

  c. Regardless of the configurations of team roles/functions within an individual setting, societal and regulatory mandates expect designated accountability and responsibility for the health services provided, including outreach, diagnosis, treatment, and follow-up.

D. Ambulatory care typically includes the family or significant other in care practices, while mindful of and careful to preserve the patient's right to privacy and confidentiality.

  1. The family is usually the individual patient's major support system.

2. Providing appropriate information and support to the patient's caregiver(s) enhances their ability to sustain the patient in acute, chronic, or terminal stages of health.
3. Giving information and support to patients and their caregivers includes addressing cultural, language, and other differences, and closing gaps where disparities occur.

Current Trends Impacting Ambulatory Care And Nursing Practice

Organizational preparation to accommodate new trends in society and the health care environment is imperative because these trends affect health care organizations and nursing practice. These trends, or mega issues, while broad and sweeping, make demands and will bring changes to ambulatory care organizations and the nurses who practice in them (Futch & Phillips, 2003).

A. Increased life expectancy: The life span of both men and women has increased due to new treatments and advancing technology.
   1. Definitions of the term "elderly" will change.
   2. Incidence of chronic disease will rise.
   3. Care at the end of life will assume prominence.
B. Environmental threats: The world has become a global community; events far and near require local responses. Terrorism, war, new diseases emerging from mutating microbes, and occurrences of environmental cataclysms threaten personal and community safety and health.
   1. Rapid responses and preparation for imminent danger, imperative in an uncertain world, will require revisions of organizational disaster plans.
   2. Alternative therapies and isolation techniques will be used as current vaccines, and antibiotics may not be effective on new diseases.
   3. New forms of warfare will require acquiring new knowledge and clinical skills.
C. Increased legislation and regulation: The level of federal and state regulation of health care is higher now than at any other time in our history and is likely to escalate.
   1. The *Health Insurance Portability and Accountability Act of 1996* (HIPAA) mandates

that organizations securely procure, transmit, and house personal health information (PHI).
   2. The Center for Medicare and Medicaid Services (CMS) has instituted managed care programs for vulnerable populations (such as frail older adults).
   3. States are increasingly mandating managed care for Medicaid beneficiaries including persons with disabilities.
   4. CMS and state Medicaid agencies oversee the quality of care and performance improvement in managed care plans that serve Medicare and Medicaid beneficiaries.
   5. CMS and state Medicaid agencies audit claims on a regular basis to detect fraud and abuse of benefits and services.
   6. Health care report cards for the public's use are disclosing how well health care organizations deliver quality health care and improve health outcomes.
   7. The *Balanced Budget Act of 1997* requires compliance with diverse regulations.
E. Ethical integrity in business and clinical practices is a prominent issue as health care organizations grapple with instituting compliance programs that address regulatory requirements.
   1. Organizations are developing codes of conduct for assuring that clinical practices and business decisions are ethically based on principles of integrity.
   2. Health care organizations need to build public trust and confidence that they are doing the right thing, the right way, the first time.
   3. Accountability to consumers and payers is a primary focus.
   4. Research-based guidelines are serving as the basis for clinical interventions.
   5. Evolving technology and expanded life expectancy pose complex ethical dilemmas (Futch & Phillips, 2003).
F. Advancing technology is occurring rapidly, bringing new capabilities to health care providers and health delivery systems.
   a. Diagnostic and therapeutic technological advances require the development of new clinical and organizational practices.
   b. Information technological progress has

introduced new ways of documenting and retrieving health information for clinicians and organizations.

c. Communications technology that allows long-distance diagnosis, monitoring, and treatment is beginning to revolutionize the way care is provided.

Nursing and Nursing Care Delivery Models in Ambulatory Care

Nursing models in ambulatory care have developed and evolved along with the changing concepts about health and their application in health care organizations and emerging societal and health industry trends. While a number of diverse models of nursing care delivery exist, professional ambulatory nursing practice is predicated on a theoretical base of knowledge that grows through evidence-based research and adherence to professional standards of practice and guidelines for clinical care.

A. Nursing knowledge serves as the foundation and is the source of continued expansion of professional ambulatory care nursing practice.
   1. The theoretical base of nursing knowledge is acquired in educational settings (such as accredited schools and colleges of nursing).
   2. This knowledge grows in professional practice through four major mechanisms:
      a. Utilizing research-based evidence found in nationally and/or professionally approved guidelines and protocols (Pravikoff, Tanner, & Pierce, 2005).
      b. Conducting and/or utilizing the findings of quality studies for improving professional nursing, health care delivery, and consumer health outcomes.
      c. Participating in continuing nursing educational programs, such as:
         (1) Formal college or university courses of study.
         (2) Certification in nursing or allied health specialties.
         (3) Professional conferences and seminars.
         (4) Current textbooks.
         (5) Literature reviews to gather evidence in libraries or Web-based resources.

d. Applying professional standards – Standards of practice published by professional nursing organizations.
   (1) American Academy of Ambulatory Care Nursing (AAACN):
      (a) *Ambulatory Care Nursing Administration and Practice Standards* (AAACN, 2004).
      (b) *Telehealth Nursing Practice Administration and Practice Standards* (AAACN, 2004).
   (2) Other professional nursing organizations:
      (a) *Code of Ethics for Nurses with Interpretive Statements* (American Nurses Association [ANA], 2001), *Nursing Scope and Standards of Practice* (ANA, 2004a), *Nursing's Social Policy Statements* (ANA, 2003), and *Scope and Standards for Nurse Administrators* (ANA, 2004b).
      (b) Standards published by nursing specialty organizations, such as the Oncology Nursing Society.

B. Nursing care delivery models in ambulatory care use the nursing process in all nurse-client interactions. The diverse models of nursing care delivery are classified in three major categories: facilitating access to care, direct intervention, and care coordination.
   1. Access models – These types of nursing models function to ensure that consumers have access to the health care system for care and questions.
      a. Nurse-triage services in clinics and offices are examples of access models that require expert assessment skills, critical thinking, and problem-solving skills, as well as the ability to deal with diverse and often serious acute or chronic health conditions.
      b. Telehealth nursing practice is a subspecialty nursing domain that pervades ambulatory nursing practice in all settings.
         (1) The two general categories of telehealth nursing practice settings are:
            (a) Centralized call centers – Formal settings where nurses

ensure consumers have access by telephone to appropriate health care services.

  (b) Decentralized telephone practice – Nurses maintain telephone communication with individuals and families regarding their health care inquiries and concerns as a part of their daily practice regardless of the practice setting.

(2) Nursing roles in telehealth include the ability to:

  (a) Triage queries from clients about health problems that may range from emergency or urgent situations to routine.

  (b) Assist the caller to access the appropriate provider.

  (c) Provide information about diagnostic test results.

  (d) Call pharmacies with prescriptions.

  (e) Give medical and health care advice according to standardized protocols.

  (f) Conduct follow-up inquiry and evaluation after treatment.

(3) Standards of telehealth nursing practice were developed and published first by AAACN in 1997.

c. Parish nursing is an example of an access model where nurses are available within a religious or faith community.

(1) Philosophically, parish nursing promotes the health of a faith community by working with the clergy and staff to integrate the theological, sociological, and physiological perspectives of health and healing into liturgies, and service provided for the congregation (O'Brien, 1999).

(2) History: Parish nursing, as it is evolving in America today, can trace its roots to Europe.

  (a) Groups such as the German Christian deaconesses (Gemeindeschwestern) were active in the 19th century.

  (b) U.S. contemporary parish nursing was instituted during the mid-1980s by Granger Westberg, a Lutheran pastor, as an outgrowth of a holistic health center project funded jointly by the Kellogg Foundation and the University of Illinois College of Medicine (O'Brien, 1999).

(3) Parish nurses serve as volunteers or paid staff, affiliated with a specific church or with a specific health care institution in partnership with a local church.

(4) Parish nurses visit individuals and families in homes, churches, hospitals, extended care facilities, and other community sites.

(5) Parish nurse roles focus on integrating the spiritual and religious dimensions with wellness, illness, and adaptation to chronic disease.

(6) Roles can vary by individual practice but generally include:

  (a) *Health counselor* – Answers health questions; provides grief/bereavement assistance and counseling for marriage and family problems, substance abuse, dysfunctional behaviors, and other personal needs.

  (b) *Health educator* – Conducts health screenings and wellness activities (for example, age-specific health programs), maintains a health-related library and pamphlet file, expands understanding about the role of the parish nurse.

  (c) *Health facilitator* – Trains volunteers to assist in family crises, refers individuals and families to community resources, facilitates small groups (single parents, marriage encounter, loss support), participates in healing services, and coordinates outreach efforts.

(d) *Liaison* to health services and professionals in the local community (for example, works in partnership with and as a referral source to physicians and public health nurses) (O'Brien, 1999).

2. Direct intervention models – This second general category of nursing models in ambulatory care includes those that provide direct nursing care. These include the following care delivery systems.

   a. *Nursing centers or nurse-managed clinics* are both a concept and a place (Frenn, Lundeen, Martin, Riesch, & Wilson, 1998).

      (1) Conceptual definitions of nursing centers have two basic dimensions:
          (a) That the nursing care is directly accessible to the client, family, or community.
          (b) That all nursing practice is directly controlled by nurses.

      (2) Geographically, nursing centers operate within a specific locale.

      (3) Classified in three types (Reisch, 1992):
          (a) Community health and institutional outreach models: Can be freestanding or institution-sponsored.
              (i) Provide primary care services to medically underserved populations.
              (ii) Use a multidisciplinary staff.
              (iii) Are funded by diverse public and private sources.
          (b) Wellness and health promotion models: Based on community needs with services developed to focus on promoting health.
              (i) Services often delivered where groups gather (work, school, church, shelters).
              (ii) Often viewed as alternatives to traditional health care delivery.
          (c) Faculty practice, independent practice, and nurse entrepre-

neurship models: Include agencies and services owned and operated by nurses (Frenn et al., 1999).

   b. *Advanced practice nurses (APNs)* – Nurses educated, certified, and licensed as nurse practitioners, nurse midwives, and/or clinical specialists who provide medical and nursing care to defined populations of patients; usually, but not necessarily allied with, a physician's practice depending on state practice laws.

   c. *Clinical registered nurses* in medical offices or clinics (hospital-based, HMO, community sites, etc.) – Function according to the practices of the institution in which they are employed.

      (1) Triage patient problems and needs in face-to-face and telephone encounters.

      (2) Monitor patient conditions and health status.

      (3) Perform nursing therapies for treatment of illness/disease (intravenous therapy for dehydration, medication administration, immunizations, etc.).

      (4) Educate patients and families about managing their disease (diabetes, asthma, heart disease, behavioral problems, etc.).

      (5) Communicate health information between physicians and patients (follow-up reports on laboratory/ radiology findings, changes in medications or therapies, etc.).

      (6) Assist patients and families to access other relevant providers (such as specialist referrals, diagnostic studies, other treatments including physical, occupational, or speech therapy, etc.).

3. Care coordination, also known as case or care management – This is the third category of nursing care delivery models found in ambulatory settings.

   a. Definition of *case/care management*: Case management is a collaborative process of assessment, planning, facilitation, and advocacy for options and services to meet an individual's health needs through communication and available resources to promote quality cost-effective outcomes (Case Management Society of America, 2002).

b. Case management emerged first in the early 1900s with services provided by public health nurses and social workers who coordinated services in the public sector.

c. The current evolution of formalized care coordination or care/case management evolved in the 1970s:

   (1) Public sector – Medicare and Medicaid demonstration projects employed nurses and social workers to coordinate services for persons in categorically defined groups (low income, mentally ill, frail older adults, etc.)

   (2) Private sector – Workman's compensation insurers and re-habilitation companies employed nurses to manage cases and vocational placement.

d. Case management roles include (Case Management Society of America, 2002):

   (1) Client assessment.

   (2) Planning – Establish an evidence-based, appropriate, fiscally responsible plan of care based on client needs.

   (3) Facilitation – Coordinate, communicate, and collaborate with the patient and family, service providers, and payers to achieve goals, report progress, and maximize client outcomes.

   (4) Advocacy – Promote understanding and respect for the patient's and family's beliefs, value systems, and decisions.

e. Types of care coordination or care/case management models: Can be classified in several ways.

   (1) Institution-based vs. outpatient settings.

   (2) Individual case focus vs. population

focus (for example, geriatrics, special needs, pediatrics).

   (3) Disease management models: Those that deal with specific disease (for example, diabetes, asthma, behavioral and mental health disorders, etc.).

f. Care coordination or care/case management consist of two major dimensions: Utilization review and the care/case management process (Forbes, 1999).

   (1) Utilization management – The management and "evaluation of the medical necessity, appropriateness, and efficiency of the use of health care services, procedures, and facilities under the auspices of the applicable health benefit plan" (Carneal, 1998, p. 20).

   (a) Historically conceptualized and operationalized as the review of hospital medical records for appropriate lengths of stay.

   (b) Currently expanded from the ambulatory perspective to include evaluating:

   (i) The best type of institution to provide the care (hospital, subacute facility, home, etc.).

   (ii) The type of provider required to provide appropriate care (physician, advanced practitioner, nurse, pharmacist, nutritionist, etc.).

   (c) A tool of utilization management is the review of the clinical situation and/or the medical record. Reviews are conducted in different time frames (Shi & Singh, 1998).

   (i) *Prospective utilization review* is performed before the care is delivered using guidelines to determine appropriateness.

   (ii) *Concurrent utilization review* occurs during the course of health care utilization (for example, hospitalization), and plans are developed for appropriate, timely discharge from services.

    (iii) *Retrospective utilization review* occurs after the service has been consumed in efforts to determine improved utilization, often profiling and comparing practices among different providers.

  (d) Evaluation of optimal utilization is dependent on a number of factors:

    (i) Severity and acuity of the presenting situation.

    (ii) Skill and competence of the provider(s).

    (iii) Type of therapy or intervention required.

    (iv) Consumer preference.

(2) The case/care management process itself has multiple dimensions:

  (a) Client identification and selection.

  (b) Problem identification.

  (c) Planning.

  (d) Monitoring.

  (e) Evaluation of progress toward achieving goals (Case Management Society of America, 2002; Powell 2000b)

g. *Care coordination* – A type of nursing practice that encompasses case/care management principles and processes but functions more intensively across a wider spectrum of providers and resources.

(1) Care coordination seeks to achieve the optimal cost-effective use of scarce resources by helping individuals obtain appropriate health services, but also encompasses coordinating social and life support services that meet the unique needs of individuals at a given point in time or across the life span (Powell, 2000a).

(2) Care coordination models are most often seen operating in vulnerable populations (for example, frail older adults or persons with disabilities).

h. A conceptual model of case/care management and care coordination for organizations includes the following dimensions (see Figure 3-1 for a conceptual diagram of health care coordination):

(1) Specify a clear vision statement that contains expected outcomes, goals, and specific objectives relevant to:

  (a) Managing the disease or presenting situation.

  (b) Improving health outcomes.

  (c) Reducing costs.

(2) Designate the multidisciplinary team of providers or network of providers and provide them with clearly written roles, functions, and responsibilities.

  (a) Core providers: Those primarily responsible and accountable for coordinating access to appropriate utilization of health services.

  (b) Resource providers: Those used on an *ad hoc* or referral basis.

(3) Establish written standards for the case/care management or care coordination processes that include:

  (a) Clinical guidelines for care using evidence-based sources (Pravikoff et al., 2005).

  (b) Program management protocols: Methods used in program operations (such as policies and procedures).

(4) Implement a well-formulated quality assurance and performance improvement program and system.

  (a) Specify indicators that measure success.

  (b) Establish monitoring, tracking, and evaluation systems.

Figure 3-1

Conceptual Diagram: Health Care Coordination

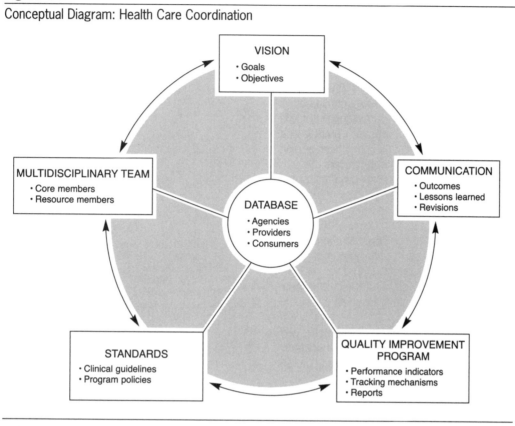

Source: Developed by Margaret Mastal. Adapted from AAACN/ANA (1997, p. 45).

(c) Disseminate relevant, user-friendly reports that support informed decision making.

(5) Execute a planned, clear system of communication that addresses modes of team member interactions, the reporting of outcomes, and the revisions needed to improve outcomes (AAACN/ANA, 1997).

(a) Establish a written, individualized plan of care that addresses the patient's unique health problems, treatment goals, therapeutic interventions, and expected outcomes.

(b) Specify how changes in the patient's status are communicated among team members (written and verbal).

(c) Identify systematic evaluation periods and revisions to the plan of care.

(d) Establish timelines for the collection and reporting of data and information (such as patient outcomes, costs, etc.).

(6) Establish and maintain an accurate, formal database.

(a) The database must minimally contain:

(i) Demographic and credentialing information about agencies and providers.

    (ii) Demographic and clinical information about consumers, both at the individual and population levels.

    (iii) Patient service utilization and financial information.

  (b) The database optimally will be:

    (i) Electronic for ease of data retrieval and reporting.

    (ii) Have capabilities to link with other databases for use across the consumer's life span.

C. Evolving concepts of health coupled with societal and health industry trends expand notions of health beyond curing or treating illness and disease. Expansions include emphasizing disease prevention and health promotion for both individuals and populations, and are refashioning the face of ambulatory care.

  1. These concepts have spurred the emergence of new expectations and practices for providers and consumers across diverse outpatient settings.

  2. Multidisciplinary teams of providers, partnering with consumers, focus on individuals and populations more holistically, and address wellness, disease prevention, recovery from acute illness, adaptation to chronic disease, and palliation with dignity at the end of life.

  3. Changes in the health care environment have presented new, expanded, evolving roles for the nurse as an integral member of the provider team, the health care organization, and the consumer community.

References

American Academy of Ambulatory Care Nursing (AAACN). (2004a). *Ambulatory care nursing administration and practice standards.* Pitman, NJ: Author.

American Academy of Ambulatory Care Nursing (AAACN). (2004b). *Telehealth nursing practice administration and practice standards.* Pitman, NJ: Author.

American Academy of Ambulatory Care Nursing (AAACN)/ American Nurses' Association (ANA). (1997). *Nursing in ambulatory care: The future is here.* Washington, DC: American Nurses Publishing.

American Nurses Association (ANA). (2004a). *Nursing scope and standards of practice.* Silver Spring, MD: Author.

American Nurses Association (ANA). (2004b). *Scope and standards for nurse administrators* (2nd ed.). Washington, DC: Author.

American Nurses Association (ANA). (2003). *Nursing's social policy statement.* Silver Spring, MD: Author.

American Nurses Association (ANA). (2001). *Code of ethics for nurses with interpretive statements.* Silver Spring, MD: Author.

Bedlak, A.K. (1996). A new approach to primary nursing. *AAACN Viewpoint, 18*(1), 10.

Carneal, G. (1998). Getting accredited. *Continuing Care, 17*(10), 18-24, 42.

Case Management Society of America. (2002). *Standards of practice for case management.* Little Rock, AR: Author.

Forbes, M.A. (1999). The practice of professional nurse case management. *Nursing Case Management, 4*(1), 28-33.

Frenn, M., Lundeen, S.L., Martin, K.S., Riesch, S.K., & Wilson, S.A (1998). Symposium of nursing centers: Past, present and future. *Journal of Nursing Education, 35*(2), 4-62.

Futch, C., & Phillips, R (2003). The mega issues of ambulatory care nursing. *Nursing Economic$, 21*(3), 140-142.

Gulzar, L. (1999). Access to health care. *Image, 31*(1), 13-19.

Haas, S., & Hackbarth, D. (1995). Dimensions of the staff nurse role in ambulatory care: Part II – Comparison of role dimension in four ambulatory settings. *Nursing Economic$, 13*(3),152-165.

Hackbarth, D. (1995). Institute of Medicine revises definition of primary care. *AAACN Viewpoint, 17*(4), 1, 4.

Institute of Medicine (IOM). (1978). Primary health care defined. In: *A manpower policy for primary health care: Report of a study* (pp. 15-28). Washington, DC: National Academies Press.

Institute of Medicine (IOM). (1996). *Primary care: America's health in a new era.* Washington, DC: National Academies Press.

McDonald. G., & Bunton, R. (1992). Health promotion: Discipline or disciplines? In R. Bunton & G. McDonald (Eds.), *Health promotion: Disciplines and diversity* (pp. 1-9). London: Routledge.

Morgan, I.S., & Marsh, G.W. (1998). Historic and future health promotion contexts for nursing. *Image: Journal of Nursing Scholarship, 30*(4), 379-383.

O'Brien, M.E. (1999). *Spirituality in nursing.* Sudbury, MA: Jones and Bartlett.

Powell, S.K. (2000a). *Case management: A practical guide to success in managed care.* Philadelphia: Lippincott, Williams & Wilkins.

Powell, S.K. (2000b). *Advanced case management outcomes and beyond.* Philadelphia: Lippincott, Williams & Wilkins.

Pravikoff, D.S., Tanner, A.B., & Pierce, S.T. (2005). Readiness of U.S. nurses for evidence-based practice. *American Journal of Nursing, 105*(9), 40-51.

Riesch, S.K. (1992). Nursing centers. In J.J. Fitzpatrick, A. Jacox, & R.L. Taunton (Eds.), *Annual review of nursing research* (Vol.10) (pp. 145-162). New York: Springer Publishing.

Shi, L., & Singh, D.A. (1998). *Delivering health care in America: A systems approach.* Gaithersburg, MD: Aspen.

U.S. Department of Health and Human Services (DHHS). (1991). *Healthy people 2000: National health promotion and disease prevention objectives.* DHHS Publication No. (PHS) 91-50213. Washington, DC: Author.

U.S. Department of Health and Human Services (DHHS). (1999). *Web site of the Secretary's Council on National Health Promotion and Disease Prevention Objectives for 2010.* Retrieved May 15, 2006, from http://www.health.gov/healthypeople

U.S. Department of Health and Human Services (DHHS). (2000). *Healthy people 2010: Understanding and improving health.* Washington, DC: Author.

U.S. Surgeon General. (1979). *Healthy people: The Surgeon General's report on health promotion and disease prevention.* Washington, DC: United States Public Health Service.

Williams, S.J. (1993). Ambulatory health services. In S.J. Williams, & P.R. Torrens (Eds.), *Introduction to health services.* New York: Delmar.

World Health Organization (WHO). (1978). *Primary health care. Report of the international conference on primary health care.* Alma Ata, USSR. Geneva: Author.

World Health Organization (WHO). (1987). Ottawa charter for health promotion. *Health Promotion, 1*(4), iii-iv.

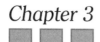
The Context of Ambulatory Care Nursing

This test may be copied for use by others.

COMPLETE THE FOLLOWING:

Name: _____

Address: _____

City: _____ State: _____ Zip: _____

Preferred telephone: (Home)_____ (Work)_____

E-mail_____

AAACN Member Expiration Date: _____

Registration fee: AAACN Member: $12.00
                   Nonmember: $20.00

Answer Form:

1. If you applied what you have learned from this activity into your practice, what would be different?

_____

_____

_____

Evaluation	Strongly disagree				Strongly agree
2. By completing this activity, I was able to meet the following objectives:					
a. Trace the evolutionary changes of the concept of health from the early 1900s to the present time.	1	2	3	4	5
b. Discuss the application of health concepts in the ambulatory care environment.	1	2	3	4	5
c. Discuss the effects of consumerism on health care providers and organizations.	1	2	3	4	5
d. Identify major societal and health care industry trends and their impact on the ambulatory care environment.	1	2	3	4	5
e. Describe diverse nursing care delivery models in ambulatory settings.	1	2	3	4	5
3. The content was current and relevant.	1	2	3	4	5
4. The objectives could be achieved using the content provided.	1	2	3	4	5
5. This was an effective method to learn this content.	1	2	3	4	5
6. I am more confident in my abilities since completing this material.	1	2	3	4	5

7. The material was (check one) ___new ___review for me.

8. Time required to read this chapter: _____minutes

I verify that I have completed this activity: _____
                                                            Signature

Comments: _____

_____

_____

Objectives

This educational activity is designed for nurses and other health care professionals who practice in ambulatory care. For those wishing to obtain CE credit, an evaluation follows. After studying the information presented in this offering, you will be able to:

1. Trace the evolutionary changes of the concept of health from the early 1900s to the present time.
2. Discuss the application of health concepts in the ambulatory care environment.
3. Discuss the effects of consumerism on health care providers and organizations.
4. Identify major societal and health care industry trends and their impact on the ambulatory care environment.
5. Describe diverse nursing care delivery models in ambulatory settings.

Posttest Instructions

1. To receive continuing education credit for individual study after reading the article, complete the answer/evaluation form to the left.

2. Detach and send the answer/evaluation form along with a check or money order payable to the *American Academy of Ambulatory Care Nursing (AAACN)*, East Holly Avenue Box 56, Pitman, NJ 08071–0056.

3. Test returns must be postmarked by August 1, 2011. Upon completion of the answer/evaluation form, a certificate for **1.5** contact hour(s) will be awarded and sent to you. Should the material contained in this chapter become outdated prior to the above expiration date, AAACN reserves the right to withdraw this CE test.

This activity is co-provided by the *American Academy of Ambulatory Care Nursing (AAACN)* and Anthony J. Jannetti, Inc. (AJJ). AJJ is accredited as a provider of continuing nursing education by the American Nurses' Credentialing Center's Commission on Accreditation (ANCC-COA). AAACN is a provider approved by the California Board of Registered Nurses, provider number CEP 05336.

This article was reviewed and formatted for contact hour credit by Sally S. Russell, MN, CMSRN, AAACN Education Director; and Candia Baker Laughlin MS, RN, C, Editor.

Chapter 4

The Ambulatory Care Team

Susan M. Paschke, MSN, RN, BC, CNA

Objectives

Study of the information presented in this chapter will enable the learner to:

1. Identify the professional and non-professional roles of those working in ambulatory care.
2. Describe a typical ambulatory care team and the evolving role of the professional nurse as team member and team leader.
3. Discuss strategies to improve collaboration and build effective teams.
4. Describe priority management or throughput in ambulatory care.
5. Discuss supervision and delegation as skills required by the professional ambulatory care nurse.

Key Points

1. The professional nurse plays a pivotal role in the provision of ambulatory care.
2. Ambulatory care teams are multidisciplinary, and they include the patient and family or significant others.
3. Teams develop when members collaborate, communicate, and demonstrate support, respect, and trust.
4. Priority management insures that the patient receives the right care in the right place at the right time.
5. The professional nurse maintains responsibility and accountability for tasks that are delegated.

Ambulatory care continues to grow as a specialty within the practice of nursing, and new and innovative roles for all members of the health care team are developing as care of the patient continues to shift to the outpatient setting. The coordinated, interdisciplinary provision of comprehensive health care by a team of providers with the inclusion of the patient or client and significant others is the basis of ambulatory care. Comprehensive care includes health promotion, disease prevention, health education, and management of symptoms and disease processes. The professional nurse is the team member most qualified to effectively coordinate these various aspects of care so that the team can work in partnership to fully maximize the benefit to the patient. In order to accomplish this, professional nurses must be comfortable with the collaborative nature of ambulatory care, understand how to prioritize nursing interventions, and develop and improve skills in supervision and delegation to other members of the team. Physicians, physician's assistants (PAs), and advanced practice nurses, such as nurse practitioners (NPs), make decisions about the care patients receive, but the professional nurse "coordinates care with the patient, providers, and other members of the interdisciplinary team" (Koloroutis, 2004, p. 96).

Caregiver Roles in Ambulatory Care

Nursing practice in ambulatory care is differentiated by the qualifications of the nurse and the other caregivers and the role of the nurse in different settings. The professional nurse always maintains the responsibility, authority, and accountability for the provision of nursing care. Unlicensed assistive personnel (UAPs), such as nursing assistants or medical assistants, fulfill roles of low complexity. Licensed practical or vocational nurses (LPNs/LVNs) assume additional responsibilities while functioning under state nurse practice acts. The roles of team leader, triage nurse, manager of a nurse-run clinic, or case manager are most appropriately filled by professional registered nurses (American Academy of Ambulatory Care Nursing [AAACN], 2004b).

A. Distinguishing the role of the professional registered nurse (RN) within the ambulatory care setting is difficult for the following reasons:

1. Nurses in ambulatory care function as members of a multidisciplinary team in which the role of the professional nurse is still evolving and may change frequently.
2. In ambulatory care settings, not every patient requires nursing care (AAACN, 2004b).
3. Professional and nonprofessional disciplines practice simultaneously, often providing similar or overlapping services.
4. Care requirements and cost containment are key determinants of the level of the caregiver who provides services or performs a given role.

B. Role definition.
   1. The roles of all members of the health care team in the ambulatory care setting are constantly changing based on patient needs and regulatory requirements.
   2. Roles in the health care workforce are influenced by social values, costs, political forces, government, and expectations of the health care system (Jacox, 1997).
   3. Roles can be competitive and collaborative as evidenced by:
      a. The role of the physician demonstrates more interdependence than independence, and more collaboration than hierarchy (Koloroutis, 2004).
      b. Nurse practitioners (NPs), other advanced practice nurses (APNs), and physician assistants (PAs) are assuming responsibilities for patient care that were previously performed only by physicians (Hermann & Zabramski, 2005).
      c. Professional nurses coordinate and manage the care of patients as case managers and triage nurses in nurse-run clinics.
      d. LPN/LVNs and UAPs are performing many of the less complex tasks originally performed by the professional nurse.

C. The role of the professional nurse.
   1. Nursing has a unique role in ambulatory care.
   2. The professional nurse provides direct care to the patient in addition to providing coordination of care to ensure that:
      a. Appropriate care is provided across the multidisciplinary team.
      b. The patient progresses through the system appropriately.
      c. Referrals for needed services are initiated.
      d. Education on self-care management, health promotion, and disease prevention is provided.
      e. Case management for high-risk patients is planned.
   3. Telehealth nursing practice is the practice of nursing using the nursing process to provide care to individuals or defined patient populations via a telecommunication device. It includes the provision of patient care, health education, patient advocacy, and coordination of care (AAACN, 2003).
      a. Professional nurses provide care, advice, direction, and education to patients via the telephone and other devices.
      b. Only professional registered nurses can assess patients. Other levels of caregivers are able gather information or collect data, but it remains the role of the professional nurse to analyze the situation and determine the next steps in the nursing plan of care.
   4. The professional nurse demonstrates leadership skills necessary to ensure that:
      a. Care is provided efficiently.
      b. Multidisciplinary aspects of care are integrated.
      c. The environment is safe and secure to meet the patient's needs.
      d. Daily operations of the clinical area function effectively.

Ambulatory Care Team

The pivotal member of the ambulatory care team is the patient. The team is comprised of the patient and his or her family, and/or significant others partnered with any group of health care workers who provide care in an outpatient setting. As a team, they collaborate to ensure that assessments are multidisciplinary, develop a treatment plan to assure that care is continuous, and coordinate the use of resources in providing patient care. The team recognizes that the patient determines acceptance of and compliance with treatment plans (AAACN, 2004b).

A. Members of the ambulatory care team include:
1. Physicians.
2. Nurse practitioners (NPs) and other advanced practice nurses (APNs).
3. Physician's assistants (PAs).
4. Registered nurses (RNs).
5. Licensed practical or vocational nurses (LPN/LVNs).
6. Unlicensed assistive personnel (UAPs).
7. Clerical and secretarial support personnel.
8. Professionals and nonprofessionals from other disciplines such as pharmacy, respiratory, occupational or physical therapy, social work, nutrition, psychology, etc.

B. Ambulatory care can be provided in a variety of settings (see Chapter 2, *The Ambulatory Care Practice Arena*).

C. Primary care teams.
1. A primary care team consists of a primary care provider aligned with a group of other health care practitioners. The primary care team is responsible for:
   a. Providing comprehensive health care to a patient and/or a group of patients.
   b. Serving as the point of access to the system.
   c. Providing quality care in the most cost-effective manner possible.
   d. Focusing on self-care management, health promotion, and disease prevention.
2. Roles of team members in primary care. Disciplines most commonly included as core members of the primary care team are:
   a. *Physicians/NPs/APNs/PAs* – Providers of care responsible for delivery of comprehensive general health care to a group of patients ensuring that care is coordinated and consolidated within the primary care team.
   b. *Social workers* – Provide psychosocial assessments, ongoing counseling, and treatment; they serve as consultants on psychosocial issues to other team members.
   c. *Dietitians* – Perform nutritional screening and/or assessment; develop, imple-

ment, and educate the patient and family members regarding the nutrition therapy plan.
   d. *Pharmacists* – Educate patients about medications including expected outcomes, side effects, precautions, interactions, and reactions.
   e. *Psychologists* – Serve as mental health resources to assist with assessment and treatment of patient conditions.
   f. *Therapists (respiratory, physical, occupational)* – Treat a variety of patient conditions and educate patients regarding ongoing care at home.
   g. *Clerical support* – Register patients, set up clinics, schedule appointments, contact patients, and retrieve medical records and other pertinent information to enable providers to deliver care.
   h. *Nursing personnel (RNs, LPN/LVNs, UAPs).*

D. Nurses in ambulatory care settings provide primary care, or they may provide care in clinics or settings based on medical specialty or patient diagnosis.
1. Nurses play an integral role as members of the primary or specialty care team.
2. The professional staff nurse provides direct care as well as coordination of care for the patients on the team, ensuring continuity and appropriateness of care.
3. Nurses have the ability to perform many of the roles of other members of the team, such as nutrition education, psychosocial support, and clerical duties, in the event that these team members are not available.
4. Roles specific to the professional nurse include:
   a. Telephone triage/advice/screening.
      (1) Use of formalized triage protocols for specific complaints to determine the most appropriate course of action.
         (a) Immediate intervention – Emergency department or urgent care.
         (b) Intervention within 24 hours.
         (c) Routine appointment.
      (2) Difficulties arise when patients pres-

ent multiple complaints, have complex medical history, or are poor historians – Protocols may not relate to the symptoms.

(3) Assessment, judgment, and critical thinking skills are necessary for this role.

b. Hands-on, face-to-face patient care.

(1) Care and treatment of scheduled patients.

(2) Triage and care of walk-in patients.

(3) Management of emergencies.

c. Referrals to other members of the health care team or to community services, such as home care, assisted living facilities, or nursing homes.

d. Case management – "A collaborative process that assesses, plans, implements, coordinates, monitors, and evaluates options and services to meet an individual's health needs through communication and available resources to promote quality, cost-effective outcomes" (Marquis & Huston, 2003, p. 216).

(1) The professional nurse possesses the appropriate knowledge, judgment, and skill to coordinate the care of the patient across the continuum of care.

(2) Not every patient requires case management.

e. Supervision of LPN/LVNs and UAPs – Includes monitoring, evaluation, education, and delegation.

f. Patient advocacy – See Chapter 9, *Patient Advocacy*.

g. Demand management – Providing the right care in the right place at the right time.

(1) Focuses on using alternatives, such as telephone advice and complementary services, including health promotion or screening programs.

(2) Educates patients regarding chronic disease management, self-care, and wise consumerism.

h. Health education – Teaching the patient and family to safely care for themselves

outside of and between visits to the health care setting.

(1) Includes assessment of the patient's readiness to learn; physical, emotional, or cultural barriers to learning; preference for method of learning; and should include the patient's response to the educational session (JCAHO, 2005).

(2) Includes information on disease, treatments, medication, self-care management, lifestyle risk factors, and community resources.

(3) Focuses on health promotion and disease prevention for both individuals and groups.

(4) Intervenes based on objectives set forth in *Healthy People 2010* (U.S. Department of Health and Human Services, 2000).

(5) Educates in congruence with nursing theory.

(a) Dorothea Orem's theory of self-care – Nursing action compensates for patients' self-care limitations.

(b) Virginia Henderson's theory – The role of the nurse is to support the patient in meeting health needs until he or she is able to do for him or herself.

(c) Both relate to the concepts of health promotion and health maintenance, and reinforce the individual's and family's responsibility for health care and encourage participation of family members and significant others whenever possible.

(6) Evaluates the need for end-of-life planning – Educates patients about their rights to plan for medical care and provides information regarding advance directives (for example, living wills, durable power of attorney for health care, and treatment preferences).

i. Quality improvement activities.

(1) Quality improvement opportunities

may be identified by any member of the health care team.

    (2) Patient outcomes are key indicators.

    (3) Measuring or monitoring the contributions of nursing to patient outcome creates accountability for nurses as professionals. Indicators include:

      (a) Accessibility and timeliness of care.

      (b) Telephone access to care.

      (c) Access to specialists for complex health-related issues.

      (d) Availability of preventive services.

      (e) Outcomes of nursing interventions, including patient education.

      (f) Patient satisfaction (Marquis & Huston, 2003).

  5. The professional nurse must recognize that his or her knowledge and understanding of all aspects of a patient's care do not mandate that the nurse perform all of the care. Rather, this knowledge identifies the nurse as the person most qualified to:

    a. Coordinate the care of the patient.

    b. Delegate appropriate tasks to appropriate team members.

    c. Utilize leadership and delegation skills to ensure a collaborative team effort and a smooth flow of daily operations. (Kramer& Schmalenberg, 2003).

Collaboration

Collaboration is the working of like-minded people toward a common goal (Boswell & Cannon, 2005). "There is an agreement to pursue a common purpose and a sharing of knowledge to resolve problems, decide issues, and set goals within a structure of collegiality" (Rowland & Rowland, 1997, p. 50).

A. Collaboration requires knowledge sharing and joint responsibility for patient care (Lindeke & Sieckert, 2005).

  1. Physicians and other providers determine the medical plan of care and share the responsibility for delivery of health care services with other professionals on the health care team.

  2. Collaboration and cooperation is essential.

  3. All disciplines concur and agree on who will provide what for the patient.

  4. The common goal is the provision of cost-effective quality care.

B. Key behaviors that enhance collaboration and team building (Boswell & Cannon, 2005).

  1. Networking is the exchange of information or services among individuals, groups, or institutions, drawing from the experiences of others as resources and support.

  2. Leadership (see Chapter 12, *Leadership*)

    a. Inspiring others to devote time, energy, and resources toward a desired outcome (Buonocore, 2004).

    b. Motivating others to achieve outcomes that exceed expectations.

    c. Developing shared vision with focus on goals.

    d. Developing others.

    e. Promoting trust as an underlying value and behavior.

  3. Vision is a core set of principles that guides the group toward a common goal or mission.

B. Characteristics of a collaborative team (Gardner, 2005).

  1. Consensus regarding goals, values, and vision is evident.

  2. Roles and responsibilities are defined.

  3. Specific tasks and relevant time frames are identified.

  4. Monitors are in place to evaluate team performance.

  5. Practice/process parameters have been established (such as conflict resolution, decision-making).

  6. Open, honest communication is practiced.

  7. Team members discuss problems, concerns, issues, etc.

  8. Mutual trust, respect, and support are evident.

  9. Diversity is acknowledged and valued.

  10. Responsibility and accountability are shared.

  11. Financial issues, which affect the team, are discussed.

  12. Data, reports, and analyses are shared with

all team members.
D. Team member characteristics:
    1. Professionally competent.
    2. Contributes to the function of the team.
    3. Values contribution of each team member.
    4. Recognizes individual strengths, abilities, and talents, as well as those of team members.
    5. Accepts own role and responsibilities.
E. Barriers to collaboration
    1. Hierarchical culture of health care.
    2. Failure to acknowledge diversity.
    3. Independence vs. interdependence and interdisciplinary relationships.
    4. Lack of effective communication.
    5. Uncertain commitment or competence of team members.
    6. Lack of trust.
F. Strategies for effective team building in ambulatory care
    1. Appreciate unique knowledge of contributing members.
    2. Develop a shared goal or outcome.
    3. Maintain the patient as focus.
    4. Develop clear role definitions and expectations.
    5. Avoid blaming and encourage dialogue – Agree to disagree at times.
    6. Communicate, communicate, communicate!

Priority Management

Priority management is the ability to manage and direct patient access and flow for effective and efficient clinical operations (Weinstein, 2004).
A. Operational issues include:
    1. Those with acute or urgent problems are triaged and treated quickly and efficiently.
    2. Patients are seen as close to their appointment time as possible to avoid delays and wait time.
    3. All patients receive the appropriate level of care in the appropriate setting.
B. Operational challenges include:
    1. Walk-in patients.
    2. Late patients and/or "no shows."
    3. Add-on patients.
    4. Acutely ill patients.
    5. Emergencies.

C. Strategies to maintain optimum flow.
    1. Identify the nature of the patient visit and assign the patient to the most appropriate caregiver or member of the team.
    2. Assure that resources needed for each visit are immediately available.
    3. Focus nursing interventions on those patients or groups of patients with complex nursing needs.
    4. Delegate tasks with low complexity to assistive personnel.

Delegation and Supervision

According to the American Nurses Association (1997), delegation is the transfer of responsibility for the performance of a task from one person to another. The professional nurse uses delegation to ensure that routine tasks are performed by others, thereby allowing the nurse to handle complex problems or those that require a higher level of expertise. Delegation can also be used as a learning opportunity or as a challenge for growth and development of the other person.
A. Delegation is a learned skill and improves with practice (Marquis & Huston, 2003).
B. Common mistakes in delegating include:
    1. Under-delegating due to:
        a. Lack of trust in subordinates to do the job.
        b. Fear of resentment from subordinates.
        c. Lack of experience in delegation.
    2. Over-delegating due to:
        a. Insecurity in performance of the task.
        b. Overly relying on exceptionally competent employees – May lead to burnout and decreased productivity.
    3. Improper delegation.
        a. Delegation to the wrong person, at the wrong time, for the wrong reason (Cohen, 2004).
        b. Delegation of tasks beyond the capability of the person.
        c. Delegation of decision making without adequate information.
C. Delegation to unlicensed assistive personnel (UAPs).
    1. Definition of UAP – A person trained to function in an assistive role to the professional

nurse for the provision of patient care activities as delegated by the nurse.

2. Rising health care costs, downsizing, and the implementation of new care models has resulted in an increase in the use of UAPs. UAPs can perform tasks and non-nursing functions thus enabling the professional nurse to perform nursing functions. This leads to the appropriate increased use of well-trained, competent, lower-cost personnel.

3. Delegation of tasks can increase the liability to the professional nurse. The professional nurse:
   a. Must provide supervision to employees to whom tasks are delegated.
   b. Must be aware of training, experience, and skills of the person, including job description.
   c. Maintains responsibility and accountability for tasks that are delegated but is not held liable if the UAP is negligent, provided that the UAP received training and is deemed competent. However, the nurse can be held liable for his or her lack of competence in performing the duties of supervision (Rowland & Rowland, 1997).
   d. May not delegate tasks or activities that rely on the nursing process or require specialized skill, knowledge, and professional judgment.
   e. Must understand the state Nurse Practice Act regarding delegation.

D. Delegation algorithm (Johnson, 1995) – Series of questions to assist with appropriate delegation to UAPs:
   1. Is the task within the scope of nursing practice? If no, the task cannot be performed or delegated by the professional nurse.
   2. Does the task require nursing knowledge, skill, or independent judgment? If yes, the task cannot be delegated.
   3. Is the task within the level of educational preparation and demonstrated competence of the person to whom it is delegated? If no, the task cannot be delegated.
   4. Is the professional nurse available to supervise? If no, the task cannot be delegated.
   5. Is the patient's condition such that someone other than a professional nurse can perform

the task? If no, the task cannot be delegated.
   6. Does the task involve initial assessment, analysis, development of a plan of care, or evaluation of patient progress?
      a. If yes, the task cannot be delegated.
      b. If no, the task can be delegated.

E. Supervision.
   1. Definition – Having the direction and oversight of the performance of others (Marquis & Huston, 2003).
   2. Supervision is a role expectation for all professional nurses.
   3. Supervision ensures that UAPs perform activities safely and appropriately. The supervising nurse:
      a. Evaluates the method and effectiveness of communication of the activity.
      b. Determines the extent of supervision necessary.
      c. Evaluates the outcome.
   4. With the increased number of UAPs, professional nurses who were trained under the primary nursing model may not have the skills or experience in delegation and supervision required to fulfill the supervisory role (Anthony, Standing, & Hertz, 2000). Concerns include:
      a. Discomfort in giving feedback, both negative and positive.
      b. False ideas about legal responsibilities related to supervision.
   5. The role of the professional nurse in ambulatory care will require development of the following skills:
      a. Ability to direct and guide other professional members on their team, as well as LPNs and UAPs.
      b. Supervision, direction, monitoring, and evaluation of the progress and completion of the task.
      c. Evaluation of patient outcomes.
      d. Evaluation of staff satisfaction.
   6. Strategies for effective supervision of unlicensed assistive personnel (UAP).
      a. Know the assistive workers, their role expectations, and their levels of competence. The best way to accomplish this is to consistently assign the assistive worker to the same nurse and the same

team(s) and/or clinic(s) (Anthony, Casey, Chau, & Brennan, 2000).

b. Allocate time for supervision and for evaluating the progress of care delivery. Time for oversight of the work of UAP must be built into the care model so that work performance can be observed and timely performance feedback given.

c. Allow for open lines of communication.

   (1) The professional nurse supervising UAPs must be willing to recognize the importance of open, respectful, constructive communication.

   (2) When conflict occurs, communication should be non-confrontational and focus on actual occurrences, behaviors, and job expectations.

d. Adhere to patient care and work performance standards. The professional nurse in a supervisory role must serve as a role model and adhere closely to the standards of care and the mission of the institution in which he or she works.

e. Give timely feedback, both positive and negative.

   (1) Personnel, especially those in new positions, should be made aware of their progress.

   (2) UAPs should be encouraged to offer feedback and suggestions about operational issues.

F. The role of the nurse manager or nurse executive is to:

1. Support the professional nurse in the role of supervisor.

2. Assure appropriate training and skill development in supervision to meet job requirements.

3. Assess job satisfaction and promote retention in the supervisory role.

References

American Academy of Ambulatory Care Nursing (AAACN). (2003). *Telehealth nursing practice core course manual.* Pitman, NJ: Author.

American Academy of Ambulatory Care Nursing (AAACN). (2004a). *Telehealth nursing practice administration and practice standards.* Pitman, NJ: Author.

American Academy of Ambulatory Care Nursing (AAACN). (2004b). *Ambulatory care nursing administration and practice standards.* Pitman, NJ: Author.

American Nurses Association (ANA). (1997). *Position statement: Registered nurse utilization of unlicensed assistive personnel.* Retrieved May 26, 2006, from http://www.nursing world.org/readroom/position/uap/uapuse/htm

Anthony, M.K., Casey, D., Chau, T., & Brennan, P.F. (2000) Congruence between registered nurses' and unlicensed assistive personnel perception of nursing practice. *Nursing Economic$, 18*(5), 285-293.

Anthony, M.K., Standing, T., & Hertz, J.E. (2000). Factors influencing outcomes after delegation to unlicensed assistive personnel. *Journal of Nursing Administration, 30*(10), 474-481.

Boswell, C., & Cannon, S. (2005). New horizons for collaborative partnerships. *Online Journal of Issues in Nursing, 10*(1), 3.

Buonocore, D. (2004). Leadership in action: Creating a change in practice. *AACN Clinical Issues, 15*(2), 170-181.

Cohen, S. (2004). Delegating vs. dumping: Teach the difference. *Nursing Management, 35*(10), 14, 18.

Gardner, D.B. (2005). Ten lessons in collaboration. *Online Journal of Issues in Nursing, 10*(1), 2.

Herrmann, L.L., & Zabramski, J.M. (2005). Tandem practice model: a model for physician- nurse practitioner collaboration in a specialty practice, neurosurgery. *Journal of the American Academy of Nurse Practitioners, 17*(6), 213-219.

Jacox, A. (1997). Determinants of who does what in health care. *Online Journal of Issues in Nursing,* Retrieved February 27, 2006, from www.nursingworld.org/ojin/tpc5/tpc5_1.htm

Johnson, E.M. (1995). Assistive personnel in ambulatory care. *AAACN Viewpoint, 17*(3), 1.

Joint Commission on Accreditation of Healthcare Organizations (JCAHO). (2005). *Hospital accreditation standards.* Oakbrook Terrace, IL: Author.

Koloroutis, M. (2004). *Relationship-based care: A model for transforming practice.* Minneapolis, MN: Creative Healthcare Management.

Kramer, M., & Schmalenberg, C. (2003). Securing "good" nurse-physician relationships. *Nursing Management, 34*(7), 34-38.

Lindeke, L.L., & Sieckert, A.M. (2005). Nurse-physician workplace collaboration. *Online Journal of Issues in Nursing, 10*(1), 5.

Marquis, B.L., & Huston, C.J. (2003). *Leadership roles and management functions in nursing: Theory and application* (4th ed.). Philadelphia: Lippincott.

Rowland, H.S., & Rowland, B.L. (1997). *Nursing administration handbook* (4th ed.). Gaithersburg, MD: Aspen.

U.S. Department of Health and Human Services. (2000). *Healthy people 2010: Understanding and improving health.* Washington, DC: Author.

Weinstein, S. (2004). Strategic partnerships: Bridging the collaboration gap. *Journal of Infusion Nursing, 27*(5), 297-301.

Additional Readings

McConnell, C.R. (2005). Larger, smaller, and flatter: The evolution of the modern health care organization. *Health Care Manager, 24*(2), 177-188.

Pender, N.J., Murdaugh, C.L., & Parsons, M.A. (2002). *Health promotion in nursing practice* (4th ed.). Upper Saddle River, NJ: Prentice Hall.

Potter, P., & Grant, E. (2004). Understanding RN and unlicensed assistive personnel working relationships in designing care delivery strategies. *Journal of Nursing Administration, 34*(1), 19-25.

Reed, P.G., Crawford Shearer, N.B., & Nicoll, L.H. (2003). *Perspectives on nursing theory* (4th ed.). Philadelphia: Lippincott.

The Ambulatory Care Team

This test may be copied for use by others.

COMPLETE THE FOLLOWING:

Name: _____

Address: _____

City: _____ State: _____ Zip: _____

Preferred telephone: (Home)_____ (Work)_____

E-mail_____

AAACN Member Expiration Date: _____

Registration fee: AAACN Member: $12.00
                     Nonmember: $20.00

Answer Form:

1. If you applied what you have learned from this activity into your practice, what would be different?

_____

_____

_____

Evaluation

	Strongly disagree				Strongly agree
2. By completing this activity, I was able to meet the following objectives:					
a. Identify the professional and non-professional roles of those working in ambulatory care.	1	2	3	4	5
b. Describe a typical ambulatory care team and the evolving role of the professional nurse as team member and team leader.	1	2	3	4	5
c. Discuss strategies to improve collaboration and build effective teams.	1	2	3	4	5
d. Describe priority management or through-put in ambulatory care.	1	2	3	4	5
e. Discuss supervision and delegation as skills required by the professional ambulatory care nurse.	1	2	3	4	5
3. The content was current and relevant.	1	2	3	4	5
4. The objectives could be achieved using the content provided.	1	2	3	4	5
5. This was an effective method to learn this content.	1	2	3	4	5
6. I am more confident in my abilities since completing this material.	1	2	3	4	5

7. The material was (check one) ___new ___review for me.
8. Time required to read this chapter: _____minutes

I verify that I have completed this activity: _____
                                                        Signature

Comments: _____

_____

_____

Objectives

This educational activity is designed for nurses and other health care professionals who practice in ambulatory care. For those wishing to obtain CE credit, an evaluation follows. After studying the information presented in this offering, you will be able to:

1. Identify the professional and non-professional roles of those working in ambulatory care.
2. Describe a typical ambulatory care team and the evolving role of the professional nurse as team member and team leader.
3. Discuss strategies to improve collaboration and build effective teams.
4. Describe priority management or through-put in ambulatory care.
5. Discuss supervision and delegation as skills required by the professional ambulatory care nurse.

Posttest Instructions

1. To receive continuing education credit for individual study after reading the article, complete the answer/evaluation form to the left.

2. Detach and send the answer/evaluation form along with a check or money order payable to the *American Academy of Ambulatory Care Nursing (AAACN)*, East Holly Avenue Box 56, Pitman, NJ 08071–0056.

3. Test returns must be postmarked by August 1, 2011. Upon completion of the answer/evaluation form, a certificate for **1.4** contact hour(s) will be awarded and sent to you. Should the material contained in this chapter become outdated prior to the above expiration date, AAACN reserves the right to withdraw this CE test.

This activity is co-provided by the *American Academy of Ambulatory Care Nursing (AAACN)* and Anthony J. Jannetti, Inc. (AJJ). AJJ is accredited as a provider of continuing nursing education by the American Nurses' Credentialing Center's Commission on Accreditation (ANCC-COA). AAACN is a provider approved by the California Board of Registered Nurses, provider number CEP 05336.

This article was reviewed and formatted for contact hour credit by Sally S. Russell, MN, CMSRN, AAACN Education Director; and Candia Baker Laughlin MS, RN, C, Editor.

Chapter 5

Practice/Office Support

Cindy Angiulo, MSN, RN, C

Elizabeth Dickey, MPH, RN, FNP

Objectives

Study of the information presented in this chapter will enable the learner to:
1. Schedule patients efficiently.
2. Design productive spaces and workflow.
3. Enhance patient and staff safety, and improve the patient care environment.
4. Reduce environmental hazards and risks in work settings.

Key Points

1. Nurses working in ambulatory care must fully comprehend the intricacies of the scheduling system because the degree to which that system functions effectively has profound effects on work volume and work flow.
2. Nurses play a major role in facility planning, design, and oversight, and those in provider roles need an awareness of how space affects productivity, quality of care, and satisfaction on the part of patients and staff.
3. Nurses in ambulatory settings have accountability for proactive evaluation of patient care environments and for the development of safety and infection control plans, ongoing monitoring, and implementation of process improvements.
4. Nurses in ambulatory care are accountable to assure safe handling, inventory control, and appropriate charging of patient care equipment and supplies.

The quality of patient care provided in any ambulatory setting is as dependent on the soundness of the delivery systems and environmental supports as it is on the skills and abilities of providers. Nurses play a key role in assuring quality; therefore, this chapter outlines important aspects of patient intake and scheduling, facility design and workflow, and environmental management, the latter now largely a matter of regulatory compliance.

Scheduling

Scheduling is the prearranged timing of patient visits intended to reduce waiting time for patients and providers. The type of clinic practice often determines how scheduling is designed. Efficient scheduling will enhance utilization of support staff, space, and ancillary services (such as lab and radiology), and will improve visit planning with regard to financial matters, prior tests and reports, and specific patient preparation. Nurses working in ambulatory care, whether as providers or supporters of that care, must fully comprehend the intricacies of the scheduling system because the degree to which that system functions effectively has profound effects on work volume and work flow. Scheduling has a major effect on patient satisfaction because as the point of entry for patients, it reflects the competency of the practice's communication system. As such, it is a key ingredient in the operational and financial success of a practice (Ross, Williams, & Pavlock, 1998). Appropriate and timely scheduling also reflects the provider's commitment to facilitate access to care (Delio, 2005).

A. Scheduling types (Barnett & Mayer, 1992).
  1. Type of visit.
    a. New patient vs. established patient.

b. Advance appointment vs. same-day appointment vs. walk-in.
c. Primary care vs. specialty care.
d. Type of specialty and/or requirement for procedures.
e. Provider-requested (professional referral) vs. patient-initiated (self-referral).

2. Type of scheduling.
   a. Set time (for example, 4 patients: 9:00, 9:15, 9:30, 9:45) vs. block time (for example, 4 patients: all at 9:00).
   b. Fixed time increments (for example, 1:00, 1:15, 1:30, 1:45) vs. varied time increments (for example, 1:00, 1:05, 1:10, 1:20, 1:40).
   c. Individual (for example, one patient per time slot) vs. group (for example, several patients per time slot).
   d. Provider-specific (for example, appointment with Dr. Smith) vs. clinic-specific (for example, appointment with pediatric clinic).
   e. Open/advanced access (provides a wide range of appointments for any type of patient to be seen any time of day) (Delio, 2005).
   f. Centralized scheduling vs. decentralized scheduling.

B. Provider variables.
   1. Type of provider (for example, internist vs. general surgeon; nurse practitioner vs. nurse educator).
   2. Personal traits.
      a. Fast vs. slow worker.
      b. Early, on-time, late starter.
      c. No lunch, short lunch, long lunch.
      d. Needs no support, some support, a lot of support.
      e. Beginner vs. experienced practitioner.
   3. Provider-specific show rate (for example, do not double-book procedures with 90% to 100% show rates).
   4. Specialist-specific issues.
      a. Appropriateness of referral vis-à-vis lack of referral.
      b. Completeness of prior workup.
      c. Previsit planning requirements.
   5. Providers' overall schedule and availability.
      a. On-call requirements.

b. Meeting requirements.
c. Teaching schedules (such as the need for coordination between attending, resident, and medical students).
d. Planned leaves of absence (such as vacation, continuing education).
e. Hourly limits on resident's time.

C. Patient variables.
   1. Urgency of problem and/or followup.
      a. Medically urgent.
      b. Medically non-urgent.
      c. Followup is time-sensitive.
      d. Followup is not time-sensitive.
   2. Newness of the problem.
      a. New patient/new problem.
      b. New patient/existing problem.
      c. Established patient/new problem.
      d. Established patient/existing problem.
   3. Database requirements.
      a. Complete history and physical vs. focused history and physical.
      b. Existence/availability of prior databases/test results.
      c. Need for pre-visit triage and/or assessment.
   4. Special needs.
      a. Foreign language and/or American Sign Language (ASL) interpreters.
      b. Physical limitations including wheelchair users and blind patients.
      c. Acutely ill or debilitated patients using stretchers.

D. Support variables.
   1. Staff.
      a. Number available (ratio of supporters/providers).
      b. Teamed or unteamed.
      c. Type and mix of staff (RN, LPN, NA/MA/technician).
   2. Space.
      a. Number of examination rooms available (ratio of rooms per provider).
      b. Examination room configuration vis-à-vis visit type (room is properly sized and equipped for the type of visit conducted).
      c. Essential clinic services space (such as lab, radiology, cardiac testing, fetal testing).
      d. Procedure, observation, and/or recovery space available.

3. Business variables.
   a. Insurance verification/authorization.
   b. Closed vs. open practice (for example, accepting new patients or restricted to established patients).
4. Other.
   a. Special equipment availability.
   b. Test results; consult reports availability.
E. Scheduling system features and qualities (Ross et al., 1998).
   1. Computerized systems should include:
      a. Search capability by:
         (1) Provider.
         (2) Patient.
         (3) Clinic.
         (4) Day/date/time.
      b. Interface with patient registration, financial eligibility, and charging system.
      c. Coordination and linkage of two or more visit types or services.
      d. Generation of clinical orders associated with specific visit types.
      e. Provision for sequencing of appointments that need to be done in a specific order.
      f. Twenty-four hour interdepartmental access and scheduling capacity.
      g. A trigger for medical records, radiology and test results retrieval.
      h. Generation of various warnings and safety alerts (for example, patient allergies, critical lab values, security alerts, duplicate procedures).
      i. Allocation of essential resources (for example, assure availability of specific individuals, space, and/or equipment).
      j. Management of waiting lists.
   2. All systems should be:
      a. Flexible in response to:
         (1) Varying demand.
         (2) Special needs/requests.
      b. Realistic (based on actual experience as well as targeted goals).
F. No-shows, cancellations, and late arrivals.
   1. Preventive strategies.
      a. Pre-visit calls to new patients.
      b. Reminder calls to all patients.
      c. Policies for handling chronic no-show patients including termination of care.

   d. Appointment time tailored to the patient's schedule.
   2. Management strategies that enhance scheduling.
      a. Medical records reviews.
      b. Followup calls.
      c. Re-appointing processes/policies.
      d. Outreach to high-risk patients.
      e. Late arrival process/policy.
      f. Statistical monitoring.

Facility Design and Workflow

The location and design of an ambulatory care facility can make or break a practice. The overall facility must be accessible to patients and staff (parking is a big issue); convenient to home, work, and hospitals; project a positive, healthy image; be capable of expansion and functional change; and support good flow and productivity. Space size is not as important as functionality (Delio, 1999). It is important to decrease unnecessary variation in facility design and workflow to enhance productivity and reduce costs. Nurses play a major role in facility planning, design, and oversight, and those in provider roles need an awareness of how space affects productivity, quality of care, and satisfaction on the part of patients and staff. Basic concepts of facility design might include small work units, maximum flexibility, confidentiality, optimal visibility, circular flow, minimal distance to tasks, and the ability to move staff and functions closer to patient/provider interaction (Delio, 1999). All facilities must be *Americans with Disabilities Act* (ADA) compliant (American Institute of Architects [AIA], 2001).
A. Pre-assessment.
   1. Review the following practice processes before attempting facility design or redesign (Redling, 2002).
      a. Telephone volume.
      b. Staffing levels.
      c. Medical record storage and retrieval.
      d. Provider work relative-value units per clinical session.
      e. Patient waiting times.
      f. Patient volume per provider.
      g. Hours of operation.
   2. Complete an environmental scan of current

and projected ambulatory care market-expanding programs and referral sources.

B. Location issues (Barnett & Mayer, 1992).
  1. Accessibility.
     a. Traffic and congestion patterns.
     b. Adequate, close-in parking provided at the rate suggested for each different type of facility (AIA, 2001) or regulated by local code.
     c. Conveniently accessible via public transportation.
     d. Near home, office, shopping district, community center, or retirement/extended care facilities.
     e. In compliance with the *Americans with Disabilities Act* (ADA-P.L.#101-336, 1990) (U.S. Congress, 1990), state and local regulations.
  2. Visibility.
     a. Adequate signage.
     b. Easy entry and egress.
  3. Area safety.
     a. Safe neighborhood.
     b. Adequate police, fire, and security protection.
     c. Well-lighted area.
     d. Secure entryways and limited access.
  4. Image.
     a. Not in proximity to noisy, dangerous, odorous, or otherwise offensive business or industry.
     b. Clean.
     c. Low clutter.
     d. Environmentally congruent.
  5. Expandability.
     a. For building expansion.
     b. For parking expansion.

C. Layout and design issues (AIA, 2001). All areas should include privacy for patients throughout the care process, including appropriate levels of acoustical and visual privacy, and dignity.
  1. Reception/main waiting.
     a. Patient entryway separate from staff entry.
     b. Warm, welcoming space with easy access to reception and information.
     c. Private, confidential, and secure areas for patient registration, insurance authorization, financial discussions, and

payment transactions.
     d. Main waiting/reception areas sized to accommodate patients, family, and/or friends. Smaller waiting areas help discourage long waits. Separate adults from children, and separate patients with communicable illnesses from others. Private areas for patients who require anonymity (such as staff members, individuals with disfigurements, cosmetic surgery patients).
     e. Security protection as required in certain areas (for example, bullet-proof glass enclosures, panic buttons, video cameras, lock-down capabilities).
     f. Sufficient number of public restrooms without passing through patient care or staff work areas.
     g. Sufficient number of telephones, and Internet connectivity where appropriate.
  2. Exam/direct care space. All areas should have rest rooms separate from public use areas and be easily located to permit access from patient care areas without passing through public areas.
     a. Triage/discharge space.
        (1) Provide confidentiality (soundproof, doors close).
        (2) Locate triage between waiting area and exam area.
        (3) Accommodate patient plus one adult or two children, and an interpreter.
        (4) Limit clutter and equipment to reduce distraction.
        (5) Separate telephone triage space from onsite triage space.
        (6) Provide storage space for brochures and education materials in rooms that are regularly used for patient education, discharge, and/or teaching. May also need space for TV monitor, DVD/VCR, and computer.
        (7) Design triage areas for ease of documentation and to accommodate computer connections.
     b. Vital sign and measurement areas: These functions may be performed in the triage/interview room, in the examination room, or in an area specially

designed for this purpose. The following apply regardless of location.

    (1) Accommodate use of automatic BP monitors, pulse oximeters, wide platform digital scales (pediatric digital scales when appropriate).

    (2) Pay attention to ergonomics to foster productivity.

    (3) Provide hooks and/or counters for patient clothing, purses, etc., and a place to sit if taking off shoes prior to weighing.

c. Examination rooms.

    (1) Minimum of two per provider, higher for certain specialties (such as obstetrics, orthopedics, dermatology).

    (2) Minimum floor area of 80 net sq. ft. with appropriate clearance at each side and foot of examination table.

    (3) Configured for stretcher access, if required (AIA, 2001).

    (4) Handwashing stations provided.

    (5) Standardized room design and layout to the extent possible.

    (6) Multipurpose examination rooms (serves different providers/different functions) preferred over single purpose (specific provider/specific function).

    (7) Designed for visual privacy during disrobing and examination, soundproofed for communication.

    (8) Clustered in twos, threes, or fours, depending on minimum number per provider. Consider proximity to provider office, nursing area, and consultation rooms.

    (9) Address infection control and safety issues (such as sharps containers and disposal of hazardous waste).

    (10) Designed to lighten or darken as needed.

    (11) Have flag or light system to facilitate internal communication (for example, clean/dirty, occupied by patient only, patient and provider, or patient and assistive staff, and assistance needed).

    (12) Contain adequate seating for provider, patient, parent or companion, and interpreter.

    (13) Contain adequate storage/counter space for essential supplies and equipment.

    (14) Have appropriate and limited art, signage, or instructional material on walls.

    (15) Have adequate writing and/or computer space.

    (16) Address ergonomic requirements of various examinations.

d. Treatment/procedure rooms for minor medical/surgical procedures.

    (1) Number of procedure/treatment rooms dependent on specialty.

    (2) Minimum floor area of 120 net square feet.

    (3) Room dimensions not less than 10 ft. with appropriate configuration for stretcher access (AIA, 2001).

    (4) Room arrangement provides a minimum clearance of 3 ft. at each side and at the foot of the table (AIA, 2001).

    (5) Handwashing station provided.

    (6) Emergency power equipment available.

    (7) Room design and layout standardized to the extent possible.

    (8) Designed for proximity to key equipment and supplies, ease of circulation of two or more staff members, and generally equipped with oxygen, monitoring equipment, and crash cart.

    (9) Spot lighting is essential; consider dimmer capabilities.

    (10) Rooms often double as observation areas, so they are best located in close proximity to nursing stations and restrooms.

e. Protective environment/airborne infection/isolation rooms (AIA, 2001).

    (1) Need determined by an infection control risk assessment.

    (2) When required, rooms must comply with state regulations.

f. Nursing/support staff stations.
    (1) Close proximity to examination room clusters and procedure areas.
    (2) Designed not to be magnet area for all staff. Often best to decentralize.
    (3) Sufficient counter space for computers and writing, computer screen privacy, paper and forms storage.
    (4) Easy access to medications, biologicals, supplies, and frequently used equipment.
    (5) Private area for reviewing medical records, test results, entering data into patient registers/logs, and telephoning patients.

g. Special work/storage areas.
    (1) Medication room/storage area in secured area with refrigeration, handwashing areas, and preparation counters.
    (2) Clean utility for storing clean and sterile supplies.
    (3) Soiled utility for separate collection, storage, and disposal of soiled materials.
    (4) Lab room/work area for in-office lab procedures, microscopic examination of specimens with appropriate disposal facilities.
    (5) Secure storage rooms for supplies and equipment. Size and design vary according to specialty.

h. Shared/multipurpose work areas.
    (1) Documentation, dictation, telephone and computer access, space that is private, soundproof, and close to examination rooms.
    (2) Fax and copy room that is private and soundproof.
    (3) Provider office space (private or shared) that has restricted access, soundproofing for telephone calls, and computer connections.
    (4) Nurse office space for visit/care planning, patient education, and record reviews.

i. Interior patient sub-waiting areas essential for clinics where waits are common between triage/intake, examination, lab/X-ray, or procedures.

4. In-house lab/X-ray.
    a. Short distance from clinic area to clinic-based phlebotomy.
    b. Have processes to transmit results and diagnostic images to work areas and examination and procedure rooms.
    c. Sub-waiting area(s) and separate restroom(s).

5. In-house pharmacy.
    a. Confidential area for discussion of medications.
    b. Workspace with computer connections.
    c. Proximity to medical records area is desirable when pharmacist fills prescription directly from the record.
    d. Separate windows for drop-off, pick-up.
    e. Private consult rooms to educate patients about proper drug/device use.
    f. Secure area with restricted access to pharmacy staff.

6. Medical records.
    a. Adjacent to clinic area or designed for quick movement of records to and from the clinic.
    b. Work space for providers and nurses to document and review records.
    c. Restricted access to all except records staff.
    d. Expandable space crucial (or remote storage plan) so long as paper records are maintained.

7. Business office – Close physical proximity to medical records is highly desirable because coding/billing clerks often need to review patient records.

8. Administrative office – Can be located away from the clinic area but be onsite so administrative personnel are available to staff and patients.

9. Staff lounges.
    a. Close proximity to the clinic enhances productivity and encourages staff to take breaks.
    b. Should not be visible or accessible to patients.

10. Maintenance/cleaning/refuse areas.

a. Clinic staff should know how to access these areas or contact area-specific personnel to perform these functions.

b. Medical waste has specific handling, disposable, recycling issues (see *Environmental Management* section later in this chapter).

11. Other design/layout considerations.

a. Space planning and scheduling should be linked to provider/staff hiring and scheduling.

b. Support staff can better manage a group of examination rooms when they have direct visual control of those rooms.

c. Providers and support staff need proximity or devices that ease communications between individuals and from the front to the back office.

(1) Patient arrival/status notification.

(2) Pagers for staff and patients.

(3) Annunciator panels, call lights, status lights/flags.

d. Separate clinic entrance and egress improve flow. Discharge planning/exit discharge consult rooms are located near point of egress.

e. Use of computers in the clinical areas will continue to increase many-fold. New construction and renovation should anticipate the space, wiring/wireless requirements, and related needs of computerization.

f. Proximity and speed of elevators in multi-story facilities affect how quickly patients can move from area to area.

Environmental Management

Appropriate management plans assure a safe, accessible, effective, and functional environment of care. Ambulatory settings present special challenges due to patient mix, especially in waiting areas; the nature of undiagnosed conditions; and the movement of patients through multiple areas of the ambulatory care environment (Association for Professionals in Infection Control and Epidemiology, Inc. [APIC], 2005). Nurses in ambulatory settings have accountability for proactive evaluation of patient care environments and for the development of safety and infection control plans, ongoing monitoring, and implementation of process improvements (Joint Commission on Accreditation of Healthcare Organizations [JCAHO], 2005a).

A. Safety.

1. Recognize factors that affect patient safety.

a. Physical disability.

b. Mental status and judgment.

c. Medication effects.

d. Fall risk.

2. Assess need for furnishings and equipment suitable for population served.

a. Age/size appropriate.

(1) Child safety (such as electrical outlet covers).

(2) Elder safety (such as heavy, non-moveable chairs).

(3) Safety for large/obese patients (such as oversized chairs, scales, and wheelchairs).

(4) Safety for patients at risk for falls (such as gate belts and table straps).

b. Specialty specific.

(1) Rehabilitation patients (such as wheel chair accessible).

(2) Orthopaedic patients (such as higher seating).

(3) Immunocompromised patients (such as HEPA air filtration).

(4) Disabled and geriatric patients (such as adjustable examination tables that lower).

3. Initiate fall prevention strategies to reduce injuries (JCAHO, 2005b).

a. Population-specific evaluation.

b. Staff and patient education.

c. Fall risk patient assessment scale.

d. Identification of high-risk patients.

e. Use of appropriate safety equipment (see #4 below).

4. Equip environment to promote staff/patient safety.

a. Patient transfer and lift devices.

b. Powered examination/procedure tables.

c. Wheelchair-accessible scales.

d. Gate belts, procedure table straps.

e. Hallway safety rails.

f. Call lights in bathrooms, procedure areas, observation/recovery areas.

5. Develop plans to monitor/control recalled medications, products, and medical devices, and report safety-related events (U.S Food and Drug Administration [FDA], 2005).

6. Standardize disinfection and sterilization procedures (refer to *Management of Equipment and Supplies* later in this chapter).

7. Develop hazardous materials and waste management plans.

    a. Identify types of hazardous materials and waste (for example, chemicals, air pollutants/gases/vapors, blood-soiled items, and energy sources/lasers/X-ray equipment).

    b. Identify handling, storage, labeling, using, and disposing procedures consistent with applicable law and regulation (such as NIOSH and state OSHA; see Chapter 15, *Regulatory Compliance and Patient Safety*).

    c. Provide staff orientation, education, and competency assessment for maintenance/management of hazardous materials and waste.

    d. Use appropriate precautions when working with potentially harmful chemicals.

    e. Implement emergency procedures for exposures to spills. Have spill kits readily available.

    f. Develop performance improvement/preventive actions for subsequent.

8. Assure reporting, investigation, improvement/prevention actions for all incidents of injury, property damage, exposure, and occupational illness.

B. Security.

1. Establish systems to control access.

    a. Monitor facility entrances and parking areas.

    b. Provide vehicular access to emergency/urgent care areas.

    c. Secure surgical/procedure areas including specialized equipment (such as laser equipment).

    d. Secure prescription pads, needles, and medications including sample medications and controlled substances.

2. Assure patient and staff/provider identification.

    a. Patient identification at point of service.

    b. Assign at least two patient identifiers (neither to be related to room number) whenever administering medications/blood products, obtaining blood/specimens for clinical testing, or doing any treatments/procedures (JCAHO, 2005b).

    c. Photo identification and appropriate attire/presentation for staff/providers.

3. Recognize security emergencies and implement emergency plan response.

    a. Escalating/aggressive patient behavior/suicide risk patients.

    b. Patients with possession of weapons (such as guns, knives, pepper spray).

    c. Bomb threats (such as knowledge of questions to obtain information that may help identify the caller).

4. Maintain security preparedness for man-made and natural disasters.

C. Medical emergencies.

1. Ensure staff competence in recognizing acute changes in the patient's condition.

2. Ensure appropriate placement of age-specific medical equipment and medication doses to institute emergent patient care (such as crash cart, resuscitation equipment, transport gurney).

3. Provide staff orientation and education.

    a. Role and responsibilities during emergencies.

    b. Skills required.

    c. Competency assessment/reassessment.

    d. Ongoing performance evaluation/scheduled drills.

4. Initiate emergent treatment/cardiac/respiratory/resuscitation.

5. Complete documentation for:

    a. Patient's medical record.

    b. Patient transfer communication.

    c. Risk management/incident reporting.

6. Assure inspection/oversight of medical equipment (refer to the *Management of Equipment and Supplies* section later in this chapter).

D. Infection control.
  1. Recognize health exposure risks and presence of infection.
    a. Symptoms of infection (such as wound drainage, jaundice, diarrhea, respiratory secretions).
    b. Airborne diseases (including chicken pox, measles, tuberculosis, SARS, Avian Influenza, and other foreign, emerging, or potentially re-emerging [such as smallpox] diseases).
    c. High-risk body fluids (such as needle sticks, splash to mucous membranes [eyes, nose, mouth]).
  2. Provide staff orientation/ongoing education.
    a. General infection control principles and clinic-specific procedures.
      (1) Disease transmission.
      (2) Standard precautions.
      (3) Enhanced precautions.
      (4) Respiratory hygiene.
      (5) Employee safety.
    b. Competency assessment.
    c. Ongoing education with annual update on changing infection control requirements.
  3. Clinic-specific environmental infection control policies and procedures (University of Washington Medical Center, 2004).
    a. Patient waiting areas.
      (1) Encourage patients with communicable diseases to stay at home if they can be managed safely by telephone communication.
      (2) Provide signage to encourage reporting of symptoms to receptionist/nurse upon check-in.
      (3) Immediately remove patients and family members with obvious symptoms/diagnosed infection/immunosuppression to examination area.
      (4) Schedule patients with airborne diseases at the end of the day.
      (5) Explain purposes of isolation/procedures to patient and/or family member (such as respiratory hygiene).
    b. Examination rooms.
      (1) Clean examination room between patients (such as changing table

paper, removing soiled equipment/linen, and disinfecting soiled surfaces).
      (2) Clean examination tables, counter tops, treatment carts, and floors daily.
      (3) Bring services/equipment to patient in examination area to prevent the spread of disease to other facilities (for example, restroom, lab, pharmacy).
      (4) Disinfect patient care equipment between patients.
      (5) Close room occupied by a patient with an airborne infection for a prescribed time based on number of air exchanges required, and disinfect before placing another patient in the room.
    c. Equipment and supplies.
      (1) Separate all clean and soiled supplies/linen.
      (2) Disinfect/re-sterilize soiled and/or outdated equipment according to clinic-specific policies and procedures.
      (3) Discard disposable equipment after each use into designated waste receptacles.
      (4) Use safer sharps and needleless system technologies.
      (5) Discard syringes, needles, glass vials, and all other sharps into appropriate sharps containers.
      (6) Disinfect all patient care equipment between uses (such as electronic thermometers, handpieces, stethoscopes).
      (7) Use disposable thermometers on infection/isolation patients.
      (8) Label sterile solutions for irrigation and discard 24 hours after opening or sooner.
      (9) Follow prescribed reprocessing/high-level disinfection procedures for fiberoptic endoscopes and accessories.
    d. Refrigerators and freezers.
      (1) Separate medication, food, and

specimen storage.
  (2) Maintain temperature within safe range.
  (3) Monitor temperature daily and record on a log (manually or central process).
  (4) Implement immediate actions when temperature is out-of-range.
  (5) Clean and defrost at regular intervals.
4. Prevention of infectious disease transmission.
  a. Assure hand hygiene compliance (Centers for Disease Control and Prevention [CDC], 2002).
  b. Avoid direct contact with blood, respiratory or excretory secretions, wound drainage, aerosols, or contaminated articles/patient belongings.
  c. Practice standard precautions for all patients.
  d. Provide equipment and protective apparel appropriate in type and size to clinic-specific activity (JCAHO, 2005a).
    (1) Disposable masks, gowns, gloves.
    (2) Protective eyewear, face shields.
    (3) Personal respiratory protection (for example, minimum OSHA requirement for masks/respirators).
    (4) Isolation sign.
    (5) Examination room with sink (splash-guards when appropriate) and door.
    (6) Portable HEPA tent transport system or high-filtration mask for the patient with potential or newly diagnosed airborne communicable disease.
  e. Use appropriate containers to hold contaminated items for transport, disposal, reprocessing (such as covered metal containers for speculums, endoscope containers).
5. Postexposure treatment.
  a. Implement emergency procedures; administer first aid for exposures.
  b. Develop post-exposure prophylaxis procedure and monitoring program (per CDC recommendations).
6. Reportable diseases.

  a. Obtain current list of reportable diseases as regulated by local, state, and federal health agencies.
  b. Ensure mechanism for timely reporting.
  c. Document in patient/employee medical record.
7. Surveillance monitoring (APIC, 2005).
  a. Identify and track infections associated with clinic-specific patient care/treatment (such as urinary tract infections after instrumentation, gastroenteritis after endoscopy, surgical wound infections).
  b. Ensure patient followup on signs of infection and laboratory results reporting (such as urine, throat, wound cultures).
  c. Develop ongoing quality monitoring program using results to educate staff, and develop/modify policies and procedures.
E. Emergency preparedness.
1. Identify specific procedures in response to internal and external disasters (for example, fire, explosion, earthquake, hurricane, terrorism).
2. Define facility's role in community-wide disaster.
3. Provide staff orientation and education.
  a. Role and responsibilities during emergencies.
  b. Skills required.
  c. Competency assessment.
  d. Ongoing performance evaluations/scheduled drills.
4. Establish communication systems and back-up plans during disasters/emergencies.
5. Develop plans to obtain disaster supplies and equipment.
6. Develop primary and alternative evacuation plans including access to transport equipment.
7. Establish plans for utilities disruption/failure.
  a. Alternative sources of essential utilities (such as emergency power, telecommunications, water, steam).
  b. Emergency procedures for system failures.
  c. Location of emergency shut-off controls.
  d. Process for repair services.

Management of Equipment and Supplies

This is the process to establish and maintain medical equipment and supplies including a plan to promote safe and effective use of equipment, staff competency assessment and education, and cost-effective purchasing. Nurses in ambulatory care are accountable to assure safe handling, inventory control, and appropriate charging of patient care equipment and supplies.

A. Selecting medical equipment and supplies.
    1. Equipment and supply function(s).
    2. Risks associated with use.
    3. Maintenance requirements.

B. Ordering/purchasing of equipment and supplies.
    1. Purchasing specifications and sole source requirements.
    2. Shared purchasing contracts ("group buying") to ensure the best possible cost.
    3. Service/maintenance contracts and warranties.
    4. Expedited delivery of urgently needed equipment/supplies.

C. Controlling inventory.
    1. System to monitor current supply "stock on hand" such as:
       a. Description.
       b. Quantity.
       c. Lot number.
       d. Expiration date.
    2. Ability to limit inventory to preserve financial investment (Delio, 1999).
       a. Agreements for standardization.
       b. Frequent ordering/purchasing.
       c. Designated "par levels."
       d. Expedited delivery processes.
    3. Accessible internal ordering vendor information.
    4. Storage areas that are in close proximity to point of care.

D. Staff orientation/ongoing education.
    1. Learning requirements and competency assessment process for use of equipment.
    2. Training, technical skills, and current competency as part of the privileging/credentialing process.
    3. Initial and recurring staff training/reassessment on equipment/supply changes.
    4. Training on emergency procedures in an event of failure/user error.

E. Ongoing assessment and monitoring for safe and functional equipment (University of Washington Medical Center, 2004).
    1. Responsibility assigned for oversight of medical equipment including:
       a. Policy and procedures.
       b. Equipment maintenance/management plan.
       c. Required inspection labeling.
    2. Initial inspection of all powered medical equipment for compliance with appropriate specifications prior to initial use. Label applied indicating date inspected.
    3. Routine preventive maintenance through:
       a. Scheduled inspections.
       b. Ongoing repair/replacement of existing equipment.
    4. Systems for monitoring equipment.
       a. Staff checking equipment before use to ensure good operating condition (for example, no frayed electrical cords, no evidence of physical damage).
       b. Staff schedule for checking of all critical alarms (such as working conditions and audibility).
       c. Action plans for hazard alerts and recall notification.
    5. Report equipment problems, failures, and user errors as required by the *Safe Medical Device Act of 1990* (FDA, 2005).
    6. Availability of back-up equipment (such as battery-operated equipment for emergency conditions).

F. Charging for supplies.
    1. Determine costs of individual medical/surgical supplies.
    2. Develop charge schedule based on applicable reimbursement coding/standardize charges across facility.
    3. Institute standard charging process.
    4. Determine review schedule for supply charges.

G. Storage.
    1. Ensure appropriately sized storage located in close proximity to point of care (refer to *Facility Design and Workflow* earlier in this chapter).

2. Control access to sterilized equipment/storage of expensive equipment.
3. Use exchange carts to reduce restocking labor costs.
4. Enclose/cover areas for linen storage.
5. Preassemble surgical trays/case carts for specialty-specific procedures and locate near point of care.

H. Recycling.
   1. Identify what can be safely recycled.
   2. Provide staff education.
   3. Provide appropriate, labeled containers.
   4. Ensure shredding of confidential papers.
   5. Arrange for regular pick-ups and disposal.

References

American Institute of Architects (AIA). (2001). *Guidelines for design and construction of hospitals and health care facilities.* Washington, DC: Author.

Association for Professionals in Infection Control and Epidemiology, Inc. (APIC). (2005). *APIC text of infection control and epidemiology.* Washington, D.C.: Author.

Barnett, A.E., & Mayer, G.G. (1992). *Ambulatory care management and practice.* Gaithersburg, MD: Aspen.

Centers for Disease Control and Prevention (CDC). (2002). *Guideline for hand hygiene in health care settings. MMWR, 51*(RR-16), 1-56.

Delio, S.A. (1999). *The perfect practice.* Englewood, CO: Medical Group Management Association.

Delio, S.A. (2005). *The efficient physician: Seven guiding principles for a tech-savvy practice* (2nd ed.). Englewood, CO: Medical Group Management Association.

Joint Commission on Accreditation of Healthcare Organizations (JCAHO). (2005a). *Comprehensive accreditation manual for hospitals: The official handbook, update 2.* Oakbrook Terrace, IL: Author.

Joint Commission on Accreditation of Healthcare Organizations (JCAHO). (2005b). *Hospital accreditation standards, national patient safety goals.* Oakbrook Terrace, IL: Author.

Redling, R. (2002). *Size matters: Measure twice, cut once. MGMA Connexion 2*(7), 37-38.

Ross, A., Williams, S.J., & Pavlock, E.J. (1998): *Ambulatory care management* (3rd ed.). Albany, NY: Delmar.

U.S. Congress. (1990). *Americans with disabilities act of 1990, 42 U.S.C.A. § 12101 et seq.* (West 1993).

University of Washington Medical Center. (2004). *Administrative policies and operating procedures.* Seattle, WA: Author.

U.S. Food and Drug Administration (FDA). (2005). *How to report problems with products regulated by FDA.* Retrieved September 12, 2005, from http://www.fda.gov/opacom/backgrounders/problem.html

Additional Reading

The Society for Healthcare Epidemiology of America. (2004). *Practical handbook for healthcare epidemiologists* (2nd ed.). Thorofare, NJ: Slack Inc.

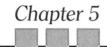
Practice/Office Support

This test may be copied for use by others.

COMPLETE THE FOLLOWING:

Name: _____

Address: _____

City: _____ State: _____ Zip: _____

Preferred telephone: (Home) _____ (Work) _____

E-mail _____

AAACN Member Expiration Date: _____

Registration fee: AAACN Member: $12.00
                     Nonmember: $20.00

Objectives

This educational activity is designed for nurses and other health care professionals who practice in ambulatory care. For those wishing to obtain CE credit, an evaluation follows. After studying the information presented in this offering, you will be able to:

1. Schedule patients efficiently.
2. Design productive spaces and workflow.
3. Enhance patient and staff safety, and improve the patient care environment.
4. Reduce environmental hazards and risks in work settings.

Answer Form:

1. If you applied what you have learned from this activity into your practice, what would be different?

_____

_____

_____

Evaluation	Strongly disagree				Strongly agree
2. By completing this activity, I was able to meet the following objectives:					
a. Schedule patients efficiently.	1	2	3	4	5
b. Design productive spaces and workflow.	1	2	3	4	5
c. Enhance patient and staff safety, and improve the patient care environment.	1	2	3	4	5
d. Reduce environmental hazards and risks in work settings.	1	2	3	4	5
3. The content was current and relevant.	1	2	3	4	5
4. The objectives could be achieved using the content provided.	1	2	3	4	5
5. This was an effective method to learn this content.	1	2	3	4	5
6. I am more confident in my abilities since completing this material.	1	2	3	4	5

7. The material was (check one) ___new ___review for me.

8. Time required to read this chapter: _____minutes

I verify that I have completed this activity: _____
                                              Signature

Comments: _____

_____

_____

Posttest Instructions

1. To receive continuing education credit for individual study after reading the article, complete the answer/evaluation form to the left.

2. Detach and send the answer/evaluation form along with a check or money order payable to the *American Academy of Ambulatory Care Nursing (AAACN)*, East Holly Avenue Box 56, Pitman, NJ 08071–0056.

3. Test returns must be postmarked by August 1, 2011. Upon completion of the answer/evaluation form, a certificate for **1.5** contact hour(s) will be awarded and sent to you. Should the material contained in this chapter become outdated prior to the above expiration date, AAACN reserves the right to withdraw this CE test.

This activity is co-provided by the *American Academy of Ambulatory Care Nursing (AAACN)* and Anthony J. Jannetti, Inc. (AJJ). AJJ is accredited as a provider of continuing nursing education by the American Nurses' Credentialing Center's Commission on Accreditation (ANCC-COA). AAACN is a provider approved by the California Board of Registered Nurses, provider number CEP 05336.

This article was reviewed and formatted for contact hour credit by Sally S. Russell, MN, CMSRN, AAACN Education Director; and Candia Baker Laughlin MS, RN, C, Editor.

Chapter 6

Health Care Fiscal Management

Linda D'Angelo, MSN, RN, MBA, CMPE

Objectives

Study of the information presented in this chapter will enable the learner to:
1. Explain the financial environment of health care.
2. Acquire knowledge of common revenue sources.
3. Apply knowledge of managed care financial principles in daily practice as well as mechanisms to ensure quality and appropriate care.
4. Acquire knowledge of common coding systems.
5. Use resource management in daily practice.
6. Gain an understanding of the business of health care and its relationship to the budgeting process.

Key Points

1. Nurses have significant opportunity to impact the cost of an admission, a case, or a visit through proactive continuum of care guidelines, preventive health, and disease management programs.
2. Managed care presents new opportunities for nurses to use knowledge and skills to improve care for patients.
3. Understanding health care financial management, including resource management, program planning, and budget management, is an important knowledge base for all nurses.
4. There are many ways in which nurses contribute to the financial health of an organization.

In today's health care economic environment, ambulatory care nurses must understand the economics of health care and appreciate their role in controlling costs. The magnitude of public expenditures for health care has resulted in significant growth in the government's role in financing and regulating health care. Decisions made by nurses not only affect the financial viability of the organizations for which they work, but may directly affect the financial well-being of their patients. Ambulatory care nurses must make point-of-care changes quickly to foster cost-effective care delivery. This chapter will provide ambulatory nurses with a basic knowledge of health care finance and will allow them to knowledgeably and actively participate in providing cost-effective patient care services.

In this chapter, the ambulatory care nurse will acquire knowledge of commonly used financial terms and acronyms applicable in the work setting. The nurse will gain understanding of basic financial concepts, such as revenue stream, cost accounting, cost benefit analysis, managed care concepts, and coding and reimbursement mechanisms. The nurse will also gain insight into how personal performance affects business viability and acquire addi-

tional knowledge of resource management principles. The nurse's awareness of clinical behavior's impact on the cost of health care services is essential in the ambulatory care environment. Failure to understand and apply clinical guidelines and decision pathways may result in otherwise avoidable emergency department visits, hospitalizations, and other costly interventions. The ambulatory care nurse's specific role in the continuum of care focuses on the integration of the plan of care, measurement of results (outcomes), and education of patients, and it also ensures access to care. These activities result in lower costs, higher quality, and continuous improvements in care management and care delivery.

Financial Environment of Health Care Organizations

Cleverley (2003) explains that a health care organization as a provider of health services will be financially viable if it receives revenues from services provided in an amount equal to or greater than the dollars expended to provide the services. Patient service revenue represents the amount that results from the provision of patient care services. Other sources of revenue may include government payments at the local, state, or federal level for servuces such as educational programs and research or foundation grants.

A. Fee setting or costing allows organizations or providers the opportunity to recover the cost of rendering a service. Direct and indirect costs must be identified prior to establishing fees.

   1. Direct costs can be traced to a specific service provided. Examples of direct costs are nursing salaries, supplies, and medications.

   2. Indirect costs are not usually attributable to a single service or item. The cost of employee salaries in the business office, rent, and parking expenses are examples of indirect costs.

   3. Desired net income must be determined prior to setting fees.

      a. Net income equals the amount of income, allowing for noncollectible amounts or bad debt, after expenses are paid.

      b. The sum of net income for all goods and services provided equals the net income for the overall business.

      c. Net income is used to develop new programs, fund capital expenses (such as information technology systems or building projects), contribute to retained earnings for operations in future years, or is paid out as profits or dividends to shareholders in a for-profit health care entity.

B. Revenue is the total return or income produced from a given source. The rapidly changing health care environment and a payer (health plan) focus on controlling costs can directly affect an organization's revenue stream or sources and amounts of revenue. Medicare, Medicaid, and other insurance types have coverage limits and payment levels that change frequently and can significantly affect the revenue stream.

   1. A charge or fee for a service often does not reflect the actual amount collected. The actual amount received is commonly referred to as the collectible.

      a. Bad debt occurs when an insurer, an employer, or a patient does not pay a bill.

   b. Usual, customary, and reasonable (UCR) amount is a method used to determine if a fee is usual, customary, and reasonable.

      (1) Usual refers to fees normally charged by a doctor or health care provider for a service.

      (2) According to Kelley (2004), customary is based on a percentile of aggregated fees charged in a geographic area for the same service. When a health insurance plan pays 80% of an organization's fee based on a usual and customary fee schedule, the unpaid amount is often not collectible.

      (3) An insurer will pay the lower of the usual and customary fee unless a reasonable fee adjustment is warranted, based on documented special circumstances of a case (Kelley, 2004).

   c. Discounts are often negotiated by health care organizations to secure a contract with another organization. This provides some assurance of business volume. An example is a physical examination performed by a nurse practitioner for a particular company according to a sole provider agreement.

Revenue Sources

The major payers of ambulatory health care services are the primary revenue sources for most organizations.

A. Governments (federal, state, and local) fund or provide health plans.

   1. Medicare: Government plan that provides some type of coverage for hospital expenses (Part A) and physician services (Part B) for individuals over 65 and other qualifying individuals (managed care Medicare programs are covered later in this chapter in the section, *Managed Care Concepts*).

   2. Medicaid: A plan jointly funded by federal and state governments, introduced in 1966 to cover poor individuals and managed independently by each state.

3. TriCare: A federal program providing coverage to families of active duty military personnel, military retirees, spouses, and dependents which has replaced the Civilian Health and Medical Program of the United States (CHAMPUS).
4. The Indian Health Service and the federally supported Community Health Center programs: Provide government funding for health care for specific populations.
5. Other: Some states and local governments provide additional limited coverage of health services based on need or qualification.
B. Private insurance: Private insurance includes both commercial indemnity plans and managed care plans. Individual or employer chooses type of insurance (such as Blue Cross/Blue Shield, Prudential). There are a variety of private insurance plans.
   1. Commercial indemnity plans: A type of insurance contract in which the insurer pays for care received up to a fixed amount per encounter or episode of illness. For example, in an 80/20-indemnity plan, the insurer would pay 80% of UCR. The insured individual would be responsible for 20% or remainder of the fee.
   2. Managed care plans: For example, the insurer may offer health maintenance plans (HMOs), preferred provider organization plans (PPOs), or point of service plans (POS) (these will be described under *Managed Care Concepts* later in this chapter).
C. Fee-for-service: Reimbursement method in which payment is made for each service or item. May drive up costs because it encourages a doctor or an organization to provide more medical care by paying for each service provided. Examples include preoperative chest X-rays and annual cholesterol screening, which may not be indicated by history and clinical findings.
D. Employer-provided insurance: May elect to offer health plan choices or provide an employer-funded plan where the company bears the risk. Often contracts with an outside organization to manage the plan, a third-party administrator.
E. Private pay: Individual pays for health care services he or she receives.

F. Out-of-pocket expense: The portion of health care cost for which the individual is responsible. Could be 100% if an uncovered service such as cosmetic or plastic surgery is performed, If the individual has no insurance or the portion that is not paid by the insurance plan under which an individual is covered, then 100% is out-of-pocket.
G. Copayment: Out-of-pocket expense paid by an individual for a specific service defined in the insurance plan. For example, 20% of charges for care or $10 per visit may be charged to the individual.
H. Deductibles: The amount an insured individual is responsible to pay before insurance pays. For example, an individual may have a $200 deductible for hospitalization before the remainder of the hospital stay is covered.

Managed Care Concepts

Kongstvedt (2004b) describes managed care as a system that combines financing and care delivery through comprehensive benefits delivered by selected providers and financial incentives for enrolled members to use these providers. The goals of managed care are quality, cost-effectiveness, and accessibility to health care. It is a coordinated system of health care that achieves outcomes (reduced utilization and improved population health) through preventive care, case management, and the provision of medically necessary appropriate care.
A. Prepaid health insurance: A fixed amount is paid to the contracted provider of care each month for each enrollee for specific services defined by the health care plan. For example, radiology services may be contracted at specific rates for enrollees in a plan.
B. Capitation: A method for funding expenses of enrollees in prepaid health care plans that pays providers a fixed fee per member regardless of whether or not service is provided.
   1. The provider is responsible for delivering or arranging the delivery of all services required under the conditions of the provider contract.
   2. For example, a plan that pays a per member per month (PMPM) amount to a physician group to provide primary care services for each enrollee in the plan.

3. Efforts to reduce duplication and control costs create new professional demands on ambulatory nurses, emphasizing efficient resource allocation, coordinated care planning, and outcomes assessment.

C. Managed care plans: Different types of managed care plans define where patients may receive the most cost effective care, which providers are included, and how expenses will be paid.

1. Preferred provider organization (PPO): A program in which contracts exist between the health care plan and care providers at a discount for services. Typically, the plan provides incentives for patients to utilize in- network providers as opposed to non-participating providers (independent/noncontracted) through decreased copayments. Kongvstedt (2004a) describes network providers as those health care professionals who are contracted through a health care plan to deliver health care to subscribers.

2. Point of service (POS): A plan that defines service providers in the service area outside of the usual preferred provider network. According to Kongstvedt (2004b), an insured patient pays an increased premium with more out-of-pocket expenses. Service providers are providers outside the network, contracted to provide specialty services such as invasive cardiology.

3. Health maintenance organization (HMO): There are two possibilities.

   a. A health care plan may place risk on the providers for medical expenses. In this instance, providers are encouraged to provide appropriate medical services but not medically unnecessary services in exchange for larger premiums. The risk lies in the fact that the provider may deliver services for which he or she may not be paid. For example, the provider may not be fully paid if he or she did not achieve certain predefined quality outcomes (such as immunization or mammography screening targets).

   b. A health plan that uses physicians as gatekeepers. In this model, the patient chooses a primary care provider (PCP) who is responsible for all aspects of care management and who must authorize (gatekeeper) or give permission for referral to other providers.

      (1) PCPs are often paid a panel management fee and have financial incentives for providing more comprehensive services within the provider's own practice. Physicians may receive a standard amount, $2 to $10 per member per month, to actively manage the care for the panel population by offering special programs or services based on the panel's clinical conditions or demographics (for example, cholesterol screening for hypertensives, retinal screening for diabetics).

      (2) Many HMOs have open access, allowing patients to see specialists within the network without the primary care physician's approval.

4. Independent practice association (IPA): Kelley (2004) defines an IPA as a legal entity whose members are independent physicians or physician groups who contract with the IPA for the purpose of having the IPA contract with one or more HMOs. The HMOs contract with an IPA for provision of services for their members for a negotiated fee.

5. Physician hospital organization (PHO): Legal organizations often developed for purposes of contracting with managed care plans. A PHO links physicians to specific hospitals for hospitalization care.

6. Medicare managed care: Instead of the traditional fee-for-service payments, reimbursement is paid on a capitated, per enrollee basis each month.

   a. A fee scale is set based on the average adjusted per capita cost (AAPCC) that has been historically paid in a given region or county for Medicare-eligible enrollees (Cleverley, 2003).

   b. The Centers for Medicare and Medicaid continues to refine the reimbursement methodology in an attempt to make managed care options attractive to Medicare eligible seniors as well as providers.

7. Medicaid managed care: Managed care plans for Medicaid enrollees are relatively new and are experiencing significant difficulty with both patient care coordination and costs management.

D. Mechanisms to ensure quality and appropriateness.

1. Health Plan Employer Data and Information Set (HEDIS®).

   a. Measures plan performance against plan predictions and performance targets (such as cervical cancer screening rates or mammogram rates).

   b. Employers may choose not to enter into contracts with health plans if performance goals are not met.

2. Precertification: The process of obtaining authorization or certification from a health care plan for routine hospital admissions, referrals, procedures, or tests.

   a. Ambulatory care nurses are commonly involved in obtaining precertification or authorization from health care plans for coverage approval for costly procedures (such as surgery and MRIs) or for out-of-network referrals.

   b. Enables review for clinical appropriateness for the procedure against standards and ensures the service is provided in the most cost-effective, appropriate setting (such as ambulatory surgery center vs. inpatient admission and main operating room).

3. Concurrent review: Case management of costly cases is often performed by nurses to ensure hospitalized patients are being managed most efficiently relative to length of stay and discharge planning needs. Case management is a method for managing the provision of health care to members/patients with catastrophic or high-cost medical conditions. The focus is on coordinating the care to improve the continuity and quality of care, as well as lower costs.

4. Care delivery: Nurses providing care – right patient, right setting, right care, right provider, at the right time.

   a. Care delivery systems are financially stronger when efficiencies are maximized.

   b. Disease management: Method that utilizes standardized care plans based on evidence and best practices to manage patients with chronic conditions.

      (1) Provides uniform care and ensures patients are being properly managed.

      (2) Diabetes care, hypertension management, and anticoagulation clinics are examples in which better care can be provided at less cost with guidelines, through programs, or by case management.

   c. Health promotion/wellness education is key to promoting healthier patients. Self-care promotion provides opportunities for nurses.

   d. Case management for specific populations and care management over time provides enhanced opportunities for nurses to affect (decrease) total cost of care for an episode or condition by early detection of impending health crisis and early intervention. Examples such as congestive heart failure monitoring via home care or telephone decrease hospital admissions or emergency department visits.

Coding

Coding is a standard method used to report patient care services provided to private or government health plans in order to receive payment.

A. The Centers for Medicare and Medicaid Services (CMS), formerly called The Health Care Financing Administration (HCFA), within the U.S. Department of Health and Human Services determines the standard rules and reporting mechanisms for health care services.

1. This oversight group initially introduced a view that payment for inpatient Medicare enrollees should be derived from a cost-based reimbursement system.

2. Due to escalating costs driven by fee-for-service payment methodology (without quality, appropriateness, or utilization controls), HCFA (now CMS) switched to diagnostic-related groups (DRGs) in 1983, paying a

fixed amount for defined hospital services based on diagnosis-related levels of service provided, length of stay, or cost of care.

3. It was expected that hospitals would improve operational efficiencies, provide quality care, and maintain financial viability.

B. Diagnostic-related groups (DRGs) is a system for classifying hospital inpatients into groups requiring similar quantities of resources according to characteristics such as diagnosis, age, procedure, complications, and comorbidities.

1. The care costs of DRGs are estimated.

2. Advances in technology and reduced payments from HCFA/CMS have had significant effects on hospital lengths of stay resulting in lesser costs assigned to DRGs.

3. This cycle has produced system-wide ramifications including a marked shift in care setting from inpatient to ambulatory environments.

4. Ambulatory care nurses have a significant opportunity to affect the cost of an inpatient admission, a case, an encounter, or a service.

    a. Preadmission and preprocedure patient education and discharge planning begin with the ambulatory nurse.

    b. Proactive planning with the patient and family ensure more efficient processes and allow shorter lengths of stay and faster recovery periods for patients.

C. Resource-based relative value system (RBRVS) is a classification system that attempts to assign within a defined setting the resource requirements based on weights according to relative cost of each service.

1. RBRVS has been used by HCFA/CMS since 1992 for determining payment to physicians for services provided to Medicare enrollees.

2. Relative value unit (RVU) was established by HCFA/CMS to approximate the work (physician knowledge skill and judgement), practice expense, and malpractice expense for the delivery of physician services.

    a. For every procedure, these three components reflect the value of a particular service, which make up a classification unit (code) in the RBRVS.

    b. According to Cleverley (2003), each RVU is multiplied by a region-specific price index to reach the reimbursement rate for a particular service that is paid by HCFA/CMS.

D. HCPCS is the acronym for the Health Care Financing Administration (HCFA) Common Procedure Coding System.

1. HCPCS is a uniform method for health care providers and medical suppliers to report professional services, procedures, and supplies to health care plans.

2. HCPCS allows for consistent communication of services provided.

3. HCPCS ensures validity of profiles for the classification system and fee schedules through standardized coding. HCPCS also enhances education and research by providing local, regional, and national data comparisons.

4. The *Physicians' Current Procedural Terminology (CPT), CPT 2005* (2004), is published by the American Medical Association and is the internationally recognized coding system for reporting medical services and procedures. Nurses use CPT coding guidelines for reporting services provided by nurses. The insurance carrier determines if a nurse is an eligible billing provider. There are three levels of HCPCS CPT codes.

    a. CPT Level I.

        (1) Evaluation and management (E&M): Category of CPT codes that represent non-procedural provider encounters (such as an office visit for an earache, a blood pressure monitoring, or a comprehensive medical examination).

        (2) 99211: Minimal office visit for an established patient. It is the only code that a nurse can bill independent of a physician encounter. An example is an office visit for a 20-year-old female who receives an allergy vaccine injection and is observed by a nurse. The assessment and plan of care must be documented for the nurse to bill independently utilizing this code.

    b. CPT Level II: Represents alphanumeric codes established for services and items not listed in CPT I such as supplies and drugs. An example is 90746 Hepatitis B vaccine, adult dose.

c. CPT III represents alphanumeric codes established by individual state Medicaid carriers to cover services not listed in Level I or II.

5. ICD 9: *International Classification of Diseases, 9th Revision, Clinical Modification* (ICD 9-CM) 6th ed., published by the U.S. National Center for Health Statistics (2003), is the internationally recognized system for the purposes of international morbidity and mortality reporting. In the U.S., it is used for coding and billing purposes.
   a. CMS requires the use of ICD 9-CM codes on claims submitted by health care providers.
   b. The numerical code must represent an accurate translation of the diagnostic statement or terminology documented by the provider and may be a sign, symptom, or condition.
   c. Coders are individuals who are used by many health care organizations.
      (1) Coders are responsible for providing an accurate picture of the patient's condition using numerical codes to translate the physician's documentation into billable services.
      (2) They may only apply standardized codes to information that is documented.
   d. Electronic coding systems: Electronic systems (computers) translate physician online documentation in clinical information systems into billable service codes.
6. Documentation: Medical terminology describing the reason for a patient's encounter must appear on a source document.
   a. Source documents include any documentation of a patient encounter.
   b. Encounter forms, emergency reports, billing forms, and patient records are examples of source documents that may vary from facility to facility.

7. Compliance: The provider of health care services must follow standard coding guidelines and be prepared to provide documentation of the service provided. Failure to do so could result in allegations of fraud and significant monetary fines, and may result in loss of licenses by hospitals.

E. Additional classification systems for reimbursement of ambulatory visits or encounters were originated in the 1990s in the public sector as an attempt by government to control costs and quality through fixed pricing.
   1. Ambulatory patient groups (APGs): Patient classification system designed to explain amount and type of resource used in ambulatory care visit; forerunner to the more commonly used Ambulatory Patient Classifications (APCs).
   2. APCs were adopted in 2000 by CMS for outpatient prospective payment in hospital outpatient departments and ambulatory surgery centers. Kongstvedt (2004a) describes APCs as similar to DRGs for hospitals.
      a. APCs are based on procedures rather than diagnoses.
      b. APCs provide for severity adjustment.
      c. More than one code may be billed if more than one procedure is performed; however, additional charges are discounted.

Resource Management

Resource management is an organization's ability to effectively manage its resources, people, capital, equipment, and supplies. Beyers (2004) suggests that in today's environment, adjusting resource use to match fluctuating patient census and ensuring adequacy of supplies and equipment is an ongoing activity. Baker (2004) describes the nurse's role in staffing and inventory management to control resource expense.

A. Non-labor resource management: Management of clerical and medical-surgical supplies, linen, pharmaceuticals, and durable medical equipment affects unit costs. Nurses can have great opportunity to contribute to management of daily operational cost when they take an active role and interest in understanding how supply or linen usage or staffing patterns affect costs. Over-ordering and overstocking leads to waste when supplies sit unused on shelves or expire before use.

1. Inventory management via par levels: Minimum supply levels are determined and maintained to ensure a short shelf life while meeting user demand.
2. Product evaluation: A standard methodology adopted by organizations to ensure cost-effective purchasing decisions of supplies and other equipment.
    a. Product evaluation involves choosing the least expensive alternative that achieves desired results (outcomes) vs. personal preferences.
    b. Product evaluation may be accomplished by the committee using studies (product trials within the institution) and literature reviews.
3. Trending and tracking: Tracking sheets are used to monitor volume and frequency of use of specific items or supplies.
    a. Invoices are provided by suppliers when supplies are received and should be matched against those items ordered or requested.
    b. Budget variance reports identify variances in dollars over or under projected amounts.

B. Labor resource management: Managing numbers and levels of staff and the hours they are paid typically has greater cost implications than non-labor resource management.
1. Practice efficiency: Staffing for the right level of care and volume.
    a. Length of encounter, waiting times, delay in process, downtime (no-shows, vacant appointments, hold times) can increase the need for support staff.
    b. Efficient management of phone calls, scheduling of procedures, and organizing workflow to meet customers' needs will lead to more cost effective staffing.
2. Appropriate staffing: The right person, based on educational preparation and licensure, assigned to do the work that must be performed at the right time.

Budget

Budgeting is a logical way for a health care organization to plan for and manage its processes. Strategic, longer-term plans drive operational or shorter-term budget cycles.

A. Planning: A process used to develop specific courses of action to attain organization's goals and objectives. Budget planning can be defined as the process by which organizational plans are expressed in dollars and cents.
1. Planning is a formalized process in most organizations and key to health care organizations' financial viability.
2. Budgets are built on historical performance: Projected numbers of visits, number of encounters, or number of patients in a physician's panel for which he or she will receive capitated fees may be used in planning revenues and expenses.
3. Budget planning requires goals, which are broad statements indicating what is to be achieved, and objectives, which are more specific statements of what is to be achieved within a specific time period.
4. Budgets forecasts anticipated revenues associated with anticipated expenses.
5. Benefits of planning a budget:
    a. Promotes effective decision-making.
    b. Allows one to consider alternatives.
    c. Specifies major assumptions (for example, rate of inflation) and fee increase estimates.
    d. Uses financial and statistical indicators that allow both operations and productivity to be monitored.

B. Financial reports: Expenses budgeted (planned) and actual (incurred) are reported and the volume of activity measured (visits or procedures).
1. Reports typically include productivity indicators (for example, paid man-hours per visits).
2. Hospital referral report: Tracks hospital admission days and charges to reconcile with practice.
3. There are many other types of financial reports.

C. Programming: Determines the programs an organization will offer to reach its stated goals and objectives.
1. Feasibility study is completed to determine how feasible it is to offer or continue offering

a program or service. This might include market studies, patient interest surveys, facility requirements, and identification of similar programs in the area.

2. Cost benefit analysis: A formal financial analysis completed by organizations to determine the cost of a program and projected revenues, and to identify and quantify program benefits. It includes assumptions about specific expenses and potential revenue based on projected volumes (Cleverley, 2003). Analysis is usually completed before starting a new program or service and may be included in the feasibility study.

D. Types of budgets: The most common budgets are capital and operating budgets.

1. Capital budget: Departments usually forecast or estimate capital needs (generally, high-cost items or expenses) for the coming year translated into dollars; includes such items as new and replacement equipment, facility renovation, new technology, and other items that may be paid for over several years.

2. Operating budget: Includes statistical, revenue, and expense budgets (Cleverley 2003).

    a. Statistical budget provides measures of workload or activity for each responsibility center or service provided.

    b. Expense budget is a projection of expected costs allocated to a specific program or service based on anticipated volume of activities (for example, payroll and supplies expense). It includes allocation of direct identifiable costs related to a specific program budget and allocation (assignment) of indirect costs, such as building and equipment, depreciation, and bad debt estimates.

    c. Revenue budget is a projection of expected revenues associated with a specific program or service, based on volumes projected in the statistical budget.

E. Accounting: The financial services or accounting department collects and reports information on revenues and expenses of a specific department or program.

F. Analysis: Analysis of budget includes reporting, trending, and tracking results; report analyzing.

1. Critical success factors are defined by management. These are the essential factors needed in order to continue in the business or to continue providing a service or a program.

2. Key performance indicators: Balanced approach to planning and forecasting; process of measuring organizational performance against plan. Ensures the ultimate financial success of the organization. Goals help to provide organization focus. Kedrowski (2003) describes the balanced scorecard/report card approach being used by many ambulatory care organizations which incorporate a variety of measures to help them improve quality at lower costs.

    a. In addition to profitability, areas for indicator determination may include non-financial measures, such as access to care, utilization and productivity, and quality in service. Examples:

        (1) Profitability: Achieve X % net revenues after expenses.

        (2) Access to care: Consult request turnaround time.

        (3) Utilization and productivity: Support staff full time equivalents (FTEs) per provider FTE.

        (4) Quality in service: Immunization rates.

    b. Variance reports: Demonstrate differences between actual results compared to the plan.

References

American Medical Association (AMA). (2004). *Physician's current procedural terminology, CPT 2005, standard edition.* Chicago, IL: Author.

Baker, J. (2004). *Health care finance: Basic tools for nonfinancial managers.* Boston, MA: Jones and Bartlett.

Beyers, M. (2004). The management of nursing services. In L. Wolper (Ed.), *Health care administration* (4th ed.) (pp.348-372). Boston, MA: Jones and Bartlett.

Cleverley, W. (Ed.). (2003). *Essentials of health care finance* (5th ed.). Boston, MA: Jones and Bartlett.

Kedrowski, S. (2003). Performance measures in ambulatory care. *Nursing Economic$, 21*(4), 188-193.

Kelley, M. (2004). Physician practice: Organization and operation. In L. Wolper (Ed.), *Health care administration* (4th ed.) (pp. 843-870). Boston, MA: Jones and Bartlett.

Kongstvedt, P. (2004a). *Managed care: What it is and how it works* (2nd ed.). Boston, MA: Jones and Bartlett.

Kongvstedt, P. (2004b). *Managed health care.* In L. Wolper (Ed.), *Health care administration* (4th ed.) (pp. 547-584). Boston, MA: Jones and Bartlett.

U.S. National Center for Health Statistics. (2003). *International classification of diseases, 9th revision, clinical modification* (6th ed.). Hyattsville, MD: Author.

Additional Readings

Barr, K. (2004). Ambulatory care. In L. Wolper (Ed.), *Health care administration* (4th ed.) (pp. 507-546). Boston, MA: Jones and Bartlett.

Dasco, S. (2002). *Managed care answer book* (5th ed.). New York: Aspen.

Laughlin, C. (1999). Federal reimbursement for services: A primer for ambulatory care nurses. *AAACN ViewPoint, 21*(5), 8-9.

Mundinger, M. (2004). Essential health care: Affordable for all? *Nursing Economic$, 22*(5), 239-244.

Nolin, J. (2005). Redirecting health care spending: Consumer-directed health care. *Nursing Economic$, 22*(5), 251-253.

Health Care Fiscal Management

This test may be copied for use by others.

COMPLETE THE FOLLOWING:

Name: _____

Address: _____

City: _____ State: _____ Zip: _____

Preferred telephone: (Home)_____ (Work)_____

E-mail_____

AAACN Member Expiration Date: _____

Registration fee: AAACN Member: $12.00
                   Nonmember: $20.00

Answer Form:

1. If you applied what you have learned from this activity into your practice, what would be different?

   _____

   _____

   _____

Evaluation	Strongly disagree				Strongly agree
2. By completing this activity, I was able to meet the following objectives:					
a. Explain the financial environment of health care.	1	2	3	4	5
b. Acquire knowledge of common revenue sources.	1	2	3	4	5
c. Apply knowledge of managed care financial principles in daily practice as well as mechanisms to ensure quality and appropriate care.	1	2	3	4	5
d. Acquire knowledge of common coding systems.	1	2	3	4	5
e. Use resource management in daily practice.	1	2	3	4	5
f. Gain an understanding of the business of health care and its relationship to the budgeting process.	1	2	3	4	5
3. The content was current and relevant.	1	2	3	4	5
4. The objectives could be achieved using the content provided.	1	2	3	4	5
5. This was an effective method to learn this content.	1	2	3	4	5
6. I am more confident in my abilities since completing this material.	1	2	3	4	5

7. The material was (check one) ___new ___review for me.
8. Time required to read this chapter: _____minutes

I verify that I have completed this activity: _____
                                              Signature

Comments: _____

_____

_____

Objectives

This educational activity is designed for nurses and other health care professionals who practice in ambulatory care. For those wishing to obtain CE credit, an evaluation follows. After studying the information presented in this offering, you will be able to:

1. Explain the financial environment of health care.
2. Acquire knowledge of common revenue sources.
3. Apply knowledge of managed care financial principles in daily practice as well as mechanisms to ensure quality and appropriate care.
4. Acquire knowledge of common coding systems.
5. Use resource management in daily practice.
6. Gain an understanding of the business of health care and its relationship to the budgeting process.

Posttest Instructions

1. To receive continuing education credit for individual study after reading the article, complete the answer/evaluation form to the left.

2. Detach and send the answer/evaluation form along with a check or money order payable to the *American Academy of Ambulatory Care Nursing (AAACN)*, East Holly Avenue Box 56, Pitman, NJ 08071–0056.

3. Test returns must be postmarked by August 1, 2011. Upon completion of the answer/evaluation form, a certificate for **1.5** contact hour(s) will be awarded and sent to you. Should the material contained in this chapter become outdated prior to the above expiration date, AAACN reserves the right to withdraw this CE test.

This activity is co-provided by the *American Academy of Ambulatory Care Nursing (AAACN)* and Anthony J. Jannetti, Inc. (AJJ). AJJ is accredited as a provider of continuing nursing education by the American Nurses' Credentialing Center's Commission on Accreditation (ANCC-COA). AAACN is a provider approved by the California Board of Registered Nurses, provider number CEP 05336.

This article was reviewed and formatted for contact hour credit by Sally S. Russell, MN, CMSRN, AAACN Education Director; and Candia Baker Laughlin MS, RN, C, Editor.

Chapter 7

Informatics

Ida M. Androwich, PhD, RN, BC, FAAN

Objectives

Study of the information presented in this chapter will enable the learner to:

1. Define the concept of nursing informatics as it applies to ambulatory care nursing.
2. Understand the benefits and requirements for a computerized patient record (CPR).
3. Identify criteria for evaluating computer technology for use in the ambulatory care setting.
4. Articulate the importance of standardized languages, particularly focusing on the Nursing Minimum Data Set (NMDS) nursing elements (diagnosis, intervention, outcome, and intensity).
5. Describe the potential of clinical decision support systems (CDSS) and evidence-based practice (EBP) to manage performance outcomes and enhance clinical care.
6. Understand current issues relating to privacy and confidentiality of medical record information.

Key Points

1. It is essential for ambulatory care nurses to understand nursing informatics and be informed users of information technology.
2. Nurses are surrounded with an overwhelming increase in technological capabilities.
3. Today more than ever, every nurse practicing in ambulatory care settings must be familiar with a range of health care information technology applications.
4. An information system must be capable of providing information to a provider at the point of care to assist in care decision-making about the present encounter, as well as being able to capture data and information that can be aggregated to inform future encounters.
5. Nursing informatics applications are in all areas of nursing: clinical practice, administration, education, and research.
6. Nurses who have information science and computer science expertise combined with their health care expertise are uniquely positioned to assume leadership roles in translating the information needs of patient caregivers to those designing the actual systems to capture patient care data.
7. Because of the power and potential of automated, computer-based documentation, the translation of nursing documentation from the paper record to the electronic record involves more than merely translating what was done on paper to the computer.

Nurses have long demonstrated the ability to accept and incorporate new technology into their professional practice. David Brailer, the National Health Information Technology Coordinator, calls nurses "early adopters" and states that their input is essential to the realization of the nation's health information goals (Taylor, 2005, p. 2). Consequently, it is essential for ambulatory care nurses to understand nursing informatics and be knowledgeable users of information technology. The term nursing informatics came into being during the tech-

nology explosion. Technology, the practical application of science, can be classified as either information-oriented or therapeutic in use. Therapeutic technologies in the ambulatory care setting could include laser and cryosurgery, pharmacotherapeutics, and magnetic resonance imaging (MRI), as well as various electronic monitoring devices and the electronic health record (EHR). Information technologies can be classified as either information-producing or information-managing. Nurses are surrounded with an overwhelming increase in technological capabilities: Web-based information retrieval and storage, telehealth delivery modes for patient education, and clinical decision support systems that automate care processes. Teich and Wrinn (2000) describe information systems of the future in which the review of results, electronic records, referral processing, secure messaging, order entry for prescriptions and tests, and decision support in the form of alerts are possible. The development and use of these systems will likely affect the role elements of the nurse in ambulatory care settings. With many of the coordination of care activities that would normally belong to the registered nurse becoming automated, how will the ambulatory care registered nurse of the 21st century reshape the role? Kerfoot (2000) identifies a technical intelligence quotient as a survival skill for the new millennium. She defines technical intelligence quotient as not merely being aware of how a specific technology works, but as understanding the relationships among the technology, the users, and the affected systems, and how they interact to produce outcomes (Kerfoot, 2000).

This chapter focuses on developing a basic understanding of information technology applications, and the issues associated with using technology to meet patient needs and enhance health care delivery in the ambulatory care setting. Today more than ever, every nurse practicing in ambulatory care settings must be familiar with a range of health care information technology applications. Ambulatory care nurses also need to understand how to best use informatics and technology to improve the quality of patient care and support professional practice. They must also leverage the information available through technology to evaluate potential risks to their patients, patient populations, and practice environment.

Definition of Nursing Informatics and Applications

A. Nursing informatics is defined by the American Nurses Association (ANA) as "A specialty that integrates nursing science, computer science, and information science to manage and communicate data, information, and knowledge in nursing practice" (ANA, 2001, p.46).

B. Conceptual basis for the understanding of information technology (Graves & Corcoran, 1989).
   1. Information is derived from data (basic facts

or observations) that is organized in such a manner as to have meaning to the user.
   2. Knowledge is an evaluation or recognition of something with familiarity that is gained through experience that can put the information to use.

C. Over the past two decades, professional nursing has recognized the importance of informatics in the health care arena.
   1. Automated systems in health care have existed for over 35 years (Saba & McCormick, 2006) and were initially developed to meet the financial need for reimbursement. As early as the 1980s, nurses began to recognize that relevant patient information could be obtained using information technology that would support patient care delivery, nursing service administration, nursing education, and nursing research.
   2. Information systems deal with data that has been structured and named so that they can be counted. What has no name cannot be counted and consequently has no impact. What is named incorrectly or incompletely, when counted, leads to irrelevant information prohibiting practical use or a sensible interpretation.
   3. Information systems that support nursing practice require the incorporation of clinical knowledge/clinical content (see Figure 1). The system must be capable of providing information to a provider at the point of care to assist in care decision-making about the present encounter, and also be able to capture data and information that can be aggregated to inform future encounters.
   4. Nursing informatics applications are in all areas of nursing: clinical practice, administration, education, and research.
      a. Nursing practice activities are supported by computers and include:
         (1) Generation of patient-focused work lists.
         (2) Computer-generated care plans, ideally incorporating evidence-based content at the point of care to support decisions.
         (3) Transmission of orders to ancillary departments.

Figure 7-1.

Role of Knowledge in Care Process and Information Systems

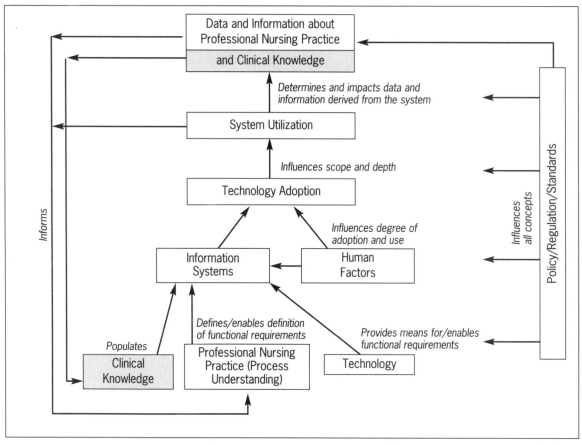

Source: Androwich et al., 2003.

(4) Scheduling procedures.

(5) Retrieving test results.

(6) Charting medications and treatments.

(7) Changes in the plan of care.

(8) Documentation in discharge summaries.

(9) Monitoring of patients through devices.

(10) Providing reminders and alerts.

b. Nursing administration information system applications are designed to meet the following data needs (Simpson & Weaver, 2006):

(1) Allocating resources (staffing and scheduling, patient classification, acuity, inventory, patient billing, budgeting and payroll, nursing intensity, claims processing, and referrals).

(2) Ensuring that practice standards are established and implemented (quality assurance/outcomes management, regulatory reporting, consumer surveys, evidence-based practice).

(3) Evaluating care delivery models (personnel files, risk pooling, costing nursing care, case mix).

(4) Collaborating and planning (forecasting and planning, preventive

maintenance, unit activity reports, utilization review, shift summary reports, census).

   (5) Planning, organizing, implementing, and controlling the care of individuals and aggregates (computer-based patient records, poison control, allergy and drug reactions, incident reports, communication networks, training and education).

  c. Nursing education applications include:
   (1) Computer-assisted instruction.
   (2) Computer-adaptive testing.
   (3) Distance learning.
   (4) Internet resources.
   (5) Computerized tracking of competencies.

  d. Nursing research areas supported by information technology include:
   (1) Computerized literature searches.
   (2) Complex statistical analysis of data.
   (3) Standard languages documentation strategy development.
   (4) Population-based decision support.

5. Nurses who have information science and computer science expertise combined with their health care expertise are uniquely positioned to assume leadership roles in translating the information needs of patient caregivers to those designing the actual systems to capture patient care data.

6. All nurses need to be able to translate the data/information provided by existing systems and to evaluate it to promote improved patient care.

The Computerized Patient Record

The computerized patient record (CPR), or the electronic health record (EHR) as it is now called, is an "electronic patient record that resides in a system specifically designed to support users by providing accessibility to complete and accurate data, alerts, reminders, clinical decision support systems, links to medical knowledge, and other aids" (Institute of Medicine [IOM], 1991, p. 6).

A. Uses of an EHR (adapted from the IOM CPR Report).
   1. Document services provided.

2. Foster continuity of care (serves as a communication tool).
3. Describe diseases and causes (supports diagnostic work).
4. Support decision-making about diagnosis and treatment of patients.
5. Facilitate care in accordance with clinical practice guidelines.
6. Generate reminders (such as preventive or health maintenance action needed).
7. Allocate resources and assess workload.
8. Analyze trends and develop forecasts.

B. Requirements of an EHR (adapted from IOM [1991] CPR Report):
   1. Record content.
      a. Uniform core data elements (refer to the section on *Nursing Minimum Data Set in Ambulatory Care* later in this chapter).
      b. Standardized coding systems and formats.
      c. Common data dictionary.
      d. Information on outcomes of care and functional status.
   2. Record format: Integrated record with all providers, disciplines, and sites of care included.
   3. System performance standards for an EHR.
      a. Rapid retrieval.
      b. 24-hour access.
      c. Easy data input.
      d. Available at convenient places.
   4. Linkages.
      a. With other information systems (such as laboratory, radiology, and pharmacy).
      b. With relevant literature (refer to the section on *Decision Support Systems* later in this chapter for bibliographic database and Web site examples).
      c. With other institutional databases and registries.
      d. Electronic transfer of billing information.
   5. Intelligence.
      a. Decision support (refer to the section on *Decision Support Systems* later in this chapter).
      b. Clinician reminders.
      c. Customizable alert or alarm systems (for example, for allergies and drug interactions).
   6. Reporting capabilities.
      a. Standard clinical reports.

b. Customized reports.
c. Derived documents (such as insurance forms and mandated reports).
d. Trend reports and graphics.
7. Control and access: Safeguards against violations of confidentiality and unauthorized use.
8. Training and implementation.
   a. Minimal training required for system use.
   b. Graduated implementation possible.
C. Because of the power and potential of automated, computer-based documentation, the translation of nursing documentation from the paper record to the electronic record involves more than merely translating what was done on paper to the computer.
D. Nursing Information Data System Evaluation Center (NIDSEC) (ANA, 1997) is a program established in 1995 by the ANA Board of Directors.
1. The mission of NIDSEC is to develop and disseminate standards pertaining to information systems that support the documentation of nursing practice and to evaluate voluntarily submitted information systems against these standards.
2. This mission supports the long-term goal of widespread integration of ANA-recognized languages for nursing into nursing practice, education, administration, and research.
3. NIDSEC Standards (ANA, 1997) focus on four dimensions of nursing data sets and the information systems containing them.
   a. Nomenclature (the actual terms used) – Includes ANA recognized terminologies.
   b. Clinical content – Linkages among terms.
   c. Clinical data repository – How the data are stored and made accessible for retrieval.
   d. General system characteristics – Such as performance and attention to security and confidentiality.
4. These standards are published by American Nurses Publishing and entitled *NIDSEC Standards and Scoring Guidelines* (ANA, 1997) and can be obtained from the American Nurses' Association. NIDSEC standards and scoring guidelines are currently under revision and are planned to be published in 2006.

Evaluation

Evaluating computer technology, particularly software, for use in ambulatory care settings is an important role of the nurse manager or unit leader.
A. A major reason for dissatisfaction with software applications is unmet expectations on the part of the user. This often occurs because the ability to communicate between the domain expert in the problem domain (the nurse in the clinical area) and the domain expert in the solution domain (the programmer) is poor.
B. Questions that should be addressed before purchasing any software include:
1. How much flexibility is in the software? Is it possible to customize?
2. Can the software be modified if situations change?
3. What type of technical support and training are available? How much will they cost?
4. Will this software interface with other existing software, both internal to the organization and external, with contracted service software (such as billing agencies)? What will it take in terms of programming to build interfaces? Is the software compatible with existing hardware?
5. What is the plan for upgrades? How much will they cost?
6. Is the system equipped with adequate back up? Is there adequate security (sign-on codes or passwords)?
7. Is the system user-friendly? This entails screen design, commands, menus, and navigation throughout the program. For example, can screens be skipped for a simple entry, or does the program require a lock-step, screen-by-screen approach? Can the user go back and edit one data element without redoing the entire entry?
8. What industry standards does the software meet? For example, Health Language 7 (HL7) is the accepted standard for messaging in health care.
9. Is the software capable of producing useful reports for analysis of patient care or fiscal data?

Nursing Minimum Data Set in Ambulatory Care

A. The nursing minimum data set (NMDS) includes 16 data elements that must be collected by all nurses, for all patient encounters, across all settings (Werley & Lang, 1988).
  1. Patient elements.
    a. Age.
    b. Gender.
    c. Unique patient identifier: May be medical record number, social security number, or another unique means of patient identification.
    d. Payment mechanism: Insurance coverage or reimbursement information.
    e. Medical diagnosis: Typically coded in ICD9 coding.
    f. Disposition: Refers to discharge status, not as relevant to ambulatory care setting; Useful information for ambulatory care would include living arrangements (for example, lives alone, etc.).
  2. Facility.
    a. Facility identifier: Facility type or provider code.
    b. Dates of care: In ambulatory care, pertains to encounter date.
    c. Unique provider identification: This is new for nursies to have a unique provider number and with automated or computerized documentation is often the sign-on ID.
  3. Nursing care provided.
    a. Nursing diagnosis.
    b. Nursing intervention.
    c. Nursing outcome.
    d. Nursing intensity.
B. Allows for aggregation and comparison of nursing practice across settings.
C. The NMDS data elements have many elements in common with the *Uniform Hospital Discharge Data Set* (UHDDS) and the *Uniform Ambulatory Care Discharge Data Set* (UACDDS) (National Committee on Vital Health and Statistics, 1996).
D. The NMDS is designed so that a comparison of patient-centered data can be made to evaluate the effectiveness of nursing interventions across practice settings, specialties, specialty settings, and geographic boundaries.

E. The UACDDS is similar to UHDDS but is based on a patient encounter, not on an admission.
F. Other data elements are incorporated into the UACDDS (such as living arrangements of the patient, patient's support systems, medications, and patient's ability to manage activities of daily living).

Standardized Languages

"If you cannot name it, you cannot teach it, research it, practice it, finance it, or put it into public policy." – Norma Lang, PhD, RN, FAAN (Lang, 1998).

A. Unified, not necessarily uniform, languages are necessary to document and use the nursing elements in the NMDS (diagnosis, intervention, outcomes, and intensity).
B. To support the use of multiple vocabularies and classification schemes, the ANA formed a committee in 1986 to set criteria for an accepted nursing language and to approve languages meeting the criteria.
C. The ANA Committee on Nursing Practice Information Infrastructure (CNPII), formerly the Steering Committee on Databases to Support Nursing Practice, proposes policy and program initiatives regarding nursing classification schemes, uniform nursing data sets, and the inclusion of nursing data elements in national databases.
D. The committee recommended that the profession work toward the development of a unified nursing language system that would allow linking or mapping of similar terms, retaining the integrity and purpose of each specific scheme/vocabulary. This unified system would facilitate development, analysis, and use of nursing data sets.
E. The committee also developed specific criteria for vocabularies to meet to be eligible for recognition. These criteria include:
  1. Be clinically useful for making diagnostic, intervention, and/or outcome decisions.
  2. Go beyond an application or synthesis/adaptation of vocabularies/classification schemes currently recognized by ANA, or present explicit rationale why it should also be recognized.
  3. Be stated in clear and unambiguous terms, with terms precisely defined.

4. Have been tested for reliability of the vocabulary terms.
5. Have been validated as useful for clinical purposes.

F. As of January 2006, 13 languages have met these criteria and have been approved by the ANA. They include the following (contact information is available from http://www.nursing world.org/nidsec/classlst.htm).

1. North American Nursing Diagnosis Association's (NANDA) nomenclature for nursing diagnosis.
   a. Used by nurses to document nursing diagnoses in all settings where nursing care is delivered.
   b. Classified under 9 patterns of human response to illness and life transitions.
   c. Contains 150 nursing diagnoses with accompanying etiologies, risk factors, and defining characteristics.
   d. NANDA holds copyright.

2. Nursing Interventions Classification (NIC), developed by a team at the University of Iowa led by McCloskey and Bulechek, is a taxonomy for classifying nursing interventions.
   a. Used by nurses in all settings where care is delivered to document nursing interventions.
   b. The 4th edition (2004) contains 514 interventions.
   c. The 3-level taxonomy contains domains, classes, and interventions.
   d. Both direct and indirect care interventions are included.
   e. Mosby publishes and holds copyright.

3. Clinical Care Classification (CCC) (formerly Home Health Care Classification [HHCC]), Saba's Georgetown System for Patient Problems, Interventions, and Outcomes.
   a. Used by health care agencies in providing health care services.
   b. Diagnosis and interventions vocabularies are structured identically, and modifiers are used to evaluate outcomes of conditions.
   c. The diagnoses and interventions are classified according to 21 care components with 182 diagnoses and 198 interventions.

d. The system is not copyrighted.

4. Omaha, the Omaha VNA's system for problems, interventions, and outcomes.
   a. Used by nurses to describe and document care in community settings.
   b. Contains 40 nursing problems (diagnoses) and a number of associated nursing interventions and outcomes (composed of knowledge, behavior, and status subscales).
   c. The system is not copyrighted.

5. Nursing Outcomes Classification (NOC) developed by a team led by Johnson, Maas, and Moorhead at the University of Iowa.
   a. Used by nurses to document patient outcomes sensitive to nursing care.
   b. The 3rd edition (2003) contains 330 outcomes for individual patients, families, and caregivers. Each outcome has a Likert-type scale to measure the degree to which the patient has attained that outcome.
   c. Mosby publishes and holds copyright for this classification.

6. Nursing Management Minimum Data Set (NMMDS) developed by Delaney and Huber.
   a. Used by managers in all nursing care settings.
   b. Contains 17 defined data elements.
      (1) Environment (9 elements – for example, patient population, volume, care delivery model, etc.).
      (2) Nurse resources (4 elements – for example, manager demographic profile, nursing care staff demographic profile, staffing).
      (3) Financial resources (4 elements – for example, payer type, budget expenses, etc.).
   c. NMMDS is copyrighted by Delaney and Huber.

7. Ozbolt's Patient Care Data Set (PCDS).
   a. Used by nurses to document care in all settings but primarily developed for the acute care setting.
   b. Comprised of nursing diagnoses (many are from NANDA and the HHCC), patient care actions, and nursing outcomes.

c. Organized around the 20 care components of the HHCC with two additional
components for the acute care setting.
d. Ozbolt/Vanderbilt University holds copyright.

8. Perioperative Nursing Data Set (PNDS) developed by the Association of Operating Room
Nurses (AORN).
a. Used by perioperative registered nurses
and surgical service managers in a variety of perioperative settings.
b. Contains a set of specific NANDA-
approved diagnoses (N = 68), 127 nursing interventions, and 29 nursing outcomes, all specific to the perioperative
setting.
c. AORN holds the copyright for this data
set.

9. Systematic Nomenclature for Medicine –
Reference Terminology (SNOMED-CT®)
(College of American Pathology).
a. A comprehensive, multiaxial nomenclature classification system.
b. Created for the indexing of the entire
medical and health care vocabulary.

10. Nursing Minimum Data Set (described above).

11. International Classification of Nursing (ICNP®)
(International Council of Nursing [ICN]).
a. A combinatorial terminology for nursing
practice that facilitates cross-mapping of
local terms.
b. Represents nursing phenomena (diagnoses), nursing activities (interventions),
and nursing outcomes that nurses use
across the world in all settings of care.
c. Has been translated into many languages.
d. Version 1 was introduced in 2005.

12. ABC Codes – Describe alternative medicine,
nursing, and other integrative practices, incorporating the best applications from complementary and alternative medicine.
a. ABC codes are 5-character alphabetic
symbols that represent health care products and services.
b. Designed to fill gaps created by other
coding structures.

13. Logical Observation Identifiers Names and
Codes (LOINC®).

a. LOINC codes are universal identifiers for
laboratory and other clinical observations.
b. LOINC codes are designed to be used to
transmit/exchange health care information.

G. Standardized languages can be used for:
1. Outcomes data collection, retrieval, analysis.
2. Decisions about care management.
3. Quality management and improvement.
4. Decision support.
5. Statistical and epidemiologic reporting (vital
statistics, tumor registries).
6. Administration (billing, cost data).

H. In conclusion:
1. Vocabulary is an urgent issue in nursing and
nursing informatics.
2. Vocabulary is central to the integration of
patient care data and research.

Documentation Strategies

A. Health professionals document care for many
reasons:
1. To communicate care provided to all
providers.
2. To provide continuity of care; to ensure a historical, narrative record of an episode or
episodes of care and the patient's responses to treatment.
3. To document care provided or not provided
for legal reasons.
4. To facilitate reimbursement (Turley, 1996).

B. In general, there are two approaches to automated nursing documentation – The established
nursing process approach and the newer interdisciplinary critical pathway/protocols approach.
1. The nursing process approach is based on
the traditional paper forms used by nurses.
This format addresses multiple functions.
a. Documents nursing admission assessment.
b. Documents discharge instructions via
menu lists.
c. Generates a nursing work list with routinely scheduled activities related to care of
each patient.
d. Documents specific data such as vital
signs, weights, and intake and output
measurements.

e. Provides standardized care plans for nurses to be individualized for patients.
f. Documents nursing care in the progress note format.
g. Documents medication administration via medication administration records (MARs).
2. Critical pathway/protocols approach, an approach particularly popular with the rise of managed care, is an interdisciplinary approach to documentation and is based on use of critical pathways or protocols to structure documentation.
a. The provider selects one or more critical pathways for the patient.
b. Standard MD or other order sets are included in pathway and are automatically processed.
c. The system is capable of tracking variances from anticipated care (critical pathway) and is able to aggregate variance information for analysis by the provider.
d. This provides a feedback loop, and the information is used to improve care and client outcomes.

Decision Support Systems (DSS)

Nurse leaders are constantly challenged to keep up with the rapidly growing and constantly changing information base relevant to their practice. Computers can assist in this process by bringing necessary information to the practicing nurse in forms that will leverage the information-seeking and decision-making processes. These systems provide decision support in the form of bringing evidence, expertise, and scarce resources to the provider at the point of care. Nurse leaders must use all available evidence to increase the probability of "doing the right thing." In the future, institutions will be successful in delivering quality care to the extent that they have comparable, reliable, relevant data for cost, utilization, and outcome studies for guideline development, performance management, and identification of best practices (Androwich & Kraft, 2006).
A. An automated decision support system provides an ambulatory nurse with a tool that enhances the nurse's ability to make effective and timely decisions in semi-structured, uncertain situations.

B. Structure of any decision support system includes:
1. Some type of user interface that facilitates or triggers inquiries.
2. A knowledge base (database) containing expert information organized to promote decision-making.
3. Inference engine with analytic models that can generate alternative solutions.
C. An example of how a decision support system might operate in a clinical setting is the scheduling of immunizations.
1. The system would ask you to input the child's age, weight, immunization history, and other pertinent facts.
2. The database would use the information provided to compare with accepted practice standards contained in the knowledge base.
3. Then, the algorithm in the inference engine would be used to provide a recommendation for the next immunization to be scheduled.
D. Characteristics of a decision support system include:
1. Organizes and interprets large amounts of data.
2. Standardizes decision-making criteria.
3. Provides expert level assistance to novice.
4. Allows for capturing (extracting and documenting) knowledge of experts.
E. A goal is to develop an intelligent health care system – A learning organization that promotes a culture of knowledge and empowerment among its members.
F. The computer has virtually unlimited storage and great information processing capability, whereas man has limited storage and memory, but much experience, knowledge, intuition, and judgment. We must build on both the strengths of man and the computer (Weed, 1997).
G. The trend in ambulatory patient care is to organize care around targeted patient populations (such as high-cost or high-volume). Care planning relies upon identification of best practice models from the literature that derives recommendations from large population studies.
H. Population-based decision support is one form of a decision support system. In these situations, data from a number of patients are aggregated and used to provide information to support patient care for individual patients. These sys-

tems are essential for disaster preparedness in that they enable the early detection of trends via syndromic surveillance, as well as providing resource management and decision support in actual disasters (O'Carroll, Yasnoff, Ward, Ripp, & Martin, 2003). The term syndromic surveillance applies to surveillance using health-related data (typically symptom clusters) that precede a given diagnosis and signal a sufficient probability of a number of cases or a potential population outbreak that would warrant further response. Though historically the syndromic surveillance has been used to target the investigation of potential cases, public health officials are increasingly exploring the usefulness of syndromic surveillance methods in detecting outbreaks associated with bioterrorism (Haas & Androwich, 2006).

I. Evidence-based practice is the "integration of the best research evidence with clinical experience and patient values to facilitate clinical decision making" (Sackett, Strauss, Richardson, Rosenberg, & Haynes, 2000). This same principle can be used in planning care for patient populations. Evidence-based nursing sources of evidence include:
1. Computerized literature databases, such as the Cumulative Index of Nursing and Allied Health Literature (CINAHL) (http://www.cinahl.com) and the National Library of Medicine's (NLM) Medline (http://www.nlm.gov).
2. On-line, published, systematic evidence reviews include the Cochrane Collaboration (http://www.cochrane.org/index0.htm), the Agency for Healthcare Quality and Research (AHRQ)(http://www.ahcpr.gov), Zynx Health (http://www.zynx.com) for interdisciplinary plans of care, and CINAHL's Clinical Innovations Database (CCID) (http://www.cinahl.com).

J. The goal of evidence-based practice is to provide rigorous answers for clinical questions (see Chapter 13, *Evidence-Based Practice*).
1. For patients – What is the best care option?
2. For providers – How am I doing? How am I doing compared to others (inside and outside the system)?
3. For the ambulatory care nursing professional – How can I improve?

Telehealth Issues

A. Telehealth can be defined as the use of modem telecommunications and information technology to provide health care to individuals at a distance and to transmit information to provide care.

B. Issues to be addressed in light of the increased use of distance technology for patient education, clinical diagnosis, and therapeutic interventions include:
1. Provider credentialing – With the advent of telephone nursing practice and distance telehealth media, the importance of ensuring competence and accountability, in many cases across state lines or national borders, requires thoughtful consideration.
   a. The National Council of State Boards of Nursing (NCSBN) (2005) adopted a system of mutual recognition via interstate compact that allows a single licensure system for nurses practicing in more than one state (physically or electronically).
   b. The issue of multistate licensure continues to be dynamic and will need creative resolution to protect both the public and members of the health care professions.
   c. By the year 2005, 18 states had adopted the interstate compact with legislation pending in other states.
2. Information quality – Few standards are available for providers and consumers to use to evaluate the quality of information that is offered on the Internet.
3. An ambulatory care nurse can use the AAACN metric to evaluate information for use and should also teach patients to be savvy information consumers.
4. The AAACN metric (Androwich, 1999):
   a. **A**ccuracy – How valid and reliable does this information seem? Is it consistent with "mainstream" knowledge or is it apparent? If no, why not?
   b. **A**uthorship – What is the expertise and credibility of author(s)? Does the author of the information have a commercial interest in the product referenced? If so, is the commercial relationship explicit? With what organization(s) is the author or site associated? Are they credible?

c. **A**ttribution – Is the information referenced? Are the citations reliable, and do they include experts in the area?

d. **C**urrency – How dated is the information? When was the information posted?

e. **N**ursing Practice Relevance – Is this important to my patients? Is it a POEM? (Patient-Oriented Evidence that Matters – matters because it will require practice change.)

5. The overall soundness of a source is evaluated based on the above criteria.

Privacy and Confidentiality/Standards/Accreditation

A. *The Health Insurance Privacy and Portability Act of 1996* (HIPPA) provides safeguards for patient health care data (U.S. Congress, 1996; U.S. Department of Health and Human Services, 2003). At minimum, this means that measures are in place to protect against:

1. Unauthorized access and harm to patient care data (system security).

2. Accidental or intentional disclosure to unauthorized persons or unauthorized data alteration (data security).

3. Transmission of sensitive information to unauthorized recipients (data confidentiality).

4. Assurance of consistency and accuracy of data stored in data-based systems (data integrity).

B. At the Federal level, the National Committee on Vital and Health Statistics (NCVHS) has been charged by Congress with providing recommendations related to the nature, characteristics, quality, and degree of security needed for various types of data elements. All ANA-approved nursing vocabulary developers have testified at NCVHS. NCVHS deals with all issues that pertain to:

1. National health information infrastructure (NHII).

2. Population health data.

3. Data quality.

4. Standards and security.

5. Privacy and confidentiality.

6. Interoperability (the ability to share data and information electronically).

7. Recommendations for personal health records (http://www.ncvhs.hhs.gov/050909lt.htm).

C. Joint Commission on Accreditation of Healthcare Organizations (JCAHO) has standards that relate to information and the use of information in patient care. Some of these involve:

1. Measures that protect information confidentiality, security, and integrity (user access, retrieval of information without compromising security or confidentiality, written policies controlling patient records, and guarding records and information).

2. Uniform definitions and methods for data capture to facilitate data comparison within and among health care organizations.

3. Education on principles of information management and training for system use.

4. Accurate and timely transmission of information (24-hour availability, minimal delay of order implementation, pharmacy system designed to minimize errors, and quick turnaround of test results).

5. Integration of clinical and non-clinical systems.

6. Client-specific data information: System collects and reports individual data and information that can be used to support practice, aid research, and support decision-making.

7. The aggregation of data/information: System generates reports that support care, improve performance, support operations, and research.

8. Knowledge-based information: Literature is available in print or electronic form.

9. Comparative data: System can provide information useful for comparison.

References

American Nurses Association (ANA). (2001). *The scope of practice for nursing informatics.* Washington, DC: American Nurses Publishing.

American Nurses Association (ANA). (1997). *NIDSEC standards and scoring guidelines.* Washington, DC: American Nurses Publishing.

Androwich, I. (1999). Evidence-based practice: Harvesting the evidence. *Chart* (March), 5.

Androwich, I., Bickford, C., Button, P., Hunter, K., Murphy, J., & Sensmeier, J. (2003). *Clinical information systems: A framework for reaching the vision* (p. 53). Washington, DC: American Nurses Publishing.

Androwich, I., & Kraft, M. (2006). Incorporating evidence: Use of computer-based clinical decision support systems for health care professionals. In V. Saba & K. McCormick (Eds.), *Essentials of nursing informatics* (pp. 167-179). New York: McGraw-Hill.

Graves, J., & Corcoran, S. (1989). The study of nursing informatics. *Image, 21*(4), 227-231.

Haas, S., & Androwich, I. (2006). Ambulatory care nursing: Challenges for the 21st century. In P. Cowen & S. Moorhead (Eds.), *Current issues in nursing* (7th ed.). In press.

Institute of Medicine (IOM). (1991). *The computer-based patient record: An essential technology for health care.* Washington, DC: National Academy Press.

Joint Commission on Accreditation of Healthcare Organizations (JCAHO). Retrieved January 22, 2006, from http://www.jointcommission.org/Standards

Kerfoot, K. (2000). TIQ (Technical IQ): A survival skill for the new millennium. *Nursing Economic$, 18*(1), 29- 31.

Lang, N. (1998, March). *Language, classification, and data. A powerbase for clinical practice: If you cannot name it...* Paper presented at the annual meeting of the American Academy of Ambulatory Care Nursing, Atlanta, GA.

National Committee on Vital and Health Statistics (NCVHS). (2005). *Letter report on Personal Health Record (PHR) systems.* Retrieved January 22, 2006, from http://www.ncvhs.hhs.gov/050909lt.htm

National Committee on Vital and Health Statistics (NCVHS). (2005). *NCVHS 2003-2004 report.* Retrieved January 22, 2006, from http://www.ncvhs.hhs.gov/03-04rpt.pdf

National Committee on Vital and Health Statistics (NCVHS). (1996). *Core data elements: Report of the National Committee on Vital and Health Statistics.* Retrieved May 2, 2006, from http://www.ncvhs.hhs.gov/ncvhsr1.htm#Review

National Council of State Boards of Nursing. (2005). *Nurse licensure compact.* Retrieved July 1, 2005, from http://www.ncsbn.org

O'Carroll, P., Yasnoff, W., Ward, M.E., Ripp, L., & Martin, E. (Eds.). (2003). *Public health informatics and information systems.* New York: Springer.

Saba, V., & McCormick, K. (Eds.). (2006). *Essentials of nursing informatics.* New York: McGraw-Hill.

Sackett, D.L., Strauss, S.E., Richardson, W.S., Rosenberg, W.M.C., & Haynes, R.B. (2000). *Evidence-based medicine: How to practice and teach EBM.* London: Churchill Livingston.

Simpson, R., & Weaver, C. (2006). Administrative applications of information technology for nurse managers. In V. Saba & K. McCormick (Eds.), *Essentials of nursing informatics* (pp. 445-456). New York: McGraw-Hill.

Taylor, N. (2005). National health IT coordinator applauds nurses as early adopters. *Nursing Management 36*(10), 2-6.

Teich, J., & Wrinn, M. (2000). Clinical decision support systems come of age. *MD Computing, 17*(1), 43-46.

Turley, J. (1996). Toward a model of nursing informatics. *Journal of Nursing Scholarship, 28*(1), 309-313.

United States Congress. (1996). *Public law 104-191: Health Insurance Portability and Accountability Act of 1996.* Retrieved May 2, 2006, from http://www.aspe.hhs.gov/admnsimp/pl104191.htm

United States Department of Health and Human Services Office of Civil Rights (OCR). (2003). *OCR summary of the HIPAA privacy rule.* Retrieved January 22, 2006, from http://www.hhs.gov/ocr/hipaa/privacy.html

Weed, L. (1997). New connections between medical knowledge and patient care. *BMJ, 315*, 231-235.

Werley, H., & Lang, N. (1988). *Identification of the nursing minimum data set.* New York: Springer.

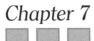
Informatics

This test may be copied for use by others.

COMPLETE THE FOLLOWING:

Name: _____

Address: _____

City: _____ State: _____ Zip: _____

Preferred telephone: (Home)_____ (Work)_____

E-mail_____

AAACN Member Expiration Date: _____

Registration fee: AAACN Member: $12.00
                     Nonmember: $20.00

Answer Form:

1. If you applied what you have learned from this activity into your practice, what would be different?

_____

_____

_____

Evaluation	**Strongly disagree**				**Strongly agree**
2. By completing this activity, I was able to meet the following objectives:					
a. Define the concept of nursing informatics as it applies to ambulatory care nursing.	1	2	3	4	5
b. Understand the benefits and requirements for a computerized patient record (CPR).	1	2	3	4	5
c. Identify criteria for evaluating computer technology for use in the ambulatory care setting.	1	2	3	4	5
d. Articulate the importance of standardized languages, particularly focusing on the Nursing Minimum Data Set (NMDS) nursing elements (diagnosis, intervention, outcome, and intensity).	1	2	3	4	5
e. Describe the potential of clinical decision support systems (CDSS) and evidence-based practice (EBP) to manage performance outcomes and enhance clinical care.	1	2	3	4	5
f. Understand current issues relating to privacy and confidentiality of medical record information.	1	2	3	4	5
3. The content was current and relevant.	1	2	3	4	5
4. The objectives could be achieved using the content provided.	1	2	3	4	5
5. This was an effective method to learn this content.	1	2	3	4	5
6. I am more confident in my abilities since completing this material.	1	2	3	4	5

7. The material was (check one) ___new ___review for me.

8. Time required to read this chapter: _____minutes

I verify that I have completed this activity: _____
                                              Signature

Comments: _____

_____

_____

Objectives

This educational activity is designed for nurses and other health care professionals who practice in ambulatory care. For those wishing to obtain CE credit, an evaluation follows. After studying the information presented in this offering, you will be able to:

1. Define the concept of nursing informatics as it applies to ambulatory care nursing.
2. Understand the benefits and requirements for a computerized patient record (CPR).
3. Identify criteria for evaluating computer technology for use in the ambulatory care setting.
4. Articulate the importance of standardized languages, particularly focusing on the Nursing Minimum Data Set (NMDS) nursing elements (diagnosis, intervention, outcome, and intensity).
5. Describe the potential of clinical decision support systems (CDSS) and evidence-based practice (EBP) to manage performance outcomes and enhance clinical care.
6. Understand current issues relating to privacy and confidentiality of medical record information.

Posttest Instructions

1. To receive continuing education credit for individual study after reading the article, complete the answer/evaluation form to the left.

2. Detach and send the answer/evaluation form along with a check or money order payable to the *American Academy of Ambulatory Care Nursing* (AAACN), East Holly Avenue Box 56, Pitman, NJ 08071–0056.

3. Test returns must be postmarked by August 1, 2011. Upon completion of the answer/evaluation form, a certificate for **1.5** contact hour(s) will be awarded and sent to you. Should the material contained in this chapter become outdated prior to the above expiration date, AAACN reserves the right to withdraw this CE test.

This activity is co-provided by the *American Academy of Ambulatory Care Nursing* (AAACN) and Anthony J. Jannetti, Inc. (AJJ). AJJ is accredited as a provider of continuing nursing education by the American Nurses' Credentialing Center's Commission on Accreditation (ANCC-COA). AAACN is a provider approved by the California Board of Registered Nurses, provider number CEP 05336.

This article was reviewed and formatted for contact hour credit by Sally S. Russell, MN, CMSRN, AAACN Education Director; and Candia Baker Laughlin MS, RN, C, Editor.

Chapter 8

Legal Aspects of Ambulatory Care Nursing

Rachel Nosowsky, JD

Objectives

Study of the information presented in this chapter will enable the learner to:
1. Describe the regulation of nursing practice generally.
2. Identify legal requirements for and liability issues related to telehealth nursing practice.
3. Understand various laws related to patient rights.
4. Understand the purpose of clinical documentation, record retention requirements, and related legal issues.
5. Describe negligence and sources of professional liability.
6. Identify circumstances under which information must be reported to legal authorities or others.
7. Understand the purpose and implications of the fraud and abuse laws.
8. Explain workplace regulatory compliance issues.

Key Points

1. Health care is governed by laws from many sources.
2. Nursing practice is regulated by state "practice acts."
3. Several legal problems may arise in the practice of telehealth nursing.
4. Patients have rights reflected in the Patient Self Determination Act, HIPAA, EMTALA, state regulations for consent and advance directives, and other statutes and case law.
5. Laws require complete and accurate documentation of health care services.
6. Nurses are legally responsible for their own actions, and for reporting incompetent or otherwise inappropriate behavior of other professionals.
7. Nurses are required to comply with workplace regulations, such as those from EEOC and OSHA.

The health care industry is one of the most heavily regulated in the United States today. Every aspect of clinical practice is affected by a complex web of laws, regulations, and judicial (court) and administrative (government agency) decisions. Among other things, these rules and legal precedents define the scope of nursing practice, protect patient rights, impose clinical standards, and regulate billing and reimbursement activities. Violation can hurt patients, and in some cases, result in civil or even criminal liability. Therefore, It is critical to understand what these laws and regulations are and how they affect ambulatory nursing practice.

The purpose of this chapter is to provide nurses with a basic understanding of some of the many legal issues that arise regularly in the practice of nursing and particularly in ambulatory care settings. Because the laws and regulations that affect nursing differ significantly from state to state, and policies designed to facilitate compliance in a local context vary across institutions, it is critical for every ambulatory care nurse to become familiar with the state laws and institutional policies and procedures that may apply to his or her practice.

Understanding the Law

The law, defined broadly, is a group of rules and standards developed by legislatures, administrative agencies, and courts that governs the conduct of individuals and institutions within a community. The practice of health care is governed by federal, state, and in some cases, local laws. Health care providers enter into contracts or adopt institutional policies and procedures that serve as additional standards with which they are expected to comply and against which their conduct or practice is measured.

A. Sources of law.
1. Constitutions (federal, state).
2. Statutes or codes.
   a. Federal laws.
      (1) Usually passed by Congress and signed by the President.
      (2) Compiled into the United States Code.
   b. State laws.
      (1) Usually passed by state legislatures

and signed by governors, or enacted by popular vote through referenda or voter initiatives.

(2) Compiled into various state codes.

(3) Vary from state to state.

3. Regulations.

   a. Rules promulgated by federal agencies (such as the U.S. Department of Health and Human Services [DHHS] or the Securities and Exchange Commission [SEC]) and state agencies (such as state health departments and insurance commissioners).

   b. Supplemented by formal and informal agency guidance.

      (1) Written interpretive guidelines that describe how agencies enforce the law.

      (2) User manuals and program memoranda.

      (3) Congressional testimony by agency representatives.

      (4) Other official communications.

4. Judicial and administrative agency action.

   a. Court decisions and court orders issued as a result of criminal enforcement or civil litigation (rules or standards developed by courts over time are referred to as "common law").

   b. Administrative agency decisions and orders issued in connection with disputes among private parties or arising from agency enforcement of regulations.

5. Contracts.

   a. Legal agreements among two or more parties.

   b. May be enforced by courts, or in some cases, through private arbitration proceedings.

B. Types of law.

1. Criminal law.

   a. Defined by statute; supplemented by regulations; interpreted by judges.

   b. Violation may be punished by fines and/or imprisonment, depending on the seriousness of the offense.

   c. Sources of investigation and enforcement.

      (1) Federal agencies (such as the U.S. Department of Justice, U.S. Food &

Drug Administration).

      (2) State agencies (such as the attorney general, state police).

      (3) Local authorities.

   d. Examples of conduct that may violate criminal laws.

      (1) Practice of nursing without a license.

      (2) Illegal prescription or use of controlled substances; drug diversion.

      (3) Fraud.

      (4) Assisted suicide.

      (5) Failure to report child or elder abuse, or neglect.

2. Civil law.

   a. Defined by statute, regulation, and common law; interpreted by administrative agencies and judges.

   b. Violation can be punished by fines, civil penalties, damages, or other sanctions including suspension or revocation of licensure.

   c. Sources of enforcement.

      (1) Federal agencies (for example, the DHHS).

      (2) State agencies (for example, state health departments or insurance commissioners).

      (3) Private parties (for example, patients harmed by negligent care; employees hurt by discriminatory practices or violation of workplace safety rules).

   d. Examples of conduct that may be the subject of civil disputes.

      (1) Malpractice/professional negligence or misconduct.

      (2) Violation of legal or ethical standards protecting patient rights (some patient rights laws, like HIPAA, may be enforced criminally depending on the circumstances).

      (3) Improper claims or reimbursement.

      (4) Breach of contract.

Regulation of Nursing Practice

The practice of medicine, nursing, and other health professions is defined and regulated at the state level by a combination of laws and regulations usually referred to as "Practice Acts."

A. Practice acts.
   1. Each state enacts and administers its own laws and regulations.
      a. Rules vary from state to state.
      b. The National Council of State Boards of Nursing (2000; 2004) has developed a model law and model regulations governing the practice of nursing.
   2. Usually enforced by oversight boards (for example, "Board of Nursing") created under the acts.
      a. Members are designated in different ways depending on the state (may be chosen by public officials or professional societies, or designated automatically based on office/affiliation).
      b. Responsible for investigating complaints and concerns raised by patients, colleagues, and others, and for disciplining unprofessional, unethical, and incompetent individuals.
      c. Involved at varying levels in health professional recovery programs for nurses and other licensed individuals with mental health or substance abuse problems.
   3. Often supplemented by general requirements in broader "occupational codes" that apply to all health professionals.
B. Purposes and functions of practice acts.
   1. Define practice for nursing and establish scope and standards of practice.
   2. Protect public from unsafe practice/practitioners.
   3. Promote competent practice by qualified professionals; protect title of "nurse" from improper use by unqualified individuals.
   4. Establish education, training, and administrative requirements for licensure.
C. Practice across state lines.
   1. Situations.
      a. Physical practice in multiple locations (for example, in two cities that straddle a state border on opposite sides, or in multiple locations as a traveling nurse).
      b. Telephone or Internet-based triage or case management, in which patients in multiple states may seek health care information and advice.
      c. Telehealth services, through which patients are assessed and even treated remotely using high-tech devices (like computerized stethoscopes, otoscopes, and ophthalmoscopes), as well as equipment that images, digitizes, and transmits radiology studies.
   2. Many states prohibit and even criminalize the practice of nursing without a current local license.
      a. State boards, which have the responsibility for protecting patients who live in their states, generally take the position that the practice of nursing occurs wherever the patient is located at the time of service.
      b. Requirements for licensure vary. In some cases, it may be necessary to hold separate licenses in multiple states. Some states have created alternative processes.
         (1) Some states permit the practice of nursing by "endorsement," which requires that nurses submit their licenses and other information to the local board for approval, a cumbersome and expensive process, particularly for those who practice in many states.
         (2) Some states adhere to a "mutual recognition model," such as the interstate compact.
   3. Interstate compacts.
      a. Enacted in less than half the states.
      b. Features of interstate compacts.
         (1) Allow nurses to practice across state lines, physically or electronically, unless under discipline or a monitoring agreement that restricts interstate practice. Nurses are licensed where they live (the "home state").
         (2) A nurse who practices in states other than the home state (called "remote states") under a compact must comply with the laws and reg-

ulations of each state.

(3) Discipline in a remote state does not necessarily result in discipline in the home state, but information is shared across jurisdictions, and discipline in one state may lead at least to investigation in others.

c. Most states that have adopted the compact have adopted a version that applies only to RNs and LPNs/LVNs. Advanced practice nurses do not need to reapply for an RN license in one of these compact states but may need to complete special applications and fulfill other requirements for advanced practice nursing.

d. As of late 2005, only two states (Iowa and Utah) had agreed to mutually recognize advanced practice nurses, and there was no date set for implementation of the advanced practice nurse compacts.

4. The law is still in flux, and rules are changing constantly; it is important for nurses to check on the rules of any state in which they plan to practice, whether by physical presence or remotely.

D. Delegation of authority.

1. Some states allow licensed practitioners to delegate their authority to perform certain services to other licensed or unlicensed practitioners.

2. Where this occurs, a physician (for example) may delegate clinical tasks not usually within the scope of a nurse's practice to a nurse or other individual who has appropriate education, experience, and expertise.

a. Delegation usually must be recorded in writing.

b. The delegating health professional (the physician, in this example) remains ultimately responsible for the service.

E. Credentialing and peer review.

1. Credentialing.

a. Review and verification of credentials (education, training, licensure, certification, experience) of nurses. In some cases (such as most nursing homes and an increasing number of other health care facilities), this includes performing criminal background checks.

b. Credentialing occurs upon employment, and in most cases, at designated intervals, often on a 2-year cycle.

c. Depending on the institution, credentialing may occur through standard clinical credentialing processes used for medical staff credentialing or through equivalent human resources processes.

2. Peer review.

a. Process of reviewing and assessing the clinical competence and conduct of health professionals on an ongoing basis.

b. An integral part of quality assessment and improvement processes.

c. Should occur regularly and on an ad hoc basis in response to complaints, concerns, and serious adverse events.

3. Confidentiality of credentialing and peer review information.

a. The process of credentialing and peer review is privileged in most states – third parties have no right (or very limited rights) to access it.

b. The federal *Patient Safety and Quality Improvement Act of 2005*, P.L. 109-41, provides additional federal protection for some peer review and quality improvement activities.

c. To protect the peer review privilege, information about the process should always be maintained confidentially and not be voluntarily disclosed to third parties (except the institution's agents and representatives) or to anyone without a need to know.

Telehealth Nursing Practice and Related Liability Issues

Health care is increasingly practiced by telephone, over the Internet, and through other non-traditional media, rather than in person. Health care facilities, managed care organizations, individual physician practices, and other organizations regularly hire nurses to triage incoming calls, dispense general health care advice, and even assist in managing complex conditions, such as heart failure and diabetes.

Figure 8-1.

Safeguards Against Legal Problems Resulting From Telephone Triage

- Use medically approved protocols to establish a standard of care. Do not deviate from the protocols unless changes are in writing and approved by the appropriate medical authority.
- Document the call and advice provided. For example, if a suit is filed 3 years later claiming the nurse did not advise the mother appropriately, the nurse's position is much more defensible if the documentation shows that protocols were followed and appropriate advice was given.
- Provide callers with an option to seek medical attention sooner if they do not agree with the advice or if the condition persists or worsens.
- Develop a mechanism to regularly review documentation and advice for consistency, accuracy, and quality.
- Orient and train staff in telephone triage protocols, policies and procedures, phone encounter techniques, dealing with difficult calls, and documentation.
- Measure outcomes. Conduct regular consumer satisfaction surveys. Followup promptly on problems and quality issues.
- Establish a positive helping relationship at the outset of the call. The average call lasts approximately 6 minutes. The effectiveness of this short encounter is often dependent on skillful communication. The initial contact can often make or break the caller's confidence and satisfaction with the telephone interaction.
- Encourage the caller to briefly describe the problem and its duration, onset, and location; past medical history medications; and allergies. Be sure to obtain the age of the person with the problem.

- Use terminology the caller can understand. Avoid medical jargon as much as possible.
- Listen carefully to the caller and avoid jumping to conclusions. Callers may mask their real concern for fear of embarrassment, particularly regarding sensitive issues such as sexually transmitted infections or mental health problems.
- Try to talk to the person with the problem, directly if possible. Direct communication is usually more reliable and inclusive than secondhand information.
- Thoroughly assess the problem before determining an action plan. The caller may underplay the symptoms and want reassurance that the problem is insignificant.
- Pay attention to the degree of anxiety and concern expressed by the caller. Remember the telephone nurse is at a disadvantage and cannot see or touch the person. If the caller is emphatic that the person is ill even though protocols may recommend home care measures or observation while waiting for an appointment, encourage the caller to seek medical attention sooner. It is better to be overly cautious than to miss a serious condition.
- Always provide the caller with the option to call back or seek medical attention if the condition persists or worsens or new symptoms develop.
- Attend conferences, workshops, and continuing education offerings to establish competency in communication skills, assessment, and telephone triage to reduce the risk of medical-legal problems.

Source: Briggs, 1997. Reprinted with permission from Lippincott, Williams & Wilkins.

A. Licensure concerns.
   1. Practice across state lines (for example, if patients call in from out of state) may be unlawful and may even be criminally prosecuted.
   2. Managing risk.
      a. Review the requirements in each state where services will be performed or patients reside.
      b. It may be necessary to become licensed in more than one state.
B. Professional liability concerns.
   1. Increased difficulty in gathering relevant information and communicating effectively with patients and caregivers.
   2. See Figure 8-1 for examples of methods to reduce legal exposure.
C. General rules for verbal orders (orders given by physicians and executed by nurses).
   1. May be for medication, treatment, intervention, or other patient care.
   2. Should be limited to urgent situations where immediate written or electronic communication is not feasible; should not be used frequently or as common practice for the convenience of physicians.

3. Documentation guidelines for the nurse receiving the verbal order.
   a. Write legibly.
   b. Include date and time.
   c. Include any information relevant to the order, including patient name, relevant history, information documenting the need for and appropriateness of ordered treatment or service, etc.
   d. Include a note that the order was received by phone (for example, "t.o." for "telephone order").
   e. Have the order authenticated in writing or electronically by the ordering physician very shortly after the order is executed, usually no later than the next encounter with the patient or within 48 hours, whichever is sooner.
      (1) If the ordering physician is unavailable, the covering physician may countersign.
      (2) Medicare regulations prohibit a nurse practitioner, physician's assistant, etc. from authenticating a physician's verbal order.
4. Managing risk in the use of verbal orders.
   a. Ask any relevant questions.
   b. Read the content of the order back to the ordering physician before hanging up.
   c. Reduce the order to writing and sign the order.
   d. Ensure that the ordering (or covering) physician has countersigned the order within the prescribed timeframe.

Informed Consent

Informed consent is the process by which a patient is provided relevant information about a proposed procedure, test, or course of treatment; given an opportunity to ask questions; and asked to voluntarily agree. The process of informed consent generally must be documented either on a form designed for that purpose or in the patient's medical record, depending on the nature of the service and the jurisdiction where the service is provided.
A. General rules *(Patient Self Determination Act of 1990).*

1. Competent adult patients are legally entitled to accept or decline recommended medical treatments.
2. Provision of care without consent may be professionally unethical, create professional liability, and in egregious cases, be viewed as civil or criminal battery.
3. Limited exceptions are recognized in most states and include:
   a. Emergency treatment.
   b. Involuntary commitment for psychiatric evaluation and treatment.
   c. Testing of patients for serious communicable diseases after possible transmission (for example, accidental blood exposure).
4. Duty to obtain informed consent.
   a. Rests with the primary provider.
   b. If the provider is a physician, the physician may delegate the task to a nurse with adequate education and experience to communicate the information to the patient or patient's representative and to answer questions he or she may have.
B. Elements of informed consent.
1. Defined by law, regulation, accreditation requirements, and institutional policy.
2. Required elements generally include at least the name of the patient; description of the service to be provided and by whom; identification of risks (including probability, if known), potential benefits, available alternatives (including no treatment), and expected outcomes; time and date; and when consent is written, signature of the patient or parent/legal guardian, and of the person administering the consent.
3. Other information.
   a. Depending on the procedure, there may be special requirements for disclosure, for example:
      (1) HIV/AIDS testing.
      (2) Genetic testing.
      (3) Elective termination of pregnancy.
      (4) Sterilization.
   b. Courts have held that a health professional has a duty to disclose positive HIV/AIDS status to a patient before performing any invasive treatment.

c. Some states have laws requiring disclosure of certain types of conflicts of interest or financial relationships with health care providers to whom a patient may be referred.

C. Form of consent.
1. Requirements vary.
2. When obtained verbally, consent should be documented in the medical record.
3. Written informed consent may be required in some cases, including high-risk procedures, HIV/AIDS testing, and genetic testing.
4. Good documentation of consent, particularly when signed by the patient (or surrogate), may help reduce professional liability exposure.

D. Minors and consent.
1. The age of "majority" (when a person is considered an adult) varies by state and sometimes by circumstances, but often is 18.
2. In general, a minor (a person who has not attained the age of majority) may not consent to their own health care unless:
   a. Legally emancipated (for example, declared independent of parents by court order).
   b. Otherwise recognized to have the capacity to make adult decisions (common examples include adolescents who are married or who are on active duty in the armed forces).
3. Many, but not all, states have adopted by statute or regulation exceptions to facilitate access to sensitive services including:
   a. Pregnancy/prenatal care; birth control.
   b. Mental health.
   c. Substance abuse.
   d. Serious communicable diseases such as HIV/AIDS and other sexually transmitted diseases (STDs).
   e. "Mature minor" rule for these or other types of services.
4. Generally, a parent, person acting in loco parentis (in the place of the parents) or legal guardian must consent to health care services in any other circumstances.

E. Incompetent adults.
1. An adult patient is usually presumed to be competent unless a court decides otherwise.

2. A person may be incompetent if they lack the ability or capacity to understand the information presented to them about their condition, or the consequences of their decisions. This may occur due to acute or chronic conditions, such as:
   a. Mental retardation.
   b. Dementia.
   c. Brain damage.
   d. Stroke.
   e. Unconsciousness.
3. State law determines who can act as a surrogate decision-maker when a patient is found incompetent. In many cases, state law designates the specific order of preference.
4. Examples of surrogate decision-makers include:
   a. Patient advocate/attorney-in-fact (see below under advance directives/power of attorney).
   b. Legal guardian.
   c. Next-of-kin (closest competent adult relative).

F. Advance directives.
1. Most states recognize one or more forms of advance directives, which allow competent adults to make certain kinds of health care decisions in advance of an acute (such as a car accident) or chronic (for example, Alzheimers or cancer) incapacity, thus ensuring that their wishes are respected even if they are unable to communicate them directly.
2. Types of advance directives:
   a. Living will – Written statement describing the kind of care the patient does and does not want; usually is very specific regarding different types of available treatments including ventilator, dialysis, nutrition, and hydration, etc.
   b. Durable power of attorney for health care – Document naming another individual, usually a relative or close friend (sometimes referred to as a "patient advocate"), as the person empowered to make health care decisions on the patient's behalf if/when the patient becomes incompetent.

c. DNR – "Do not resuscitate" order instructing medical personnel to refrain from using heroic measures to save a life after cardiopulmonary failure.

3. Typically must be in writing, voluntarily signed by the patient while competent, and witnessed or notarized.

Privacy and Other Patient Rights

Protection of patient privacy has long been a central ethical obligation of health care practitioners. Today, many laws, accreditation requirements, and professional ethical standards require nurses and other health care providers to take steps to protect patient privacy and other patient rights. Privacy protections addressed in these standards include protecting confidentiality of medical information, notifying patients of provider privacy practices, and ensuring patient access to their health information.

A. Privacy and confidentiality.
1. Federal law establishes a "floor" for privacy protection through the *Health Insurance Portability and Accountability Act of 1996* and implementing privacy and security regulations (together, referred to as HIPAA).
2. HIPAA applies to all health plans, health care clearinghouses, and those health care providers (including nurses) who bill electronically for their services.
3. HIPAA basics.
   a. Patients have a right to control their information.
   b. Patients must "authorize" use or disclosure of their health information except in limited situations.
   c. Exceptions to the authorization requirement include:
      (1) Use of information for patient care (treatment), claims and payment, and core health care operations.
      (2) Mandatory public health disclosures, such as:
         (a) Abuse, neglect, domestic violence.
         (b) HIV/AIDS diagnosis.
         (c) Cancer diagnosis.
         (d) Immunization.
      (3) De-identification of health information

for later use.
      (4) Certain uses and disclosures for research activities.
      (5) Disclosures required by law (for example, in response to a court order or a law enforcement agency demand).
   d. Special protections apply to psychotherapy notes (process notes created by mental health professionals and separated from the regular medical record).
   e. Patients have other rights, including the right to notice of privacy practices, the right to access their records, the right to request special confidentiality protections, the right to amend inaccurate records, and the right to information about some disclosures made without their authorization.
4. State laws also regulate use and disclosure of health information. In addition to general protections that may be more restrictive than HIPAA, many states grant special protection to information about:
   a. STDs or serious communicable diseases, such as HIV/AIDS.
   b. Tests or diseases that may create employment or insurance risks for patients, such as genetics testing or cancer diagnoses.
   c. Mental health or substance abuse diagnosis and treatment.

B. Other patient rights (vary by state and institution):
1. Consideration, respect for individual dignity.
2. Non-discrimination.
3. Adequate, appropriate care.
4. Access to information about their condition, plan of care, chances of recovery, and responsible providers.
5. Adequate and appropriate pain and symptom management.
6. Clear communications in a language and manner understandable to the patient.
7. Refusal of treatment.
8. Involvement in own care and decisions where feasible.
9. Freedom from physical and emotional abuse.
10. Freedom from physical and chemical

restraints except in very limited circumstances authorized by law, accreditation
standards, and institutional policies.
11. Making complaints or grievances.
12. Refusal to participate in experimental treatments or procedures.
13. Receipt of financial information (bill, sources
of financial assistance).
14. Information about rights and responsibilities.

Emergency Medical Treatment and Active Labor Act (EMTALA)

In 1986, Congress passed the *Emergency
Medical Treatment and Active Labor Act* (EMTALA)
to ensure patient access to emergency services
regardless of ability to pay. EMTALA and similar state
laws around the country (also known as "anti-dump-
ing" statutes) help ensure timely public access to
emergency treatment and safe delivery of newborns.
A. Application.
   1. Law applies to hospitals with emergency
      departments. Medicare participating hospi-
      tals without dedicated emergency depart-
      ments have more limited requirements.
   2. Law protects all patients, regardless of
      Medicare status, insurance coverage, or ability
      to pay, who:
      a. Come to emergency departments
         requesting emergency exams or treat-
         ment, or
      b. Appear for unscheduled visits to ambula-
         tory units (such as psychiatry or labor
         and delivery) of the hospital that regularly
         provide emergency care.
   3. Law includes protections for providers who
      refuse to authorize a transfer of an unstable
      patient and for hospital employees who
      report violations.
B. An emergency medical condition covered by
   EMTALA is a medical condition manifesting itself
   by acute symptoms of sufficient severity (including severe pain) such that the absence of immediate medical attention could be reasonably
   expected to result in:
   1. Placing the health of the patient (or in the case
      of a pregnant woman, the health of the woman
      or her unborn child) in serious jeopardy.
   2. Serious impairment to bodily functions.

3. Serious dysfunction of any bodily organ or
   part.
4. Active labor is considered an emergency
   medical condition. Any woman who presents
   with contractions is considered to be in
   potentially active labor and must be given an
   appropriate medical screening exam.
C. Requirements when a patient presents to the
   emergency department.
   1. Hospital must provide an appropriate med-
      ical screening exam (MSE) and relevant ancil-
      lary services to determine whether an emer-
      gency medical condition exists.
   2. If the hospital determines the individual has
      an emergency medical condition, the hospi-
      tal must do one of the following:
      a. Provide further examination and stabiliz-
         ing treatment as necessary to stabilize
         the condition.
      b. If reasonably unable to do so (such as
         lack of expertise), arrange for the transfer
         of the patient to an appropriate facility.
   3. Hospital may not delay MSE or stabilizing
      treatment to inquire about insurance or pay-
      ment status.
   4. Transfer rules.
      a. Transferring hospital must provide the
         necessary medical treatment within its
         means to minimize the risk to the health
         of the patient.
      b. Transferring hospital must provide the
         patient's relevant medical records to the
         receiving hospital.
      c. Transfer must be performed by compe-
         tent staff and with appropriate medical
         supplies.
      d. Hospital may not transfer an unstable
         patient unless:
         (1) Patient requests the transfer in writ-
             ing after being informed of the hos-
             pital's obligations and risks of the
             transfer.
         (2) Physician or other qualified medical
             personnel certifies that the benefits
             of care to be received at the receiv-
             ing facility outweigh the risk to the
             patient of undergoing transfer.
      e. The receiving hospital must accept the
         patient if it has specialized capabilities

or facilities necessary to treat the patient and sufficient capacity to do so.

5. The patient may refuse to accept treatment or transfer, but the hospital must attempt to document such refusal.

D. EMTALA imposes numerous additional administrative requirements impacting institutional policies and procedures, and imposes stiff penalties for non-compliance.

E. Advanced practice nurses and EMTALA.
   1. EMTALA generally recognizes the role of "Qualified Medical Professionals" (QMPs) (including advanced practice nurses) in delivering health care.
   2. Current regulations and interpretive guidance generally allow a QMP (for example, a nurse midwife) to conduct a medical screening examination.
   3. For a woman having contractions, a physician rather than the QMP must certify false labor to determine that no medical emergency exists (for example, that the patient is not in active labor).

Abandonment

A practitioner-patient relationship is established when a patient seeks health care services and the practitioner agrees to provide them. There are limitations on a practitioner's ability to refuse to provide services. In emergency situations, for example, the practitioner's agreement may not be necessary. Moreover, a practitioner generally may not discriminate against patients based on statutorily or contractually protected classifications (such as sex, race, religion, national origin, or insurance status).

A patient may terminate his or her relationship with a provider (including an advanced practice nurse) at any time. The provider, however, has legal and ethical obligations to facilitate continuity of care and avoid harm caused by prematurely terminating a relationship.

A. Provider's responsibilities when a patient terminates.
   1. If further treatment is needed, inform the patient of the risks of termination of care.
   2. Refer the patient to an alternative provider, if requested.
   3. Provide copies of patient records to the new

provider to facilitate continuity of care.
   4. Document the fact that the patient requested termination of the relationship, preferably on a form signed by the patient, or if not feasible, then in a written verification letter sent to the patient.
   5. If a patient is instructed to followup but fails to show up for appointments or call, reasonable attempts should be made to contact the patient and provide the information listed above.

B. Circumstances under which a provider may terminate.
   1. Provider becomes unavailable to provide further treatment due to relocation, illness, injury, or disability.
   2. Patient is disruptive or refuses to cooperate with treatment plans.
      a. Termination is not automatic.
      b. To avoid an abandonment claim, attempt a behavioral contract and document instances of noncompliance before terminating the relationship.
   3. Reasons for establishing the relationship have been resolved.
      a. Example: A pregnant patient delivers. After post-partum checkup, the provider has no obligation to provide ongoing gynecological services nor to provide maternity care for a subsequent pregnancy.
      b. Instructions should be provided to the patient for any additional necessary followup care.
   4. The provider has inadequate credentials or scope of practice to address patient's needs.
      a. Example: A primary care nurse practitioner is unable to provide a needed surgical intervention.
   5. The patient is unwilling or unable to pay for further treatment (except when EMTALA applies – see above).

C. The provider's responsibilities when terminating the relationship are to minimize liability.
   1. Notify the patient in writing by certified mail/return receipt requested.
   2. Give the reason(s) for the withdrawal of care.
   3. Identify a qualified substitute or an organiza-

tion where qualified substitutes may be found. If the relationship is being terminated because specialized care is required, refer the patient to a provider of the specialized service.

4. Provide the patient with sufficient time to find an alternative provider.
5. Offer to be available to the patient for a specified period (typically no less than 30 days) to avoid a gap in services before a relationship is established with the alternative provider.
6. Inform the patient that treatment will be provided in an emergency until a new provider is found.
7. Offer to transfer medical records.

D. Interruptions in service.
1. The provider may be temporarily unavailable due to vacation, meetings, or illness.
   a. Replacement should be arranged, if feasible.
   b. The patient should be informed of alternatives.
2. Two patients may require care at the same time.
   a. The provider must prioritize each patient's needs.
   b. One patient must not be abandoned entirely to attend to another.

E. Home health care settings.
1. Home nursing services may be discontinued when:
   a. Source of payment no longer exists.
   b. Environment is unsafe for the ambulatory care nurse.
   c. The physician orders to terminate care if no longer medically necessary.
2. If home health services are discontinued, documentation generally should include:
   a. Notice to the patient and physician.
   b. Alternative measures taken to prevent endangerment to the patient, such as identification of alternative and accessible community resources.

F. Penalties for abandonment.
1. Malpractice liability (or in some states, potentially other theories of liability, such as breach of contract).
2. Licensing sanctions.

Legal Aspects of Clinical Documentation

Complete and accurate documentation of health care services is required by federal and state law, accreditation requirements, professional standards, and industry practice. The quality of documentation may affect the outcome of a professional liability case. Nurses, like other health care practitioners, may be held liable for inappropriate treatment as a result of inadequate documentation.

A. The value of accurate and complete documentation.
1. The medical record provides legal proof of the type and quality of nursing care provided to patients.
2. The medical record can be used by attorneys to help analyze the merits of a malpractice claim and as a defense to claims of negligence or intentional misconduct.
3. The medical record is often necessary to support third-party reimbursement.

B. Elements of good documentation (applicable laws, accreditation, and licensing standards may require more or different elements depending on the circumstances).
1. Patient's symptoms, using patient's words in "quotation marks" where appropriate.
2. Objective observations.
3. Identification and analysis of any patient problems.
4. Nursing actions taken (for example, treatment plan, procedures performed, drugs prescribed or dispensed).
5. Patient's response.
6. Signature and date.

C. Characteristics of good documentation:
1. Factual.
2. Objective – Void of personal opinions or observations unrelated to the care of the patient.
3. Accurate.
4. Consistent.
5. Timely.
6. Complete – In a large organization, records generally should not be maintained in decentralized shadow files accessible only by the nurse or team within that unit.

D. Guidelines for creation and maintenance of records:
1. Always use ink, never erasable media.
2. Never erase or delete an entry unless required by law.

a. If an error occurs, draw a line through the error and write "error" above it with your initials.
b. For electronic documents, do not destroy the only electronic record. If it is inaccurate, flag it, archive it, or find some other way to notify the user that it is not to be relied upon.
3. Always use the appropriate form.
4. In a paper record, document on each line without leaving spaces between entries.
   a. Document an omission as a new entry.
   b. Avoid adding to a previously written entry.
5. Use standard abbreviations and avoid abbreviations prohibited by law, accreditation standards, or institutional policy.

E. Electronic documents and records.
1. Congress, federal agencies, and many states have adopted laws and issued regulations permitting health care providers to create and maintain documents solely in electronic form.
2. Examples.
   a. *Electronic Signatures in Global and National Commerce Act* ("eSIGN") – A federal law.
   b. *Uniform Electronic Transactions Act* ("UETA") – A model law adopted by many states.
   c. Food and Drug Administration, 21 C.F.R. part 11 (regulations on use of electronic signatures and records).
3. Laws have specific requirements regarding security of record-keeping systems and authentication of users and user signatures.
4. Minimal security measures should always be in force, including:
   a. Avoid maintaining medical records on personal computers or devices that may be susceptible to tampering, intrusion, or theft.
   b. Back up files regularly.
   c. Maintain up-to-date anti-virus and anti-spyware applications on the computer you use.
   d. Never share a user identification code, password, or other access code with anyone.

e. Report any equipment theft, potential intrusion, or improper password use promptly to institutional officials, or if you are unaffiliated with an institution, to local law enforcement personnel.

F. Document retention and destruction.
1. All types of legal rules and precedents govern the retention and destruction of medical and administrative records of health care providers and institutions including;
   a. Privacy laws.
   b. Tax laws.
   c. Food and drug laws (including laws regulating clinical research).
   d. Rules of evidence.
   e. Court or administrative decisions.
2. Rule of thumb for health care records.
   a. Retain for at least 6 years.
   b. Many laws, regulations, institutional policies, and contract requirements demand even longer periods, especially related to the care of children.
   c. Minors' health care records should be retained at least 6 years or until age 21, whichever is longer. Records for a minor who never becomes competent (for example, due to mental status) may need to be retained for life.
3. Contracts may call for return or destruction of records, but laws, regulations, and institutional policies may demand otherwise.
4. Institutional policies may require destruction of records after a certain amount of time has elapsed to address storage capacity, security, and other problems.
5. Never destroy documents when on notice of a claim or lawsuit to which the documents are relevant.
   a. The court may draw a negative inference against the former holder of the record and assume that the documents would have been supportive of the other party's case.
   b. Depending on how egregious inappropriate destruction may be, the court may hold the person who destroyed the records in contempt and may assess significant penalties.

Professional Liability/Malpractice

Nurses are responsible and may be held personally liable for their own actions, and in many circumstances, have a legal and ethical obligation to report incompetent nursing practice.

A. Professional negligence defined (four elements).
1. A duty of care is owed to the patient.
   a. Requires that the nurse had established a relationship with the patient. Depending on the circumstances, relationships may be established inadvertently (for example, when a stranger seeks health care advice during a social gathering).
   b. Duty is defined by reference to what a reasonably prudent ambulatory care nurse would have done under similar circumstances.
2. The nurse breached that duty.
   a. His or her actions deviated from the standard of care.
   b. Examples of breach of a duty of care:
      (1) Failure to use sterile technique during a dressing change.
      (2) Failure to follow an established medical protocol.
      (3) Practice beyond scope of the individual's education and experience (even if within the scope of Practice Act).
      (4) Failure to disclose, such as failure to report an adverse reaction to the administration of a drug or failure to report an error.
3. The patient suffered damages.
   a. Physical injury.
   b. Psychological injury.
   c. Financial loss.
4. The nurse's breach of duty of care "proximately" caused the patient's damages.
   a. There is a reasonably direct relationship between the nurse's action or inaction and the patient's injury.
   b. "But for" the nurse's action or inaction, the patient would not have been harmed.
B. Sources of claims and litigation.
1. Poor or unexpectedly adverse outcomes.
2. Most do not result in litigation.

a. According to at least one older study conducted by the Secretary's Commission on Medical Malpractice (Health, Education and Welfare), more than half of claims were based on minor or emotional issues, not major adverse events such as death or disability (Atchinson et al., 2001).
b. Relationship between provider and patient is often more important than actual outcome of treatment (Hickson, Clayton, Githens, & Sloan, 1992; Hickson et al., 1994)
3. Some reasons that patients file lawsuits include:
   a. Significant injury requiring future medical and other costs.
   b. Need for answers.
   c. Perceived· rude or unsympathetic providers.
   d. Poor communications resulting in unreasonable expectations on the part of the patient.
4. Specific issues include:
   a. Inadequate or inappropriate assessment.
   b. Inadequate informed consent process and documentation (such as failure to fully disclose risks and alternatives to proposed treatment).
   c. Failure to observe and communicate changes in patient's condition.
   d. Failure to question potentially inappropriate orders.
   e. Medication administration errors.
   f. Inadequate or incomplete documentation of services provided.
   g. Non-compliance with standard of care.
   h. Ethical violations, including violation of patient·privacy.

Reporting Mandates

Federal and state laws and institutional policies require nurses and others to report incompetent, unethical, unprofessional, and other inappropriate behavior, as well as disciplinary actions undertaken to address such conduct and successful malpractice claims.

A. Federally required reporting.
   1. Adverse professional review actions and professional liability payments.
      a. Reportable events include:
         (1) Suspension or revocation of licensure.
         (2) Limitation, restriction, suspension, or revocation of clinical credentials through credentialing or peer review activities related to professional competence or conduct, including incompetent clinical care or unethical conduct.
         (3) Malpractice payments.
      b. Mandatory reporting for physicians.
      c. Permissive reporting for nurses.
   2. Health care fraud.
B. State law-required reporting.
   1. Reporting requirements generally apply both to licensed facilities employing health care practitioners and to licensed practitioners themselves.
   2. Reportable events related directly to health care professionals may include:
      a. Adverse professional review actions, and in some cases, professional liability payments.
         (1) Usually mandatory for all licensed practitioners.
         (2) Reports may trigger licensing board investigations.
      b. Incompetent practice or practice outside the scope of a license.
      c. Substance abuse and controlled substance violations.
      d. Mental impairment.
      e. Privacy breaches and other unethical conduct.
      f. Fee-splitting, kickbacks, and other potentially abusive activities.
      g. Criminal convictions.
   3. Failure to report a reportable event may, in and of itself, trigger adverse licensure action.
C. Public health reporting.
   1. Federal and state law includes mandates for reporting information that may impact the public health.

   2. Examples of required public health reporting.
      a. Serious communicable diseases.
      b. Cancer diagnoses.
      c. Abuse, neglect, or domestic violence.
      d. Gunshot wounds or other evidence of violent criminal activity.
      e. Defective devices.

Fraud and Abuse

Many federal and state laws have been enacted to protect the government and taxpayers from unscrupulous contractors and patients from incentives to provide unnecessary and sometimes dangerous health care services (or to fail to provide necessary services). A few of these laws are summarized below.

A. False Claims Acts.
   1. Federal law originally enacted in the 1800s to combat defense procurement abuses in the Civil War era.
   2. Prohibits any entity from making a "false claim" to a government entity to induce undeserved payment. Applies even if the government suffers no actual damages.
   3. Private citizens may sue on behalf of the government, even if the government does not want to pursue the case.
   4. Law includes whistleblower protection provisions designed to encourage reporting of abusive organizations and individuals.
B. Prohibitions on kickbacks and referrals.
   1. Laws and regulations prohibit the solicitation, receipt, or offer of a payment of a kickback, bribe, or other type of payment, whether cash or in kind, in return for referring a patient for an item or service for which payment may be made under a federal health care program (Medicare, TRICARE, etc.).
   2. Federal anti-self referral law ("Stark") applies only to referrals made by physicians to certain designated health care services in which they or their immediate family members have a financial interest.
   3. Many states have adopted equivalent schemes to offer additional protection to Medicaid programs.

4. Kickbacks or referrals may sometimes result in false claims.
C. If one has financial relationships with referral sources or is a source of referrals to another health care provider, he or she should check with legal counsel to make sure those relationships comply with the fraud and abuse laws.
D. Other offenses.
   1. Government has many other ways to prosecute misconduct.
   2. Examples include health care fraud, mail fraud, wire fraud, and false statements.

Workplace Issues (EEOC, OSHA)

Nurses and nurse managers are required to comply with regulations providing for equal opportunity and safety in the workplace. The Equal Employment Opportunity Commission (EEOC) is a federal agency that issues and enforces regulations concerning workplace discrimination. The Occupational Safety and Health Administration (OSHA) is responsible for enforcing laws and regulations on workplace safety.
A. EEOC.
   1. Responsible for enforcement of various anti-discrimination laws:
      a. *Civil Rights Act,* prohibiting employment discrimination based on race, color, religion, sex, or national origin.
      b. *Equal Pay Act,* requiring equal pay for men and women doing substantially similar jobs.
      c. *Age Discrimination in Employment Act,* prohibiting discrimination based on age of employees who are 40 years of age or older.
      d. *Americans With Disabilities Act,* prohibiting discrimination based on disability if the prospective employee or employee can perform the work with "reasonable accommodation."
   2. Establishes rules for receiving and acting on complaints, including:
      a. Jurisdiction.
         (1) Except for *Equal Pay Act* violations, most violations of anti-discrimination laws must be filed with EEOC before going to court.
         (2) Failure to file with EEOC may result in loss of legal rights.
      b. Time limits.
         (1) General rule: Complaints must be filed within 180 days of an alleged violation.
         (2) Time limit may be extended to 300 days if the discrimination is covered by state or local anti-discrimination laws.
      c. Process.
         (1) EEOC investigates the complaint to determine whether the facts seem to support a violation of the law. Followup may occur when the case is not clear-cut.
         (2) EEOC may act as a mediator if charging party and employer both agree.
         (3) If mediation is not pursued or is unsuccessful, EEOC may dismiss the charge.
            (a) EEOC may file a lawsuit on behalf of the employee.
            (b) EEOC may issue a "right to sue" letter that allows the employee to file a lawsuit within 90 days.
   3. Remedies to discrimination, after a finding of discrimination by a court, may include:
      a. Accommodation of the employee, as needed.
      b. Hiring, promotion, or reinstatement.
      c. Payment of money damages including back pay or front pay necessary to make the victim "whole" (place the victim in the position he or she would have had if not for the discrimination).
      d. Payment of attorneys' fees, expert witness fees, court costs.
      e. Payment of punitive damages if the employer acted with malice or reckless indifference (not available against employers that are federal, state, or local governments).
      f. Other corrective action.
B. OSHA – Branch of U.S. Department of Labor.
   1. Responsible for enforcement of workplace safety laws (*Occupational Safety and Health Act),* and development and enforcement of related regulations.

a. Federal, state, and local government employers are exempt, though many states and local governments have adopted similar laws and created similar agencies.

b. Accreditation organizations also have adopted workplace safety standards with which accredited organizations must comply.

2. Establishes rules for safety standards and for receiving and investigating complaints.

3. Health care applications.

a. Universal precautions to protect health care workers from exposure to blood and body fluid-borne pathogens, such as:
(1) Hepatitis B virus (HBV).
(2) HIV/AIDS.

b. Radiation safety.

c. Drug and chemical safety.

d. Individual workplace safety issues (physical exposures due to ergonomics issues, lifting, etc.).

e. Facility guidelines (fire safety, personal security).

4. Violations.

a. Violations may be identified by complaints, incidents, or whistleblowers.

b. Citations or penalties will vary depending on the seriousness of the offense.

c. Violation citations must be posted at the worksite.

d. Employers may contest citations.

References

Atchison, D., Dabelstein, L., et al. (2001). *Nursing-legal survival: A risk management guide for nursing*. Oak Brook, IL: University HealthSystem Consortium.

Briggs, J.K. (1997). *Telephone triage protocols for nurses*. Philadelphia: Lippincott, Williams, & Wilkins.

Hickson, G.B., Clayton, E.W., Githens, P.B., & Sloan, F.A. (1992): Factors that prompted families to file medical malpractice claims following perinatal injuries. *Journal of the American Medical Association, 267*(10), 1359-1363.

Hickson, G.B., Clayton, E.W., Entman, S.S., Miller, C.S., Githens, P.B., Whetten-Goldstein, K., et al. (1994). Obstetricians' prior malpractice experience and patients' satisfaction with care. *Journal of the American Medical Association, 272*(20), 1583-1587.

National Council of State Boards of Nursing. (2000). *Nurse licensure compact information*. Retrieved February 6, 2006, from http://www.ncsbn.org/nlc/index.asp

National Council of State Boards of Nursing. (2004). *Model nursing act and rules*. Retrieved February 6, 2006, from http://www.ncsbn.org/regulation/nursingpractice_nursing_practice_model_act_and_rules.asp

Additional Readings

Brantley, D., Laney-Cummings, K., & Spivack, R. (2004). *Innovation, demand and investment in telehealth*. Washington, DC: U.S. Dept. of Commerce, Office of Technology Policy.

Center for Telemedicine Law. (2003). *Telemedicine licensure report*. Washington, DC: Department of Health and Human Services.

Guido, G.W. (2005). *Legal and ethical issues in nursing*. Upper Saddle River, NJ: Prentice Hall.

Hutcherson, C.M. (2001). Legal considerations for nurses practicing in a telehealth setting. *Online Journal of Issues in Nursing, 6*(3), 4.

Legislative Coalition of Virginia Nurses. (1998). *Multi-state nurse license recognition*. Retrieved February 6, 2006, from http://www.virginianurses.com/coalition/Multi_StateLic.htm

Reid, A.J. (2001). *Law all nurses should know*. Retrieved February 6, 2006, from http://www.continuingeducation.com/nursing/lawstoknow/index.html

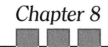
Legal Aspects of Ambulatory Care Nursing

This test may be copied for use by others.

COMPLETE THE FOLLOWING:

Name: _____

Address: _____

City: _____ State: _____ Zip: _____

Preferred telephone: (Home)_____ (Work)_____

E-mail_____

AAACN Member Expiration Date: _____

Registration fee: AAACN Member: $12.00
                   Nonmember: $20.00

Answer Form:

1. If you applied what you have learned from this activity into your practice, what would be different?

   _____

   _____

   _____

Evaluation	Strongly disagree				Strongly agree
2. By completing this activity, I was able to meet the following objectives:					
a. Describe the regulation of nursing practice generally.	1	2	3	4	5
b. Identify legal requirements for and liability issues related to telehealth nursing practice.	1	2	3	4	5
c. Understand various laws related to patient rights.	1	2	3	4	5
d. Understand the purpose of clinical documentation, record retention requirements, and related legal issues.	1	2	3	4	5
e. Describe negligence and sources of professional liability.	1	2	3	4	5
f. Identify circumstances under which information must be reported to legal authorities or others.	1	2	3	4	5
g. Understand the purpose and implications of the fraud and abuse laws.	1	2	3	4	5
h. Explain workplace regulatory compliance issues.	1	2	3	4	5
3. The content was current and relevant.	1	2	3	4	5
4. The objectives could be achieved using the content provided.	1	2	3	4	5
5. This was an effective method to learn this content.	1	2	3	4	5
6. I am more confident in my abilities since completing this material.	1	2	3	4	5

7. The material was (check one) ___new ___review for me.
8. Time required to read this chapter: _____minutes

I verify that I have completed this activity: _____
                                              Signature

Comments: _____

_____

_____

Objectives

This educational activity is designed for nurses and other health care professionals who practice in ambulatory care. For those wishing to obtain CE credit, an evaluation follows. After studying the information presented in this offering, you will be able to:

1. Describe the regulation of nursing practice generally.
2. Identify legal requirements for and liability issues related to telehealth nursing practice.
3. Understand various laws related to patient rights.
4. Understand the purpose of clinical documentation, record retention requirements, and related legal issues.
5. Describe negligence and sources of professional liability.
6. Identify circumstances under which information must be reported to legal authorities or others.
7. Understand the purpose and implications of the fraud and abuse laws.
8. Explain workplace regulatory compliance issues.

Posttest Instructions

1. To receive continuing education credit for individual study after reading the article, complete the answer/evaluation form to the left.

2. Detach and send the answer/evaluation form along with a check or money order payable to the *American Academy of Ambulatory Care Nursing (AAACN)*, East Holly Avenue Box 56, Pitman, NJ 08071–0056.

3. Test returns must be postmarked by August 1, 2011. Upon completion of the answer/evaluation form, a certificate for **1.6** contact hour(s) will be awarded and sent to you. Should the material contained in this chapter become outdated prior to the above expiration date, AAACN reserves the right to withdraw this CE test.

This activity is co-provided by the *American Academy of Ambulatory Care Nursing (AAACN)* and Anthony J. Jannetti, Inc. (AJJ). AJJ is accredited as a provider of continuing nursing education by the American Nurses' Credentialing Center's Commission on Accreditation (ANCC-COA). AAACN is a provider approved by the California Board of Registered Nurses, provider number CEP 05336.

This article was reviewed and formatted for contact hour credit by Sally S. Russell, MN, CMSRN, AAACN Education Director; and Candia Baker Laughlin MS, RN, C, Editor.

Chapter 9

Patient Advocacy

E. Mary Johnson, BSN, RN, CNA

Objectives	Key Points
Study of the information presented in this chapter will enable the learner to:	1. Ethical and advocacy principles are connected through a framework of agreed concepts and actions taken on the part of an individual, an institution, and/or professional organizations.
1. Describe the context of ethical concepts and advocacy behavior in nursing practice.	2. Today's health care system presents challenges on many fronts that require advocacy for patient/family.
2. Discuss the importance of nursing leadership to advocacy, patient relations, and risk management.	3. The advocacy for patients/families is best done when linked to education about both health/disease management and the health care system itself.
3. Describe specific applications of advocacy behaviors in ambulatory nursing practice, including individual, organizational, and community initiatives.	4. There are future advocacy opportunities for nurses in ambulatory care.

The absence of health (illness) often initiates people into the use of health care systems. Many, if not most, individuals have a limited view and understanding of how today's health care industry works, but they hold high expectations for its abilities and promise. This knowledge deficit can become apparent when illness and its unknown outcomes create a sense of vulnerability for individuals. The relationship between the patient and the health care team has always been described as fiduciary, meaning a relationship built on a public confidence involving trust. This trust is translated by patients and the public to mean that the health care team will act in the best interest of the patient. It is within this trust and commitment as a profession that nursing frames decision-making and advocacy behaviors in response to the needs of patients and families. Further, when expectations or needs are not met, nurses are also committed to assuring patient safety and comfort, and to working to mitigate damage and prevent further problems. This issue goes beyond individual actions and incorporates supporting institutional programs of managing risks that exist in health care settings. The nurse advocates for patients, individually and collectively, through analyzing risks both retrospectively and prospectively, and in applying principles of Improving Organizational Performance (IOP).

Perhaps never in the history of the modern day health care system has the emphasis been greater than now for nurses to recognize and act as patient advocates. Identifying when and how, exploring who and what can be done as implementers of health care, may be the most critical skill nurses offer to patients.

Ethical and advocacy principles are connected through a framework of agreed concepts and actions taken on the part of an individual, an institution, and/or professional organizations. The mission of the American Academy of Ambulatory Care Nursing (AAACN) is to advance and influence the art and science of ambulatory care nursing practice (AAACN, 2004). Within the *Ambulatory Care Nursing Administration and Practice Standards* is the conceptual framework of ambulatory nursing practice (AAACN, 2004). This includes specific reference to role knowledge and skill dimension of advocacy for all patient populations. Philosophically and organizationally, these public documents are congruent with nursing's commitment as a profession. An accepted principle of biomedical ethics includes the concept that professions must possess the knowledge, skill, and diligence to uphold the moral and legal standards of due care. Understanding how the nursing profession performs this role through ethical decision-making and advocacy behaviors is fundamental to the nursing practice in ambulatory care (Johnson, 2000).

A. Historical context of patient advocacy – According to Virginia Henderson (1961), the clinical definition of nursing is "to assist the individual, sick or well, in the performance of those activities contributing to health or its recovery (or to a peaceful death) that he would perform unaided if he had the necessary strength, will, or knowledge, and to do this in such a way as to help him gain independence as rapidly as possible" (p. 42).

1. The nursing profession is:
   a. An essential part of society.
   b. Dynamic and reflects the changing nature of societal need.
   c. "Owned by society" in the sense that a "profession acquires recognition, relevance, and even meaning in terms of its relationship to that society, its culture and institutions, and its other members" (American Nurses Association [ANA], 2003).

2. Authority for the practice of nursing.
   a. Based on a social contract that acknowledges professional rights and responsibilities, as well as mechanisms for public accountability (ANA, 2003).
   b. Based on specific state nurse practice acts.
   c. Based on accepted standards of practice.
   d. Based on applicable federal, state and regulatory rules.

3. People seek the services of nurses to:
   a. Obtain information and treatment in matters of health and illness.
   b. Resolve problems or manage health-promoting behaviors.
   c. Identify both short and long-term health goals.
   d. Act as advocates for people dealing with barriers encountered in obtaining health care (ANA, 2001).

4. Performance of the advocacy role in ambulatory setting through:
   a. Providing patient education.

   b. Providing access to care.
   c. Providing ongoing assessment of patient.
   d. Providing continuity of care.
   e. Providing informed decision-making.
   f. Providing mechanisms to measure patient satisfaction.
   g. Reporting patient complaints, errors in care, and near-misses.
   h. Participating in risk management programs and initiatives.

5. *Nursing Administration and Practice Standard* – Ethics and Patients Rights (VI) (AAACN, 2004) states that nursing staff members will:
   a. Support a process of informed decision-making by the patient/family.
   b. Recognize the responsibility among patients, families, and other members of the health care team in all phases of health care delivery.
   c. Educate to enable patients and families to enable them to and make informed decisions.

6. Linkage of advocacy, ethics, and risk management
   a. *Advocacy* – Act or process of advocating or supporting (a cause or proposal) on behalf of another (Steinmetz, 1997). This definition of advocacy is similar to that found in the conceptual framework for ambulatory care nurses. The *Ambulatory Care Nursing Conceptual Framework* defines advocacy as compassion, caring, and emotional support (Haas, 1998).
   b. *Ethics* – A branch of philosophy dealing with the values related to human conduct, with respect to the rightness or wrongness of certain actions and to the goodness and badness of the motives and ends of such actions; a set of moral principles or values, the principles of conduct governing an individual or a group (Steinmetz, 1997).
   c. *Risk management* – An organization-wide program to identify risks, control occurrences, prevent damage, and control legal liability: it is a process where-

by risks to the institution are evaluated and controlled (Velianoff & Hobbs, 2000). Service recovery programs and application of JCAHO's National Patient Safety Goals (NPSG) represent risk management practices within organizations.

7. The linkage of ethics and advocacy principles for ambulatory care nursing practice is in recognizing (understanding) that ethics provide a conceptual framework, and advocacy consists of the appropriate actions (behaviors) in implementing decisions made on behalf of patients. The linkage of advocacy to risk management programs is through leadership actions that seek to support IOP initiatives leading to quality care delivery and a safe working environment.

B. Present context of patient advocacy – Today's health care system presents challenges on many fronts that require advocacy for patient/family:

1. Scientific advancement in medicine in the past decade.
   a. Potential availability and application of advancements (for example, genome project, improved transplantation options, research protocols, microscopic endoscopy applications, telehealth medicine).
   b. Allocation and rationing of medical advancements can occur as a result of:
      (1) Geographic location.
      (2) Cost to payer.
   c. Institutional decision-making, as affected by cost/benefit analysis about specific therapies and experimental procedures to be offered. Incorporated within this analysis needs to be a process for adjudicating differences of plans of care available to patients (such as the decision about when to provide services of a generalist versus a specialist).

2. Financial issues.
   a. Governmental initiatives/decisions.
      (1) Medicare/Medicaid programs: Promotion of managed care systems to elderly and poverty level populations.
      (2) Consolidated Omnibus Reconciliation Bill of 1986 (COBRA):

Progressively decreased payments for health care delivery requiring decision-making about types of services that institutions will provide to consumers.

(3) Corporate compliance: The health care industry continues to develop and implement systematic processes for measuring adherence to internal and external indicators of compliance with acceptable standards. Institutional oversight for measurement and improving processes is appropriate (for example, research activities, billing practices).

(4) Pay for performance – Established goals of individual or institutional performance that may be rewarded via financial and/or other incentives.

b. Private sector insurers.
   (1) Shrinking fee-for-service market because of higher individual cost; this type of insurance plan has allowed for more choices by the individual about health care options.
   (2) Proliferation of managed care insurance products has accrued throughout the country, including high-risk Medicare and Medicaid HMO plans.
      (a) Failure of these ventures has also occurred, resulting in decreased access for Medicare and Medicaid populations.
      (b) An HMO's decision-making approval processes can create a moral dilemma for health care providers. Decisions about what testing and consulting services are needed are frequently challenged/denied by HMOs.

c. Business sector issues.
   (1) Increased premiums, putting coverage at risk.
   (2) The institution's evaluation and decisions about insurance plan options offered to staff, based upon possible risk and responsibility.
   (3) Employers' hiring decisions, which may be based in part on health sta-

tus of potential candidates (history of smoking, morbid obesity).

   (4) Demand for quality care for insured employees which may require institutional accountability for care delivery by providers.

   (5) Increased co-pays for individual employees, which may result in delays in seeking health care, putting health at risk.

   (6) Operational challenges, including redesign of ambulatory care operations practice patterns, primarily as a result of compressed length of stay (LOS) in hospitals.

     (a) Increased volume in ambulatory settings because of decreased LOS.

     (b) Increased acuity in ambulatory care because of decreased LOS.

     (c) Increased availability and incorporation of new technology.

     (d) Increased referral for home care and long-term care.

3. Political response to today's health care market focused on recognizing and providing solutions involving:

  a. Securing long-term funding of Medicare/Medicaid programs.

  b. Promoting of managed care initiative including:

    (1) Defining clinical outcomes.

    (2) Application of professional practice guidelines.

    (3) Ensuring ongoing, documented quality processes and measurements.

  c. Increasing access to health care systems.

  d. Providing services to aging U.S. population/demographics ("Baby Boomers").

  e. Providing Patient's Bill of Rights legislation (proposed).

  f. The number of uninsured Americans is currently at 45.8, and twice that number are underinsured (Center for American Progress, 2005).

  g. Implementing a national Prescriptive Drug Plan (Part D) for Medicare and Medicaid population(s), with choice and access, are proving to be costly and confusing.

4. Quality assessment and performance improvement.

  a. Evaluation beginning with patient rights/responsibilities (autonomy).

  b. Balance between cost and quality of care delivered (justice).

  c. Assessment, analysis, and management of patient care risks.

  d. Nursing identification of and participation in evaluation of quality issues.

  e. External review agencies perform reviews and monitor activities to assure consistent and reliable care (refer to Chapter 15, *Regulatory Compliance and Patient Safety*).

  f. Internal review systems, including risk management program(s), are integrated into IOP (JCAHO, 2004) that begin at:

    (1) Clinic/unit level.

    (2) Department level.

    (3) Institutional level.

     (a) Leadership responsibility/decisions as to what areas of improvement will be reviewed and supported with resources.

     (b) Risk management program(s) responsibilities include:

      (i) Risk identification.

      (ii) Loss of prevention and reduction, including incident report and investigation.

      (iii) Insurance claims management.

      (iv) Administering workers' compensation and handling legal issues or legal defense coordination.

      (v) Liability assessment of contracts.

      (vi) Risk management education.

      (vii) Handling product recall and safe medical devices issues.

     (c) Ensuring compliance with accreditation standards, regulatory mandates, and governmental rules and laws (Velianoff & Hobbs, 2000).

(d) Leadership has oversight responsibility to ensure that changes focus on improvement of care for patients, visitors and staff, and effectiveness in those being evaluated.

C. Advocacy opportunities – The advocacy for patients/families is best done when linked to education about both health/disease management and the health care system itself.

1. Empowerment of the patient and family to make informed decisions.

   a. Until early 1990s, health care providers often encouraged patients to have symptoms evaluated through an office visit. This did little to affirm and reassure the decision-making of the patients and families, and it promoted vulnerability, viewing medicine as mystifying and maybe even magical.

   b. Currently, the shift is toward a partnership between providers and educated patients (Linnell, 1998).

      (1) Shift recognizes reality of care being episodic and frequently provided by patient and/or family.

      (2) Shift requires education of patients/families to evaluate and manage illnesses through a combination of self-care, telehealth management, and office visits.

      (3) Shift requires education of patient/family to support their ability to assimilate, interpret, and evaluate information for decision making. The availability of Internet technology can help improve the understanding of patient/family of basic disease process and treatment options (Sennett, 2000).

2. Clinical operations must be designed to safely respond to the new flow patterns and be monitored for their responsiveness.

   a. Timely and accurate reporting of adverse reactions and incident reports both internally and externally (as required).

   b. Increased outreach efforts within the community. For example, influenza vaccine administration at schools, churches, etc.

   c. Flexible hours for delivery of services (for example, primary care clinics/pediatric clinics that are open 7 days per week; retail business(es) that offer limited primary care services; independent advanced practice nurse corporations that offer care).

3. Nurses' role in advocacy behaviors is based on assessment of patient needs, including increased awareness of domestic violence, elder and child abuse, National Patient Safety Goals (NPSG), recognition and decision-making when things go wrong, and on organizational systems available to provide care. Skills required include:

   a. Expert clinical assessment skills.

      (1) Telephone triage.

      (2) Telephone management/case management: Often proactive in focus.

      (3) Office visit: Consistent assessment and reassessment.

   b. Expert intervention skills.

      (1) Understanding disease process, disease management, family dynamics, and community resources.

      (2) Understanding basic survival skills in disease management.

      (3) Lifestyle skills: Current adaptation to health challenges.

      (4) Health promotion: Proactive, holistic approach to lifestyle.

      (5) Understanding of State Board of Nursing rules and regulations of professional practice.

      (6) Recognition and appropriate response to changes in system(s) that create risk to patient/family or staff.

   c. Confident decision-making skills.

   d. Partnering skills with patients/families/health care team.

   e. Knowledge of mechanisms to coordinate care across institutions/community to provide continuity.

   f. Awareness of the fiscal impact of care decisions.

4. The nurse plays a central role in working with patients/families to assure the right:

a. Access.
b. Provider.
c. Time frame.
d. Level of care.

5. Patient satisfaction measurement is a subjective data collection that responds to the perception of care delivered, understanding that perception is reality to the patient.
   a. Measurement indicators.
      (1) Patient survey feedback at provider level, unit level, institutional level.
      (2) Accreditation bodies review findings and institutional response to these findings.
      (3) Third party payers' response to care provided.
      (4) Complaint resolution process in place. Units/institutions need to create atmosphere of objectivity and specific processes for this to happen. Recognizing own values and biases of health care personnel.
      (5) IOP activities at the unit level that measure patient satisfaction and compliance with NPSG.
      (6) Employee satisfaction evaluation.
   b. Customer service.
      (1) Patient perception is reality: Do not underestimate this concept in terms of marketing and public relations.
      (2) Treat each patient and family with dignity and courtesy. The nurse needs to recognize his or her own beliefs/values. This includes the patient's family and the larger community.
   c. Techniques: Promoting advocacy and patient relations.
      (1) Acknowledge individuality and autonomy.
      (2) Acknowledge issues and responsibilities.
      (3) Be aware of verbal and non-verbal behaviors.
      (4) Provide patient relations – Service recovery programs (pro-active approach).
         (a) Cleveland Clinic Heart Protocol (Cleveland Clinic, 2004).
            (i) Hear the message.
            (ii) Empathize with the patient.
            (iii) Acknowledge the issue.
            (iv) Demand for quality care for insured employees requires institutional accountability for care delivery by providers.
            (v) Respond.
            (vi) Thank the patient for the opportunity to be of service.
         (b) Formal Ombudsman program.
         (c) Patient service representative acts as liaison to patient/family during care delivery.
         (d) Institutional Web site that educates the public about nursing's professional services and programs involving patient care.

D. Future advocacy opportunities for nurses in ambulatory care.
   1. Challenge to advocate related to:
      a. Current cost containment focus.
      b. Bottom-line decisions.
      c. Episodic nature of patient visits.
   2. Need to create opportunities for nurses to demonstrate leadership about matters such as patient complaints, IOP results, risk management initiatives, and program changes.
      a. Leadership voice in operational decisions (for example, begins at unit level and includes evaluation of current services provided and the ability to add additional new program development).
      b. Voice in health care resources/allocation (such as the evaluation of appropriate equipment, space, personnel, and systems to meet changing practice).
      c. Opportunities observed in other professionals.
         (1) Identify centers of excellence with quality outcomes.
         (2) Apply appropriate adaptation of results for specific environments.
         (3) Network with other professionals (for example, Leapfrog Group, IOM reports of health care delivery system in America).
      d. Must help patients/families understand

their rights and responsibilities in participating in the health care system (for example, build trusting partnerships, explain choices available).

e. Shared responsibility between patient/family and health care team.

    (1) Empowerment of patient/family through education.

    (2) Awareness of JCAHO intent regarding patients' rights standard.

E. Leadership coordination – Skills necessary to organize and manage an undertaking, while moving forward on agreed goals. Ambulatory care nurses can apply these skills in their work setting and the community to benefit patients.

1. Understanding community resources related to disaster planning, importance of self-management by patients/families of basic needs (food, clothing, medications).

2. Consider process for integrating the *Patient Self-Determination Act of 1991* (Rouse, 1991).

    a. Requires that patients are asked about and given the opportunity to decide their advance directive as relates to health care decisions. This is mandated for acute care, skilled nursing home health care, hospice care, long-term care, and HMO settings.

    b. Not required by federal act in the ambulatory setting; however, the primary care provider should have this discussion as part of the health care partnership/relationship, preferably over time and before a health care crisis occurs for the patient (Johnson, 2000).

    c. Promotes respect and value of the individual patient.

3. Participate in the design and implementation of an institutional system that provides consistent documentation of advance directives in patient record. Although this is extremely challenging, it is becoming more important as a result of increasing complexity of systems serving patients.

4. For selected ambulatory patients requiring an acute care episode, begin discharge planning in ambulatory setting (such as crutch walking for joint replacements, teaching patient/family infusion services, introduction to specific durable medical equipment that may be required in the plan of care used in certain procedures).

5. Promote increased communications between ambulatory/acute care/home care settings to improve the continuity of care for patients.

    a. Meet periodically with providers to promote understanding of how systems work and can improve to benefit all.

    b. Ensure flow of written communication regarding the plan of care including new technologies (such as fax, electronic medical record compatibility).

6. External environment.

    a. Community education/involvement in promoting understanding of how the health care system works.

        (1) Schools: Local systems and colleges (for example, work with the school board to promote preventive health curriculum).

        (2) Advocacy resources.

            (a) Internet (such as Advocacy in Ambulatory Care – Patient Advocate Foundation [www.patientadvocate.org], Caring Conversations [www.practical-bioethics.org], National Committee for Quality Assurance [www.ncqa.org], Institute of Medicine [www.iom.edu]).

            (b) State insurance departments.

            (c) Centers for Medicare and Medicaid Services (CMS) (www.cms.gov).

            (d) American Hospital Association/Society for Healthcare Consumer Advocacy.

            (e) Professional organizations/societies.

            (f) American Association of Retired Persons (AARP).

        (3) Church community (including parish nursing programs where available).

    b. Professional organizations/political activism.

        (1) Professional organizations support the nurse's ability to advocate.

            (a) Create standards of care to

benefit patients.

(b) Provide ongoing education for nurses.

(c) Publish journals and texts to support care of patients.

(2) Professional organizations advocate directly.

(a) Support lobbying efforts.

(b) Propose public policy related to care.

c. Create business opportunities.

(1) Intermediary between patients and insurance company.

(2) Roles within managed care organizations in quality management – Specifically, evaluating indicators of quality as they relate to subscribers.

(3) Independent consultant: Based on recognized expertise (such as redesign, accreditation process, clinical medical information system design (MISD) systems, research, and risk management/quality measurement).

References

American Academy of Ambulatory Care Nursing (AAACN). (2004). *Ambulatory care nursing administration and practice standards* (5th ed.). Pitman, NJ: Author.

American Nurses Association (ANA). (2003). *Nursing's social policy statement* (2nd ed.) (p. 2). Washington, DC: American Nurses Publishing.

Center for American Progress. (2005). *News about the ininsured*. Retrieved June 5, 2006, from http://www.american-progress.org/site/apps/s/custom.asp?c=biJRJ8OVF&b=1 415323

Cleveland Clinic. (2004). *Cleveland Clinic heart protocol*. Cleveland, OH: Author.

Haas, S. (1998). Ambulatory care nursing conceptual framework. *AAACN Viewpoint, 20,* 16-17.

Henderson, V. (1961). *Basic principles of nursing care*. London: International Council of Nursing.

Johnson, E. (2000). Advocating for patients. *AAACN Viewpoint, 22,* 1, 6-7.

Joint Commission on Accreditation of Healthcare Organizations (JCAHO). (2004). *Hospital accreditation standards (HAS), standards, intent*. Oakbrook Terrace, IL: Author.

Linnell, K. (1998). Patient health education in the changing ambulatory care environment. *AAACN Viewpoint, 20,* 1-6, 8.

Rouse, F. (1991). Patients, providers, and the PSDA. Patient Self-Determination Act. *Hastings Center Report, 21*(5), S2-S3.

Sennett, C. (2000). Ambulatory care in the new millennium: The role of consumer information. *Quality Management in Health Care, 8*(2), 82-87.

Steinmetz, S., et al. (Eds.). (1997). *Random House Webster's unabridged dictionary* (2nd ed.). New York: Random House.

Velianoff, G.D., & Hobbs, G.R. (2000). Quality improvement and risk management. In D. Huber (Ed.), *Leadership and nursing care management* (pp. 609-630). Philadelphia: W.B. Saunders.

Additional Readings

Cantone, L. (1999). Corporate compliance: Critical to organizational success. *Nursing Economic$, 17,* 15-19, 52.

Iglehart, J. (1999). The American health care system-expenditures. *New England Journal of Medicine, 340,* 70-71.

Savage, T. (1999). Ethics, the outpatient pediatric nurse and managed care. *Pediatric Nursing, 25,* 197-207.

Savage, T. (2000). *Ambulatory care in the new millennium: The role of consumer information*. Aspen Publishers, Inc.

Vitanza, A . (2000, March 6). Guardian angels aid those lost in medical maze. *Healthcare Monitor, 1,* 9.

Patient Advocacy

This test may be copied for use by others.

COMPLETE THE FOLLOWING:

Name: _____

Address: _____

City: _____ State: _____ Zip: _____

Preferred telephone: (Home)_____ (Work)_____

E-mail_____

AAACN Member Expiration Date: _____

Registration fee: AAACN Member: $12.00
                   Nonmember: $20.00

Objectives

This educational activity is designed for nurses and other health care professionals who practice in ambulatory care. For those wishing to obtain CE credit, an evaluation follows. After studying the information presented in this offering, you will be able to:

1. Describe the context of ethical concepts and advocacy behavior in nursing practice.
2. Discuss the importance of nursing leadership to advocacy, patient relations, and risk management.
3. Describe specific applications of advocacy behaviors in ambulatory nursing practice, including individual, organizational, and community initiatives.

Answer Form:

1. If you applied what you have learned from this activity into your practice, what would be different?

_____

_____

_____

Evaluation

	Strongly disagree				Strongly agree
2. By completing this activity, I was able to meet the following objectives:					
a. Describe the context of ethical concepts and advocacy behavior in nursing practice.	1	2	3	4	5
b. Discuss the importance of nursing leadership to advocacy, patient relations, and risk management.	1	2	3	4	5
c. Describe specific applications of advocacy behaviors in ambulatory nursing practice, including individual, organizational, and community initiatives.	1	2	3	4	5
3. The content was current and relevant.	1	2	3	4	5
4. The objectives could be achieved using the content provided.	1	2	3	4	5
5. This was an effective method to learn this content.	1	2	3	4	5
6. I am more confident in my abilities since completing this material.	1	2	3	4	5

7. The material was (check one) ___new ___review for me.
8. Time required to read this chapter: _____minutes

I verify that I have completed this activity: _____
                                        Signature

Comments: _____

_____

_____

Posttest Instructions

1. To receive continuing education credit for individual study after reading the article, complete the answer/evaluation form to the left.

2. Detach and send the answer/evaluation form along with a check or money order payable to the *American Academy of Ambulatory Care Nursing (AAACN)*, East Holly Avenue Box 56, Pitman, NJ 08071–0056.

3. Test returns must be postmarked by August 1, 2011. Upon completion of the answer/evaluation form, a certificate for **1.2** contact hour(s) will be awarded and sent to you. Should the material contained in this chapter become outdated prior to the above expiration date, AAACN reserves the right to withdraw this CE test.

This activity is co-provided by the *American Academy of Ambulatory Care Nursing (AAACN)* and Anthony J. Jannetti, Inc. (AJJ). AJJ is accredited as a provider of continuing nursing education by the American Nurses' Credentialing Center's Commission on Accreditation (ANCC-COA). AAACN is a provider approved by the California Board of Registered Nurses, provider number CEP 05336.

This article was reviewed and formatted for contact hour credit by Sally S. Russell, MN, CMSRN, AAACN Education Director; and Candia Baker Laughlin MS, RN, C, Editor.

Chapter 10

Staffing and Workload

Sheila A. Haas, PhD, RN, FAAN
Clare E. Hastings, PhD, RN, FAAN

Objectives

Study of the information presented in this chapter will enable the learner to:
1. Discuss methods of determining staffing requirements and skill mix in ambulatory care nursing.
2. Compare and contrast staff recruitment and retention strategies in ambulatory care settings.
3. Discuss common methods of monitoring productivity in ambulatory care nursing.
4. Enumerate the issues and challenges with staffing and workload in ambulatory care nursing.

Key Points

1. There are many complex factors and no readily applied formulas or tools for determining staffing in ambulatory care.
2. Recruitment involves seeking, attracting, and selecting qualified candidates for positions available in a cost-effective manner.
3. Retention is maintaining qualified persons in positions.
4. Ambulatory care is expanding and will require more nurses. New recruitment strategies must be considered.
5. Measuring productivity in nursing is difficult, but role clarity is important in improving productivity.

The needs of ambulatory care patients are increasingly complex and the demands for care are more intense today because of both demographics and changes in length of stay for hospitalized patients. Methods of determining staffing requirements and skill mix in ambulatory care nursing have become a major concern for nurses working in ambulatory care settings. Visit volume is no longer a good predictor of the number and type of staff needed to care for ambulatory patients. Instead, numbers and types of nursing staff must be sufficient to serve both the number of patients and the complexity of their needs. Recruiting and orienting ambulatory care nurses have become more difficult challenges as well. Ambulatory care nurses have traditionally had hospital nursing experience prior to hire into ambulatory care. As nurses are aging and retiring directly from acute care, and as the nursing shortage deepens, fewer experienced hospital nurses are available to work in ambulatory care settings. Ambulatory care nurses must give much more attention to the recruitment and retention of nurses.

Determining Staffing and Skill Mix in Ambulatory Care

A. Definitions.
   1. *Staffing* is the process of assessing patient care needs, and determining and providing the appropriate number and mix of nursing personnel to meet patients' requirements for care and desired quality outcomes.
   2. *Workload* refers to the amount and difficulty of patient care and related activities that nurses must complete in a specified period of time.
   3. *Skill mix* refers to the number and types of nursing personnel assigned to care for a given patient population.
   4. *Nursing personnel* typically providing nursing care in ambulatory settings include:
      a. Registered nurses (RNs).
      b. Licensed practical nurses/licensed vocational nurses (LPNs/LVNs).
      c. Unlicensed assistive personnel (UAP).
         (1) Nurse aides/nursing assistants (NAs).
         (2) Medical technicians or medical assistants (MTs or MAs).

          (3) Receptionists.
          (4) Clerks.
    d. Advanced practice nurses (APNs).
        (1) Nurse practitioners (NPs).
        (2) Certified nurse midwives (CNMs).
        (3) Certified registered nurse anesthetists (CRNAs).
        (4) Clinical nurse specialists (CNSs).

5. *Mid-level providers* are defined in managed care organizations as APNs and physician assistants (PAs).
6. *Staffing ratio* is the ratio of nursing personnel to required activities.
    a. In inpatient settings, staffing ratios most often reflect the number of patients assigned to a nurse for a given period of time or nursing hours per patient day.
    b. In ambulatory care settings, staffing ratios may be expressed in terms of the ratio of nurses to providers rather than patients.
7. *Full-time equivalent (FTE)* refers to a full-time position or combination of positions that is equal to 40 hours of work per week.
8. *Provider* refers to a licensed practitioner such as a physician or nurse practitioner.
9. *Intensity* of both patients and nursing care is a term that has varying definitions in the literature.
    a. Verran (1981) defined ambulatory nursing intensity as a combination of nursing care complexity and the time needed to do complex work.
    b. Currently, to validate a definition of ambulatory nursing intensity, a Delphi study is being conducted on the dimensions of ambulatory nursing intensity (Haas, Hackbarth, Cullen, & Androwich, 2000).
    c. Ambulatory patient intensity is defined by Cusack, Jones-Wells, and Chisholm (2004) as the patient's degree of illness as well as the complexity of the tasks required to provide care.

B. A staffing process consists of:
1. A precise statement of the mission of the organization and the services that the patient and/or patient caregiver can expect, including the standards of care.
2. Determination of the nursing care delivery model (for example, primary nursing care, team, modular, case management).
3. Determination of patient population care needs.
4. Use of a specific method to determine the number and types of staff required to provide care.
5. Determination of environmental factors that influence staffing (such as, geographic layout, resources readily available, physician expectations).
6. Development of assignment patterns for staff using established health care setting personnel guidelines, policy statements, and procedures, as well as professional standards.
7. Determination of the scheduling process and procedures.
8. Evaluation of quality of care provided and judgment reflecting the impact of staffing via process and outcomes measures.

C. Factors influencing staffing.
1. Payer mix and market factors.
    a. Level of managed care and capitation that alters incentives for various care delivery modes.
        (1) Under capitation, each patient visit adds cost.
        (2) Under capitation, cost is split among MD, RN, other ancillary staff, and overhead.
        (3) Under capitation, the value of the RN is in decreasing the cost per covered life including reducing the number/cost of visits.
2. The process of care delivery.
    a. Patient flow through the facility.
    b. Volume of services provided.
    c. Provider roles and practice styles.
    d. Use of midlevel providers.
    e. Availability, competency, and number of UAPs.
    f. Integration of services along the continuum of care.
    g. Availability of consult and support services.
3. Types of patient encounters.
    a. Scheduled vs. unscheduled.
    b. New vs. return and/or follow-up visits.

  c.   Office visit vs. procedure-based.
  d.   Education or counseling visit.
  e.   Telecommunication contact.
  f.   Referral.
4. Requirements per patient encounter.
  a.   Time required for encounter.
  b.   Intensity or level of skill required of provider and support staff.
  c.   Both time and intensity important.
5. Interdisciplinary team function (Hastings, 1997; Hastings & Haas, 1998).
  a.   Non-physician staff seen as augmenting/extending MD role.
  b.   Non-physician staff seen as value-added providers of service.
6. Provider-perceived (MD, APN, PA) needs for support staff.
  a.   Prior to visit.
  b.   During visit.
  c.   Following visit
  d.   Telephone support requirements.
7. Legacy from inpatient staffing models.
  a.   False assumption that each visit requires nursing care.
  b.   Unnecessary application of inpatient standards for assessment and observation.
8. Use of benchmarking or comparative data to set staffing levels.
  a.   Based on what exists in current practice, not necessarily what should be.
  b.   Often difficult to find appropriate comparisons because practices and settings may vary even in the same specialty.

D. Nursing intensity systems for ambulatory care.
  1. They are in developmental stages.
  2. Their purpose is to differentiate:
     a.   Types of visits.
     b.   Types of providers needed.
     c.   Number of nursing personnel needed including requirements for specialized competencies.
  3. Types of nursing intensity systems.
     a.   *Prototype intensity systems* involve categorizing patients/patient visits into four or five categories that describe care, complexity, time required, and nursing intensity. These categories:
        (1) Are based on the clinical character-

istics of patients presenting for care, including patient expectations and reason for visit.
        (2) Are based on role dimensions and can dictate required nursing care needed (such as teaching, care coordination, advocacy based on role dimensions).
        (3) Can be used to describe visit types and time.
        (4) Can be built to predict types (RN, LPN, UAP) of personnel needed.
     b.   *Factor-based intensity systems* involve use of indicators describing patient characteristics or nursing interventions that are summed to derive the time and complexity of care required. These indicators:
        (1) Are based on activities and time needed to perform each activity needed for care.
        (2) Can predict staff time required but usually do not predict type of nursing personnel needed.
  4. In ambulatory care, nursing intensity systems are not used prospectively for staffing on a day-to-day basis because of visit volume but rather are used for trending retrospectively.
     a.   Visit volume may vary significantly day to day and week to week, making one day's staffing data difficult to use as a predictor.
     b.   It takes a large variation in individual patient intensity or number of visits overall to make a difference in staffing requirements.
     c.   There is no fixed "capacity" in an outpatient setting that corresponds to the bed capacity on an inpatient unit.
  5. Ideal patient intensity systems (Cusack et al., 2004):
     a.   Reflect true patient care intensity.
     b.   Project accurate staffing patterns and patient care requirements.
     c.   Are user friendly.
     d.   Facilitate collaboration on administrative and clinical decisions.
     e.   Adapt to multiple settings.

f. Increase staff satisfaction because workload is acknowledged.

6. Outcomes of implementing a patient intensity system in ambulatory care (Cusack et al., 2004).

   a. Helps nurses articulate direct and indirect patient care needs.

   b. Assists with resource allocation.

   c. Assists with use of critical thinking skills to distinguish between system and staffing issues.

   d. Nurse managers use the tool to evaluate the need for additional FTEs and to improve performance.

7. Issues with nursing intensity systems in ambulatory care that should assist with determining staffing.

   a. *Validity:* All classification systems are dependent on instruments to measure nursing intensity. These are only valid if they truly measure or capture what they are supposed to measure: the work that nursing personnel does with patients in ambulatory care.

      (1) No generally accepted definition or measure of nursing intensity in ambulatory care.

      (2) Role ambiguity in nursing in ambulatory care continues.

   b. *Reliability:* Any instrument designed to determine nursing or patient intensity in ambulatory care must be used consistently by everyone; data must be reproducible (Jones, Cusack, & Chisholm, 2004); it must be user friendly and easy to use with a large visit volume.

   c. *Automation:* Given the visit volume in many ambulatory care areas, a nursing intensity system must be computerized and must have sufficient capacity to handle large volumes of data (Jones et al., 2004).

Recruitment and Retention of Nurses in Ambulatory Care

A. Definitions.

   1. *Recruitment* involves seeking, attracting ("selling the organization"), and selecting qualified candidates for positions available in a cost-effective manner.

   2. *Retention* is maintaining qualified persons in positions.

B. Requirements for recruitment and retention.

   1. Planning for numbers and types of personnel, as well as where and how to best look for new hires.

   2. Developing relationships with potential sources of new hires (for example, schools of nursing).

   3. Attention to recruitment, even during times of perceived surplus nursing personnel (shortages are cyclical).

   4. Cooperation throughout the organization to be successful; current employees "sell" the organization.

   5. In ambulatory care, recruitment entails overcoming myths and stereotypes.

      a. Ambulatory care nursing is "a piece of cake," "easy," "a vacation" compared to inpatient nursing.

      b. Ambulatory care is the place to go for straight day shifts, no evenings, nights, or weekend shifts (no longer true).

C. Recruitment planning includes:

   1. Developing a position description including responsibilities, accountabilities, and required qualifications (accurate position descriptions are more likely to result in a good match).

   2. Identifying all relevant sources of potential candidates including the use of summer internships for student nurses.

   3. Determining the optimal mode of communicating vacancies (such as personnel communication, internal and external Web postings, letters, ads).

   4. Ensuring that all recruitment communication is in compliance with internal and external policies on recruitment.

   5. Validating that the compensation package is appropriate for the position and the marketplace.

   6. Coaching current employees regarding recruiting, selling, and selecting candidates.

   7. Evaluating responses to the recruiting effort and modifying it as needed.

D. Variables affecting recruitment.

1. Competitiveness of salaries and benefits, as well as perceptions of salary compression over time (perception that nurses' salaries have not consistently increased as have those of other occupational groups).
2. Position of the unit or facility in comparison to other local settings.
   a. Is the position in a clinical setting affiliated with a hospital or a multi-hospital system?
      (1) If yes, what are the incentives or disincentives for transitioning to ambulatory care?
      (2) If no, how competitive are employment options compared to local hospital-based settings?
   b. How rare are the competencies required for the position?
   c. What is the availability of seasoned ambulatory care staff to orient a new person?
3. Available supply of qualified nursing personnel.
   a. In a poor national economy, nurses tend to work more, as the economy improves, nurses may work fewer hours.
   b. Fewer young nurses are available as a result of:
      (1) Decreased enrollments related to a perceived surplus of nurses in the early 1990s.
      (2) Attraction of other careers open to young people.
      (3) Nursing faculty shortage, so fewer nurses can be educated.
   c. The mean age of ambulatory care nurses is 44.3 years (U.S. Department of Health and Human Services [DHHS], Division of Nursing, 2004).
   d. Size of the applicant pool is also influenced by specific position qualifications. Often see increased demand for specialty-prepared nurses (OR, ER, critical care).
   e. Proximity to schools of nursing.
4. Available resources for advertisements, literature, and recruiter visits to career days.
5. Attractiveness of the work setting and perceptions about the safety of the work environment.
6. Reputation of the organization regarding past employment practices and quality of patient care.
7. Values related to scheduling, time available for leisure.
8. Status of national and local economy.
9. Reputation for work group cohesiveness.

E. Factors that attract professional nurses to ambulatory care (Hackbarth, Haas, Kavanagh, & Vlasses, 1995).
   1. Hours and schedules without rotating shifts.
   2. Challenging nature of the work (variety, rapid pace).
   3. Working with clients and families over a long period of time.
   4. Nature of the work.
   5. Seeing outcomes of care.
   6. Autonomy in practice.
   7. Coworker relationships.
   8. Teaching and health promotion.

F. Current status of ambulatory nurse satisfaction – Ambulatory care nurses report the highest levels of satisfaction with their jobs despite salaries for nurses employed in ambulatory care settings below the mean for every type of position (DHHS, Division of Nursing, 2004).

G. Recruitment issues for ambulatory settings.
   1. With hospital nursing shortages and consequent salary and shift incentives, as well as nurses retiring directly from acute care positions, fewer recruits will come to ambulatory care with inpatient experience.
   2. Ambulatory care is expanding and will require more nurses. New recruitment strategies must be considered, such as providing ambulatory settings as student clinical sites and recruiting the best and brightest.

H. Recruitment strategies for ambulatory care nursing.
   1. Enhance understanding of all nurses of the ambulatory care nurse role.
   2. Participate in venues (such as certification) that provide overt recognition of ambulatory care nurse expertise.
   3. Increase ambulatory care nurse participation in professional nursing organizations.

I. Retention in ambulatory care nursing positions.
   1. Requires planning.
   2. Factors that increase likelihood of retention:
      a. A planned orientation to each ambulatory care nursing role.
      b. A planned preceptor, coaching, and

mentoring program for new recruits.
c. A planned continuing development program for employees.
d. A recognition program for individual contributions and accomplishments.
e. Collegial working relationships.
f. A salary and benefits that are perceived as equitable with inpatient nursing.
g. Flexible or self-scheduling.
h. Less role ambiguity, role stress, or role overload.
i. Trust in the organization.
3. Cost effective because turnover:
a. Involves recruitment, orientation, and development costs.
b. Affects productivity.
c. Affects quality of care.

Productivity Monitoring in Ambulatory Care

A. Definitions.
1. *Productivity* in nursing is described as a measure of the efficiency with which labor and materials are converted into service or care (Edwardson, 1985), or the volume of output related to the amount of resources consumed/used to produce the specified output/services.
2. *Productivity Ratio:* Productivity = output/ input (Chamberlain, 1965).
3. *Output* is the product or service expressed in terms of dollars that is statistically adjusted to eliminate the effects of inflation.
4. *Input* is the dollar cost of person-hours needed to produce a product or service.
5. *Nursing outcome classification* (NOC) involves a systematic use of standards and language that identifies patient outcomes, indicators, and measurements that are responsive to nursing interventions (Johnson & Maas, 1997).
6. *Traditional nursing productivity ratio* is hours of care required that is multiplied by quality and divided by hours of care expended (Dennis, Dunn, & Benson, 1980).
7. *Efficiency* is a measure of how well work is done with respect to the use of worker time, materials, capital, or other resources (Ruh, 1982). Often, efficiency is measured by

budget variances for personnel and supplies.
8. *Effectiveness* is a measure of how well the work meets or exceeds stated goals or standards.
9. *Outcomes* are used synonymously with results achieved from planned or unplanned interventions.
10. *Nursing-sensitive ambulatory outcomes* are changes in the actual or potential health status, behavior, or perceptions of individuals, families, or populations that can be attributed to nursing interventions provided in an ambulatory care setting in which client-nurse contacts may be single or intermittent contacts of 23 hours or less.
B. Issues with measuring productivity in nursing.
1. Often no physical product is created in nursing. Once the service is performed, the evidence disappears (Ruh, 1982).
2. Marked discretion in professional nursing work (planning, assessment, and evaluation) is difficult to measure.
3. Continued difficulty with measuring quality in ambulatory care; often only measure easily quantifiable variables (such as immunizations).
C. Current measures of productivity in ambulatory care.
1. Focus is on outcomes such as:
a. Cost of care.
b. Financial performance (cost per procedure).
c. Satisfaction of patients and staff.
d. Health status.
e. Incidence of complications.
f. Access and availability: time to next appointment.
g. "Report card" measures: immunization rates, mammogram rates.
h. Visit volume.
2. Little work on measurement of process productivity.
a. Concern with increasing expectation that providers see more patients per hour is that outcomes may not be as good because the care process is shortened.
b. Much ambiguity as to who should be involved in the care process.
D. Approaches to productivity improvement in

ambulatory care.
1. Role clarity for nursing personnel.
   a. Use personnel at levels consistent with their competence and education.
   b. Provide orientation and continuing education for staff.
   c. Involve nursing personnel in evolution of roles.
2. Appropriate staffing ratios to achieve efficiency and effectiveness.
   a. Staffing ratios will differ related to patient population being served (for example, oncology patients requiring high-tech, teaching, and care coordination dimensions of nursing care will require more RNs and fewer UAPs in ambulatory care settings).
   b. Collaboration among nursing staff working with a given patient population such that each knows own scope of practice and works effectively as a team player.
3. Use and evaluate effectiveness incentives to enhance productivity such as gain sharing, which is a program where employees receive a portion of revenues gained as monies saved through specified efforts of employees.
4. Use automation to enhance effectiveness: the computerized patient record, databases.
5. Use of standardized nursing languages: North America Nursing Diagnosis Association (NANDA), Nursing Intervention Classification (NIC), Nursing Outcome Classification (NOC), Omaha System, and Saba Home Healthcare Classification B (see Chapter 7, *Informatics*) to capture data on nursing process and outcomes.
6. Use performance appraisal and coaching to enhance effectiveness.

Issues and Challenges with Staffing And Workload

A. Assumption that methods used in inpatient settings will work as well in ambulatory care mandates that nurses:
   1. Develop, implement, and evaluate a simple yet valued and reliable nursing or patient intensity system for ambulatory care to track

and trend the demand for numbers and types of ambulatory care nursing personnel.
2. Develop, implement, and evaluate process and outcome measures that demonstrate the impact of different nursing staff mixes.
3. Develop, implement, and evaluate ambulatory care productivity measures.
   a. Measures need to capture the unique contribution of nurses and other providers on the interdisciplinary team.
   b. Data should be easily entered, preferably as a part of routine documentation.
      (1) Embed the nursing minimum data set elements in encounter form data.
      (2) Embed NIC and NOC coding in nursing documentation (Johnson & Maas, 1997).
      (3) Include intensity measurement as a part of clinical documentation or as a part of the appointment scheduling process.
   c. Select measures of processes and outcomes over which providers (nurses) have control.
   d. Select measures that are easily understood by those being evaluated.
   e. Select measures that are compatible with corporate mission and measures.
B. The characteristics of ambulatory care nursing have changed as patients coming to ambulatory settings are sicker and there has been an increase in capitation that alters the incentives for providers and requires that we:
   1. Develop, implement, and evaluate strategies to enhance work group effectiveness.
   2. Develop, implement, and evaluate staffing ratios for specific patient populations.
   3. Develop, implement, and evaluate orientation programs and competency assessment for ambulatory care nursing personnel.
   4. Develop retention strategies that assist with retention of competent nursing personnel.

References

Chamberlain, N. (1965). *The labor sector*. New York: McGraw-Hill.

Cusack, G., Jones-Wells, A., & Chisholm, S. (2004). Patient intensity in an ambulatory oncology research center: A step forward for the field of ambulatory care. *Nursing Economic$*, *22*(2), 58-63.

Dennis, L., Dunn, M., & Benson, G. (1980). *An empirical model for measuring nursing in acute care hospitals.* Chicago: Medicus Systems.

Edwardson (1985). Measuring nursing productivity. *Nursing Economic$*, *3*(1), 9-14.

Haas, S., Hackbarth, D., Cullen P., & Androwich, I. (2000). *Defining nursing intensity in ambulatory care.* Presentation at Midwest Nursing Research Symposium, Cleveland, OH.

Hackbarth, D., Haas, S., Kavanagh, J., & Vlasses, F. (1995). Dimensions of the staff nurse role in ambulatory care: Part I – Methodology and analysis of data on current staff nurse practice. *Nursing Economic$*, *13*(2), 89-98.

Hastings, C. (1997). The changing multidisciplinary team. *Nursing Economic$*, *15*(2), 106-108, 105.

Hastings, C., & Haas, S. (1998). *Update on the AAACN/MGMA staffing study, and Strategies for managing patient satisfaction.* Presented at the American Academy of Ambulatory Care Nursing 23rd Annual Conference, Atlanta, GA.

Johnson, M., & Maas, M. (1997): *Nursing outcomes classification (NOC): Iowa outcomes project.* St. Louis: Mosby.

Jones, A., Cusack, G., & Chisholm, L. (2004). Patient intensity in an ambulatory oncology research center: A step forward for the field of ambulatory care – Part II. *Nursing Economic$*, *22*(3), 120-123.

Ruh, W. (1982). The measurement of white collar productivity. *National Productivity Review*, Autumn, 16-26.

U.S. Department of Health and Human Services (DHHS), Division of Nursing. (2004). *National sample survey of registered nurses.* Rockville, MD: Health Services and Resource Administration, Bureau of Health Professionals, Division of Nursing.

Verran, J. (1981). Delineation of ambulatory care nursing practice. *Journal of Ambulatory Care Management, 4*(2), 1-13.

Additional Readings

American Academy of Ambulatory Care Nursing (AAACN). (2005). *Ambulatory care staffing: An annotated bibliography.* Pitman, NJ: Author.

Fey, M.K., & Miltner, R.S. (2000). A competency-based orientation program for new graduate nurses. *Journal of Nursing Administration, 30*(3), 126-132.

Haas, S. (1992). Coaching: developing key players. *Journal of Nursing Administration, 22*(6), 54-58.

Hastings, C. (1995). Orientation and competency assessment in ambulatory care, Presented at the AAACN Workshop: *Role transitions into ambulatory care nursing.* Orange, CA, & Oakland, CA, November.

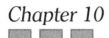
Staffing and Workload

This test may be copied for use by others.

COMPLETE THE FOLLOWING:

Name: _____

Address: _____

City: _____ State: _____ Zip: _____

Preferred telephone: (Home)_____ (Work)_____

E-mail_____

AAACN Member Expiration Date: _____

Registration fee: AAACN Member: $12.00
                    Nonmember: $20.00

Answer Form:

1. If you applied what you have learned from this activity into your practice, what would be different?

_____

_____

_____

Evaluation	Strongly disagree				Strongly agree
2. By completing this activity, I was able to meet the following objectives:					
a. Discuss methods of determining staffing requirements and skill mix in ambulatory care nursing.	1	2	3	4	5
b. Compare and contrast staff recruitment and retention strategies in ambulatory care settings.	1	2	3	4	5
c. Discuss common methods of monitoring productivity in ambulatory care nursing.	1	2	3	4	5
d. Enumerate the issues and challenges with staffing and workload in ambulatory care nursing.	1	2	3	4	5
3. The content was current and relevant.	1	2	3	4	5
4. The objectives could be achieved using the content provided.	1	2	3	4	5
5. This was an effective method to learn this content.	1	2	3	4	5
6. I am more confident in my abilities since completing this material.	1	2	3	4	5

7. The material was (check one) ___new ___review for me.

8. Time required to read this chapter: _____minutes

I verify that I have completed this activity: _____
                                                          Signature

Comments: _____

_____

_____

Objectives

This educational activity is designed for nurses and other health care professionals who practice in ambulatory care. For those wishing to obtain CE credit, an evaluation follows. After studying the information presented in this offering, you will be able to:

1. Discuss methods of determining staffing requirements and skill mix in ambulatory care nursing.
2. Compare and contrast staff recruitment and retention strategies in ambulatory care settings.
3. Discuss common methods of monitoring productivity in ambulatory care nursing.
4. Enumerate the issues and challenges with staffing and workload in ambulatory care nursing.

Posttest Instructions

1. To receive continuing education credit for individual study after reading the article, complete the answer/evaluation form to the left.

2. Detach and send the answer/evaluation form along with a check or money order payable to the *American Academy of Ambulatory Care Nursing (AAACN)*, East Holly Avenue Box 56, Pitman, NJ 08071–0056.

3. Test returns must be postmarked by August 1, 2011. Upon completion of the answer/evaluation form, a certificate for **1.4** contact hour(s) will be awarded and sent to you. Should the material contained in this chapter become outdated prior to the above expiration date, AAACN reserves the right to withdraw this CE test.

This activity is co-provided by the *American Academy of Ambulatory Care Nursing (AAACN)* and Anthony J. Jannetti, Inc. (AJJ). AJJ is accredited as a provider of continuing nursing education by the American Nurses' Credentialing Center's Commission on Accreditation (ANCC-COA). AAACN is a provider approved by the California Board of Registered Nurses, provider number CEP 05336.

This article was reviewed and formatted for contact hour credit by Sally S. Russell, MN, CMSRN, AAACN Education Director; and Candia Baker Laughlin MS, RN, C, Editor.

Telehealth Nursing Practice

Carole A. Becker, MS, RN

Traci S. Haynes, MSN, RN, CEN

Objectives

Study of the information presented in this chapter will enable the learner to:

1. Define telehealth nursing practice.
2. Discuss the scope of telehealth nursing practice, its purpose, and its role within ambulatory care nursing.
3. Describe the core dimensions fundamental to telehealth nursing practice.
4. Discuss the use of decision support tools for assessment and care management.
5. Describe the professional competencies of telehealth nursing practice.
6. Identify risk management strategies that support the safe practice of telehealth nursing.
7. Recognize nursing intervention classifications (NIC) and nursing outcome classifications (NOC) for telehealth nursing.

Key Points

1. Telecommunication technology in health care includes telephones (including telephony), computers, the Internet, interactive video, and teleconferencing.
2. A relationship is created between the consumer and the nurse with each telehealth encounter, and the nurse has a duty to provide safe and effective care.
3. Telehealth nursing follows the nursing process with emphasis on assessment and communication skills.

This chapter will describe telehealth nursing and its support of improved access, quality, and cost-efficiency of health care delivery, regardless of whether the setting is a centralized call center or any decentralized ambulatory practice setting. Consumers seek assistance in making health care decisions, finding answers to their health care questions, learning more about self-management of specific conditions, and receiving emotional support. Telehealth nursing practice supports the achievement of the six specific Institute of Medicine (IOM) aims for health care quality improvement (safe, effective, patient-centered, timely, efficient, and equitable) (Institute of Medicine, 2001). Today, telehealth nursing practice is recognized as a nursing subspecialty by the American Academy of Ambulatory Care Nursing (AAACN) and the American Nurses Association (ANA) (AAACN, 2005).

Telehealth Nursing Practice Defined

A. Definitions approved and adopted by the Telehealth Nursing Practice Special Interest Group (Greenberg, Espensen, Becker, & Cartwright, 2003).

1. *Telehealth:* "The delivery, management, and coordination of health services that integrate electronic information and telecommunications technologies to increase access, improve outcomes, and contain or reduce costs of health care." *Telehealth* is used as an umbrella term to describe the wide range of services delivered across distances by all health-related disciplines.

2. *Telehealth nursing:* "The delivery, management, and coordination of care and services provided via telecommunications technology within the domain of nursing." Telehealth nursing is a subset of telehealth, encompassing all types of nursing care and servic-

es delivered across distances. Telehealth nursing is a broad term encompassing practices that incorporate a vast array of telecommunications technologies (for example, telephone, fax, electronic mail, Internet, video monitoring, and interactive video) to remove time and distance barriers for the delivery of nursing care.

3. *Telephone nursing:* "All care and services within the scope of nursing practice that are delivered over the telephone." A component of telehealth nursing practice restricted to the telephone.

4. *Telephone triage:* "An interactive process between nurse and client that occurs over the telephone and involves identifying the nature and urgency of client health care needs and determining the appropriate disposition." A component of telephone nursing practice that focuses on assessment and prioritization and referral to the appropriate level of care.

B. Evolution of telehealth nursing practice.

1. The word triage originated from the French word "trier," which means to pick or sort. It was used by the French military to designate where wounded soldiers would be sent. Later, the U.S. military used the term "triage" to identify a sorting station for wounded solders, who would then be transported to secondary facilities (Newberry, 2003).

2. An often-repeated story identifies the first telehealth interaction occurring during a telephone call by Alexander Graham Bell. He was calling for Mr. Watson, his assistant, to come and help him with an injury to his hand.

3. In the last half of the 1970s, health maintenance organizations (HMOs) began using telephone triage and advice services as a "gatekeeping" effort to control patients' access to care.

4. In the early 1980s, hospital marketing departments began providing physician and service referral, class registration, and consumer health education along with triage and advice services to attract and retain market share.

5. The proliferation of managed care organizations further expanded telehealth services for:

a. Demand management.
b. Recertification and referral authorization.
c. Customer services providing information and assistance regarding benefits, eligibility, and assistance with provider relations.
d. Member services including enrollment, health risk appraisals, and primary care provider selection (Briggs, 2002).

6. Increased incidence of chronic illness, rising health care costs, and increased emphasis on the delivery of quality health care have motivated the development of services that incorporate telehealth nursing as a care delivery strategy.

a. Disease management.
b. Care management.
c. Case management.
d. Clinical prevention services.

Scope of Practice for Telehealth Nursing Practice

State boards of nursing define the scope of nursing practice for each state. It is important for registered nurses to be familiar with the nurse practice act and the rules and regulations in the practice of nursing in their state of residence. A scope of practice statement describes the who, what, where, when, why, and how of nursing practice (ANA, 2004).

A. Experienced registered nurses deliver telehealth nursing care in all settings of ambulatory care as well as in formal call center programs. They utilize their knowledge and apply the nursing process to meet the actual or potential health needs of clients. They are supported by telecommunication technology and decision support tools to provide care 24/7.

B. The purpose of telehealth nursing practice.

1. Improve access to health care for individuals, groups, and specific patient populations at risk.

2. Improve the quality of health care outcomes through patient-centered, collaborative care.

3. Improve the cost efficiency of care delivery by meeting the needs of patients with timely and appropriate resources.

Standards of Telehealth Nursing Practice

Standards are authoritative statements the nursing profession uses to describe the responsibilities for which its practitioners are accountable. Standards reflect the values and priorities of the profession. They provide direction for professional nursing practice and a framework for the evaluation of this practice. Standards of professional nursing practice describe a competent level of nursing practice and professional performance common to all registered nurses (ANA, 2004).

A. Standards relevant to telehealth nursing.
1. Legal standards: State nurse practice acts and the rules and regulations for the practice of nursing.
2. Professional standards pertaining to telehealth nursing practice. Developed by accrediting professional organizations and applied to general or specialty practice.
    a. *Telephone Nursing Practice Administration and Practice Standards* were first published in 1997 by AAACN. They were reviewed and broadened in 2001, and re-titled *Telehealth Nursing Practice Administration and Practice Standards* to reflect advancement of practice. They were last revised and published in 2004.
    b. General standards applicable to telephone nursing: American Association of Office Nurses (AAON), *Office Nursing Practice Standards for Quality Care of Patients* (Jones, 2004).
    c. Position statement applicable for telephone nursing: Emergency Nurse Association (ENA), *Position Statement Telephone Advice*, developed in 1991, most recently revised in 2001 (ENA, 2001).
    d. Position statement applicable for telehealth nursing: National Association of School Nurses (NASN), *Position Statement Use of Telehealth in the Practice of School Nursing*, developed in 2002 (NASN, 2002).
3. Regulatory standards.
    a. Developed by local and state health departments and federal agencies, such as *Americans with Disabilities Act* (ADA) and *Occupational Safety and Health Administration* (OSHA).
    b. Developed by national organizations such as:
        (1) Joint Commission for Accreditation of Healthcare Organizations (JCAHO) *2005-2006 Standards for Ambulatory Care* (JCAHO, 2005).
        (2) American Accreditation Healthcare Commission/URAC (2005) has developed *Health Call Center Accreditation Standards* for organizations that provide clinical triage and health information services (American Accreditation Healthcare Commission/URAC, 2005).
4. Organizational standards.
    a. Define performance expectations for the telehealth practice nurse within the organizational structure.
    b. Organizational standards include:
        (1) Policies and procedures.
        (2) Position descriptions.
        (3) Performance standards.
        (4) Standards of care.
        (5) Decision support tools.

Core Dimensions Fundamental to Telehealth Nursing Practice

While core dimensions provide a basis for all nursing practice, telehealth nursing has its own unique dimensions that set it apart from other nursing subspecialties. The most notable difference in telehealth nursing practice is not being in the physical presence of the patient. This results in adaptation of the nursing process, with increased emphasis on assessment and communication skills.

A. Dimensions of telehealth nursing practice.
1. Systematically assesses patient needs using decision support tools and clinical judgment.
2. Builds rapport and trust quickly to assess patient/caller's needs and to determine urgency in time-limited encounters.
3. Applies relevant communication techniques utilizing telecommunication devices to interact and educate patients.
4. Facilitates collaboration for the planning of care with patients, their support systems, and providers of health care.

5. Documents the telecommunication interaction.
6. Utilizes telecommunication technology to provide patient care.
7. Demonstrates knowledge of legal issues specific to telehealth nursing practice.
8. Evaluates outcomes of telehealth practice using quality measurements.
9. Maintains confidentiality of telehealth encounters (AAACN, 2003).

B. The nursing process in telehealth nursing practice – The nursing process consists of interrelated steps that provide the blueprint for consistent care delivery in all patient settings, including telehealth. It promotes humanistic outcome-focused, cost-effective care (Alfaro-Lefevre, 2002). AAACN has developed a model that illustrates the interactive, circular relationship of the nursing process for telehealth nursing practice (see Figure 11-1). The core reflects the interaction between the nurse and the patient/caregiver. The nurse prioritizes the urgency of the situation based on assessment data, utilizes decision support tools, and collaborates with other health care professionals and the patient/caregiver to develop a plan of care, implement appropriate interventions, and evaluate the outcome (AAACN, 2003).

Figure 11-1

Model of Telehealth Nursing Practice

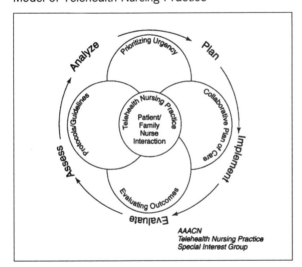

AAACN
Telehealth Nursing Practice
Special Interest Group

1. Assessment – Data collection.
   a. The reason for the call or patient's chief complaint.
   b. Medical history – Confirming diagnosed health care problems, allergies, prescribed and over-the-counter medications, and alternative therapies.
   c. History of symptoms and associated symptoms.
   d. Focused assessment of the patient's actual or potential health needs.
2. Analyze and plan – Continually analyze the data gathered to develop an effective plan of care.
   a. Use decision support tools to prioritize the triage category (such as emergent, urgent, non-urgent).
   b. Reference other resources as appropriate and/or collaborate with others.
   c. Determine the disposition of the patient based on acuity of symptoms (for example, 911, emergency department, walk-in clinic, self care) and nursing diagnosis.
3. Implementation – Putting the plan into action.
   a. Define plan that is patient-centered.
   b. Carry out the interventions that are in control of the nurse (such as transferring calls to 911, scheduling of provider appointment).
      (1) Facilitate follow-up care and coordinate resources (such as referrals).
      (2) Provide information and education (such as providing home care measures for symptoms).
   c. Intervention carried out by the patient/caregiver.
      (1) Nurse utilizes communication/counseling skills that induce actions to achieve desired outcomes.
   d. Documentation of nursing process.
4. Evaluation – Achievement of expected outcome.
   a. Patient's understanding, acceptance, and implementation of the plan of care, including when to call back for further intervention.
   b. Follow-up actions and plans of the nurse.
   c. Analyze/re-evaluate effectiveness of each step of the nursing process.

Telehealth Assessment

Registered nurses do not medically diagnose but assess patients and make critical decisions regarding appropriate care. Assessing patients in most practice settings involves face-to-face interactions in which the nurse is able to use all sensory input (auditory, visual, olfactory, and tactile), along with both verbal and non-verbal communication. The assessment of patients using telecommunication devices is unique because the locus of assessment changes. Additionally, the nurse must be sensitive to verbal and emotional cues communicated through speech as well as the presence of background sound (AAACN, 2003).

A. The locus of assessment shifts to the patient/caregiver.
   1. The nurse must guide the patient in assessing symptoms.
      a. The nurse needs to listen, interpret, and direct the patient during the assessment process.
      b. The patient is an active partner in the assessment and is the primary assessor (for example, the patient must actively determine the site of pain and describe the location to the nurse).
      c. There must be clear delineation between the patient being an active participant in assessment and the patient self-diagnosing.
   2. The locus of assessment may not be with the patient, but with the caller/caregiver who is with the patient.
      a. The caregiver becomes the eyes and ears for the nurse.
      b. The nurse directs the caregiver to describe what they observe.
B. The locus of care is not physically with the nurse. The patient/caregiver carries out interventions appropriate for the assessed needs.
C. The telecommunication encounter is time-limited.
   1. The communication must be focused upon moving the caller to the next best step or level of intervention.
   2. The nurse must focus on the most important needs of the encounter.
   3. Extensive needs of a caller/patient may indicate that an in-person assessment is required.

Telehealth Communication

The key to the telehealth assessment is the interaction with the patient or caregiver. The nurse must develop a partnership in order to initiate interactive health care management. Interactions are brief, with communication techniques focusing on obtaining detailed information without the use of tactile or visual senses.

A. The nurse directs the caller to examine self or the patient.
   1. The caller uses techniques provided by the nurse.
   2. The nurse interprets the caller's description of symptoms, location, and appearance.
B. The nurse must establish trust immediately to elicit accurate information.
   1. Identifies self to caller with name and title.
   2. Identifies the patient by name, and if the patient is not the caller, the relationship to the caller.
   3. Identifies the patient's relationship to the provider (for example, established patient or new patient).
C. The nurse demonstrates expert communication skills.
   1. Uses open-ended and close-ended questions appropriately.
   2. Uses active listening techniques.
   3. Seeks the reason for the call from the patient's/caller's perspective and identifies preferences.
   4. Identifies any hidden agendas for the call (such as exploring why the caller is really calling and what the caller expects to achieve/obtain from the interaction).
   5. Clarifies the caller's statements to understand his or her descriptions.
      a. Directs the caller to clarify location of symptoms by instructing to point to the area and describe in relation to well-known anatomical part (for example, the "belly button").
      b. Asks the caller to quantify and qualify symptoms by using pain scales, common sizes (such as pea size, quarter size).

6. Utilizes terminology consistent with the patient/caller's level of comprehension.

7. Utilizes counseling skills such as motivational interviewing or positive reframing to support self-management behaviors.

D. The nurse manages multiple symptoms' presentations or co-morbidity.

1. Hearing the caller describe multiple symptoms.

2. Identifying primary symptoms and secondary symptoms.

3. Sorting and prioritizing these symptoms.

4. Discouraging caller's self-diagnosis and/or bias toward treatment.

E. The nurse maintains confidentiality of interactions.

1. Patient interactions take place in a private environment away from other patients, visitors, and inappropriate personnel.

2. Disclosure statements are signed by patients before information is provided to family members or others. Care of minor children or incompetent adults is handled according to legal statutes and institutional policy (see Chapter 8, *Legal Aspects of Ambulatory Care Nursing*).

3. Records of calls are safeguarded against breach in confidentiality and in accordance with HIPAA.

Decision Support Tools

A decision support tool is a plan or guide for the assessment and management of an actual or potential health problem(s) for individuals, groups, or at-risk populations to reduce the risk of omissions and increase the predictability of desired outcomes. Decision support tools support, but do not replace, the use of the nursing process and critical thinking skills used by the telehealth nurse to meet the unique needs of a patient and his or her preferences, given the situation and available resources. Protocols, guidelines, algorithms, and care pathways are some of the terms used as descriptors for decision support tools.

A. Desirable attributes of evidence-based guidelines (IOM, 1990).

1. *Validity* – Result in desired health and cost management outcomes.

2. *Reliability* – Given like or similar clinical presentation, other clinicians concur with the content and process.

3. *Applicability* – Explicitly describes the population to which they apply.

4. *Flexibility* – Identifies specific clinical cautions for patient populations.

5. *Clarity* – Unambiguous language and precise definitions of terms.

6. *Multi-disciplinary input* – Participation by representatives of key affected groups in the development and review.

7. *Scheduled review* – Defined review cycle.

8. *Documentation* – Citation of references, assumptions, procedures, and analytic methods must be documented and described.

B. Purpose and benefits of using decision support tools for assessment, triage, and care management of patients.

1. Provide safe, effective, appropriate care and disposition for the actual or potential health needs of individuals, groups, or patient populations.

2. Provide standardization of care to achieve desired outcomes.

3. Improve efficiency of assessment process.

4. Decrease omissions or harmful practices.

5. Facilitate the ease, efficiency, and retrievability of appropriate documentation.

6. Support evidence-based interventions.

7. Reduce liability risk.

8. Meet accreditation standards.

9. Enhance evaluation of performance.

C. Content and structure of decision support tools.

1. Symptom-based or condition-specific. Not intended to medically diagnose, but to evaluate acuity of symptoms and facilitate appropriate care to improve health outcomes.

2. Description of the scope of guideline subject, defining what it does and does not include.

3. Overview or background information, discussing pertinent clinical indicators, risk factors, and assessment parameters for the subject.

4. Sequenced assessment questions to determine clinical needs and urgency of symptoms. Organized in groupings designating acuity level (for example, emergent, urgent, non-urgent, self care).

5. Clinical alerts that define or clarify the assessment parameters to increase reliabili-

ty. Clinical alerts also include pertinent clinical information such as age-specific risk factors, unusual presentations, or clinical rationale to support clinical judgment.

6. Self care measures that provide detailed information on first aid or self care to manage or resolve symptoms.

7. Defined directions for the patients/callers regarding "watchful waiting" or warning signs that describe symptoms to watch for and stated timeframes for seeking care if these symptoms occur, worsen, or do not improve.

8. Disposition information describing the appropriate site, provider, and timeframe of care, for example:
   a. *Emergent* – 911 or emergency department.
   b. *Urgent* – Seek medical care within the next 4 to 6 hours.
   c. *Non-urgent* – Ranging from seek medical care within 24 hours to home/self care.

9. Reference list citing sources used to develop the guideline.

D. Common ambulatory care situations utilizing guidelines.
   1. Telephone triage, counseling, and education programs.
   2. Case management and disease management services; may include use of home monitoring devices.
   3. Crises lines for suicide prevention, child abuse, etc.
   4. Hot lines or support lines for HIV/AIDS, substance abuse, etc.
   5. Ambulatory procedures and examinations (such as ocular examinations, auditory evaluation, glucose tolerance testing).
   6. Anticipatory guidance counseling sessions.
   7. Perioperative care.
   8. Post-hospitalization follow-up.

E. Perceived disadvantages of using guidelines for assessment, triaging, and care of patients in a telehealth situation.
   1. For professional registered nurse.
      a. Focus on single condition or symptom. Co-morbidity increases complexity of nursing intervention.

      b. Requires in-depth training and experience to become proficient.
      c. Patient interaction is more structured than an impromptu interaction.
   2. For physician/provider.
      a. Perceived loss of control for each patient's plan of care.
      b. Conflict in allowing professional registered nurse empowerment in assessment and triage decisions.
   3. For administration.
      a. Concern of guidelines being expensive to develop, maintain, or purchase.
      b. Concern of risk management issues if guidelines are not strictly followed by all nurses.

Professional Competencies

Defined competencies for telehealth nursing practice identify the behaviors and outcomes specific to providing efficient, effective, evidenced-based care (AAACN, 2004). Competencies should be measurable and include:

A. Professional knowledge – A minimum of 3 to 5 years of applicable clinical nursing experience is the industry average before employment in a telehealth nursing position (AAACN, 2005).
   1. Call processing: Manages clinical calls using the nursing process.
   2. Assessment: Demonstrates critical thinking skills in assessing covert and overt parameters relevant to the needs of the caller.
   3. Age-specific competencies: Provides care consistent with the functional requirements of the person's developmental age.
   4. Cultural awareness: Provides culturally sensitive care to diverse populations.
   5. Interventions and outcomes: Uses clinical judgment and effective interventions to enhance patient/client outcomes.

B. Interpersonal skills.
   1. Trust relationship: Establishes a trust relationship to elicit accurate patient/caller information.
   2. Communication skills:
      a. Uses effective interpersonal communication skills to engage in, develop, and disengage in a therapeutic interaction.

      b. Uses communication skills to facilitate collaboration, such as negotiation, conflict resolution, group decision making, etc.

    3. Counseling skills: Utilizes counseling skills to facilitate patient self-management behaviors, such as motivational interviewing, positive reframing, etc.

    4. Customer service: Applies customer service skills when interacting with a caller.

C. Technical skills.

    1. Telecommunication technologies: Adapts to equipment and demonstrates efficient use of technology devices to perform role.

    2. Software programs: Understands, selects, and uses relevant software programs appropriately.

    3. Care management and analysis: Uses selected program decision support tools to address caller/patient needs in order to identify actual and potential health risks.

D. Documentation of telehealth encounters: Documents telecommunications encounters that reflect care specific to the actual or potential health needs of the caller/patient.

E. Personal and professional development: Accepts personal responsibility for maintaining and improving the knowledge and skills necessary to assess, triage, and manage patients.

    1. Core education is included in the *AAACN Telehealth Nursing Practice Core Course* (TNPCC) (AAACN, 2003).

    2. The Telephone Nursing Practice Certification Examination requires 2 years of experience in telephone nursing, which comprises a minimum of 2,000 hours (National Certification Corporation [NCC], 2005).

    3. Researching and defining practice as further concepts in medical and nursing management are developed, including personal health management, disease management, quality management, and outcome management.

    4. Remaining abreast of telehealth changes and recommending improvements for practice.

    5. Advancing telehealth nursing by demonstrating professional clinical knowledge, critical thinking, participating in quality improvement, and utilizing research related to clinical practice.

F. Resource management: Internal and external resource utilization. Locates and utilizes appropriate resources to meet the needs of caller/patient.

G. Practice and administrative issues: Practices in accordance with an ethical, legal, and organizational framework that ensures the caller's/ patient's interest and well being are met (AAACN, 2005).

Risk Management and Quality Improvement Strategies for Telehealth Nursing Practice

With the initiation of each telehealth encounter, a relationship is created between the consumer and the nurse, and the nurse has a duty to provide safe and effective care. It is expected that the nurse will provide a level of care that would be given by a reasonable, prudent nurse under the same or similar circumstances. Published professional standards, such as *the Telehealth Nursing Practice Administration and Practice Standards* (AAACN, 2004), define the responsibilities for which its practitioners are accountable. There are inherent risks with all clinical practice, and in a highly litigious environment, it is important to consider proactive strategies to reduce risk and to minimize potential liability associated with telehealth practice.

A. Program planning needed to meet quality standards.

    1. Define program mission and goals.

    2. Define roles and responsibilities consistent with state practice acts and professional standards.

    3. Develop policies and procedures specific to telehealth services to promote standardization that include, but are not limited to:

      a. Management of emergencies or at-risk situations (potential suicide, violence and abuse, childbirth, any basic life support situation, calls from minors, reportable conditions, etc.).

      b. Call management processes, such as maintaining confidentiality, dealing with anonymous callers or those refusing to provide information, timeframe for returning calls/delay of care, inability to contact patient/caller, second or third-party calls, dealing with non-compliant callers or repeat callers, access to emergency medical services, etc.

c. Knowledge and appropriate use of approved guidelines, including how to manage callers with multiple symptoms, overriding dispositions, presenting symptoms not covered in a guideline, etc.

4. Assignment of a medical director or panel of physicians to review guidelines, and policies and procedures, serve as a resource for clinical issues and participate in outcome management and quality improvement processes.

B. Documentation of telehealth encounters – Thorough and accurate documentation of telehealth encounters communicates relevant patient data to other health care providers to promote continuity of care and aid collaboration. Documentation supports reimbursement for care provided, and in turn, helps define the value of telehealth services. It is also utilized by professional disciplines and accrediting agencies to judge the quality of care delivered. Complete documentation is usually described as one of the most effective ways to protect oneself from legal risk. The method and format for documenting calls is organizationally defined and should be consistently followed in daily practice.

1. Basic encounter documentation should include:
   a. Date and time of the encounter.
   b. Patient's legal name with confirmed spelling.
   c. Date of birth.
   d. Name of person calling, if other than the patient, and relationship to patient.
   e. Patient's reason for call.
      (1) In caller's own words; use quotations to indicate precise verbiage.
      (2) Stated expectations and/or perceived urgency.
   f. Phone number and location.
2. Relevant history, including diagnosed health problems and health risks, current medications and use of any alternative treatments, allergies, recent injuries, procedures, and infection or exposure to infectious disease.
3. Assessment of symptom(s), including onset, location, duration, character, effect of symptom(s) on usual activities, history of similar

symptoms, and associated or other symptoms. It is also helpful to know if any patient action has worsened or improved the symptoms.

4. Guideline selected for client's symptom(s).
5. Interventions, including suggested home care, disposition, and follow-up plans. It is important to consider any barriers that might limit the patient/caregiver's ability to carry out suggested interventions, such as comorbidity, emotional state, ability to understand, impact of symptoms on ability to carry out activities of daily living, and ability to access care. In these instances, it is imperative that clinical decisions are made to best meet the patient's needs.
6. Verification of patient's understanding and intended action.

C. Staff education and performance management processes.
1. Orientation.
2. Formal training for preceptors.
3. Competency verification.
4. Continuing education opportunities.

D. Defined quality improvement process.
1. The Institute of Medicine (2001) defined quality as "The degree to which health services for individual and populations increase the likelihood of desired health outcomes and are consistent with current professional knowledge" (p. 232).
2. Outcomes measurement simply defined is the collection and reporting of information about the relationship of interventions to the results of care. The challenge is to define and measure outcome indicators for clinical effectiveness in telehealth nursing practice and to identify action plans for improvement of care.
3. Outstanding needs:
   a. Data and format standardization to support comparisons.
   b. Longitudinal as well as episodic data.
   c. Evaluation of variables that impact results.
4. Examples of effectiveness measures focusing on nurse-sensitive outcomes:
   a. Increased compliance with treatment plans.
   b. Increased rates of age-specific immunizations.
   c. Increased participation in age-appropri-

ate health screenings.
d. Improved functional status.
e. Earlier identification of condition-specific complication.
f. Satisfaction with nursing care.

Telehealth Nursing Interventions and Outcomes

Telehealth nursing includes nursing interventions "based upon clinical judgment and knowledge that a nurse performs to enhance patient/client outcomes" (McCloskey & Bulechek, 2000).
A. Approved nursing intervention classifications (NIC) for telephone nursing (McCloskey & Bulechek, 2000).
   1. Telephone consultation.
      a. Definition: "Eliciting patients' concerns, listening and providing support, information, or teaching in response to patient's stated concerns, over the telephone" (McCloskey & Bulechek, 2000, p. 659).
      b. Activity examples: Identify self with name and credentials, inform patient about call process, establish level of caller's knowledge, provide means of overcoming identified barriers to learning.
   2. Triage: Telephone.
      a. Definition: "Determining the nature and urgency of a problem(s) and providing directions for the level of care required over the telephone" (McCloskey & Bulechek, 2000, p. 675).
      b. Activity examples: Direct, facilitate, and calm the caller; prioritize reported symptoms; use standardized symptom-based guidelines; maintain confidentiality; and discuss and resolve problems with collegial help.
   3. Telephone follow-up.
      a. Definition: "Providing results of testing or evaluating patients' response and determining potential for problems as a result of previous treatment examination, or testing, over the telephone" (McCloskey & Bulechek, 2000, p. 661).
      b. Activity examples: Obtain consent to disclose test results to non-patient, provide

information on community resources, document education-provided and resultant self-care responsibilities.
   4. Surveillance: Remote electronic.
      a. Definition: "Purposeful and ongoing acquisition of patient data via electronic modalities (telephone, video conference, e-mail) from distant locations, as well as interpretation and synthesis of patient data for clinical decision making with individuals or population" (McCloskey & Bulechek, 2000, p. 663).
      b. Activity examples: Determine the patient's health risk(s), identify data with problematic or population implications, monitor data for validity and reliability, monitor patient-coping strategies.
B. Nursing outcome classifications (NOC) that can be applied to telehealth nursing. A detailed description of the NIC/NOC system for telehealth nursing is available in the *Nursing Interventions Classification* (McCloskey & Bulecheck, 2000).
   1. Telephone consultation, examples of NOCs: Acceptance, health status, anxiety control, caregiver outcomes, compliance behavior, information processing.
   2. Telephone triage, examples of NOCs: Decision making, self-care outcomes, suicide self-restraint.
   3. Telephone follow-up, examples of NOCs: Coping, participation, health care decisions, well-being.
   4. Telephone surveillance, examples of NOCs: Risk control, risk detection (Haas & Androwich, 1999).

Operational Elements of a Telehealth Nursing Service

Each practice setting has unique services and patient populations. Key to an effective telehealth nursing service is determining its role as a value-added service in supporting the health care organization's strategic initiatives. It is therefore imperative to identify both the essential components of a telehealth nursing program as well as the demand for telehealth nursing care to provide optimal services. Additional considerations include practice setting/workspace design and technological needs.

A. Foundational components of a telehealth nursing service/program.
  1. Defined purpose and mission.
  2. Defined scope of practice.
  3. Formal orientation and continuing education.
  4. Assessment of competencies for role performance.
  5. Decision support tools.
  6. Program-specific policies and procedures.
  7. Continuous performance improvement processes.
B. Identify the demands and needs for telehealth care.
  1. Patient populations that will contact the service/provider.
  2. Patient's expectation of a telehealth service (such as symptom assessment, clarification of instructions, reinforcement of education, prescriptions).
C. Identify the specific populations being served.
  1. Special needs (such as elderly patients, oncology patients, indigent populations).
  2. Cultural issues (such as language barriers, differences in self-care management).
D. Identify the telecommunication flow and prioritization of encounter handling.
  1. Systematically sort encounters and develop internal triaging.
    a. Prioritize symptoms by acuity and handle before non-symptom/general encounters.
    b. Assessment and triage performed only by registered nurses or physicians.
    c. All personnel recognize emergency encounters and notify appropriate personnel to handle immediately.
  2. Efficiently and effectively respond to telecommunication encounters.
E. Analyze telecommunication encounter volumes.
  1. Identify peak access days and times.
  2. Identify the "waiting time" for answering the initial encounter.
  3. Identify the "holding time" after answering the encounter.
  4. Develop staffing models to meet encounter demands.
  5. Identify reasons for abandoned encounters.
  6. Identify inappropriate messaging.
F. Create methods to decrease telecommunication demand.

  1. Develop educational brochures for patients on care of illnesses.
  2. Provide ambulatory patients with written discharge instructions.
  3. Provide descriptors of when/how to contact the telehealth nursing service.
G. Determine the telehealth nursing service location/physical space.
  1. Identify the practice setting where patient confidentiality will be maintained.
  2. Identify amount of work surface and storage needed to support type of work performed.
  3. Consider sound control/noise reduction (such as height of walls if cubicle design, acoustic wall paneling).
  4. Provide overhead lighting that is non-glare as well as adjustable task lighting.
  5. Consider ergonomics when designing work space (such as seating, monitor position, keyboard).
  6. Determine type of headsets to be used if communication involves use of telephone.
H. Determine technological needs.
  1. Evaluate computer hardware/software needs to support documentation of encounter and use of decision support tools.
  2. Evaluate telecommunication device and system needs based on volume assumptions, hours of operation, and flow of encounter.

References

Alfaro-LeFevre, R. (2002). *Applying nursing process promoting collaborative care* (5th ed.). Philadelphia: Lippincott.

American Academy of Ambulatory Care Nursing (AAACN). (2003). *Telehealth nursing practice core course manual* (2nd ed.). Pitman, NJ: Author.

American Academy of Ambulatory Care Nursing. (AAACN). (2004). *Telehealth nursing practice administration and practice standards* (3rd ed.). Pitman, NJ: Author.

American Academy of Ambulatory Care Nursing (AAACN). (2005). *A guide to ambulatory care nursing orientation and competency assessment.* Pitman, NJ: Author.

American Accreditation Healthcare Commission/URAC. (2005). *Health call center accreditation program.* Retrieved September 16, 2005, from www.urac.org

American Nurses Association (ANA). (2004). *Nursing: Scope and standards of practice.* Washington, DC: Author.

Briggs, J.K. (2002). *Telephone triage protocols for nurses* (2nd ed.). Philadelphia: Lippincott.

Emergency Nurses Association (ENA). (2001). *Position statement telephone advice.* Retrieved on September 26, 2005, from http://www.ena.org/about/position/

Greenberg, M., Espensen, M., Becker, C., & Cartwright, J. (2003). Telehealth nursing practice SIG adopts teleterms. *AAACN Viewpoint, 25*(1), 8-10.

Haas S., & Androwich, I. (1999). Telephone consultation. In G. Bulechek & J. McCloskey (Eds.), *Nursing interventions: Effective nursing treatment* (3rd ed.), 670-684. Philadelphia: W.B. Saunders.

Institute of Medicine (IOM). (1990). *Clinical practice guidelines: Directions for a new program*. Washington, DC: National Academy Press.

Institute of Medicine (IOM). (2001). Crossing the quality chasm: A new health system for the 21st century. In: *Committee on good quality of health care in America*. Washington, DC: National Academy Press.

Joint Commission on Accreditation of Healthcare Organizations (JCAHO). (2005). *2005-2006 Standards for ambulatory care (SAC)*. Retrieved September 26, 2005, from http//store.trihost.com/jcaho/dept.asp?

Jones, M.A. (Ed.). (2004). *Office nursing practice standards for quality care of patients* (2nd ed.). Montvale, NJ: American Association of Office Nurses (AAON).

McCloskey, G., & Bulechek, J. (Eds.). (2000). *Nursing interventions classification (NIC)* (3rd ed.). St. Louis: Mosby.

National Association of School Nurses (NASN). (2002). *Position statement use of telehealth in the practice of school nursing*. Retrieved September 26, 2005, from http://www.nasn.org/positions/positions.htm

National Certification Corporation (NCC). (2005). *Telephone nursing practice certification exam*. Retrieved September 26, 2005, from http://nccnet.org/public/pages/index.cfm?pageid+1

Newberry, L. (Ed.). (2003). *Sheehy's emergency nursing principles and practice* (5th ed.). St. Louis: Mosby.

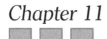

AMBP6c11

CE Answer/Evaluation Form

Telehealth Nursing Practice

This test may be copied for use by others.

COMPLETE THE FOLLOWING:

Name: _____

Address: _____

City: _____ State: _____ Zip: _____

Preferred telephone: (Home)_____ (Work)_____

E-mail_____

AAACN Member Expiration Date: _____

Registration fee: AAACN Member: $12.00
                     Nonmember: $20.00

Answer Form:

1. If you applied what you have learned from this activity into your practice, what would be different?
_____
_____
_____

Evaluation	Strongly disagree				Strongly agree
2. By completing this activity, I was able to meet the following objectives:					
a. Define telehealth nursing practice.	1	2	3	4	5
b. Discuss the scope of telehealth nursing practice, its purpose, and its role within ambulatory care nursing.	1	2	3	4	5
c. Describe the core dimensions fundamental to telehealth nursing practice.	1	2	3	4	5
d. Discuss the use of decision support tools for assessment and care management.	1	2	3	4	5
e. Describe the professional competencies of telehealth nursing practice.	1	2	3	4	5
f. Identify risk management strategies that support the safe practice of telehealth nursing.	1	2	3	4	5
g. Recognize nursing intervention classifications (NIC) and nursing outcome classifications (NOC) for telehealth nursing.	1	2	3	4	5
3. The content was current and relevant.	1	2	3	4	5
4. The objectives could be achieved using the content provided.	1	2	3	4	5
5. This was an effective method to learn this content.	1	2	3	4	5
6. I am more confident in my abilities since completing this material.	1	2	3	4	5

7. The material was (check one) ___new ___review for me.
8. Time required to read this chapter: ____minutes
I verify that I have completed this activity: _____
                                                Signature

Comments: _____
_____
_____

Objectives

This educational activity is designed for nurses and other health care professionals who practice in ambulatory care. For those wishing to obtain CE credit, an evaluation follows. After studying the information presented in this offering, you will be able to:

1. Define telehealth nursing practice.
2. Discuss the scope of telehealth nursing practice, its purpose, and its role within ambulatory care nursing.
3. Describe the core dimensions fundamental to telehealth nursing practice.
4. Discuss the use of decision support tools for assessment and care management.
5. Describe the professional competencies of telehealth nursing practice.
6. Identify risk management strategies that support the safe practice of telehealth nursing.
7. Recognize nursing intervention classifications (NIC) and nursing outcome classifications (NOC) for telehealth nursing.

Posttest Instructions

1. To receive continuing education credit for individual study after reading the article, complete the answer/evaluation form to the left.

2. Detach and send the answer/evaluation form along with a check or money order payable to the *American Academy of Ambulatory Care Nursing (AAACN)*, East Holly Avenue Box 56, Pitman, NJ 08071–0056.

3. Test returns must be postmarked by August 1, 2011. Upon completion of the answer/evaluation form, a certificate for **1.5** contact hour(s) will be awarded and sent to you. Should the material contained in this chapter become outdated prior to the above expiration date, AAACN reserves the right to withdraw this CE test.

This activity is co-provided by the *American Academy of Ambulatory Care Nursing (AAACN)* and Anthony J. Jannetti, Inc. (AJJ). AJJ is accredited as a provider of continuing nursing education by the American Nurses' Credentialing Center's Commission on Accreditation (ANCC-COA). AAACN is a provider approved by the California Board of Registered Nurses, provider number CEP 05336.

This article was reviewed and formatted for contact hour credit by Sally S. Russell, MN, CMSRN, AAACN Education Director; and Candia Baker Laughlin MS, RN, C, Editor.

The Professional Nursing Role in Ambulatory Care

Chapter 12

Leadership

Jane Westmoreland Swanson, PhD, RN, CNAA, BC

Objectives

Study of the information presented in this chapter will enable the learner to:
1. Describe an overview of leadership characteristics and transformational leadership concepts.
2. Describe the importance of collaboration in ambulatory care and colleague relationships.
3. Discuss conflict resolution and strategies.
4. Describe the program planning process for ambulatory care nursing interventions and programs.
5. Discuss various professional activities, associations, and national initiatives.

Key Points

1. Each ambulatory care nurse should be a leader, and should use a variety of leadership skills to problem solve and develop relationships with patients and staff.
2. Ambulatory care nurses should have the ability to be emotionally intelligent.
3. Leaders in ambulatory care need to spot toxic situations and initiate proactive steps to resolve them.
4. Conflict resolution and negotiation strategies are vital to the success of the organization and the well-being of the patient.
5. Strategic plans evaluate the organization and help it attain long-term goals and objectives.

Magnet hospital research indicates that a work environment that fosters professional nursing practice in which nurses are encouraged to use their expertise and judgment is an essential ingredient in increasing job satisfaction among nurses (Aiken, 2002). It is the responsibility of every nursing leader to create a supportive infrastructure that encompasses trust and accountability, whereby nurses have the autonomy to make decisions and practice nursing in accordance with professional standards. Each ambulatory care nurse needs to be a leader. Nurses should use a variety of leadership skills to problem solve and develop relationships as they care for individual patients and families, supervise the work of others, and use evidence-based practice and research process to plan and evaluate ambulatory care programs. This chapter is designed to provide the ambulatory care nurse with an outline of leadership concepts and with the knowledge and skills needed to understand and implement effective leadership and team building. Emphasis is placed on transformational leadership, team building, and collaboration to provide evidence-based practice and evaluation of ambulatory care. Further reference and additional study references are included.

Transformational Leadership In Ambulatory Care

During rapid change, there is a tendency to revert to what one knows has worked in the past. Some leaders may default to a dictatorial command and control-type leadership. However, that style of nonparticipatory leadership in decision making can result in further disengagement of workers, lack of teamwork, and less effective problem solving. A lesson learned from the military is that to make the most effective progress, one needs to engage the intelligence of everyone involved. Utilizing transformation leadership with self-managed teams is far more productive, flexible, and resilient.
A. Major tasks of 21st Century nursing leaders (Wheatley, 2005).
   1. Removing barriers to health care and problem solving.
   2. Alerting staff regarding implications of practice.
   3. Establishing safety around developing new skills and practices.
   4. Anticipating changes and trends early.
   5. Translating changes so that staff members understand the implications and their roles.
   6. Articulating organizations as living systems

where changes in one department impact reactions in other departments.

7. Developing clear core goals that are congruent with the overall mission and understood by all.
8. Demonstrating personal engagement with the changes or "walking the talk."
9. Helping others adapt to the demands of a changing health system.
10. Putting a premium on intelligent action: Individuals taking initiative and making changes.
11. Creating a work environment that is safe and that provides worker satisfaction and constantly updated, relevant information.
12. Highlighting small steps of progress and success while striving for overall change.
13. Celebrating accomplishments when goals are reached and helping to chart the next steps.
14. Recognizing that quick fixes are oxymoron.

B. Transformational leadership is a long-term process.
1. It requires enormous amounts of self-awareness and support.
2. Change requires more time than one usually wants to acknowledge.
3. Real change is usually at least a three to five-year process.

C. Leadership outcomes and maximized skills are evidenced by:
1. High-quality, evidence-based care is provided to patients and families.
2. Supervision of others' work is fostered in a collaborative, value-driven model.
3. Patient population programs involve multiple, interdependent systems with complexity-based models of design that are interdependent.
4. Services are provided efficiently to high volumes of patients in spite of unpredictable clinical and organizational issues.

D. Transformation leadership benefits over hierarchical structures (Porter-O'Grady & Mallock, 2002).
1. Focuses on potential rather than present circumstances.
2. Realizes change and circumstances are different not worse.
3. Realizes that work needs to be shared and is

collaborative, not just the efforts of one individual.
4. Requires broad-based participation.
5. Work is performed differently rather than the "perception of doing more with less."

E. Transformational leadership advantages interrelated systems: More complex and rapid change, and focusing on the potential.
1. Multifocal rather than unilateral interests and goals.
2. Strong alignment of all stakeholders versus allowing non-participation.
3. Driven by mutual interest rather than self-interest.
4. Focus on relatedness rather than function alone.
5. Outcomes-driven rather than just competitive.
6. Centered on improvement and thriving rather than survival focus.
7. Horizontal and vertical linkages rather than vertically integrated.
8. Diverse perceptions honored, yet unifying core beliefs and mutual interests shared.

Transformational Leadership Characteristics For Emotional Competence

Emotionally competent transformational leaders can connect with different groups of people in a variety of context and circumstances by increasing their emotional intelligence. Emotional intelligence is the ability to accurately perceive one's own and others' emotions, to understand the signals that emotions send about the relationship, and to manage one's own and others' emotions. (Goleman, 2004; Porter O'Grady & Mallock, 2002; Swanson, 2000; Wheatley, 2005).

A. Self awareness.
1. Recognition of feelings' impact on self, others, and job performance.
2. Comfortable discussing own strengths and areas for improvement.
3. Appreciation and acceptance of differences.

B. Mindfulness or to "be present."
1. Concentration on the present.
2. Development of deep listening skills.
3. Increased ability to detect trends or patterns.

C. Openness to new ideas.
   1. Appreciation of multiple perspectives.
   2. Development of ability to listen without judgment.
   3. Development of trust.
D. Impulse control.
   1. Ability to temper negative emotions or self-regulate.
   2. Ability to appropriately share emotions and maintain dignity.
   3. Ability to confront conflict and resolve with multiple strategies.
   4. Self-regulation and achievement motivation equal ability to overcome frustration and set backs.
E. Willingness to continually learn and unlearn.
   1. Display of humility and willingness to admit vulnerability of not knowing.
   2. Willingness to let go of old knowledge and accept new learning.
   3. Willingness to emulate best practices and incorporate into processes.
F. Will power and courage.
   1. Willingness to explore new options and take risks.
   2. Willingness to act on convictions and detect trends that are ahead of conventional practice.
   3. Display of integrity as defined by honest and moral actions.
   4. Ability to provide consistent feedback.
G. Compassionate and value driven.
   1. Ability to express sincere empathy without needing to control the situation or solution.
   2. Willingness to clarify and articulate values.
   3. Ability to empathize with others' needs, concerns, and goals.
H. Passionate optimism (Block, 2002).
   1. Enthusiasm and energy regarding work.
   2. Positive mindset.
   3. Idealism sustains our values.
   4. Pride in a job well done.
   5. Unflagging energy to improve performance.
I. Resilience and reflection.
   1. Ability to accept and manage disappointment or setbacks.
   2. Supportive of others to cope with disappointments and grieve loss.
   3. Ability to take time to nurture self and encourage others to live in balance.
   4. Ability to effectively use humor and relieve tension with mirth.

Strategies to Counter Negative Influences, Achieve Positive Outcomes, and Foster Collaboration

Working conditions in health care organizations are not always healthy, and it is important for the leader to stay open to cues of dysfunctional behaviors or toxicity. Dysfunctional behaviors make it more difficult to achieve positive outcomes and create working environments that are energizing and collaborative. The following suggestions help the leader to spot toxicity and initiate proactive steps that foster collaboration and focus upon outcomes central to the stated organizational mission and goals.

A. Keep organizational mission, vision, and values the central focus.
   1. What is the preferred outcome?
   2. Are all plans and strategies focused on the goal?
B. Discuss disagreements.
   1. Encourage voicing diverse opinions that may provide better solutions and multiple options.
   2. Encourage time for discussion, especially from the doubters.
C. Cultivate truth tellers.
   1. Ensure there are individuals present who will tell you what they really think.
   2. Create an environment where it is safe to voice unpopular or unpalatable opinions.
D. Treat others as you would like to be treated.
   1. Observe both actions and verbal responses.
   2. Set a good ethical climate.
   3. Have clear boundaries.
E. Honor your intuition.
   1. If your gut indicates you are being manipulated...you are probably right.
   2. Be honest with yourself.
F. Delegate, don't desert.
   1. Share control and empower staff.
   2. Remember who is ultimately responsible for outcome.
   3. Trust but verify progress reports.
G. Coaching to develop a framework for developing leaders (Dreyfus & Dreyfus, 1996).
   1. Novice stage (initial leadership experience).
      a. Formal education in leadership principles.
      b. Lacks leadership experience.
      c. Usually first formal leadership position.

2. Advanced beginner (active participant).
   a. Increased self-awareness but limited openness to the ideas of others.
   b. Tends to be judgmental.
   c. Increased confidence in the ability to make decisions.
   d. Unsure of the connection between the even and total assessment of the situation.
3. Competent (integrated in process).
   a. Has emerging compassion for others.
   b. Increased teamwork skills and listening ability.
   c. Improved communication and ability to provide both positive and negative feedback.
   d. Increasingly open to others' ideas.
   e. More comfortable in challenging the status quo.
   f. Better at controlling impulses and planning actions.
4. Proficient (therapeutic engagement).
   a. Emerging sense of optimism and ability to manage negative emotions.
   b. More experience in reading situations (recognizes supportive allies, hostile behaviors).
   c. Positive but realistic attitude.
5. Expert (full engagement).
   a. Demonstrates self-awareness and utilized self-assessment information to improve personal performance and team performance.
   b. Possesses and coaches others in positive outlook and workplace resilience.
   c. Provides didactic and emotional support simultaneously.
   d. Very open to others' viewpoints and ideas.
   e. Proactively seeks feedback from team members on their task processes and performance.
   f. Mentors team members and new staff.
   g. Exhibits well-developed impulse control.

Conflict Resolution, Negotiation Strategies, And Alternative Dispute Resolution

Conflict happens frequently in relationships and different perceptions. Conflict resolution has generated a body of literature and research, and many strategies for individuals confronted with conflict in the work environment, including a method known as alternative dispute resolution (ADR). A June 2002 survey about nurse-physician relationships reported, "Although respondents saw a direct link between disruptive physician behavior and nurse satisfaction and retention, the three respondent groups of administrators, physicians, and nurses differed in their beliefs about the outcomes of these conflictual situations" (Rosenstein, 2002, p. 27). Nurses scored the administrative support they received in nurses' conflicts with physicians significantly lower than either the administrators or physicians. Nurses did not feel supported in such conflicts either by their bosses or by other physicians. Nurses also feared retribution and did not believe that physician counseling processes were adequate.

A. Conflict resolution.
   1. Conflict: A situation with multiple viewpoints and where perceptions are not shared, resulting in differing outcomes.
   2. Realities can be distorted or obstructed by imbalances in power.
   3. Negotiation is a process or activity to create a range of possibilities to resolve a conflict.
B. Guidelines for creating conditions for negotiation.
   1. Develop an even playing field, although it may be very difficult to provide equal places for all parties.
   2. Acknowledge the dominant culture or world view that is present in the situation.
   3. Creating alternative solutions and a range of possibilities.
C. Conflict management strategies and outcomes.
   1. Valentine (2001) reports a synthesis of research findings about nurses' conflict management strategies as identified by use of the Thomas-Kilmann Index (TKI).
   2. The TKI is a conflict mode index that identifies preferred conflict management strategies from a set of five options: Avoiding, compromising, collaborating, competing, accommodating.

3. Conflict strategies used predominately by all categories of nurses, in order of decreasing frequency, are avoiding, compromising, and accommodating.
   a. Avoiding: One party does not pursue own concerns or those of the other party; uses withdrawal and suppression.
      (1) Useful situations: As a cool-down mechanism when confronting issues so damaging as to outweigh benefits; need for information; for trivial issues or when one party is much more powerful.
      (2) Outcomes: Lose-lose; unassertive; short-term resolution.
   b. Compromising: One party gives up something to satisfy both parties; middle position.
      (1) Useful situations: Quick fix for temporary settlement of complex issues; for inconsequential issues; when goals are important but not worth major disruption; backup when collaboration and competition fail.
      (2) Outcomes: No-win, no-lose; moderately assertive, cooperative; short-term resolution.
   c. Collaboration: One party works with the other party to find a solution that satisfies both parties; cooperative, confronting issues.
      (1) Useful situations: Merge insights from different perspectives for crucial issues; gains understanding; gains commitment for change; solves disruptive emotional issues; spreads responsibility and risk taking.
      (2) Outcomes: Win-win; fully assertive, cooperative; long-term resolution.
   d. Accommodation: One party neglects own concerns to satisfy concerns of others; emphasizes similarities, minimizes differences, self-sacrificing.
      (1) Useful situations: For routine issues; when one is wrong; when the issue is more important to the other party; when outmatched; to build credits for later use; to pre-

serve harmony; to teach others.
      (2) Outcomes; Lose-win; unassertive, cooperative, short term resolutions.
   e. Competing: One party wins, one party loses; power-oriented, high concern for self; low concern for others.
      (1) Useful situations: Quick decisions; unpopular causes: issues vital to organization; defense against people who exploit noncompetitive behaviors; knowledgeable person able to make decision.
      (2) Outcomes: Win-lose; assertive, uncooperative, short-term resolution.

D. Suggestions to utilize to increase nurse conflict resolutions strategies (Kritek, 2002).
   1. Be aware that nurses are conflict avoidant.
   2. Avoid seeking "easy" answers or simple solutions for complex issues.
   3. Recognize that conflicts are about relationships and values.
   4. Refrain from snap judgments and conduct a conflict analysis.
   5. Search for common ground, and avoid blaming and judging.
   6. Seek to clarify the situation by asking questions and evoking more information.
   7. Clarify the difference between accommodation and collaboration that smooth over a situation without resolving the conflict.
   8. Recognize some of the structure inequities designed in our health care systems that can place nurses in uneven positions in relationship to administration and physicians.
   9. Seek the widest variety of options and choices that reinforces not rushing to a quick solution or settlement; investigate the consequence of each action.
   10. Speak the truth. Keeping silent or compromising one's integrity diminishes one's authentic self and increases dissatisfaction with the profession.
   11. Become more skilled at conflict resolution and obtain training in this area.
   12. Ask peers and colleagues to critique one another's conflict skills and provide feedback on behaviors.

13. Form a coalition with other colleagues interested in improving their conflict management skills. Learn from one another and normalize dealing with conflict as a group expectation.

E. Alternative Dispute Resolution (ADR). ADR refers to an array of processes used by individuals and groups to resolve disputes, make decisions, or improve relationship outcomes.

   1. ADR approaches (Moore, 2004).
      a. Power-based: Authoritarian or authority-based that uses competition with the most powerful person winning.
      b. Rights or entitlement-based: Uses court adjudication; arbitration; are rights-based mediation based on entitlements.
      c. Interest-based: "Win-win" negotiations; also called "problem-solving" negotiation.
      d. Relational: Consider interests, rights, ethics, and power, and are involved in relationship building and other "transformative" approaches to peace building.

   2. Criteria for selection of ADR process.
      a. Negotiation: Two or more parties attempt to reach a joint decision on matters where there exists actual, perceived, or potential disagreement or conflict.
      b. Facilitation: A third party helps to coordinate and manage a group process and guide the group through tensions and conflict toward desired outcomes.
      c. Coaching: An ADR expert assists persons in expanding and applying their conflict management skills.
      d. Mediation: An impartial third party helps disputants resolve differences through a voluntary, confidential, structured discussion.
      e. Arbitration: Impartial third party reviews dispute, arguments, and evidence, and issues a decision on behalf of disputants. Decision can be binding, meaning that disputants must accept outcome, or non-binding, meaning that disputants can view decision as advisory but are not required to accept it.

Planning Ambulatory Care Nursing Interventions and Programs

The objective of planning is to produce the best possible practical plan that will achieve organizational goals and specific program objectives, *and* has the support of all the stakeholders. Significant opportunity exists to increase the productivity and effectiveness of all teams, and this is also true in ambulatory care.

A. These conditions improve team relationships:
   1. Trust among members.
   2. Sense of group identity.
   3. Sense of group efficacy or consistent goal direction.
   4. Development and coaching of leaders.

B. Strategic planning process. Strategic planning is the continuous process of systematically evaluating the nature of the ambulatory care organization, defining its long-term objectives, identifying quantifiable goals, developing strategies to reach these objectives and goals, and allocating resources to carry out these strategies. Strategic planning begins by addressing the following four questions:
   1. Situational analysis: Where are we today?
   2. Program planning: Where do we want to go?
   3. Implementation of plan: How do we get there?
   4. Program evaluation: Have we achieved the desired outcomes?

C. Characteristics of effective goals:
   1. Recognized as important.
   2. Clear and easy to understand.
   3. Documented in specific terms.
   4. Measurable and framed in time.
   5. Aligned with organizational strategy.
   6. Achievable but challenging.
   7. Supported by appropriate awards.

D. Prioritization of goals:
   1. Which goals are valued most by the organization?
   2. Which goals have the greatest impact on performance or profitability?
   3. Which of the goals are most challenging or difficult to obtain?
   4. Which goals best fit team members' talent or training?
   5. Highest priority are goals of high value and primary concern.

6. Next priority are goals of medium value and secondary importance.
7. Lowest priority goals have little value and minor importance.
8. Next step is to prioritize highest-priority goals according to most important.
E. Four steps to accomplish goals by converting to realities.
   1. Break each goal into specific tasks with clear measurable outcomes.
   2. Plan the execution of tasks with timetables to accomplish.
   3. Gather the required resources.
   4. Execute the plan.
F. General considerations involving various stakeholders with various agendas and priorities of outcomes.
   1. Are the proposed programs consistent with the organization mission and strategic goals?
   2. Are the proposed programs consistent with the values of the stakeholders?
   3. Do the plans fit within the timeframe and budget?
   4. Does the plan include consideration of all resources needed to support the program (such as money, time, staff, space, goodwill of the community, etc.)?
   5. Is the proposed program evidence-based and include latest clinical practice guidelines as standard of care?
   6. Does the plan include evaluation criteria and standards to judge success/failure based on program goals and measured outcomes?
G. Needs assessment is the first step in planning ambulatory care nursing interventions and programs.
   1. New programs may be triggered by perceived deficits in existing programs, changes in standard, or changing populations served.
   2. Program decisions reflect organizational mission and values, and have fiscal benefit.
H. Needs assessment in ambulatory care is a process to reflect the needs of the community served (Anderson & McFarland, 2005). Sources of data include:
   1. What is the history of the community and what can be gained by talking with members of the community?

2. What are the demographics of the community that can be gathered from census data from local, state, and federal agencies regarding age, sex, racial, and ethnic distribution?
3. What are the cultural and ethnicity indicators as gathered by interviews, local planning boards, and chamber of commerce?
4. What values and beliefs are held by the community or population to be served?
5. What is the physical environment impact (such as availability of housing, air quality, climate, water sources) on the population?
6. What existing health and social services and resources outside of the immediate community are available?
7. What is the economy of the population to be served with indications of employment, unemployment rates, and insurance availability?
8. What are the transportation and safety issues of the community?
9. Are there signs of political and government support?
10. Is there common communication, or will language variations be a barrier?
11. Are schools and educational resources available for distribution of information and gathering for health initiatives?
12. What recreational areas are available for children to play, and what are the major forms of recreation?
13. How do residents perceive their living conditions and community?

Designing Ambulatory Care Nursing Programs and Interventions

A. Write program goals and measurable objective based on mission of organization.
B. Criteria for a successful project.
   1. Secure approvals of stakeholders.
   2. Develop a budget and secure funding.
   3. Develop accounting, budgeting, and management information systems.
   4. Establish policy and procedures.
   5. Set standards and criteria for evaluation.
   6. Hire and train personnel.
   7. Plan marketing and celebration.

Participation in Professional Associations

Participation in professional associations is a very rewarding endeavor and helps a nurse mature in professional responsibilities and perspectives.
A. Nursing professional associations do the following:
1. Educate members.
2. Provide opportunities to present scholarly knowledge.
3. Facilitate collegiality and networking.
4. Seek to identify opportunities to be of service to the community and larger society.
5. Advocate for change, providing evidence to shape policy.
6. Develop and improve standards of practice.
7. Provide learning about diverse methods and outcomes across communities.
8. Co-create models of care delivery that remove the structural barriers to equitable health care for all.
B. Nurses in magnet-recognized organizations have been shown to value professional autonomy, control over practice, and nurse-physician collaboration much more highly than nurses in non-magnet facilities. Nurses in magnet-recognized organizations tend to have higher membership in professional organizations and be certified in their nursing specialty (Cary, 2001).
C. Professional, community, scholarly, and specialty organizations are available on a local, state, and national level. Below are a few options and web sties that provide more information.
1. American Academy of Ambulatory Care Nursing: www.aaanc.org
2. American Nurses' Association: www.ana.org
3. Sigma Theta Tau Honor Society of Nursing: www.nursingsociety.org
4. American Organization of Nurse Executive: www.aone.org
5. The Alliance of Nursing Organizations (www.nursing-alliance.org) lists a number of specialty organizations.
D. Magnet Recognition Program®.
1. In 1991, the American Nurses Credentialing Center (ANCC) developed a program to recognize health care organizations that provides the very best in nursing care and upholds the tradition within professional nursing practice.

2. The program founded 14 forces of magnetism that serve as the evidence basis for transforming the work environment and enhancing quality of nursing care. These essential characteristics are:
a. Quality of nursing leadership.
b. Flat organizational structure with decentralized decision-making.
c. Participative management style.
d. Nursing supportive personnel policies and procedures.
e. Professional model of nursing care.
f. Quality care that values patient concerns as paramount.
g. Quality improvements.
h. Adequate consultation and perceived adequate nurse staffing resources.
I. Autonomy in nursing practice.
j. Involvement of the hospital in the community.
k. Nurse as teacher.
l. Professional image of nursing and clinical competence.
m. Positive nurse-physician and interdisciplinary relationships.
n. Supportive professional development programs.

National Initiatives

In 2005, over 40 million Americans were uninsured, and millions more lack adequate care. Communities of color have a higher incidence of chronic diseases, cardiovascular disease, diabetes, cancer, violence, and HIV/AIDS that leads to high rates of morbidity and mortality. The number of nurses entering the nursing profession is not keeping pace with the number that are retiring, nor the expected forecast of aging Americans who will require health care by 2010. Also, the number of nursing school faculty who are retiring without replacements is escalating at an alarming rate. Nursing continues to seek leaders who promote and participate in groups of health professionals and consumers to reach consensus agreements on health care delivery models for medically underserved, ethnic populations, changing workforce regulations, and improving global health. National initiatives focus on strategies for improving health care delivery models, providing culturally competent care, and retaining the available supply of nurses, while striving to increase the capacity.

A. Strategies for health improvements and delivery models.
    1. Increasing attention to health care access for the working poor and uninsured.
    2. Improving access services in transportation, childcare, and social services.
    3. Advancing culturally competent health care.
B. Responses to changing workforce issues.
    1. Advocating for accessible, affordable health care with culturally competent providers.
    2. Promoting research that identifies modes of care to improve the health status of diverse populations.
    3. Increasing the number of ethnic minority nurse leaders in the areas of health policy, practice, education, and research.
    4. Increasing the number of ethnic minority nurses to reflect the nation's diverse population.
C. Nurses and nurse leaders can stay current through involvement with professional organizations, journals, and newsletters of professional organizations, computer access to listservs, professional conference attendance, and participation in political action committees.

References

Aiken, L.H. (2002). Superior outcomes for Magnet hospitals: The evidence base. In M.I. McClure & A. Hinshaw (Eds.), *Magnet hospitals revisited*. Washington, DC: American Nurses Publishing.

Anderson, E., & McFarland, J. (2005). *Community as partner: Theory and practice in nursing* (4th ed). Philadelphia: Lippincott, Williams & Wilkins.

Block, P. (2002). *The answer to how is yes*. San Francisco: Berrett-Kohler Publisher.

Cary, A. (2001). Certified registered nurses: Result of study of certified workforce. *American Journal of Nursing, 101*(1), 44-52.

Dreyfus, H.L., & Dreyfus, S. (1996). The relationship of theory and practice in the acquisition of skill. In P. Benner et al. (Eds.), *Expertise in nursing practice: Caring, clinical judgment, and ethics* (pp. 29-47). New York: Springer.

Goleman, D. (2004). What makes a leader? *Harvard Business Review, 76*(7), 93-102.

Kritek, P. (2002). *Negotiating at an uneven table: Developing moral courage in resolving our conflicts* (2nd ed.). San Francisco: Jossey-Bass.

Moore, C. (2004). *The mediation process: Practical strategies for resolving conflict* (3rd ed.). San Francisco: Jossey-Bass.

Porter O'Grady, T., & Mallock, K. (2002). *Quantum leadership: A textbook of new leadership*. Gaithersburg, MD: Aspen.

Rosenstein, A. (2002). Nurse-physician relationships: Impact on nurse satisfaction and retention. *American Journal of Nursing, 102*(6), 26-34.

Swanson, J. (2000). Zen leadership: Balancing energy for mind, body and spirit harmony. *Nursing Administration Quarterly, 24*(2), 29-33.

Valentine, P. (2001). A gender perspective on conflict management strategies of nurses. *Journal of Nursing Scholarship, 33*(1), 69-74.

Wheatley, M. (2005). *Finding our way: Leadership for an uncertain time*. San Francisco: Berrett-Keohler.

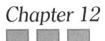
Leadership

This test may be copied for use by others.

COMPLETE THE FOLLOWING:

Name: _____

Address: _____

City: _____ State: _____ Zip: _____

Preferred telephone: (Home)_____ (Work)_____

E-mail_____

AAACN Member Expiration Date: _____

Registration fee: AAACN Member: $12.00
                    Nonmember: $20.00

Answer Form:

1. If you applied what you have learned from this activity into your practice, what would be different?

_____

_____

_____

Evaluation	Strongly disagree				Strongly agree
2. By completing this activity, I was able to meet the following objectives:					
a. Describe an overview of leadership characteristics and transformational leadership concepts.	1	2	3	4	5
b. Describe the importance of collaboration in ambulatory care and colleague relationships.	1	2	3	4	5
c. Discuss conflict resolution and strategies.	1	2	3	4	5
d. Describe the program planning process for ambulatory care nursing interventions and programs.	1	2	3	4	5
e. Discuss various professional activities, associations, and national initiatives.	1	2	3	4	5
3. The content was current and relevant.	1	2	3	4	5
4. The objectives could be achieved using the content provided.	1	2	3	4	5
5. This was an effective method to learn this content.	1	2	3	4	5
6. I am more confident in my abilities since completing this material.	1	2	3	4	5

7. The material was (check one) ___new ___review for me.

8. Time required to read this chapter: _____minutes

I verify that I have completed this activity: _____
                                                        Signature

Comments: _____

_____

_____

Objectives

This educational activity is designed for nurses and other health care professionals who practice in ambulatory care. For those wishing to obtain CE credit, an evaluation follows. After studying the information presented in this offering, you will be able to:

1. Describe an overview of leadership characteristics and transformational leadership concepts.
2. Describe the importance of collaboration in ambulatory care and colleague relationships.
3. Discuss conflict resolution and strategies.
4. Describe the program planning process for ambulatory care nursing interventions and programs.
5. Discuss various professional activities, associations, and national initiatives.

Posttest Instructions

1. To receive continuing education credit for individual study after reading the article, complete the answer/evaluation form to the left.

2. Detach and send the answer/evaluation form along with a check or money order payable to the *American Academy of Ambulatory Care Nursing (AAACN)*, East Holly Avenue Box 56, Pitman, NJ 08071–0056.

3. Test returns must be postmarked by August 1, 2011. Upon completion of the answer/evaluation form, a certificate for **1.5** contact hour(s) will be awarded and sent to you. Should the material contained in this chapter become outdated prior to the above expiration date, AAACN reserves the right to withdraw this CE test.

This activity is co-provided by the *American Academy of Ambulatory Care Nursing (AAACN)* and Anthony J. Jannetti, Inc. (AJJ). AJJ is accredited as a provider of continuing nursing education by the American Nurses' Credentialing Center's Commission on Accreditation (ANCC-COA). AAACN is a provider approved by the California Board of Registered Nurses, provider number CEP 05336.

This article was reviewed and formatted for contact hour credit by Sally S. Russell, MN, CMSRN, AAACN Education Director; and Candia Baker Laughlin MS, RN, C, Editor.

Chapter 13

Evidence-Based Practice

Beth Ann Swan, PhD, FAAN, CRNP
Rebecca Linn Pyle, MS, RN
Eileen M. Esposito, RN, C, MPA, CPHQ

Objectives

Study of the information presented in this chapter will enable the learner to:

1. Understand the meaning of evidence-based practice and performance improvement, and their application to ambulatory care nursing practice and quality care.
2. Describe the key steps of evidence-based nursing practice, discuss rating the quality and strength of the evidence, and identify strategies for facilitating evidence-based nursing practice initiatives and the use of clinical practice guidelines within an organization.
3. Discuss the differences between quality assurance and continuous performance improvement models.
4. Discuss why indicators are integral to the performance improvement process, define different types of indicators, and provide an example of each.
5. Describe the multiple factors affecting the development of a reliable and valid process to monitor competencies and outcomes.
6. Understand the relationship of varied indicators on a balanced scorecard, dashboard, or report card in reflecting the outcomes of an organization.

Key Points

1. Evidence-based nursing practice and continually improving practice performance are two critical components of professional nursing practice in all ambulatory care settings.
2. Evidence-based initiatives are often central to the performance improvement process, and the improvement process is a cornerstone of total quality management programs.

E vidence-based nursing practice and continually improving practice performance are two critical components of professional nursing practice in all ambulatory care settings. Evidence-based initiatives are often central to the performance improvement process, and the improvement process is a cornerstone of total quality management programs. This chapter is designed to provide nurses with a basic understanding of evidence-based practice and performance improvement, and the naturally occurring linkages between the two processes. Joined together, evidence-based practice and performance improvement can impact the quality of care delivered in ambulatory care settings.

Origin and Evolution of Evidence-Based Practice

A. Evidence-based practice originated in medicine to determine the effectiveness and efficiency of medical interventions (Melynk & Finout-Overholt, 2005). It is rooted in the work of A.L. Cochrane, a British epidemiologist.
   1. In the 1970s, Cochrane struggled with the efficacy of health care and challenged the public to pay only for care that had been empirically supported as effective.
   2. He strongly encouraged his colleagues to use evidence from randomized controlled trials (RCTs) to determine the effectiveness and efficiency of medical interventions.
B. Evidence-based medicine is the "conscientious, explicit, and judicious use of current best avail-

able evidence in making decisions about the care of individual patients" (Straus, Richardson, Glasziou, & Haynes, 2005, p. 3).

C. The practice of evidence-based medicine means "integrating individual clinical expertise with the best available external clinical evidence from systematic research" (Straus et al., 2005, p. 3).

D. Nursing has approximately 25 years of experience with one dimension of evidence-based nursing practice, research utilization through the Conduct and Utilization of Research in Nursing (CURN) project in the 1970s (Estabrooks, 1998).
   1. Research utilization is the use of research findings in any and all aspects of one's work (Estabrooks, 1998).
   2. Research utilization is typically based on a single study.

E. Goals of evidence-based practice.
   1. Integrating individual clinical expertise with the best available external evidence from systematic research.
   2. Reducing wide variation in practice.
   3. Eliminating worst practices.
   4. Enhancing best practice.
   5. Reducing cost and improving quality.

F. Definitions of evidence-based nursing
   1. "A process by which nurses make clinical decisions using the best available research evidence, their clinical expertise, and patient preferences in the context of available resources" (DiCenso, Cullum, & Ciliska, 1998, p. 38).
   2. "Care concerning the incorporation of evidence from research, clinical expertise, and patient preferences into decisions about health care of individuals" (Le May, Mulhall, & Alexander, 1998, p. 429).

G. Rationale for further basing ambulatory care nursing interventions on research evidence.
   1. Ambulatory care nursing interventions should be based on research evidence, and areas with identified gaps in research evidence should be further studied.
   2. Research reports, including on-line full text articles from nursing, medicine, and health care, are increasingly available and accessible.
   3. Refined criteria for appraising research findings.

4. Risk management concerns: An assumption of decreased risk when ambulatory interventions are supported by research.
5. Increased potential for better outcomes.
6. Reduction in uncertainty and variability in health care decision making.
7. Potential to reduce costs.
8. Demonstration of the value of ambulatory care nursing.
9. Potential to increase professional satisfaction.
10. Increased competitive edge.

H. Key assumptions in evidence-based practice.
   1. Clinicians directly involved in delivering patient care influence, either positively or negatively, patient outcomes.
      a. Clinicians assume full responsibility for their practice; in the case of nursing, some aspects of practice are dependent, interdependent, or independent.
      b. Clinicians draw on, as well as contribute to, a body of knowledge elucidating best evidence and optimum effectiveness (Kitson, 1997).

Key Steps of Evidence-Based Nursing Practice

Melynk and Fineout-Overholt (2005) outline the following key steps of evidence-based nursing practice.

A. Formulate the clinical question. Determine the clinical practice problem to solve and frame it as a question.
   1. Use PICO format:
      a. P – Patient population.
      b. I – Intervention of interest, or when not intervention focused, "I" can be "interest area."
      c. C – Comparison intervention or status.
      d. O – Outcome.

B. Collect the most relevant and best evidence.
   1. Where to find the best evidence.
      a. Nurses who are members of professional organizations, such as the American Academy of Ambulatory Care Nursing (AAACN), receive peer-reviewed journals and newsletters as a member benefit. These journals are usually specific to the

practice of the nurse and are an excellent source of current information.

b. Ambulatory care organizations, hospitals, and medical centers usually maintain both print libraries and access to online databases. Sample databases useful to ambulatory care nurses include:

(1) Cumulative Index of Nursing and Allied Health Literature (CINAHL): Provides comprehensive coverage of the English language journal literature for nursing and allied health disciplines.

(2) Evidence-Based Medicine (EBM) Reviews including American College of Physicians (ACP) Journal Club and Database of Abstracts of Reviews of Effects (DARE): Screens the top clinical journals, identifying studies that are both methodologically sound and clinically relevant, and provides an enhanced abstract of the chosen articles, providing a commentary on the value of the article for clinical practice.

(3) Cochrane Database of Systematic Reviews and Cochrane Central Register of Controlled Trials: Includes the full text of the regularly updated systematic reviews of the effects of health care prepared by the Cochrane Collaboration (www. cochrane.delcc/cochrane/index.htl)

(4) Campbell Collaboration Database of Systematic Reviews: Includes the full text of the regularly updated systematic reviews of the effects of interventions in the social, behavioral, and educational arena prepared by the Campbell Collaboration (www.campbellcollaboration.org/index.html).

c. National Guideline Clearinghouse (NGC): Publicly available electronic repository for clinical practice guidelines and related materials that provides online access to guidelines (http://www.guidelines.gov).

d. World Wide Web sample sites with health care information:

(1) Federal government Web sites.
   (a) National Institutes of Health: www.nih.gov
   (b) Centers for Disease Control: www.cdc.gov
   (c) Department of Health and Human Services: www.dhhs.gov
   (d) Morbidity and Mortality Weekly Report: www.edu.gov/mmwr
   (e) Health Finder: www.healthfinder.gov
   (f) Global Evidence: www.global evidence.com
   (g) Joanna Briggs Institute: www. joannabriggs.edu

(2) Professional associations.
   (a) American Nurses Association: www.ana.org or www.nursing world.org
   (b) American Academy of Ambulatory Care Nursing: www. aaacn.org
   (c) Sigma Theta Tau International: www.nursingsociety.org
   (d) Evidence-Based Nursing: www. evidencebasednursing.org

(3) Voluntary health organizations.
   (a) American Lung Association: www.ala.org or www.lungs.org
   (b) American Heart Association: www.americanheart.org
   (c) American Cancer Society: www.cancer.org
   (d) John A. Hartford Center of Geriatric Nursing Excellence (HCGNE): www.nyu.edu/nursing/

2. Levels of evidence are designed to help reviewers rate the quality and strength of the evidence.
   a. Scientific design.
   b. Statistically significant.
   c. Valid and reliable.
   d. Least amount of bias.
   e. Time controlled.
   f. Evidence of direct correlation.

3. Rating system for the hierarchy of evidence (Melynk & Fineout-Overholt, 2005, p. 10, reprinted with permission from Lippincott, Williams & Wilkins).

a. "Level I: Evidence from a systematic review or meta-analysis of all relevant randomized controlled trials (RCTs), or evidence-based clinical practice guidelines based on systematic reviews of RCTs."

b. "Level II: Evidence obtained from at least one well-designed RCT."

c. "Level III: Evidence obtained from well-designed controlled trials without randomization."

d. "Level IV: Evidence from well-designed case-control and cohort studies."

e. "Level V: Evidence from systematic reviews of descriptive and qualitative studies."

f. "Level VI: Evidence from a single descriptive or qualitative study."

g. "Level VII: Evidence from the opinion of authorities and/or reports of expert committees."

C. Critically appraise the evidence (Swan & Boruch, 2004).
 1. What is the evidence?
 2. Is the evidence valid?
 3. If valid, is the evidence important?
 4. If valid and important, can one apply this evidence when caring for your patient, family, or population?

D. Integrate all evidence with one's clinical expertise, patient preferences, and values in making a practice decision or change (Melynk & Finout-Overholt, 2005).
 1. Ethical considerations need to be explored with patients related to their treatment decisions.
 2. Health care consumers want to participate in the clinical decision-making process.

E. Evaluate the practice decision or change (Melynk & Fineout-Overholt, 2005).
 1. Did the treatment work?
 2. How effective was the clinical decision with a particular patient or practice setting?

Evidence-Based Clinical Practice Guidelines

A. Clinical practice guidelines are "statements that have been systematically developed to assist practitioners and patients in making decisions about appropriate health care for specific clinical circumstances" (Handley, Stuart, & Kirz, 1994, p. 75).

B. Guidelines have been used to accomplish two major goals:
 1. The improvement of clinical quality.
 2. The control of medical care costs.

C. "At their best, clinical practice guidelines allow for the integration of research with the clinical context, specific patient circumstances, and patient values" (Melnyk & Fineout-Overholt, 2005, p. 209).

D. Guideline development consists of a systematic review of the literature and consensus of a group of decision makers who consider the evidence and make recommendations (Melnyk & Fineout-Overholt, 2005).

E. Clinical practice guidelines can overcome the barriers to research utilization by reducing the need to access and critically appraise the literature and make general conclusions and recommendations. They do not eliminate clinical judgment regarding how well particular clients match the target population for the practice guideline (Melnyk & Fineout-Overholt, 2005).

Translating Evidence into Practice

A. "The focus of translation research has been the exploration of potentially useful strategies for enhancing the uptake or adoption of evidence and related guidelines into practice" (Stetler, 2003, p. 99).
 1. "Not all improvements in practice, or quality in general, can be achieved by inducing or exhorting individual clinicians and managers to change their own practice" (Steller, 2003, p. 98).
 2. "Evidence-based change is not likely to be sustained over time without explicit system supports" (Steller, 2003, p. 98).
 3. "Organizational context can have either a facilitative or hindering impact on the adoption of research findings" (Steller, 2003, p. 98).
 4. "The process of implementing and using research findings must be institutionalized so that evidence-based practice and related implementation efforts become part of both the organization's and the individual clinician's daily way of doing business" (Steller, 2003, p. 99).

B. Barriers to translating research into practice (Mohide & King, 2003).
   1. Workload, lack of resources.
   2. Conflicting goals and priorities in the organization.
   3. Limited access to research journals.
   4. Lack of skills to search and critique the literature.
   5. Experiential knowledge is often favored over empirical knowledge.
   6. Lack of organizational support.
   7. Communication within organizations.
   8. Complexities of organizational change.
   9. Negative viewpoints about research.
   10. Explosion of knowledge.
   11. Organization system limitations.
   12. Authority to implement findings.

C. Strategies for facilitating evidence-based practice (Funk, Tornquist, & Champagne, 1995).
   1. Creation of an environment in which nurses are comfortable questioning and evaluating current practice, seeking out research-based solutions to care problems, and testing them in trials appropriately.
   2. Support group activities, such as journal clubs and research committees, research presentations, and expert consultation.
   3. Time to read research, evaluate its applicability for the setting, and develop setting-specific protocols and pilot them.
   4. Access to journals, library searches, and photocopying.
   5. Development of nurses' research skills.
   6. Support from administrators for their belief in the value of research utilization by example and by expectations.
   7. Support of evidence-based projects through small research utilization grant funding.

Definition and Overview of Performance Improvement

A. Performance improvement is the systematic analysis of the structure, processes, and outcomes within systems for the purpose of improving the delivery of care (Joint Commission on Accreditation of Healthcare Organizations [JCAHO], 2005).

1. Performance improvement is one of the most critical endpoints in a quality model.
2. The ultimate goal of performance improvement is to determine if the desired outcome is achieved through the implementation of appropriate processes, policies, procedures, guidelines, or any combination of the above.

B. Optimal performance is doing the right thing, for the right reason, and doing it well. (Dlugacz, Restifo, & Greenwood, 2004). Aspects of performance include the timeliness, efficacy, efficiency, appropriateness, and respectfulness of care delivery in a safe environment that flows seamlessly to promote continuity of care (JCAHO, 2002).

C. Definitions of quality.
   1. The Institute of Medicine (IOM) defines quality as, "the degree to which health services for individuals and populations increase the likelihood of desired health outcomes and are consistent with current professional knowledge" (IOM, 1990, p. 21).
   2. "Quality in health care means doing the right things right and making continuous improvement...Quality helps patients achieve optimal health outcomes in an atmosphere of excellent service" (Leebov & Ersoz, 1991, p. 10).
   3. Quality management is customer focused, process oriented, and data driven (JCAHO, 2005).
   4. Regardless of how quality is defined, value is an implicit attribute (Hall, 1996).
      a. Health care value in simple terms is directly proportional to quality and inversely proportional to cost (Gerberding, 2001).
      b. Consumers are increasingly demanding the information about quality that is necessary to insure that they receive high-quality health care, and they will often seek out comparative information from publicly available sources (for example, JCAHO Quality Report, HEDIS™ Quality Compass, Healthgrades.com, etc.). Undoubtedly, consumer pressure influenced the public reporting of quality measures or core measures by Centers for Medicare and Medicaid Services (CMS) and JCAHO.

D. History of quality assurance (QA), continuous quality improvement (CQI), quality performance improvement (QPI), and total quality management (TQM).

   1. Historically, performance improvement initiatives focused on quality assurance (QA).

      a. Quality assurance relies on principles of inspection and audit. It is frequently referred to as the "bad apple" approach in which the bad apples are discarded but there is no process to assure the production of only good apples. As recently as the 1980s, health care organizations used a QA approach in meeting the accreditation requirements of JCAHO and the regulatory requirements of other agencies (National Associate for Healthcare Quality [NAHQ], 1998). Using a QA approach, health care organizations focused on the performance of individuals or specific departments and used audit methodologies to review areas of mortality review, transfusion utilization, medical record review, etc. This approach is problem-focused and tends to be defensive and reactive (Leebov & Ersoz, 1991).

   2. In 1986, JCAHO introduced a 10-step process that replaced the problem-focused QA approach with one that required systematic evaluation and monitoring of key aspects of patient care. Through the use of additional strategies, including the use of written specifications or guidelines and more rigorous statistical evaluations that focus on performance over time, the concept of continuous quality improvement (CQI) or continuous performance improvement emerged. CQI relies on the use of data, not anecdotal evidence, as the basis for comparison and performance over time, and data are tracked and trended through use of control charts and other statistical tools (NAHQ, 1998).

   3. To accomplish the transition from QA to CQI, organizations and businesses needed to adopt a new approach to both management principles and quality assessment. One of the most influential quality "gurus" in this transition process was an American named W. Edwards Deming, Ph.D. Deming believed that a culture of quality within an organization would influence the outcomes. Deming (2000) created a management philosophy based on 14 points for businesses to be competitive:

      a. Create consistency of purpose toward quality improvement.

      b. Adopt a philosophy which expects good products and services.

      c. Cease dependence on mass inspection and build quality into the product or service.

      d. Do not award business solely on price tag.

      e. Improve constantly the system of production and service.

      f. Institute on-the-job training and retraining.

      g. Institute leadership with an arm to help people and machines do better jobs.

      h. Drive out fear.

      i. Break down barriers between departments.

      j. Eliminate slogans, exhortations, and targets.

      k. Eliminate numerical quotas and management by objective, and substitute leadership.

      l. Remove barriers to pride in workmanship.

      m. Institute education and self-improvement.

      n. Take action to accomplish the transformation (NAHQ, 1998).

   4. In the 1920s, Walter Stewart introduced the concept of Plan-Do-See; Deming modified the Stewart Cycle to Plan-Do-Study-Act (PSDA), and today, the Deming Cycle includes Plan-Do-Check-Act (PDCA) (ValueBasedManagement.net). This cycle is the basis for most performance improvement programs in place today. There are variations of the acronym, but all are intended to define a process of continuous assessment, evaluation, and action.

      a. PDSA – Plan, do, study, act.

      b. Six Sigma DMAIC – Design, measure, analyze, improve, control.

      c. FOCUS-PDCA – Find a process to improve; organize a team that knows the process; clarify current knowledge; understand variation; select a potential process improvement; plan, do, check, act.

5. Deming, along with Philip B. Cosby and Joseph Juran, created a set of strategies in which the front line workers had as much input into process improvement as the managers and as such were held accountable for the outcomes of production (Juran Institute, 2003). The strategies also included soliciting and listening to the "voice of the customer" to understand requirements, needs, and desires, and aligning the performance improvement efforts with the mission, vision, and strategic plan of the organization. These strategies forced the transition from quality assurance, in which the "bad apple" is plucked from the assembly line or a poorly performing employee is removed but no other changes are made, to total quality management (TQM) or continuous performance improvement (CPI). The latter seeks to improve the quality and consistency of the product, reduce process variation, and decrease the number of defects that enter the system. Reduction of process variation is the hallmark of quality methodologies, such as Six Sigma. Performance improvement focuses on the processes of care, not the individual person's performance. This approach removes the placement of blame from a single individual and seeks to improve processes of care to assure greater success among a wider cohort of employees.

6. A classic model that acts as a mechanism to focus our quality efforts is the Donabedian (1966) quality trilogy model: Structure, process, and outcomes. Successful improvement efforts require the integration of all three. Within the quality model, structure, process, and outcome can be defined as:

a. Structure – Factors within an organization that support the delivery of quality care.
   (1) Staff credentials.
   (2) Staff abilities/competency.
   (3) Staffing ratios.
   (4) Facility design and equipment.
   (5) Administrative structures that support the delivery of care (such as policies, procedures, and guidelines).

b. Process – The work that supports delivering quality care on behalf of the patient or health care consumer.
   (1) Accurately medicating patients.
   (2) Providing patient education.
   (3) Documenting care in the health care record.
   (4) Complying with evidence that indicates care can be improved if provided a certain way (such as clinical practice guidelines).
   (5) Evaluating each clinician's competency. Competency evaluation may identify a gap or strength in an employee's critical thinking, interpersonal, or technical skills. These data, therefore, can enhance quality improvement efforts.

c. Outcome – The result of performance (or nonperformance) of a function, intervention, or process (JCAHO, 2005).
   (1) Outcomes can measure the impact of health care on individuals and populations, and may include physical health, emotional health, and even financial health.
   (2) Outcomes can also measure operational efficiency, patient and staff satisfaction, and accessibility. (JCAHO, 2002).
   (3) Outcomes are measured through the use of indicators.

E. Performance improvement (PI) indicators and measurements.

1. An indicator is a performance measure that provides an indication of an organization's performance in relation to a specified process or outcome. Performance measures include:
   a. *Clinical* measures of the patient's health or functional status.
   b. *Administrative* measures of utilization and productivity.
   c. *Operational* measures of key functions.
   d. *Perception* of care or measures of patient satisfaction (JCAHO, 2005).

2. Measurement is the process of collecting and aggregating data. There are three fundamental purposes of measurement (JCAHO, 2005).

a. *Assessing current performance –* Measurement to assess current performance is often the first step in a structured PI project. Such measurement produces data that illustrate the strengths and weaknesses of current processes and achieved outcomes, thereby providing a baseline. Practices can be "benchmarked" or compared to like practices to assess current performance in key areas.

b. *Verifying improved performance –* Measurement can also demonstrate the effectiveness of improvement actions. This helps organizations obtain a clear picture of how design changes affect processes and outcomes. For example, an organization that has added an advanced practice nurse to a group practice may use measurement to determine whether the addition has indeed met a high-volume community need, enhanced patient volume, and increased revenue.

c. *Control of performance –* Measurement can also be used to determine whether key processes are in control. It can provide an early warning system that identifies an undesirable change in performance and allow immediate corrective actions to be made. For example, an ambulatory care organization measuring waiting times may find unusually long waits outside its acceptable time frames and will allow for system improvement before the delays result in significant patient diversions to other providers.

4. How is an indicator or measure chosen?
  a. PI priorities are usually determined by the performance improvement coordinating group (PICG) or quality council and may be based on needs identified through the PI process, sentinel events, JCAHO standards compliance, Department of Health (DOH) regulations, hospital agenda, or administrative direction (NAHQ, 1998).
  b. PI priorities for a department or division are usually identified through focused review, the PI process, or through identification of clinical, operational, or administrative needs. Processes often chosen for review include:
    (1) New techniques or equipment.
    (2) High-risk.
    (3) High-volume.
    (4) High-cost.
    (5) High-risk and low-volume.

5. Basic types of indicators (JCAHO, 2005).
  a. Clinical indicators (such as pap smear, mammography, and immunization rates) reflect the adherence of the practice to known standards of care or clinical guidelines.
  b. Administrative indicators (such as revenue, expenses, etc.) reflect the practice efficiency.
  c. Operational indicators (such as visit volume data, no-shows, cancellations, etc.) are a measure of access to care.
  d. Perception of care indicators are measures of patient satisfaction and may include waiting time, attributes of caring by staff, etc.

F. Priority focus areas (PFA).
  1. Priority focus areas are processes, systems, or structures in a health care organization that significantly impact the quality and safety of care.
  2. JCAHO, through the use of data base analysis, expert literature, and expert opinion, has identified 14 PFAs that are most likely to ensure safe, high-quality care and are generally universal across health care organizations and settings (JCAHO, 2004). The 14 PFAs are:
    a. Assessment and care/services.
    b. Communication.
    c. Credentialed practitioners.
    d. Equipment use.
    e. Infection control.
    f. Information management.
    g. Organizational structure.
    h. Orientation and training.
    i. Rights and ethics.
    j. Physical environment.
    k. Quality improvement expertise and activity.
    l. Patient safety.
    m. Staffing.

3. When identifying performance improvement opportunities, it is crucial for organizations to consider the 14 PFAs in relation to their scope of services or scope of care; their high-risk, high-volume, problem-prone services; and newest technologies.

G. Balanced scorecards and dashboards.

1. Today's ambulatory organizations must consider the interrelation of the various types of indicators in reflecting the total picture of the organization. A balanced score card or dashboard is a graphic or pictorial display of the organization's indicators chosen to support the strategic plan and vision of the organization.

2. The balanced scorecard is populated with measures that reveal the interdependency of the core business values, employee values, and patient values (Castaneda-Menedez, Mangan, & Lavern, 1998).

3. The balanced scorecard allows for examination of relationships among separate indicators (care, quality, financial, operational, etc.) to assure alignment with the strategic plan.

4. Regular review of the scorecard allows for timely action plans and corrective measures to be developed to keep the organization on track with its vision for the future.

5. Key performance measures (Kedrowski & Weiner, 2003) in ambulatory care include:
   a. Access to care.
   b. Utilization and productivity.
   c. Financial operations.
   d. Quality and service (see Table 13-1).

Pay for Performance

A. As health care costs increase, consumers (including individuals, employers, and the government) demand to know how an organization is improving performance. Financial reimbursement and incentives may be tied to the organization's (and individual practitioner's) ability to meet the performance standards, benchmarks, and outcomes.

1. The demand for information about performance is driving a revolution that will profoundly affect health care providers and payers (IOM, 2002).

2. Variation in specific indicators will help consumers determine different values and will help organizations identify potential opportunities for improvement.

B. Report cards.

1. Display collected data on the indicators that affect typical patients (such as satisfaction, immunization, and Pap smear rates).

2. Report cards identify performance measures that include quality indicators (such as immunization, Pap smear, and mammogram rates), utilization indicators (such as membership, access, finances, hospital, and ER admission), and satisfaction levels.

3. Consumers use report card data to compare the performance of different organizations against a predetermined standard/best practice.

4. Report cards support consumers' informed purchasing decisions about which health plan might more closely meet their health care needs.

5. A challenge in using report cards effectively is to assure the data collection methods are standardized and relevant.

6. The data contained in report cards may be too broad to explicate the exact factors that make up the data. For example, high satisfaction scores may not lead to a better understanding of what makes the patient satisfied unless specified. Was patient satisfied with his or her care because of the low cost, fast response time to answering questions, or friendliness of staff?

7. Tools that document data on health status, which can be affected by nurses, illustrate the value nurses add to the health care equation. These data provide recognition for the contribution of nurses to quality patient care. The data must be continually refined to determine which nursing structure and processes are linked to nursing outcomes.

8. Report cards are not benchmarks. However, report card data can be used in the benchmarking process.

9. Different types of report cards have been created by different organizations to specify what indicators are most important to track or to identify information important to con-

Table 13-1.

Key Performance Measures in Ambulatory Care

Access to Care	Utilization and Productivity	Financial Operations	Quality and Service
Appointment availability; for example, next vs. 2nd or 3rd available	Space/Exam room utilization Visits per exam room	Charge timeliness and accuracy • Charge lag	Patient satisfaction
Bumped/rescheduled appointment rate	Number of specialty referrals	Co-payment and cash collection rate	Staff satisfaction
No show appointment rate	Number of ED visits	Rejection/Denial rate	PI projects; site specific
Wait time • Exam room • Waiting room	Number of visits conforming to CPT codes	Accounts receivable days	Sedation outcomes
Cancellation rate	Staff mix per visit	Insurance/registration accuracy	Immunization rates
Referral request turnaround	Staff turnover rate	Total visit volume • New patient • Urgent/walk-in visits • % change to prior year visit variance to budget	Diabetes compliance • Hgb A1C • Annual eye exams • Foot care
Consult request turnaround	Support staff FTEs per MD	Total direct cost per visit	Point of care testing compliance
Availability of urgent or walk-in appointments	Expenses per visit	Revenue and expense per visit	Population-specific guidelines, e.g. CHF, COPD, CF
Telephone access • Abandonment rate • Average time before answered • Total number of calls by agent • Response time for clinical triage	Relative Value Units (RVUs) • RVUs per visit • Total RVUs • RVU variance to budget	Billing timeliness and accuracy • Billing lag	Prevention of tobacco use

Source: Kedrowski & Weiner, 2003. Reprinted with permission from Jannetti Publications, Inc.

sumers (Lowe & Baker, 1997; Schriefer, Urden, & Rogers, 1997; Spath, 1998).

10. The Joint Commission Quality Report provides summary information for the public about the quality and safety at an accredited organization. It is created at the organizational level and is designed to allow for easy comparison of state and national information with other accredited organizations (JCAHO 2006).

11. AAACN has begun to identify national nursing indicators for report cards in the ambulatory setting (Mastal, 1999).

12. American Nurses Association (ANA) Quality

Initiatives and Indicators:
a. Patient Safety and Nursing Quality Initiative (1994).
b. National Database of Nursing Quality Indicators (NDNQI) (1997).
c. Acute Care Indicators: 10 indicators (1995).
d. Non-Acute Care Community-Based Indicators (2000a, 2000b).
e. National Center for Nursing Quality (2002).
13. Examples of different ambulatory report cards and their indicators are:
a. Health Plan Employer Data and Information Set (HEDIS®) (see Chapter 15, *Regulatory Compliance and Patient Safety*).
   (1) Emphasis is on health plan performance in managed care.
   (2) The indicators are more tangentially then directly linked to nursing (such as immunization, Pap smear, and satisfaction rates).
   (3) Data from this report card are used to determine health plan expenditures and performance accountabilities (Ribnick & Carrano, 1995).
b. Medical Outcomes Trust Short Form (MOS-SF36).
   (1) Originally developed to describe variations in physician practice styles and outcomes (Benson, 1992).
   (2) The newest version (SF-36) includes indicators that can be influenced by nursing interventions including role limitations caused by physical and emotional problems, social functioning, bodily pains, and general health perceptions.
c. Standardized Outcomes and Assessment Information Set (OASIS) for home health care.
   (1) A lengthy survey that contains predominantly functional criteria required by Medicare-certified home health agencies.
   (2) Examples of some of the functional items are activities of daily living (ADL) and intermediate activities of

daily living (IADL), integumentary, sensory, respiratory, elimination status, as well as living arrangements and supportive assistance.
   (3) Most of the items focus on long-term rather than short-term outcomes such as blood oxygen levels, and wound and infusion site infection.
d. Child Health Questionnaire (CHQ-PF50). Similar to the SF-36 but for use with pediatric patients (Rieve, 1999).

Establishing a Mechanism for the Performance Improvement Process

Mechanisms provide a structured method of analyzing care delivery structures, processes, and outcomes that result in reliable information that can be used to improve performance.
A. General mechanisms.
   1. Improving performance by reducing variation is the main focus of the total quality management (TQM) process (Carey & Lloyd, 1995). Reduction of process variation is the hallmark of quality methodologies, such as Six Sigma.
   2. Improving every aspect of performance is often not possible because of limited resources. Efforts should be concentrated on key process performance and the core requirements of the customer (Pande & Holpp, 2002).
   3. One general mechanism is to focus performance improvement (PI) efforts by identifying scopes of care, important aspects of care, and indicators of care (JCAHO, 2003).
   a. Scope of care is the organizational or professional reason for being and represents the activities performed by governance, managerial, clinical, or support staff (JCAHO 2006). The scope of care defines who you are as an organization and the purpose for being. For example, the scope of care for an ambulatory care unit might be to provide continuity of care across the lifespan to maintain and promote health.

4. Identifying, analyzing, and managing sentinel events and other incidents that put patient safety at risk is another mechanism for preventing future incidents and improving the institution's performance (JCAHO, 2005).

    a. JCAHO's Sentinel Event Policy defines events that must be reviewed (JCAHO, 2005). The institution's definition and policy may include other events, including such things as "near misses" of serious adverse events.

    b. Channels need to be in place to support reporting of such events.

    c. Thorough root cause analyses should focus on process and system elements which lead to the bad outcome, error, or near error.

    d. An action plan should be developed, documented, implemented, and measured for effectiveness.

B. Specific mechanisms. Many different specific mechanisms exist to improve quality. Each mechanism serves a different purpose in the PI process. This section discusses three of these mechanisms – Benchmarking, flowcharts, and root cause analysis.

    1. Benchmarking is a continuous measurement of a process, product, or service in comparison to those of the toughest competitor, to those considered industry leaders, or to similar activities in the organization and using the information to change/improve practices, resulting in superior performance as determined by measured outcomes (JCAHO, 2002).

        a. Three types of benchmarking.

            (1) Internal benchmarking: Process of examining internal performance and gauging improvement over time.

            (2) External or competitive benchmarking: Measurement of performance of a given organization with reliable and valid indicators, against that of another similar organization using identical indicators. Comparative reference databases (national, regional, or system level) as well as practice guidelines, critical paths, care maps®, and other recognized pro-

fessional standards of practice and care are used for benchmarking (JCAHO, 2003).

            (3) Functional benchmarking: Comparing a similar function or process, such as scheduling, in another industry.

        b. Outcomes of benchmarking (Ellis, 1995; Jefferies & Timms, 1998; Kobs, 1998; Spann, 1997).

            (1) Quality improvement and practice development are accelerated.

            (2) Quality measures are established.

            (3) Motivation and enthusiasm among staff is improved as a result of recognition and reward for achievement and success.

            (4) A structured forum for networking is provided.

            (5) A systematic process for evaluating and improving care and service delivery to patients is developed.

        c. Selecting what to benchmark (Kobs, 1998).

            (1) Ask the question, "Have the best of the best been identified in any other organization?"

            (2) Identify what services, products, and practices have been benchmarked internally and externally.

            (3) Decide which services, products, and practices, if improved, would have the most impact within your organization.

            (4) Agree on what are the most critical services, products, and practices for quality improvement.

        d. Models and processes for benchmarking (Kobs, 1998).

            (1) Follow a simple, logical sequence of activity. Keep process models simple.

            (2) Place a heavy emphasis on planning and organization of data collection and analysis.

            (3) Use customer-focused benchmarking: Identify the customer who will benefit from the improved service, products, or process.

            (4) Make benchmarking a generic process. Be consistent throughout the organization.

(5) Utilize characteristics of collaboration and interdisciplinary practices.

2. Process improvement flowcharts provide specific steps to identify opportunities for improvement and develop subsequent solutions to improve the process (JCAHO, 2002). Carey and Lloyd (1995) described a process-improvement process that includes the following steps:

a. Identify the opportunity for improvement.

b. Organize a team.

c. Flowchart the process.

d. Determine if the process is standardized – If not, standardize the process.

e. If the process is standardized, identify the important aspects of the process.

f. Select the most important aspect in the process.

g. Define what the most important aspect is and develop a plan to collect data to study the most important aspect.

h. Analyze the data collected, and determine the degree of variation in the data and whether the variation is random (occurring by chance). If the variation is not occurring by chance, a special reason may be causing the variation.

(1) Common-cause variation is variation that occurs due to chance. It represents the normal variation found in any process and is not indicative of a process that is out of statistical control (JCAHO, 2002).

(a) Example: Fluctuating oral/rectal temperatures around a set of normal limits.

(2) Special-cause variation occurs when a factor intermittently and unpredictably induces variation that is not a normal part of the process. It often appears as an extreme point beyond the control limits on a control chart, or as a specific, identifiable pattern in the data (JCAHO, 2002).

(a) Example: A temperature spike that is caused by an infection. A spike significantly higher than

most of the values would need to be questioned to determine if something unusual is occurring to cause the abnormally high temperature.

(b) Example: Patient satisfaction rates drop precipitously following a decrease in the number of clinicians who provide care, therefore causing the waiting room times to increase significantly.

(3) Different PI actions are taken depending on the type of variation.

(a) If data indicate common-cause variation is present, then the team must first decide if the degree of variation is acceptable. When using control charts to assess data, processes are considered in control when data remains within two standard deviations from the statistical mean and no data runs or trends are noted.

(i) For example, if data indicate patient satisfaction varies between 80% and 85%, the team would ask, "Is that level acceptable?", or should the team attempt to improve performance by raising the goal to 87% to 90%?

(ii) The team would also consider what factors have the greatest influence on the process.

(iii) The most important factor influencing the process is then selected and an improvement strategy is implemented.

(iv) Data are collected to determine if the intended improvement was achieved.

(v) If not, another factor is selected, actions are implemented to improve the process, and data are again collected.

(vi) When the action achieves

the intended improvement, the action becomes a permanent part of the process.

(b) If data indicate a special cause is present, the team will work to eliminate it. For example, more clinicians would need to be hired in the patient satisfaction special cause example (see h., [2b]).

(4) Root-cause analysis is a method to determine the fundamental reason that causes variation in performance (Dlugacz et al., 2004).

(a) Reactive root-cause analysis analyzes the reason for problems that have occurred.

(b) Proactive root-cause analysis analyzes opportunities for improvement before problems occur. Failure Mode Effects Analysis (FMEA) is an example of a proactive methodology for determining risk-reduction strategies in relation to potential risk factors.

(c) Key characteristics of root-cause analysis include:

(i) A focus on systems rather than individuals. When analyzing systems, the PI team would attempt to design out any flaws that lead to problems.

(ii) Analyzing special causes first, then common causes by repeatedly asking, "Can anything be causing this problem?", until no further logical answers can be found.

(d) To implement successful root-cause analyses, the basic belief must be accepted that clinicians are human and mistakes can be expected, but organizational improvement is achievable.

(e) The steps of a root-cause analysis include:

(i) Define the event – What happened?

(ii) Identify the proximate cause

– Why did this happen? Types of proximate causes may include human error, process deficiency, equipment breakdown, environmental factors.

(iii) Identify the underlying reason for the proximate cause by brainstorming to determine why the proximate cause happened.

(iv) Collect and assess data on the proximate and underlying causes.

(v) Develop and implement interim changes. If one cause might be broken equipment, the team should not wait to fix the equipment.

(vi) Identify the root cause by asking key questions including:

(A) What factors in the environment might have contributed to the errors. For example, was staffing adequate, was the activity level greater than normal, was the equipment working properly, were breaks being taken?

(B) How is the flow of communication being managed? For example, does information flow freely, accurately, clearly? Is the information accessible?

(C) Is staff competent and is a system in place to objectively assess staff competency?

(D) How is competent performance maintained?

Once the factors have been identified, a performance improvement action plan is developed and implemented. The modified processes are assessed for positive change in the outcome, and additional modifications are made as necessary to prevent future occurrences.

References

American Academy of Ambulatory Care Nursing/American Nurses Association (AAACN/ANA). (1996). *Nursing in ambulatory care: The future is here*. Washington, DC: American Nurses Association.

American Nurses Association (ANA). (1994). *Nursing sensitive quality indicators for acute care: Settings and ANA's safety and quality initiative*. Retrieved March 28, 2006, from www.nursingworld.org/readroom/fssafe99/htm

American Nurses Association (ANA). (1995a). *Implementation of nursing practice standards and guidelines*. Washington, DC: Author.

American Nurses Association (ANA). (1995b). *Manual to develop guidelines*. Washington, DC: Author.

American Nurses Association (ANA). (1995c). *Nursing care report card for acute care*. Washington, DC: Author.

American Nurses Association (ANA). (1996). *Nursing quality indicators: Definitions and implications*. Washington, DC: Author.

American Nurses Association (ANA). (1997). *The National Center for Nursing quality indicators: The National Database of Nursing Quality Indicators (NDNQI)*. Retrieved March 28, 2006, from www.nursingworld.org/quality/database.htm

American Nurses Association (ANA). (2000a). *Nurse quality indicators beyond acute care: Literature review*. Washington, DC: Author.

American Nurses Association (ANA). (2000b). *Nurse quality indicators beyond acute care: Measurement instruments*. Washington, DC: Author.

American Nurses Association (ANA). (2002). *Welcome to NCNQ and NDNQI*. Retrieved March 28, 2006, from www.ana.org/quality

Benson, D.S. (1992). *Measuring outcomes in ambulatory care*. Chicago: American Hospital Association.

Carey, R.G., & Lloyd, R.C. (1995). *Measuring quality improvement in health care: A guide to statistical process control applications*. New York: Quality Resources.

Castaneda-Menendez, K., Mangan, K., & Lavern, A. (1998). The role and application of the balanced scorecard in healthcare quality management. *Journal of Healthcare Quality, 20*(1), 10-13.

Deming, W.E. (2000). *Out of the crisis*. Cambridge, MA: The MIT Press.

DiCenso, A., Cullum, N., & Ciliska, D. (1998). Implementing evidence-based nursing: Some misconceptions. *Evidence-Based Nursing, 1*, 38-40.

Dlugacz, Y., Restifo, A., & Greenwood, A. (2004). *The quality handbook for health care organizations: A manager's guide to tools and programs*. San Francisco: Jossey-Bass.

Donabedian, A. (1966). Evaluating the quality of medical care. *Milbank Quarterly, 44*, 166-203.

Ellis, J. (1995). Using benchmarking to improve practice. *Clinical Quality Assurance, 9*(35), 25-28.

Estabrooks, C.A. (1998). Will evidence-based nursing practice make practice perfect? *Canadian Journal of Nursing Research, 30*(1), 15-36.

Funk, S.G., Tornquist, E.M., & Champagne, M.T. (1995). Barriers and facilitators of research utilization. *Nursing Clinics of North America, 30*(3), 395-407.

Gerberding, J.L. (2001). *Health care quality promotion through infection prevention: Beyond Centers for Disease Control and Prevention*. Atlanta, GA: Centers for Disease Control and Prevention.

Hall, J. (1996). The challenge of health outcomes. *Journal of Quality in Clinical Practice,16*, 5-15

Handley M.R., Stuart, M.E., & Kirz, H.L. (1994). An evidence-based approach to evaluating and improving clinical practice: Implementing practice guidelines. *HMO Practice, 8*(2), 75-83.

Institute of Medicine (IOM). (2002). In J.M. Corrigan, A. Greiner, & S.M. Erickson (Eds.). *Fostering rapid advances in health care: Learning from system demonstrations*. Washington, DC: The National Academies Press.

Institute of Medicine (IOM). (1990). *Medicare: A strategy for quality assurance* (Vol. I). Washington, DC: National Academy Press.

Jeffries, E., & Timms, L. (1998). Sharing good practice: Developing network forums. *Nursing Standard, 12*(50), 33-34.

Joint Commission on Accreditation of Healthcare Organizations (JCAHO). (2002). *Tools for performance measurement in healthcare: A quick reference guide*. Oakbrook, IL: Author.

Joint Commission on Accreditation of Healthcare Organizations (JCAHO). (2003). *Cost effective performance improvement in ambulatory care*. Oakbrook, IL: Author.

Joint Commission on Accreditation of Healthcare Organizations (JCAHO). (2004). *Tracer methodology: Tips and strategies for continuous systems improvement*. Oakbrook, IL: Author.

Joint Commission on Accreditation of Healthcare Organizations (JCAHO). (2005). *Accreditation manual for ambulatory care*. Oakbrook, IL: Author.

Joint Commission on Accreditation of Healthcare Organizations (JCAHO). (2006). *Comprehensive accreditation manual for hospitals*. Oakbrook, IL: Author.

Juran Institute. (2003). *Juran Institute's Six Sigma breakthrough and beyond: Quality performance breakthrough methods*. Columbus, OH: McGraw-Hill Professional.

Kedrowski, S., & Weiner, C. (2003). Performance measures in ambulatory care. *Nursing Economic$, 21*(4), 188-193.

Kitson, A. (1997). Using evidence to demonstrate the value of nursing. *Nursing Standard, 11*(28), 34-39.

Kobs, A. E. (1998). Getting started on benchmarking. *Outcomes Management for Nursing Practice, 2*(1), 45- 48.

Leebov, W., & Ersoz, C. (1991) *The health care manager's guide to continuous quality improvement*. Chicago: American Hospital Publishing, Inc.

Le May, A., Mulhall, A., & Alexander, C. (1998). Bridging the research-practice gap: Exploring the research cultures of practitioners and managers. *Journal of Advanced Nursing, 28*(2), 428-437.

Lowe, A., & Baker, J. (1997). Measuring outcomes: A nursing report card. *Nursing Management, 38*, 40-41.

Mastal, M. (1999). New signposts and directions: Indicators of quality in ambulatory nursing care. *Nursing Economic$, 17*(2), 103-104.

Melynk, B.M., & Fineout-Overholt, E. (2005). *Evidence-Based practice in nursing and healthcare: A guide to best practice*. Philadelphia: Lippincott Williams & Wilkins.

Mohide, E.A., & King, B. (2003). Building a foundation for evidence-based practice: Experiences in a tertiary hospital. *Evidence Based Nursing, 6*, 100-103.

National Association for Healthcare Quality. (1998). *Guide to quality management* (8th ed.). Glenview, IL: Author.

Pande, P., & Holpp, L. (2002). *What is Six Sigma?* New York: McGraw-Hill.

Ribnick, P.G., & Carrano, V.A. (1995). Understanding the new era in health care accountability: Report cards. *Journal of Nursing Care Quality, 10*(1), 1-8.

Rieve, J.A. (1999). Case identification and selection outcomes. *The Case Manager, 10*(3), 22, 25.

Schriefer, J., Urden, L.D., & Rogers, S. (1997). Report cards: Tools for managing pathways and outcomes. *Outcomes Management for Nursing Practice, 1*(1), 14-19.

Spann, K. (1997). Benchmarking: Best practices. *MEDSURG Nursing, 6*(1), 5-6, 8.

Spath, P. (1998). Quality report cards market your services. *Hospital Peer Review, 23*(12), 231-233.

Stetler, C.B. (2003). Role of the organization in translating research into evidence-based practice. *Outcomes Management, 7*(3), 97-103.

Straus, S.E., Richardson, W.S., Glasziou, P., & Haynes, R.B. (2005). *Evidence-based medicine: How to practice and teach EBM* (3rd ed.). London: Churchill Livingstone.

Swan, B.A., & Boruch, R.F. (2004). Quality of evidence: Usefulness in measuring the quality of health care. *Medical Care, 42*(2), II-12-II-20.

Value Based Management.net (2006). *The Deming cycle.* Retrieved May 16, 2006, from www.valuebasedmanagement.net/methods_demingcycle.html

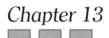
Evidence-Based Practice

This test may be copied for use by others.

COMPLETE THE FOLLOWING:

Name: _____

Address: _____

City: _____ State: _____ Zip: _____

Preferred telephone: (Home)_____ (Work)_____

E-mail_____

AAACN Member Expiration Date: _____

Registration fee: AAACN Member: $12.00
                   Nonmember: $20.00

Answer Form:

1. If you applied what you have learned from this activity into your practice, what would be different?

_____

_____

_____

Evaluation	Strongly disagree				Strongly agree
2. By completing this activity, I was able to meet the following objectives:					
a. Understand the meaning of evidence-based practice and performance improvement, and their application to ambulatory care nursing practice and quality care.	1	2	3	4	5
b. Describe the key steps of evidence-based nursing practice, discuss rating the quality and strength of the evidence, and identify strategies for facilitating evidence-based nursing practice initiatives and the use of clinical practice guidelines within an organization.	1	2	3	4	5
c. Discuss the differences between quality assurance and continuous performance improvement models.	1	2	3	4	5
d. Discuss why indicators are integral to the performance improvement process, define different types of indicators, and provide an example of each.	1	2	3	4	5
e. Describe the multiple factors affecting the development of a reliable and valid process to monitor competencies and outcomes.	1	2	3	4	5
f. Understand the relationship of varied indicators on a balanced scorecard, dashboard, or report card in reflecting the outcomes of an organization.	1	2	3	4	5
3. The content was current and relevant.	1	2	3	4	5
4. The objectives could be achieved using the content provided.	1	2	3	4	5
5. This was an effective method to learn this content.	1	2	3	4	5
6. I am more confident in my abilities since completing this material.	1	2	3	4	5

7. The material was (check one) ___new ___review for me.
8. Time required to read this chapter: _____minutes

I verify that I have completed this activity: _____

Signature

Comments: _____

_____

Objectives

This educational activity is designed for nurses and other health care professionals who practice in ambulatory care. For those wishing to obtain CE credit, an evaluation follows. After studying the information presented in this offering, you will be able to:

1. Understand the meaning of evidence-based practice and performance improvement, and their application to ambulatory care nursing practice and quality care.
2. Describe the key steps of evidence-based nursing practice, discuss rating the quality and strength of the evidence, and identify strategies for facilitating evidence-based nursing practice initiatives and the use of clinical practice guidelines within an organization.
3. Discuss the differences between quality assurance and continuous performance improvement models.
4. Discuss why indicators are integral to the performance improvement process, define different types of indicators, and provide an example of each.
5. Describe the multiple factors affecting the development of a reliable and valid process to monitor competencies and outcomes.
6. Understand the relationship of varied indicators on a balanced scorecard, dashboard, or report card in reflecting the outcomes of an organization.

Posttest Instructions

1. To receive continuing education credit for individual study after reading the article, complete the answer/evaluation form to the left.

2. Detach and send the answer/evaluation form along with a check or money order payable to the *American Academy of Ambulatory Care Nursing (AAACN)*, East Holly Avenue Box 56, Pitman, NJ 08071-0056.

3. Test returns must be postmarked by August 1, 2011. Upon completion of the answer/evaluation form, a certificate for **1.5** contact hour(s) will be awarded and sent to you. Should the material contained in this chapter become outdated prior to the above expiration date, AAACN reserves the right to withdraw this CE test.

This activity is co-provided by the *American Academy of Ambulatory Care Nursing (AAACN)* and Anthony J. Jannetti, Inc. (AJJ). AJJ is accredited as a provider of continuing nursing education by the American Nurses' Credentialing Center's Commission on Accreditation (ANCC-COA). AAACN is a provider approved by the California Board of Registered Nurses, provider number CEP 05336.

This article was reviewed and formatted for contact hour credit by Sally S. Russell, MN, CMSRN, AAACN Education Director; and Candia Baker Laughlin MS, RN, C, Editor.

Chapter 14

Ethics

Carrol Gold, PhD, RN

Objectives

Study of the information presented in this chapter will enable the learner to:
1. Define nursing ethics.
2. Differentiate ethical issues from legal issues.
3. Identify the essential requirements for ethical practice stated in the American Nurses' Association (ANA) Code for Nurses.
4. Discuss the principles that guide ethical decision making.
5. Discuss two philosophical theories used in ethical decision making.
6. Identify the critical elements in an ethical dilemma.
7. List the essential steps in the process of ethical decision making.
8. Identify ethical problems of particular concern to ambulatory nursing.
9. Appreciate the role of the nurse as advocate for patient and family in ethical dilemmas.
10. Discuss the role of the nurse in working with an ethics committee.

Key Points

1. Nursing ethics involves choosing from two or more options, none of which may be totally desirable, to guide actions within the nurses' scope of practice.
2. The ANA Ethical Code for Nurses offers specific statements regarding the nurse's duty to respect, safeguard, and protect the patient and his or her rights.
3. There are several principles that guide ethical decision making.
4. The two approaches most commonly used in ethical decision making are weighing the benefits to be gained with the resulting burden or selecting an action based on accepted duty.

Nursing practice is founded on and sustained by adherence to ethical principles. Ethical decision making involves choosing from two or more options, none of which may be entirely satisfactory or unsatisfactory. The expansion of the scope of nursing practice, technologic advances, and a wider range of options for patients and families have resulted in nurses' involvement with an increasing number of situations in which an ethical conflict is central. These situations require that nurses develop an understanding of ethical decision making and action processes, either as individuals or as a part of the health care team or ethics committee. Nurses in the ambulatory care setting are challenged by many of the same ethical concerns as inpatient nurses. However, ambulatory care nurses have additional challenges that include less direct supervision of assistive personnel; the need for shared, but protect-

ed, patient information across ambulatory units; and access issues presented by managed care protocols. In addition, patients seen in ambulatory care settings are more frail and challenged than in the past, and there are increasing concerns about social justice and the use of health care resources.

Definition of Nursing Ethics

A. Nursing ethics involves choosing from two or more options, none of which may be totally desirable, to guide actions within the nurses' scope of practice.
B. Ethics attempts to answer the question, "What ought one to do in a given situation?" (Burkhardt & Nathaniel, 2002). Ethics involves an examination of how one ought to act.

Differences Between Ethical Issues And Legal Issues

A. Ethical principles are not legally binding, although some laws are supported by ethical precepts (Hall, 1996).
   1. The patient's right to confidentiality is supported by law and by the ethical principle of confidentiality. It is an ethical violation to breech confidentiality; a patient can bring a lawsuit over violations of confidentiality.
   2. Giving preferred appointment times to patients with private insurance or who are private pay may be ethically questionable, but it does not necessarily violate law.
B. Laws and those things that are legally binding may or may not be considered ethical, based on an individual's ethical stance.
   1. Abortion and withdrawal of life support are supported in law, but may or may not be considered ethical.
   2. Denial of access to certain treatments or medications by managed care companies is, in some cases, legal, but subject to ethical concerns.

The ANA Ethical Code for Nurses

This code has specific statements regarding the nurse's duty to:
A. Respect the dignity of the individual, whatever the socioeconomic status, personal attributes, or type of health problem.
B. Safeguard the patient's right to confidentiality.
C. Protect the patient and public from unsafe or unethical practices.
D. Exercise responsibility and accountability for nursing actions.
E. Maintain own practice competencies.
F. Exercise professional knowledge and judgment in accepting and carrying out assignments and in delegating to others (ANA, 2001).

Principles That Guide Ethical Decision Making

A. *Autonomy*: Self-determination, the freedom to choose one's own course of action.
   1. Implies that one is cognitively able to exercise this right.
   2. Implies that no coercion has taken place.

B. *Beneficence*: Doing good.
   1. Requires defining what is meant by good in the situation.
   2. Requires an understanding of what is in the best interest of the patient.
C. *Nonmaleficence*: Acting in such a way that avoids harm, either intentional harm or harm as an unintended outcome.
   1. Consideration must be given to the need to sometimes do harm in order to do good. For instance, chemotherapy may have serious systemic consequences; the treatment may be as life-threatening as the illness.
   2. Consideration must be given to the benefits vs. the burden of action, which may result in unintended or secondary harm.
D. *Justice*: Fair, equitable distribution of resources.
   1. Requires recognition that resources and services are not limitless, that a system for decision making about how resources are used must be in place, and that ongoing examination of the concept of social justice in the distribution and use of health care resources must be a part of discussions.
   2. Requires that distribution of resources is based on the belief in the importance and value of each person. Each person has innate value as a human being as opposed to having some particular attribute, such as intelligence or creativity, or because they hold a particular station in life.
E. *Veracity*: Truth telling.
   1. Truth is the foundation of the development of trust between patient and nurse. All patients and/or their families, if families are acting as surrogates, are owed the duty of being informed about health conditions, treatment options, and prognoses, with as much completeness and accuracy as possible.
   2. Immediate attention, without prejudgment, must be given to situations in which a family or individual does not wish to know about a diagnosis or prognosis, in an effort to understand why a family or individual would take such a stance.
      a. Such situations should be referred for consultation with the institution's ethics committee.
      b. In the absence of such a committee,

staff may seek consultation with clergy, social services, ethics consultants from outside the system (university ethicist, for instance) or ethical resource persons from specialty or professional organizations.

F. *Confidentiality*: To protect the patient's and family's right to privacy regarding information that the nurse or institution holds regarding the patient.

   1. Sharing of information must occur only between those parties who require access to fulfill obligations to provide care, consultation, or referral.

   2. Attention must paid to electronic patient records and databases that are transferred between numerous care-delivery locations. Technology and the movement of patients through a number of ambulatory care delivery units add new burdens to the protection of confidentiality.

   3. Adherence to HIPAA requirements, the understanding of their rights and responsibilities in the health care system by patients and families, and preservation of confidentiality in the uses of patient data for Q.I. activities (Fox & Tulsky, 2005; Wolfish & Sharp, 2005).

G. *Fidelity*: Faithfulness.

   1. Involves the duty owed to patients, families, and colleagues to do what one says one will do and to consistently act in accordance with the requirements of the state's nurse practice act and the ethical standards of the profession.

   2. Requires an understanding that the privilege of using the protected title, RN, through state licensure, implies a duty owed to the citizens of the state or commonwealth issuing the license to practice. Those duties are stated in the nurse practice acts of each state (Gibson, 1993).

Philosophical Theories Used in Ethical Decision Making

Although there are a number of philosophic theories underlying ethical decision making, the two approaches most commonly used involve assessment of the consequences of an action by weighing the benefits to be gained with the resulting burden, or selecting an action based on some accepted duty. In concert with the ethical principles, the philosophic approaches structure understanding of dilemmas and assist in clarification of possible solutions to these dilemmas.

A. Utilitarianism (also known as consequence-based ethics) is the theory that seeks to choose the option that will offer the most good to the greatest number of people, increase pleasure, and avoid pain.

   1. It is also characterized by the belief that the end justifies the means.

   2. An act or decision is judged as a desirable choice based on its outcome. According to this theory, an act is ethical that brings the greatest benefit for the greatest number of people (Edge & Groves, 1994).

     a. Example: Based on the principle of beneficence, or doing good, it is permissible to administer morphine for pain relief in a terminally ill patient even though the drug may depress respirations.

     b. This involves weighing the benefit (relief from suffering) from the burden (possible hastening of death).

B. Deontology (also known as duty-based ethics) is based on the belief that there are duties to which one must be faithful and which one is obligated to carry out because these duties are owed to all human beings and because of the expectations implied by one's professional role (Edge & Groves, 1994).

   1. Decisions are made based on what are considered universally accepted rules, and every person is owed the same duty.

   2. People are ends, in and of themselves, and cannot be used to produce a specific end.

   3. Nurses are bound by their professional codes to uphold duties that honor patient autonomy, mandate truth telling, protect patient confidentiality, extend justice and fairness to all, do no harm, seek to do good, and promote well-being.

   4. Examples of deontology or duty-based ethics:

     a. The use of placebos violates the duty to be truthful. Principle: Veracity.

     b. The patient must receive the same quality of care and be offered the same services, regardless of the ability to pay or payer source. Principle: Justice.

c. It is a duty to report incidents of incompetent nursing or medical care. Principles: Veracity, fidelity, nonmaleficence.

Ethical Dilemmas

A. Ethical dilemmas exist because no clear right or wrong answers exist for the question of what one ought to do or how one ought to act in certain situations.
  1. There may be conflicts of duty or a conflict in principles.
  2. Duties of beneficence and nonmaleficence (to do good and avoid harm) can be in conflict with the duty to protect the individual's autonomy (self-determination) when a patient is restrained.
B. Ethical dilemmas differ from moral dilemmas in that for the individual, moral decisions have a clear yes/no, right/wrong answer. If an individual is very clear about what he or she considers right or wrong and there is no sense of a conflicting possibility, an ethical dilemma does not exist for that person.

Essential Steps in the Process of Ethical Decision Making

A. Gather relevant information and facts, including a narrative describing the situation. The narrative should include an identification of conflicting duties, rights, beliefs, and cultural, religious, and societal values of the parties involved (Burkhardt & Nathaniel, 2002).
B. Identify the stakeholders.
  1. Who are the people involved in the deliberations and decision-making process?
  2. Who holds the authority for making the final decision?
  3. How will the decision be made?
  4. When will the decision be made?
C. Determine the abilities of the stakeholders to make a decision.
  1. What are the developmental, cognitive, and psychologic states of the individuals who will engage in the decision-making process?
  2. Are these individuals able to engage in a deliberative, reflective process about the issues at stake?
D. Identify the desired outcome(s).
  1. Which outcomes are acceptable and which are not acceptable?
  2. What are the consequences of each alternative?
E. Decide upon what action will be taken.
  1. Who will implement the action?
  2. How will the action be implemented?
  3. When will the action be implemented?
F. Evaluate and reassess the effect of the action taken.
  1. Was the dilemma resolved to the satisfaction of the stakeholders?
  2. Has the first action resulted in a situation in which another ethical decision has arisen?

Ethical Problems of Particular Concern to Ambulatory Nursing

A. Maintain and adhere to standards of care.
  1. Observe for instances of poor judgment and incompetence of caregivers. These may be difficult to observe in ambulatory care because of the physical design of ambulatory areas, mobility of the patient group, brief length of patient interactions, and the inability to observe the actions of other professional and nonlicensed personnel.
  2. Encourage daily walking rounds through ambulatory areas.
  3. Schedule care conferences on selected groups of patients.
  4. Distribute, analyze, and provide feedback to staff on patient satisfaction surveys.
  5. Perform ongoing chart audits and quality improvement activities.
  6. Designate a professional nurse as quality control coordinator.
  7. Educate and expect staff to engage in quality improvement activities.
B. Assess for differences in the delivery of care or treatment, based on the patient's reimbursement sources.
  1. Advocate for equities within patient care system.
  2. Collaborate and network with other health care resources to provide for patient care needs.

C. Protect patient privacy and confidentiality.
    1. Create a system to protect privacy of records that are transferred from one division to another (informatics issues are discussed further in Chapter 7, *Informatics,* and HIPAA requirements are discussed in Chapter 8, *Legal Aspects of Ambulatory Care Nursing*).
    2. Orient and monitor staff to the need for telephone privacy when discussing or conversing with patients.
    3. Provide for private areas in which to interact with patients, engage in patient education, assess such information as weight or glucometer readings, or discuss treatment plans.
    4. Provide confidential check-in process and flow through settings. Avoid sign-in sheets or posted schedules that can be viewed by those without a need for such information.
D. Provide for staff mix appropriate to the intensity level of patients by instituting evidence- or research-based staffing patterns designed for ambulatory care settings (Haas & Hackbarth, 1995).

The Role of the Nurse as Advocate for Patient And Family in Ethical Dilemmas

In assisting patients and families with ethical dilemmas, the nurse is acting on the principles of beneficence, justice, and fidelity.

A. Educate patients and families about patient rights.
B. Assure that the voices of patients and families are heard, especially of those unable to articulate their own needs.
C. Identify and articulate ethical concerns as they occur in practice.
D. Assume responsibility to move ethical concerns through to a resolution, either with the unit or through involvement of an institutional ethics committee.
E. Monitor and evaluate the outcome of actions taken.

Role of Nurse in Working with an Ethics Committee

A. Ethics committees serve two major functions within health care organizations.
    1. Education of care providers within institutions regarding the ethical rights of patients, the ethical position of the institution (for example, through policies, bylaws, and guidelines), and the function of the ethics committee.
    2. Consultation on issues brought to the committee.
        a. Inform staff about the process for bringing issues to the attention of the committee.
        b. Distribute written documents describing the work and availability of the committee to providers, staff, patients, and families.
        c. Select appropriate members for the committee, including nurses, physicians, social workers, clergy, legal counsel, and administrators (Benjamin & Curtis, 1992). Multidisciplinary representation brings vital diversity of perspective to committee deliberations.
        d. Observe confidentiality in considering patient issues.
B. When an ethics committee does not exist within an organization, some sources for consultation include:
    1. The ANA *Ethics in Nursing: Position Statements and Guidelines* (2001). This document is available from the ANA, state nurses' associations, and college, university, and hospital nursing libraries.
    2. Value statements/ethics codes developed and published by specialty organizations, such as the American Association of Ambulatory Care Nursing, the American Association of Critical Care Nursing, the American Organization of Nurse Executives, and/or colleague consultants from such organizations.
    3. Colleagues in college and university nursing and/or ethics programs with expertise in health care ethics.
    4. Consultants from state nursing organizations.

5. Colleagues from organizations with ethics committees to advise on how to institute an ethics committee in one's own organization.

References

American Nurses' Association (ANA). (2001). *Ethics in nursing: Position statements and guidelines.* Washington, DC: Author.

Benjamin, M., & Curtis, J. (1992). *Ethics in nursing* (3rd ed.). New York: Oxford University Press.

Burkhardt, M.A., & Nathaniel, A.K. (2002). *Ethics and issues in contemporary nursing.* Albany, NY: Delmar.

Edge, R.S., & Groves, J.R. (1994). *The ethics of health care: A guide for clinical practice.* Albany, NY: Delmar.

Fox, E., & Tulsky, J.A. (2005). Recommendations for ethical conduct of quality improvement. *Journal of Clinical Ethics, 16*(1), 61-71.

Gibson, C. (1993). Underpinnings of ethical reasoning in nursing. *Journal of Advanced Nursing, 18*(12), 203- 207.

Haas, S., & Hackbarth, D. (1995). Dimensions of the staff nurse role in ambulatory care: Part III – Using data to design new models of nursing care delivery. *Nursing Economic$, 13*(4), 230-241.

Hall, J.K. (1996). *Nursing ethics and law.* Philadelphia: WB Saunders.

Wolfish, S., & Sharp, S.P. (2005). Readability level of HIPAA notices of privacy practices used by physical rehabilitation services. *Journal of Clinical Ethics, 16*(2), 156-159.

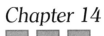
Ethics

This test may be copied for use by others.

COMPLETE THE FOLLOWING:

Name: _____

Address: _____

City: _____ State: _____ Zip: _____

Preferred telephone: (Home)_____ (Work)_____

E-mail_____

AAACN Member Expiration Date: _____

Registration fee: AAACN Member: $12.00
                    Nonmember: $20.00

Answer Form:

1. If you applied what you have learned from this activity into your practice, what would be different?

   _____

   _____

   _____

Evaluation	Strongly disagree				Strongly agree
2. By completing this activity, I was able to meet the following objectives:					
a. Define nursing ethics.	1	2	3	4	5
b. Differentiate ethical issues from legal issues.	1	2	3	4	5
c. Identify the essential requirements for ethical practice stated in the American Nurses' Association (ANA) Code for Nurses.	1	2	3	4	5
d. Discuss the principles that guide ethical decision making.	1	2	3	4	5
e. Discuss two philosophical theories used in ethical decision making.	1	2	3	4	5
f. Identify the critical elements in an ethical dilemma.	1	2	3	4	5
g. List the essential steps in the process of ethical decision making.	1	2	3	4	5
h. Identify ethical problems of particular concern to ambulatory nursing.	1	2	3	4	5
i. Appreciate the role of the nurse as advocate for patient and family in ethical dilemmas.	1	2	3	4	5
j. Discuss the role of the nurse working with an ethics committee.	1	2	3	4	5
3. The content was current and relevant.	1	2	3	4	5
4. The objectives could be achieved using the content provided.	1	2	3	4	5
5. This was an effective method to learn this content.	1	2	3	4	5
6. I am more confident in my abilities since completing this material.	1	2	3	4	5

7. The material was (check one) ___new ___review for me.
8. Time required to read this chapter: _____minutes

I verify that I have completed this activity: _____
                                              Signature

Comments: _____

_____

Objectives

This educational activity is designed for nurses and other health care professionals who practice in ambulatory care. For those wishing to obtain CE credit, an evaluation follows. After studying the information presented in this offering, you will be able to:

1. Define nursing ethics.
2. Differentiate ethical issues from legal issues.
3. Identify the essential requirements for ethical practice stated in the American Nurses' Association (ANA) Code for Nurses.
4. Discuss the principles that guide ethical decision making.
5. Discuss two philosophical theories used in ethical decision making.
6. Identify the critical elements in an ethical dilemma.
7. List the essential steps in the process of ethical decision making.
8. Identify ethical problems of particular concern to ambulatory nursing.
9. Appreciate the role of the nurse as advocate for patient and family in ethical dilemmas.
10. Discuss the role of the nurse in working with an ethics committee.

Posttest Instructions

1. To receive continuing education credit for individual study after reading the article, complete the answer/evaluation form to the left.

2. Detach and send the answer/evaluation form along with a check or money order payable to the *American Academy of Ambulatory Care Nursing (AAACN)*, East Holly Avenue Box 56, Pitman, NJ 08071–0056.

3. Test returns must be postmarked by August 1, 2011. Upon completion of the answer/evaluation form, a certificate for **1.4** contact hour(s) will be awarded and sent to you. Should the material contained in this chapter become outdated prior to the above expiration date, AAACN reserves the right to withdraw this CE test.

This activity is co-provided by the *American Academy of Ambulatory Care Nursing (AAACN)* and Anthony J. Jannetti, Inc. (AJJ). AJJ is accredited as a provider of continuing nursing education by the American Nurses' Credentialing Center's Commission on Accreditation (ANCC-COA). AAACN is a provider approved by the California Board of Registered Nurses, provider number CEP 05336.

This article was reviewed and formatted for contact hour credit by Sally S. Russell, MN, CMSRN, AAACN Education Director; and Candia Baker Laughlin MS, RN, C, Editor.

Chapter 15

Regulatory Compliance and Patient Safety

Anita Markovich, MSN, BSN, MPA, CPHQ

Candia Baker Laughlin, MS, RN, C

Objectives

Study of the information presented in this chapter will enable the learner to:

1. Identify organizations that promote patient safety and monitor health care organizations for quality.
2. Describe regulatory standards that apply to the practice of ambulatory care nursing.
3. Identify regulations related to the workplace and to employee safety.
4. Understand regulations regarding reportable diseases and conditions.
5. Provide a resource of references for guidelines to promote patient safety.

Key Points

1. Several regulating agencies oversee adherence to standards and requirements by health care organizations.
2. The Occupational Safety and Health Administration (OSHA) sets workplace safety and health standards, and inspects workplaces for compliance with those standards.
3. The *Americans with Disabilities Act* (ADA) protects persons with a disability or who have a relationship or association with an individual with a disability.
4. There are several regulations regarding reportable diseases and conditions.
5. The *Joint Commission on Accreditation of Healthcare Organizations* (JCAHO) has established and maintained standards since 1951.

In 2000, the Institute of Medicine (IOM) published a landmark book, *To Err Is Human*. This publication focused on preventable errors that occur in the health care environment. From this publication, regulatory organizations began to emphasize the importance of pursuing the highest standards of care for patient safety. Ambulatory care nurses working in a variety of health care settings are responsible for a continuous quality improvement approach to assure the prevention of errors and to promote patient safety. Regulatory requirements promote this.

Regulatory Requirements

Regulatory requirements are generated by federal and state legislative acts, by requirements of official agencies representing the public as advocates and purchasers of health care services, and by standards developed through professional organizations. Several regulatory agencies oversee adherence to standards and requirements by health care organizations.

The Occupational Safety and Health Administration

A. The *Occupational Safety and Health Act* was signed into law by President Nixon on December 28, 1970. Three agencies were created, one of which is the Occupational Safety and Health Administration (OSHA). OSHA is the enforcement arm for this act.

B. OSHA sets workplace safety and health standards, and inspects workplaces for compliance with those standards.

C. OSHA has the duty to investigate employee complaints about unsafe workplace conditions.

D. OSHA has established general standards, referred to as performance standards, that allow employers to determine their own level of compliance.

E. In some instances, OSHA will issue a directive, for example, the use of fit-tested equipment for employees exposed to communicable diseases.

F. It is the responsibility of every employer to communicate information to each employee about hazards within their workplace setting (OSHA, U.S. Department of Labor, 1996).

1. Employees have a right to know about hazardous chemical substances used in their work environment.
2. Material Safety Data Sheets (MSDS) provided by the manufacturer of the chemical or medication must be accessible to all employees by employers for each hazardous chemical in the workplace.
3. Containers of hazardous materials in the workplace must be labeled with the identity of the hazardous chemical contained and appropriate bio-hazard warnings.
4. All employees must be provided information and training where hazardous chemicals are present.

G. Other areas that OSHA addresses in the health care workplace are:
1. Bloodborne pathogen exposure and guidelines for prevention of transmission of disease.
   a. When indicated, universal precautions observed by all employees.
   b. The appropriate personal protective equipment worn by employees to prevent contact with blood or other potentially infectious material.
2. Measures to prevent the transmission of *Mycobacterium tuberculosis* by:
   a. Providing respiratory equipment or devices and training employees in their use.
   b. Tuberculin skin test screening at the time of hire and annually for employees in patient care areas.
3. Hepatitis B vaccination series available at no cost to all employees who may have occupational exposure to blood or other potentially infectious materials.
4. Post-exposure to blood or potentially infectious substances, evaluation, and follow-up according to current U.S. Public Health Service recommendations at no cost to all employees who have had an exposure incident.
5. Exposure to chemicals or radiation in the workplace including medical use of lasers.
6. Guidelines for the handling and storage of

cytotoxic drugs.
7. Infection control and medical waste including proper labeling and disposal.
   a. Regulated medical waste must be placed in marked bio-hazard containers that are closable, leak-proof during transport, and labeled for ready identification.
   b. Manifests and tracking of regulated waste in transportation.
8. Ergonomic disorders.
9. Workplace violence.

H. OSHA requires record keeping of employee injuries and illness.

I. OSHA also provides standards for workplace safety related to fire safety, utilities, electrical safety, and medical equipment.

J. Inspections may result from specific accidents, employee complaints, or as part of OSHA's system of programmed inspections.

K. Continuous education of employees promotes workplace safety and assures compliance with OSHA's standards.

Americans with Disabilities Act (ADA)

A. The *Americans with Disabilities Act* (ADA) of 1990 prohibits discrimination on the basis of disability in employment, state, and local government; public accommodations; commercial facilities; transportation; and telecommunications (42 USCA section 12182) (U.S. Congress, 1990).

B. ADA protects persons with a disability or who have a relationship or association with an individual with a disability. An individual with a disability is defined as a person with:
1. A physical or mental impairment that substantially limits one or more major life activities.
2. A record of such impairment.
3. Being regarded as having such an impairment (42 USCA 12102 [2]) (U.S. Congress, 1990).

C. Programs or activities that receive or benefit from federal financial assistance are prohibited from discriminating in the offering of their services on the basis of handicap.

D. Qualified individuals may not be denied full access to goods, services, facilities, privileges, advantages, and accommodation by any place considered an organization of public accommodation or public services because of a handicap (USCA 12182[a]) (U.S. Congress, 1990).

   1. Physicians' offices are considered facilities of public accommodation.

   2. "Handicap" includes any disability.

E. Both programs receiving federal financial assistance and programs of public accommodation are required to meet some specific standards under the ADA.

   1. Architectural standards for new and altered buildings and in newly leased facilities must be met, as described in the *Architectural Barriers Act* (ABA).

   2. Public accommodations must remove barriers in existing buildings where it is easy to do so without much difficulty or expense, given the public accommodation's resources.

   3. Auxiliary aids must be provided to persons with impaired sensory, manual, or speaking skills, where necessary to afford such persons an equal opportunity to benefit from the service in question.

F. Individuals with HIV infection are intended to be regarded as disabled under the ADA legislation, and this interpretation has been upheld by federal courts.

Regulations Regarding Reportable Diseases And Conditions

A. The Centers for Disease Control and Prevention's (CDC) National Center for Health Statistics receives reports of births, deaths, and terminations of pregnancies through state health departments.

   1. All states require reporting of a live birth regardless of length of gestation or weight.

   2. Fetal death is reportable, but the definition varies by state.

   3. Induced termination of pregnancy is reportable, and reporting is mandatory in 48 U.S. regions.

   4. Death certificates must be completed, including cause of death.

B. Clinicians and laboratories are required to report infectious diseases and other conditions (Chorba, Berkelman, Safford, Gibbs, & Hull, 1990).

   1. Authority to require notification of cases of diseases resides with state governments.

2. Reporting is important in controlling and preventing the spread of communicable diseases and in assuring appropriate medical therapy.

   a. All states and U.S. territories participate in the national morbidity reporting system.

   b. Forty-nine (49) infectious diseases and related conditions are reported either as individual cases or in the aggregate through the states and territories to the CDC in Atlanta, GA.

   c. State requirements vary in terms of which agency is to receive reports, what is to be reported, time frames for reporting, and other factors.

   d. Non-infectious diseases also regulated include diseases caused by occupational exposures, environmental diseases, and congenital or noninfectious childhood conditions.

   e. Diseases of "unknown or unusual etiology" which may evolve into identification of new diseases are also reportable.

3. The threat of bioterrorism heightens the need to make surveillance timely, specific, and responsive (M'ikanatha, Southwell, & Lautenbach, 2003).

   a. Computerization of patient and clinical laboratory data may allow for automated reporting to health departments.

   b. Refinement of automated systems is needed to:

     (1) Become appropriately sensitive.

     (2) To transmit important findings.

     (3) Avoid reporting of extraneous data.

     (4) Provide complete case information.

     (5) Facilitate use of uniform nomenclature and data standards.

     (6) Indicate adequate staffing and skill level to manage the system at the local level.

C. Reportable drug information:

   1. The *National Childhood Vaccine Injury Act of 1986* requires health care providers who administer vaccines and toxoids to report selected adverse events occurring after vaccination to the U.S. Department of Health and Human Services.

a. If the vaccines are acquired through public purchasing, reporting is made through local, county, and/or state health departments.

b. Events following receipt of privately purchased vaccines are directly reportable to the Food and Drug Administration (FDA).

2. Events following the administration of non-vaccine medications are reportable directly to the FDA.

D. Reporting of potential violent crimes, abuse, and neglect:

1. Health care agencies need policies for the identification, evaluation, management, and referral of patients suspected to be victims of violent crimes, domestic violence, or neglect, including the following (Burnett, 2004):

a. Safeguarding information and evidentiary material(s) that could be used in future actions as part of the legal process.

b. Responsibility for consents from the patient, parent, or legal guardian or compliance with other applicable laws.

c. Protecting evidentiary material released by the patient.

d. Acquiring legally required notifications and releases of information to authorities.

e. Implementing referrals to private or public community agencies for victims of abuse.

2. The health care agency and staff need to provide for the immediate safety of the patient.

3. Documentation in the medical record should describe the details of all findings, interventions, and actions.

4. Ambulatory care nurses need to be familiar with local and state laws and resources for reporting and providing care to victims of violence (Draucker, 2002).

The Joint Commission on Accreditation of Healthcare Organizations (JCAHO)

A. The Joint Commission on Accreditation of Healthcare Organizations (JCAHO) is an independent, not-for-profit organization that evaluates and accredits more than 15,000 health care programs in the United States.

B. Since 1951, the Joint Commission has established and maintained standards that improve the quality and safety of care provided by health care organizations.

C. A triennial survey of organizations seeking or maintaining accreditation is conducted through an onsite visit, and upon accreditation, an organization displays the distinctive *Gold Seal of Approval.*

D. JCAHO is governed by a 29-member Board of Commission, which includes nurses, physicians, consumers, medical directors, administrators, employers, a labor representative, health plan leaders, quality experts, health care administrators, and educators.

E. JCAHO standards address the organization's level of performance in areas such as:

1. Ethics and patient rights.
2. Assessment and provision of care, treatment, and services.
3. Medication management.
4. Surveillance, prevention, and control of infection.
5. Improving organization performance.
6. Leadership.
7. Nursing.
8. Management of the environment of care and equipment.
9. Information management.
10. Management of human resources.
11. Medical staff.

F. In ambulatory care nursing, standards under these areas would include (JCAHO, 2006):

1. Patients' rights to be involved in the decisions about their care, treatment, and services.
2. Patients' rights to informed consent.
3. Respect of patients' wishes to refuse care and end-of-life decisions.
4. Patients' rights to pain management.
5. Appropriate assessment of patients prior to and during invasive procedures and the administration of moderate or deep sedation.
6. Defined policies, procedures, and competen-

cy for carrying out waived testing.

7. Proper ordering, administration, labeling, and storage of medications.

8. Infection prevention, control, and surveillance with adherence to the CDC hygiene guidelines.

9. Data collection and analysis for performance improvement in an organization.

10. Identification and management of sentinel events.

11. Appropriate governance to ensure a patient safety program and use of clinical practice guidelines.

12. Organizational procedures that promote safety in all areas of the environment.

13. Orientation and ongoing competency of staff related to their job responsibilities and patient setting.

14. Maintaining and protecting accurate patient medical records.

G. In 2004, JCAHO proactively addressed patient safety by adding the National Patient Safety Goals, which are mandated for health care organizations and included in the survey process.

1. These goals apply to all accredited organizations.

2. The purpose of JCAHO's National Patient Safety Goals is to promote specific improvements in patient safety.

3. The National Patient Safety Goals highlight problematic areas in health care and provide evidence-based solutions to these problems.

H. Depending on the health care setting, some or all of the following National Patient Safety Goals may apply (JCAHO, 2006):

1. Improve the accuracy of patient identification with two identifiers and "time out" prior to invasive procedures.

2. Improve the effectiveness of communication among caregivers including:
   a. Read-back of verbal orders.
   b. Avoiding dangerous abbreviations.
   c. Timely reporting of critical test values.
   d. Accurate hand-off of patient information among care givers.

3. Medication safety in standardizing concentrates.

4. Educating and alerting staff about look-alike, sound-alike drugs.

5. Labeling of all medications or solutions (including oral, parenteral, topical medications); anesthetic agents and gases; radiopharmaceuticals and radiopaque contrast media; intravenous fluids; dialysis fluids; respiratory therapy agents; investigational medications; and medication samples.

6. Implement the "Universal Protocols" to prevent wrong site, wrong patient, wrong procedure surgery, including:
   a. Checklists to verify patient and procedure.
   b. Appropriate marking of sites with laterality or spinal surgery.
   c. Conducting a "time out" session prior to incision with active verification by all team members.

7. Preventing infections with:
   a. Proper hand hygiene.
   b. Reporting sentinel events related to nosocomial infections.

8. Reconciling medications across settings.

9. Implementing and evaluating a fall reduction program.

10. Reducing the risk of surgical fires.

11. Encouraging the active involvement of patients and families in their own care.

I. In 2004, JCAHO began publicizing compliance with the National Patient Safety Goals through a *Quality Report* available on the JCAHO Web site.

J. Along with other agencies and payor organizations, public reporting and comparative health care organizations' report cards have become an invitation to the public to be more informed of performance by the organizations and providers of their care, and a way to assist a person in deciding if an organization meets his or her needs.

Federal and State Regulations

A. A state's legislature is responsible for enacting general laws.

B. State agencies are empowered to enforce these laws through rules and regulations that they develop and implement.

C. State practice acts define the scope of practice of health professionals including physician, nurses, and other licensed health professionals.

D. Misconduct by health professionals must be reported to the state for investigation and evaluation of disciplinary action.

E. Hospitals and other health facilities are licensed by the state.

F. Health care organizations that participate in Medicare and Medicaid programs must meet Conditions of Participation (CoPs) and Conditions for Coverage (CfCs) which are standards that improve quality and protect the health and safety of beneficiaries.

G. State standards, rules and regulations, and conditions of participation are regularly evaluated and revised.

H. Most recently, the *Patient Safety and Quality Improvement Act of 2005* was signed on July 29, 2005, by President George W. Bush to promote a culture of safety across health care settings by establishing federal protections that encourage candid examinations of the causes of health care errors and the development of effective solutions to prevent their recurrence.
   1. Included in the bill is the option to create or become part of a Patient Safety Organization (PSO) for the purpose of continuing analyses of the underlying causes of adverse events.
   2. It is hoped that non-identifiable information will be shared among PSOs to improve practices and prevent errors.

I. Through regulatory processes, government agencies enforce standards to promote patient safety and assure the public's participation in its health care.

National Committee for Quality Assurance (NCQA)

A. NCQA is a not-for-profit, independent organization that assesses, evaluates, and publicly reports on the quality of health plans, health care provider groups, and individual physicians.

B. NCQA assesses health care quality through onsite and offsite surveys, audits, satisfaction surveys, and clinical performance measurement.

C. A range of quality evaluation programs are offered:
   1. Accreditation programs.
      a. Disease Management (DM).
      b. Human Research Protection, Inc (HRP).
      c. Managed Behavioral Healthcare Organ-

ization (MBHO).
      d. Managed Care Organization (MCO).
      e. New Health Plan (NHP).
      f. Preferred Provider Organization (PPO).
   2. Certification programs.
      a. Credentials Verification Organization (CVO).
         (1) HRP Accreditation is offered through the Partnership for Human Research Protection, Inc. (PHRP), which is a collaboration between NCQA and JCAHO.
      b. Disease Management (DM).
      c. Physician Organization Certification (POC).
      d. Utilization Management (UR) and Credentialing (CR).
   3. Physician recognition programs:
      a. Diabetes Physician Recognition Program (DPRP).
      b. Heart/Stroke Physician Recognition Program (HSRP).
      c. Physician Practice Connections (PPC).
      d. Future recognition programs are under consideration.

D. The NCQA health plan accreditation standards (NCQA, 2005) fall into the following categories:
   1. *Access and service* – Health plan provides its members with access to needed care and with good customer service.
      a. Number of primary and specialty providers are sufficient for the needs of the plan members.
      b. Grievances and appeals processes are responsive. Satisfaction surveys reflect good customer service.
   2. *Qualified providers* – Health plan activities that ensure each doctor is credentialed and qualified to provide the care.
   3. *Staying healthy* – Health plan provides activities that help people maintain good health and avoid illness.
      a. Preventive services guidelines are followed:
      b. Tests and screenings are provided, as appropriate.
   4. *Getting better* – Health plan provides up-to-date services that help people recover from illness.
   5. *Living with Illness* – Health plan supports people in managing chronic illness.

E. NCQA sponsors and maintains Health Plan Employer Data and Information Set (HEDIS®). HEDIS® is a registered trademark of the National Committee for Quality Assurance (NCQA).
   1. HEDIS® is a set of standardized performance measures designed to assure that purchasers and consumers have the information they need to reliably compare the performance of health care plans.
   2. HEDIS® assesses the quality of health plans across eight categories or domains.
      a. Access to/availability of care.
      b. Satisfaction with the experience of care.
      c. Stability of the health plan.
      d. Use of services.
      e. Cost of care.
      f. Informed health care choices.
      g. Health plan descriptive information.
   3. HEDIS® includes performance measures related to dozens of important health care issues, including, but are not limited to, the following:
      a. Advising smokers to quit.
      b. Antidepressant medication management.
      c. Beta blocker treatment after a heart attack.
      d. Breast cancer screening.
      e. Cervical cancer screening.
      f. Children and adolescent access to primary care physician.
      g. Children and adolescent immunization status.
      h. Comprehensive diabetes care.
      i. Controlling high blood pressure.
      j. Prenatal and postpartum care.

Accreditation Association for Ambulatory Health Care (AAAHC)

A. The Accreditation Association for Ambulatory Health Care (AAAHC) is a private, non-profit agency that offers voluntary, peer-based review of the quality of health care services of ambulatory health organizations, including ambulatory and office-based surgery centers, managed care organizations, as well as Indian and student health centers, among others (AAAHC, 2005).
B. Accreditation is based on a careful assessment of the organization's compliance with applicable standards.

C. AAAHC does not release information to the public about accreditation survey findings.
   1. AAAHC accreditation of certain types of ambulatory surgery centers is required or recognized in 25 states.
   2. AAAHC accreditation is required by several states for office-based surgery with certain levels of anesthesia.
   3. AAAHC accreditation for quality assurance reviews of HMOs is recognized by seven states.
D. Core standards will be applied to all types of organizations being surveyed:
   1. Rights of patients.
   2. Governance.
   3. Administration.
   4. Quality of care provided.
   5. Quality management and improvement.
   6. Clinical records and health information.
   7. Facilities and environment (FE).
E. Adjunct standards apply to organizations based on the types of services they provide (for example, urgent care centers, radiation oncology centers, and occupational health providers).

References

Accreditation Association for Ambulatory Health Care (AAAHC). (2005). *Accreditation handbook for ambulatory health care.* Skokie, IL: Author.

Burnett, L.B. (2004). *Domestic violence.* Retrieved February 24, 2006, from Emedicine.

Chorba, T., Berkelman, R.L., Safford, S.K., Gibbs, N.P., & Hull, H.F. (1990). Mandatory reporting of infectious diseases by clinicians. *Morbidity and Mortality Weekly Report, 39*(RR-9), 1-17.

Draucker, C.B. (2002). Domestic violence: The challenge for nursing. *Online Journal of Issues in Nursing, 7*(1), 2.

Institute of Medicine (IOM). (2000). *To err is human: Building a safer health system.* Washington, DC: National Academies Press.

Joint Commission on Accreditation of Healthcare Organizations (JCAHO). (2006). *Comprehensive accreditation manual for hospitals.* Oakbrook Terrace, IL: Author.

M'ikanatha, N.M., Southwell, B., & Lautenbach, E. (2003). Automated laboratory reporting of infectious diseases in a climate of bioterrorism. *Emerging Infectious Diseases, 9*(9), 1053-1057.

National Committee for Quality Assurance (NCQA). (2005). *Standards for accreditation of managed MCOs.* Washington, DC: Author.

Occupational Safety and Health Administration (OSHA), U.S. Department of Labor. (1996). *OSHA regulations (standards-29 CFR).* Washington, DC: Author.

U.S. Congress. (1990). *Americans with Disabilities Act of 1990.* S.933. Washington, DC: Author.

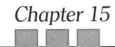

Chapter 15

CE Answer/Evaluation Form

Regulatory Compliance and Patient Safety

This test may be copied for use by others.

COMPLETE THE FOLLOWING:

Name: _____

Address: _____

City: _____ State: _____ Zip: _____

Preferred telephone: (Home)_____ (Work)_____

E-mail_____

AAACN Member Expiration Date: _____

Registration fee: AAACN Member: $12.00
                   Nonmember: $20.00

Objectives

This educational activity is designed for nurses and other health care professionals who practice in ambulatory care. For those wishing to obtain CE credit, an evaluation follows. After studying the information presented in this offering, you will be able to:

1. Identify organizations that promote patient safety and monitor health care organizations for quality.
2. Describe regulatory standards that apply to the practice of ambulatory care nursing.
3. Identify regulations related to the workplace and to employee safety.
4. Understand regulations regarding reportable diseases and conditions.
5. Provide a resource of references for guidelines to promote patient safety.

Answer Form:

1. If you applied what you have learned from this activity into your practice, what would be different?

_____

_____

_____

Evaluation	Strongly disagree				Strongly agree
2. By completing this activity, I was able to meet the following objectives:					
a. Identify organizations that promote patient safety and monitor health care organizations for quality.	1	2	3	4	5
b. Describe regulatory standards that apply to the practice of ambulatory care nursing.	1	2	3	4	5
c. Identify regulations related to the workplace and to employee safety.	1	2	3	4	5
d. Understand regulations regarding reportable diseases and conditions.	1	2	3	4	5
e. Provide a resource of references for guidelines to promote patient safety.	1	2	3	4	5
3. The content was current and relevant.	1	2	3	4	5
4. The objectives could be achieved using the content provided.	1	2	3	4	5
5. This was an effective method to learn this content.	1	2	3	4	5
6. I am more confident in my abilities since completing this material.	1	2	3	4	5

7. The material was (check one) ___new ___review for me.
8. Time required to read this chapter: _____minutes

I verify that I have completed this activity: _____
                                                        Signature

Comments: _____

_____

Posttest Instructions

1. To receive continuing education credit for individual study after reading the article, complete the answer/evaluation form to the left.

2. Detach and send the answer/evaluation form along with a check or money order payable to the *American Academy of Ambulatory Care Nursing (AAACN)*, East Holly Avenue Box 56, Pitman, NJ 08071–0056.

3. Test returns must be postmarked by August 1, 2011. Upon completion of the answer/evaluation form, a certificate for **1.4** contact hour(s) will be awarded and sent to you. Should the material contained in this chapter become outdated prior to the above expiration date, AAACN reserves the right to withdraw this CE test.

This activity is co-provided by the *American Academy of Ambulatory Care Nursing (AAACN)* and Anthony J. Jannetti, Inc. (AJJ). AJJ is accredited as a provider of continuing nursing education by the American Nurses' Credentialing Center's Commission on Accreditation (ANCC-COA). AAACN is a provider approved by the California Board of Registered Nurses, provider number CEP 05336.

This article was reviewed and formatted for contact hour credit by Sally S. Russell, MN, CMSRN, AAACN Education Director; and Candia Baker Laughlin MS, RN, C, Editor.

Chapter 16

Professional Development

Linda Brixey, RN

Michelle M. Budzinski-Braunscheidel, BSN, RN

Objectives

Study of the information presented in this chapter will enable the learner to:

1. Discuss key components of an orientation program for new staff in ambulatory care nursing roles.
2. Identify competence assessment requirements as related to accrediting agencies' standards and the essential duties of the nurse's position.
3. Discuss mandates for continuing education and professional growth and development needs.
4. Discuss continuing professional education using traditional and distance learning methods.
5. Identify the value of nursing specialty certification.
6. Describe the relationship between employee satisfaction, and retention and precepting of and by staff.
7. Discuss barriers and resources to professional nurses' self care.

Key Points

1. The orientation plan should be developed for all new staff as well as those transferring to new positions.
2. Competency assessment is not a one-time event; it is a continual process.
3. A strong preceptor program can make the new employee more successful in acclimating to the new role/position and reduce turnover.
4. Education should be available in a variety of formats, such as traditional classroom, Web-based interactive, CD-Rom, self-directed materials, and collegiate distance learning.
5. Professional certification should be encouraged and rewarded.
6. The nurse as a caregiver can be more effective and prevent burnout through consistent self-care.

Professional development is an important and ongoing process throughout one's nursing career. This chapter outlines key components of the professional development of ambulatory care nurses, including orientation of new staff, competency assessment, continuing education, professional nursing certifications, and self care of the professional nurse as a caregiver.

Orientation is a corner stone of a successful work force in ambulatory care (American Academy of Ambulatory Care Nursing [AAACN], 2005). Basic nursing skills, such as collaboration, critical thinking, and assessment, are applicable to all settings, but the way nurses exercise these skills varies. Skills, knowledge, and responsibilities outlined in a job description provide the foundation for a thorough orientation. In addition to position-specific duties, orientation provides the new employee with an introduction to the organization's culture. Orientation and competence assessment of experienced nurses new in the setting must be flexible enough to allow individualization to the nurse's position he or she will fill. Ambulatory care nurses also need to plan and prepare for integrating new graduate nurses into practice by thorough preceptoring and mentoring. New nurses need support to assimilate, find job satisfaction, and be retained by the profession. Reality shock causes many new nurses to feel vulnerable and insecure about their new profession (Lavoie-Trembley et al., 2002).

Competency assessment is a continual process, not a one-time event. A program with a single, structured plan will not fit the needs of the individual or the organization. Regulating bodies have established standards that require documented assessment of staff competence. To meet the intent of the standards, a competency assessment program should focus on verifying and validating the skills and abilities of staff to ensure that they meet the organization's standards (Summers & Woods, 2004).

Each nurse must recognize the importance of continual learning to meet the constantly changing demands of the ambulatory care setting in which he or she works and the advancement of nursing science. Many educational avenues are available to the nurse. Available options include in-services, professional books and journals, continuing nursing education (CNE) programs, and mentoring by more experienced nurses. These all work to improve skills and develop a broader knowledge base, which contribute to improved patient outcomes. Another facet of continuing education is professional nursing certification. The nurse demonstrates expert level knowledge by becoming certified in his or her specialty. Continuing professional education, whether in the traditional classroom setting or through distance learning, permits the professional nurse to expand his or her role in nursing.

Orientation

Orientation is a structured plan created by the organization to "on-board" new staff. Key components include a general organizational overview, department specifics, and individualized job duties. It is a program that is provided to new staff to smooth assimilation into a new position (Alspach, 1995). Accrediting agencies provide ambulatory care settings with standards for the expectations of an orientation.
A. Organizational components (AAACN, 2005).
　1. Human resources components.
　2. Mission, vision, and values and goals of the organization – The culture.
　3. Policies and procedures.
　4. Cultural diversity.
　5. Ethical behaviors and responses in practice.
　6. Organizational chain of command/organizational chart.
　7. Environmental health and safety.
　　a. Infection control (safety needles, communicable disease screening).
　　b. Patients rights.
　　c. Emergency preparedness (fire, weather, and disaster).
B. Department-specific job duties and responsibilities.
　1. Job description – Expectations.
　　a. Essential duties in measurable terms.
　　b. Goals of department (such as customer service targets).

　　c. Safety (such as equipment, physical environmental risks).
　　d. Required competencies – Skills, knowledge, and abilities.
　　e. Performance expectations.
　　f. Associated responsibilities.
　　g. Probationary evaluations.
　　h. Annual performance reviews.
　2. Competency.
　　a. Age-specific, disease processes, pharmacology, and other unique patient care issues for the unit's population.
　　b. Critical thinking/decision-making.
　　c. Technical skills.
　　d. Interpersonal/communication skills.
C. Position-specific duties and responsibilities.
　1. Individualized for specifics.
　2. Required competencies – Unique to the area and those needing remediation based on baseline assessments.
　3. Performance expectations.
　4. Preceptors:
　　a. Trained to facilitate new team member.
　　b. Skilled at communication techniques.
　　c. Engaged/committed to build a better team by assimilation of new staff.
D. Variety of learning experiences and in-services based on needs.
　1. Below standard or missing skills and/or competence remediation.
　2. New skills and/or competence development.
E. Regulatory requirements related to orientation.
　1. Joint Commission on Accreditation of Healthcare Organizations (JCAHO) requires organizations to have an orientation process for each individual that will:
　　a. Assess ability to perform specific responsibilities.
　　b. Be specific to job-related aspects of patient safety.
　　c. Ensure safe and effective performance of essential duties.
　　d. Provide global overview to job specifics.
　2. Accreditation Association for Ambulatory Health Care (AAAHC) requires:
　　a. Documentation of adequate orientation and training to familiarize all personnel with the organization's policies, procedures, and facilities.

b. Orientation that assesses the nurse's current ability to meet identified standards for competent performance; the assessment serves as a basis for developing an orientation plan that bridges any gap.

F. Determining quality and efficacy of orientation program.
 1. Evaluate the program by feedback from participants.
 2. Survey both participant and preceptor following precepting.
 3. Develop process improvement plan from evaluations and survey results.
 4. Benchmark best orientation practices.
  a. Benchmarking – A systematic comparison of products, services, or work processes of similar organizations, departments, or practitioners to identify best practices known to date for the purpose of continuous quality improvement.
   (1) External – Different organizations' process and procedure.
   (2) Internal – Within the organization (such as interdepartmental, location variance for process and procedure).

Competence Assessment

Competence means having the ability to demonstrate the technical, critical-thinking, and interpersonal skills necessary to perform one's job responsibilities (AAACN, 2004). JCAHO standards state that a competency program should focus on verifying and validating the skills and abilities of staff to ensure that they meet the organization's standards. The Accreditation Association for Ambulatory Health Care (AAAHC) (2005) states a similar opinion, that an organization's health care team members should have the necessary and appropriate training and skills to deliver the services provided by the organization and should be appropriately trained, qualified, and supervised. A survey by either organization requires documentation of continual competence assessment and validation (AAACN, 2005).

A. General characteristics of competency programs (Wright, 2005):
 1. Emphasize outcomes.
 2. Flexible to the needs of the employee and organization.
 3. Use self-directed activities.
 4. Use educator as a facilitator.
 5. Incorporate various learning styles.
 6. Allocate adequate time.
 7. Utilize adult learning principles.
 8. Use various verification methods including initial and ongoing assessment.
B. Establish a baseline.
 1. Self-assessment.
 2. Validator assessment.
C. Assess all skill domains.
 1. Clinical/technical.
 2. Critical thinking.
 3. Interpersonal.
D. Provide learning options, such as reading material, observation of demonstration, quizzes, tours, and individual evaluation of his or her specific practice criteria.
E. Promote professionalism.
 1. Utilizing nursing process.
 2. Maintain credentials and qualifications.
F. Focus clinical performance improvement (PI) techniques upon skills required.
G. Promote ethical behavior.
 1. Scope of practice.
 2. Legal issues.
 3. Organization's vision and goals.
H. Promote nursing leadership skills.
 1. Collaboration.
 2. Accountability.
I. Validate research results incorporated into practice.
 1. Evidence-based practice.
 2. Benchmarking.
J. Comply with regulatory mandates.
 1. Governing body rules.
 2. Risk management.
K. Assess competence related to regulatory standards by 2 methods:
 1. Provide information (such as MSDS sheets).
 2. Measure competency through a verification method, (such as return demonstration).

Precepting

The art of precepting requires more than clinical expertise. The nurse acting as a preceptor has the ability to nurture, provide acceptance, and be patient with the preceptee. Clinical expertise is important, but caring kindness is equally valuable. High-quality precepting is a key component to the success of new staff. Without it, the literature indicates increases in turnover within an organization and early nurse burnout, which may lead to nurses leaving the profession altogether (Yonge, Krahn, Trojan, Reid, & Haase, 2002). Providing a structured, well-planned, and well-supported preceptor program demonstrates a true commitment to building a strong and competent staff.

A. The preceptor's role is to:
1. Acclimate the new nurse to the new setting.
2. Acclimate the new nurse to department standards.
3. Serve as a resource for the new nurse.
4. Develop a written plan:
   a. Policies and procedures.
   b. Essential duties.
   c. Competence to be validated.
5. Provide feedback to improve preceptor program.
6. Document completion of competency validations.
7. Orient new graduate nurses.
   a. Increase understanding of the state's practice act.
   b. Develop leadership skills.
   c. Provide opportunities to lead.
   d. Encourage peer discussions.
   e. Develop critical thinking skills.
B. Training preparation for preceptor.
1. Qualifications of preceptor. The smartest and "best" nurse may not make the best preceptor.
   a. Knowledgeable in job duties.
   b. Communicates and works well with others.
   c. Open to new staff and new ideas.
2. Formal class preparation.
   a. Validates competence levels of the preceptor.
   b. Teaches adult learning principles.
   c. Reinforces good communication skills.
C. Accommodations for non-traditional precepting.
1. Cross-training to other areas.
   a. Interdepartmental – Staff are competent to support and train for a department/unit where not usually assigned.
   b. Intradepartmental – Staff are competent

to support and train team member positions.
2. One-nurse practices.
   a. Write standards of expected practice.
   b. Identify support from other staff (such as physician, office manager).
   c. Encourage the nurse to participate in a professional organization to provide a network of peers and a larger context of specialty.
3. Use of agency or per diem staff.
   a. Write a standard of expected practice and have it available.
   b. Provide formal orientation with a resource person.
   c. Maintain a working relationship with the agency or per diem pool.
      (1) Set standards of preparation/competence expectations.
      (2) Attempt to utilize same agency/per diem staff.

Continuing Professional Educational and Development

The goal of continuing education is to improve and expand the nurse's knowledge base and to allow him or her to maintain competence and further develop in a specific work setting. New graduates as well as experienced professionals benefit from continuing their education. Opportunities must meet the varied learning needs of professional nurses.

A. Agencies requiring continuing education activities for nurses:
1. Occupational Safety and Health Administration (OSHA).
   a. Blood-borne pathogens precautions.
   b. Preventing tuberculosis transmission.
   c. Handling hazardous chemicals.
2. Joint Commission on Accreditation of Healthcare Organizations (JCAHO).
   a. Staff competency for job-specific responsibilities.
   b. Care of patient standards.
   c. Population-specific competencies.
   d. Process improvement initiatives.
   e. Patient safety.
   f. Handling of medical emergencies.
   g. Fire safety.

h. Disaster management.
3. Accreditation Association for Ambulatory Health Care (AAAHC).
    a. Rights of patients.
    b. Quality of care provided – Includes staff competence.
    c. Quality management and improvement.
    d. Facilities and environment.
    e. Patient safety.
    f. Handling of medical emergencies.
    g. Fire safety.
    h. Disaster management.
    i. Health education and teaching.
4. State licensing board's rules and regulations:
    a. Some states require 20 or more continuing education hours be obtained for each register nurse's relicensure cycle.
    b. Continuing education credit may be accepted for teaching, participation in meetings, and attending academic programs, in addition to participation in continuing nursing education programs.
B. Facility-specific inservices.
    1. New equipment.
    2. Change in policy and procedure.
    3. Review of situations requiring low frequency, high-risk skills.
C. Continuing nursing education programs targeting development of skills used in the ambulatory care setting.
    1. Patient education issues.
    2. New trends in care and disease state management.
    3. Pharmacology updates.
    4. New technology.
    5. Emerging clinical practice guidelines.
D. Factors that influence one's professional continuing development.
    1. Identifying and setting short and long-term goals and objectives.
    2. Having goals that are realistic.
    3. Establishing measurable objectives.
    4. Facing and overcoming fears.
        a. Fear of failure or ridicule.
        b. Fear of inability to learn.
    5. Building confidence and self-esteem.
    6. Finding time to devote to professional goals.
    7. Personal motivation.
        a. Self-knowledge and insight.

b. Individual's desire for learning.
c. Willingness to learn and self direction.
8. Practice-related challenges.
    a. Organizational needs.
    b. Group learning.
9. Ability to access presentations, lectures, readings, online classrooms.
10. Personal learning preferences.
    a. Observation/written material – Visual learner.
    b. Doing – Psychomotor learner.
    c. Lecture/audio materials – Auditory learner.
11. Emotions (such as feelings, hope, desire).
12. Personal attributes.
    a. Interest in subject matter.
    b. Availability of time.
    c. Resources/cost.
E. Learning and professionalism is enhanced by:
    1. Critical thinking.
    2. Confidence.
    3. Positive relationships.
    4. Appropriate timing.

Distance Learning

Education for the professional nurse is an ongoing process of reflection, discovery, and adaptation that is based on beliefs, experiences, and research. Traditional classroom settings have been the standard educational model. Recent advances in technology allow creative educators to offer alternative methods for learning. Video programs, teleconferencing, and online interactions provide new resources for meeting educational needs of the professional nurse. In an age when information growth is expanding at an accelerated speed, it is difficult to keep pace. Readily available, easily accessed educational opportunities are a priority.

A. Distance learning provides access to learning modalities initially designed to reach/include persons in rural/isolated areas, providing educational opportunities/resources. Methods include:
    1. Correspondence-type courses.
        a. Individuals enroll in a correspondence course.
        b. Work on material at own pace.
        c. Submit results for grading/credit as applicable.

2. E-mail and Internet allowing for interchange with a quicker turn-around and increased teacher/learner feedback.
3. Video capabilities.
4. Video-interactive capabilities.
5. Internet access to references, persons, knowledge bases.

B. Era of information/knowledge explosion and instant communications.
1. Increasingly, viewing a college education as mastery of a body of knowledge or a complete preparation for a lifetime career is becoming outmoded. Instead, we recognize that graduates need to have acquired skills, such as critical thinking, quantitative reasoning, and effective communication, along with abilities, such as the ability to find needed information and the ability to work well with others (Twigg, 1994).
2. Increased need for learning environments and systems integration of learning.

C. Availability of learning resources.
1. Once, the cost of technology was the limiting factor.
2. Charges to cover cost (such as program cost, materials, mailing costs, computer access/cost, video/audio capability).
3. Tools are now available – Do learners have the skills to use them?
4. Learning once occurred in a "place" – The environment is changing and information can be sought wherever the tools are readily available, by those with the critical thinking skills to put the tools to use (Peterson, 2004).

D. Methods of implementation.
1. Self-initiated learning, not for credit.
2. Formalized distance learning for both continuing education credit and academic credit, established by a traditional institution of learning.
3. Universities with distance programs offer credit and even degrees via distance learning.

E. Future considerations.
1. Language assimilation.
   a. Promote and demonstrate value of bilingual students/nurses.
   b. Provide English as a Second Language (ESL) programs.
   c. Encourage language immersion programs.
2. Limits potentially placed on the Internet and access.
3. Capabilities of learners to use the tools effectively.
4. Cost implications of updates to software that is incompatible with older versions of the software.
5. Changing structure of educational environments.
6. Establishing standards for new media.
7. Evolving purposes for education tools.
8. How to validate learning and effectiveness.
9. Maintaining cost effectiveness.
10. Changing requirements and new competencies for workers, leaders.
    a. Skill sets.
    b. Communication abilities.
    c. Power.
11. Need for multiple skill sets.
12. Integration of learning and competency.
13. Utilization of method based on learner needs/requirements/time.

Professional Certification

Certification is a process that uses predetermined standards to validate and recognize an individual's knowledge, skills, and abilities in a defined functional and clinical area of specialty practice (American Board of Nursing Specialties [ABNS], 2005).

A. Numerous studies have demonstrated the positive benefits of nursing certification.
1. In 2000, the Nursing Credentialing Research Coalition identified the relationship between certified nurses and patient care quality (Cary, 2001).
2. A survey of nurse mangers demonstrated that nearly 90% of respondents clearly prefer hiring certified nurses over non-certified nurses (Niebuhr & Stromborg, in press).
3. In the same study, 58% of the nurse managers stated that they see a positive performance difference in certified nurses.
4. Additionally, an American Association of Critical Care Nurses (AACN) (2002) study demonstrated that certification has a significant positive impact on quality of patient

care and patient safety.
B. The American Board of Nursing Specialties stated the following position about nursing specialty certification on March 5, 2005 (ABNS, 2005).
1. Registered nurses should seek certification in their specialty area of practice.
2. Certified nurses should promote their certification by publicly displaying their credentials and introducing themselves as certified nurses.
3. Health care consumers should be knowledgeable of the qualifications and credentials of the registered nurses caring for them.
4. Employers should seek certified nurses for their workforce, support individuals seeking and maintaining certification, inform patients and the public about the certification status of their workforce, encourage the display of the nurses' certified credentials on identification badges, and market the accomplishments of certified nurses.
5. Specialty nursing certification is an objective measure of knowledge which validates that a nurse is qualified to provide specialized nursing care.
C. Certification in ambulatory care nursing.
1. Offered by the American Nurse Credentialing Center (ANCC) since 1999.
2. Addresses the broad scope of ambulatory care from clinics to HMOs, to group practices, to ambulatory surgery.
3. Eligibility requirements.
   a. Hold a currently active registered nurse license (Associate Degree, Diploma, Baccalaureate, or higher degree in nursing) in the U.S. or its territories, AND
   b. Have functioned as a registered nurse for 4,000 hours, with at least 2,000 of those hours within the specialty scope of practice, within the last 2 years.
4. Testing information (www.nursecredentialing.org).
D. Telehealth nursing certification.
1. Sponsored by the National Certification Corporation (NCC).
2. Eligibility Requirements:
   a. Current licensure as an RN in the U.S. or Canada.

   b. Twenty-four months specialty experience as a U.S. or Canadian RN comprised of a minimum of 2,000 hours.
   c. Employment in the specialty sometime in the last 24 months.
3. Testing information (www.nccnet.org).

Employee Satisfaction and Retention

Nurses have choices about where they work. They want to be motivated and inspired, and empowered to take initiative. The work environment should be energizing to the nurse and increase job satisfaction. The organization needs to be one for which the nurse chooses to work even when offered other opportunities. More pay, alone, may not be enticing enough to cause a satisfied nurse to make a change.
A. Characteristics of an environment that promote nurse satisfaction and retention.
1. Socialization of the nurse (Griffin, Hanley, & Saniuk, 2002).
   a. Preceptorship: Rewards and benefits are found for the preceptee and preceptor.
   b. Mentoring: Mentee develops a close bond to the mentor.
   c. Department/unit culture: Departments with fully engaged staff share comradeship and familial feelings.
2. Clarity of expectations.
   a. Clear job description.
   b. Empowerment to make decisions and prioritize work.
   c. Clear and caring leadership (especially frontline management).
3. Respect.
   a. Valued as a person.
   b. Input/opinions are sought.
   c. Meaningful work.
   d. Freedom and autonomy.
4. Collaboration among team members.
   a. Share values and mission.
   b. Share decision-making. Voices are heard.
   c. Cooperate and have supportive communications.
5. Reward and recognition (Nelson, 2005).
   a. Informal rewards, match reward to the person.
      (1) Verbal or written recognitions.

      (2) Low-cost or no-cost recognitions that reflect the individual.

      (3) Merchandise, gift certificates, theater tickets, sporting event tickets.

      (4) Time off.

   b. Formal rewards.

      (1) Organizational programs that reflect the organization's values.

      (2) Contests.

      (3) Celebrations/events.

      (4) Advancement.

6. Supported professional growth.

   a. Continuing education.

   b. Formal education.

   c. Advancement opportunities.

7. Personal growth opportunities.

   a. Meaningful work.

   b. Encouragement and mentorship by management and peers.

   c. Fostering of creativity and innovation.

B. Measurement of satisfaction.

1. Teamwork.

   a. Surveys – Find out what works and what doesn't.

   b. Evaluations.

2. Staff satisfaction.

   a. Surveys.

   b. Focus groups.

   c. Patient letters.

   d. Turn above data into action plan.

3. Leadership performance.

   a. Surveys.

   b. Focus groups.

   c. Evaluations.

Care of the Nurse Caregiver

Self-care practices used by the nurse promote harmony in mind, body, and spirit. They also aid in the prevention of illness related to depletion of energy from stressors. Nurses need skills to decide what must be fixed, nurtured, or jettisoned to remove patient-care barriers and pressures from self. These decisions enhance holistic care to others and self, providing harmony.

A. Levels of balance.

1. Harmony: Maximum potential of wellness and balance in the mental, physical, and spiritual dimensions of self-care (Dossey, Guzzetta, & Keegan, 2000).

2. Stressed or out-of-balance:

   a. Eastern philosophy definitions: Absence of inner peace.

   b. Western culture: Loss of control or harmony between mind, body, or spiritual well-being (Seaward, 1997).

3. Wound healer: Term used to describe an individual who has recognized strengths and weaknesses and is able to assist with greater self-knowledge (Achterberg, 1991).

B. Self-discovery of traits that can sabotage balance.

1. Rushed or hurried lifestyle (sometimes called "Type A personality") (Berens, 2004).

   a. Extended work hours.

   b. Time urgency: Preoccupied with time and impatient regarding waiting.

   c. Polyphasia: Engaged in multiple thoughts or activities at one time.

   d. Ultra-competitiveness: Comparing self with others to the point that peers are considered a threat.

   e. Rapid speech pattern: Often finishes sentences for other people.

   f. Manipulative control: Influences others or promotes one-upmanship.

   g. Hyper-aggressiveness and free-floating hostility: Needs to dominate others, free-floating anger erupts at trivial occurrences.

   h. Low self-esteem and perception of self-worth based on other's perceptions.

2. Codependent traits: Individuals dependent on making others dependent on them as a means of self-validation (Beattie, 1992).

   a. Traits developed in early childhood in a lifestyle or environment that is chaotic, unpredictable, or threatening.

   b. Ardent approval seeker: Seeking approval or feedback to validate efforts.

   c. Perfectionist: Extremely well-organized and in the habit of going beyond the requirements in every task.

   d. Super-overachiever: Involvement in an abundance of activities and obligated to do it all well.

   e. Crisis manager: Thrives on crisis and constantly tries to make order out of chaos.

f. Devoted loyalist: Extreme loyalty to friends and family possibly from fear of rejection or abandonment.

g. Self-sacrificing martyr: Puts everyone else first to the point of sacrificing one's own time, values, property, and even life goals.

h. Manipulator: Manages through generosity and favors.

i. Victim: In tandem with repeated acts of martyrdom, perceives that he or she never receives enough credit.

j. Inadequate: "Black cloud" of inferiority over his or her head.

k. Reactionary: Tends to overreact rather than respond to situations.

C. Traits that enhance balance and self-care.

1. Hardy personality traits: An individual who, despite stressful circumstances, appears resistant to the psycho-physiologic effects of stress and has the following three traits:

a. Commitment: Dedication to oneself, one's work, and one's family that provides the individual with a sense of belonging and life purpose.

b. Control: Empowerment or self-control that helps one overcome elements in the environment so one does not feel victimized.

c. Challenge: Ability to see change and even problems as opportunities for growth rather than threats to one's existence.

2. Self-esteem factor: A critical indication of individual's stress response (Branden, 1995).

a. Focus on action and achievement of highest potential.

b. Living consciously or living in the present moment.

c. Self-acceptance or refusal to be in an adversarial relationship with self.

d. Self-responsibility or choosing to acknowledge responsibility for one's feelings.

e. Self-assertiveness or honoring one's wants, needs, and values, and seeking appropriate ways to satisfy them.

f. Living purposefully or taking action to make one's goals happen.

g. Personal integrity or working to achieve congruence between values and actions.

D. Self-care activities that provide form and guidance for behaviors during times of regeneration and growth for mind, body, or spirit.

1. Self-care activities for the mind.

a. Dreaming.

b. Active imagination.

c. Journaling.
   (1) Gains perspective.
   (2) Allows safe venting of emotions.

d. Self-forgiveness.

e. Affirmations.

f. Using humor.

g. Time alone.

h. Reading and continual learning.

2. Self-care activities for the body.

a. Nutritious diet.

b. Exercise (such as yoga, aerobics, walking).

c. Massage.

d. Rest and relaxation.

e. Baths.

f. Deep breathing.

g. Routine check-ups, screening exams, and physical examinations.

3. Self-care activities for the spirit and emotions.

a. Time in nature.

b. Meditation or prayer.

c. Travel.

d. Solitude.

e. Journaling.

f. Reflection.

g. Crying.

h. Sabbaticals.

E. Presence: Concept has significant implications for nursing education, practice, research, and self-care. Watson (1999) defines presence as the "being" or essence of the individual and delineates three levels:

1. Physical presence: "Being there" for another through nursing interventions and providing routine tasks.

2. Psychological presence: "Being with" – The nurse uses self as an intervention tool to create a therapeutic psychological environment that meets a need for comfort and support.

3. Therapeutic presence: "Being whole" – The nurse relates to the client as a whole being, using all body, mind, emotion, and spiritual

resources.

4. Presence is a state achieved when one moves oneself to an inner reference of balance.

5. To be present implies a quality, an essence of being in the moment.

F. Benefit of self-care:
  1. Improved health.
  2. Improved job satisfaction.
  3. Improved job performance.
  4. Ability to balance personal and work life.

G. Interrelationships provide support and strengthen self esteem.
  1. Mentoring.
     a. Choosing a mentor.
     b. Goals of the relationship.
     c. Time required/invested for relationship.
     d. Communication: criticism/praise, confidence-building.
  2. Networking.
     a. Collaboration: Nurses use informed judgment, individual competencies, and qualification when seeking consultation.
     b. Accepting care responsibilities and delegation of nursing care.
  3. Friends and family provide additional support and sharing.

References

Accreditation Association for Ambulatory Health Care, Inc. (AAAHC). (2005). *Accreditation handbook for ambulatory health care.* Wilmette, IL: Author.

Achterberg, J. (1991). *Woman healer.* Boston: Shambhala.

Alspach, J.G. (1995). *The educational process in nursing staff development.* St. Louis: Mosby.

American Academy of Ambulatory Care Nursing (AAACN). (2004). *Ambulatory care nursing administration and practice standards.* Pitman, NJ: Author.

American Academy of Ambulatory Care Nursing (AAACN). (2005). *A guide to ambulatory care nursing orientation and competency assessment.* Pitman, NJ: Author.

American Association of Critical Care Nurses (AACN). (2002). *New data reveals nurse certification key component of patient safety and recruitment and retention programs (white paper).* Aliso Viejo, CA: Author.

American Board of Nursing Specialties (ABNS). (2004). *Accreditation standards.* Retrieved September 27, 2004, from http:/www.nursingcertification.org

Beattie, M. (1992). *Codependent no more: How to stop controlling others and start caring for yourself* (2nd ed.). Center City, MN: Hazelden Foundation.

Berens, L. (2004). *Understanding yourself and others: An introduction to the personality type code.* New York: Telos Publishers.

Branden, N. (1995). *The six pillars of self-esteem.* New York: Bantam.

Cary, A.H. (2001). Certified registered nurses: Results of the study of the certified workforce. *American Journal of Nursing, 101*(1), 44-52.

Dossey BM, Guzzetta, C.E., & Keegan, L. (2000). *Holistic nursing: A handbook for practice* (3rd ed.). Gaithersburg, MD: Aspen.

Griffin, M., Hanley, D., & Saniuk, C. (2002). Lightening the burden for preceptors. *Journal for Nurses in Staff Development, 18*(6), 322-326.

Lavoie-Trembley, M., Viens, C., Forcier, M., Labrosse, N., Lafrance, M., Laliberte, D., et al. (2002). How to facilitate the orientation of new nurses into the workplace. *Journal for Nurses in Staff Development, 18*(2), 80- 85.

Nelson, B. (2005). *1001 ways to reward employees* (revised). New York: Workman Publishing Co.

Niebuhr, B., & Stromborg, M. (in press). Survey of nurse managers: Perceptions of the value of specialty nursing certification. *Nursing Management.*

Peterson, T. (2004) *Peterson's guide to distance learning programs.* Lawrenceville, NJ: The Thomson Corporation.

Seaward, B.L. (2006). *Managing stress: Principles and strategies for health and well-being* (5th ed.). Sudbury, MA: Jones and Bartlett.

Summers, B., & Woods, W. (2004). *Competency assessment: A practical guide to JCAHO standards* (2nd ed.). Marblehead, ME: HCPro, Inc.

Twigg, C.A. (1994). *The need for a national learning infrastructure.* Retrieved March 20, 2006, from http://www.educause.edu/pub/er/review/reviewArticles/29516.html

Watson, J.(1999). *Postmodern nursing and beyond.* London: Churchill Livingstone.

Wright, D. (2005). *The ultimate guide to competency assessment in health care* (3rd ed.). Eau Claire, WI: Creative Health Care Management.

Yonge, O., Krahn, H., Trojan, L., Reid, D., & Haase, M. (2002). Supporting preceptors. *Journal for Nurses in Staff Development, 18*(2), 73-78.

Additional Readings

Barton, D. (2001-2005). *Engaging and retaining employee talent.* Denver, CO: Center for Talent Retention. Retrieved May 16, 2006, from http://www.keeppeople.com.

Hebda, T., Czar, P., & Mascara, C. (2005). *Internet resource guide for nurses and health care professionals* (3rd ed.). Upper Saddle River, NJ: Prentice Hall.

Herman, R.E., & Joyce, G. (2000). *How to become an employer of choice.* Winchester, VA: Oakhill Press.

Joint Commission Resources. (2005). *Assessing and improving staff competence.* CD-ROM. Oakbrook Terrace, IL: Author.

Keating, S.B. (2005). *Curriculum development and evaluation in nursing. Needs assessment.* Philadelphia, PA: Lippincott Williams & Wilkins.

Krugman, M. (2003). Evidence based practice the role of staff development. *Journal for Nurses in Staff Development, 19*(6), 279-285.

Spath, P. (2002). *Guide to effective staff development in health care organizations: A systems approach to successful training.* San Francisco: John Wiley & Sons, Inc.

Swan, B.A. (2002). Ambulatory Care nursing practice: Developing and contributing to the evidence base. *Nursing Economic$, 20*(2), 83-87.

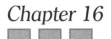
Professional Development

This test may be copied for use by others.

COMPLETE THE FOLLOWING:

Name: _____

Address: _____

City: _____ State: _____ Zip:_____

Preferred telephone: (Home)_____ (Work)_____

E-mail_____

AAACN Member Expiration Date: _____

Registration fee: AAACN Member: $12.00
                   Nonmember: $20.00

Answer Form:

1. If you applied what you have learned from this activity into your practice, what would be different?

   _____

   _____

   _____

Evaluation		Strongly disagree				Strongly agree
2. By completing this activity, I was able to meet the following objectives:						
a. Discuss key components of an orientation program for new staff in ambulatory care nursing roles.		1	2	3	4	5
b. Identify competence assessment requirements as related to accrediting agencies' standards and the essential duties of the nurse's position.		1	2	3	4	5
c. Discuss mandates for continuing education and professional growth and development needs.		1	2	3	4	5
d. Discuss continuing professional education using traditional and distance learning methods.		1	2	3	4	5
e. Identify the value of nursing specialty certification.		1	2	3	4	5
f. Describe the relationship between employee satisfaction, and retention and precepting of and by staff.		1	2	3	4	5
g. Discuss barriers and resources to professional nurses' self care.		1	2	3	4	5
3. The content was current and relevant.		1	2	3	4	5
4. The objectives could be achieved using the content provided.		1	2	3	4	5
5. This was an effective method to learn this content.		1	2	3	4	5
6. I am more confident in my abilities since completing this material.		1	2	3	4	5

7. The material was (check one) ___new ___review for me.

8. Time required to read this chapter: _____minutes

I verify that I have completed this activity: _____
                                                      Signature

Comments: _____

_____

_____

Objectives

This educational activity is designed for nurses and other health care professionals who practice in ambulatory care. For those wishing to obtain CE credit, an evaluation follows. After studying the information presented in this offering, you will be able to:

1. Discuss key components of an orientation program for new staff in ambulatory care nursing roles.
2. Identify competence assessment requirements as related to accrediting agencies' standards and the essential duties of the nurse's position.
3. Discuss mandates for continuing education and professional growth and development needs.
4. Discuss continuing professional education using traditional and distance learning methods.
5. Identify the value of nursing specialty certification.
6. Describe the relationship between employee satisfaction, and retention and precepting of and by staff.
7. Discuss barriers and resources to professional nurses' self care.

Posttest Instructions

1. To receive continuing education credit for individual study after reading the article, complete the answer/evaluation form to the left.

2. Detach and send the answer/evaluation form along with a check or money order payable to the *American Academy of Ambulatory Care Nursing (AAACN)*, East Holly Avenue Box 56, Pitman, NJ 08071–0056.

3. Test returns must be postmarked by August 1, 2011. Upon completion of the answer/evaluation form, a certificate for **1.5** contact hour(s) will be awarded and sent to you. Should the material contained in this chapter become outdated prior to the above expiration date, AAACN reserves the right to withdraw this CE test.

This activity is co-provided by the *American Academy of Ambulatory Care Nursing (AAACN)* and Anthony J. Jannetti, Inc. (AJJ). AJJ is accredited as a provider of continuing nursing education by the American Nurses' Credentialing Center's Commission on Accreditation (ANCC-COA). AAACN is a provider approved by the California Board of Registered Nurses, provider number CEP 05336.

This article was reviewed and formatted for contact hour credit by Sally S. Russell, MN, CMSRN, AAACN Education Director; and Candia Baker Laughlin MS, RN, C, Editor.

The Clinical Nursing Role In Ambulatory Care

Chapter 17

Application of the Nursing Process In Ambulatory Care

Sharon L. Lanzetta, MSN, RN, C

Objectives

Study of the information presented in this chapter will enable the learner to:

1. Outline the steps of the nursing process and how they promote critical thinking.
2. Describe the methods of assessment applicable in ambulatory care, including triage.
3. Identify knowledge necessary for technical skills applicable in the practice of ambulatory care nursing.
4. Explain how to determine if outcomes are achieved.
5. Describe the interaction of the components of the nursing process.

Key Points

1. Collaborative and multidisciplinary approaches significantly impact the role of the nurse in the provision of patient care.
2. Implementation is based on scientific principles that are congruent with the overall plan of care.
3. One goal of patient education is to empower the patient to be involved in the management of their care.
4. Outcomes are based on the established goals of care and are measured in the evaluation portion of the nursing process.
5. Health screenings involve measurements of specific physical functions to differentiate normal from abnormal physical findings.

The nursing process uses scientific reasoning and specific critical thinking to make clinical inferences about a patient's plan of care. It evaluates all aspects of nursing care in an organized fashion that promotes optimal health and quality of life in every clinical setting. By using a systematic framework, the nurse seeks information and responds to issues that affect the patient's health. The nursing process relies on cognitive, interpersonal, and psychomotor skills that are guided by professional standards and a code of ethics. Each step of the nursing process is equally important in resolving health problems.

A. The nursing process:
1. Is guided by precise, disciplined thinking.
2. Leads to accurate and complete data collection.
3. Is the organized structure and framework for the delivery of nursing care.
4. Is a systematic, problem-solving approach.
5. May not always occur in exact sequence.
6. Is not static or fixed.

B. Critical thinking – Includes diagnostic reasoning, clinical inferences, and decision-making that are outcome-focused. Nurses apply critical thinking to:
1. Ask a question.
2. Identify and question assumptions.
3. Examine the nurse's own thinking and that of others.
4. Reflect and recall other clinical situations.
5. Interpret, analyze, and evaluate.
6. Review to determine if nursing actions are based on best evidence.

C. Assessment – Uses a systematic approach to obtain data. It guides the nurse in asking pertinent questions to develop a comprehensive plan. Through the assessment process, the deliberate collection of data is obtained by interviewing, observing, and examining the patient for evidence of health problems and risk factors.
1. Assessment occurs each time a patient enters the ambulatory care system, whether in person, on the phone, through electronic communications, or via remote technological monitoring.

2. Assessment situations.
   a. Comprehensive (such as pre-admission).
   b. Problem-focused (such as symptomatic call or visit).
   c. Emergency assessment (such as triage of unconscious patient).
   d. Time-lapsed re-assessment (such as management of hypertension). Continuously monitoring responses and treatment allows for detection of any changes in the patient's health status.
3. Assessment includes:
   a. Gathering data.
      (1) Objective – Data that is observed or indirectly observed through measurements or physical examination.
      (2) Subjective – Data that is stated, described, and verified by the patient.
      (3) Interview – May be verbal and/or non-verbal.
   b. Verifying data to validate the understanding of the problem and determine that all information is factual and complete.
      (1) Confirm observations through interview and examine.
      (2) Listen to the patient and their perceptions.
      (3) Review test results and findings.
   c. Organizing/analyzing the data to prioritize potential or actual problems by clustering the data to assist with identifying problems of health or illness.
   d. Predicting, detecting, preventing, and controlling outcomes:
      (1) Consider signs and symptoms.
      (2) Consider cultural, spiritual, and environmental factors.
      (3) Recognize patient and family strengths and limitations.
   e. Documenting data to form a database to communicate with other health care professionals.
D. Triage – Based on the concept of prioritizing the needs of the patient. After immediate needs are identified, the level of treatment is further defined based upon referrals to the appropriate level of care, and the personnel and technical resources available. The ability to perform an adequate patient assessment during triage allows the nurse to perform a systematic and comprehensive approach that is critical in providing safe and effective patient care. Nurses manage collaborative problems by implementing both physician and nurse prescribed interventions to reduce further complications (Weber & Kelley, 2003). Triage includes:

1. Assessment based on interview, use of protocols, guidelines, algorithms, critical thinking, clinical judgment, and resource assessment.
2. Verification of information from database or chart.
3. Prioritization of the patient needs, specific to time.
4. Analysis/plan based on mutual decision making, collaborative plan of care.
5. Nursing interventions.
6. Determination of a disposition at the end of the triage encounter.
7. Documentation.
8. Evaluation of outcomes and quality measurements.

E. Nursing diagnoses/analysis – A statement that describes the patient's actual or potential response to a health problem that a nurse is licensed and competent to treat. The registered nurse analyzes the assessment data to determine the diagnoses or issues (American Nurses' Association [ANA], 2004). The nurse must be able to identify not only nursing problems, but also signs and symptoms that require management by a physician, an advanced practice nurse, or another member of the health care team (Alfaro-LeFevre, 2005). The North American Nursing Diagnosis Association International (NANDA-I) is recognized as the leader in development and classification of nursing diagnoses. The nursing diagnosis:

1. Analyzes data collected in the assessment for problem identification.
   a. Classifies data, grouping significant and related information.
   b. Creates a list of suspected problems.
   c. Rules out similar problems.
   d. Determines risk factors that must be managed.

e. Identifies resources, strengths, and areas for health promotion.

2. Defines the patient's problem.

   a. A nursing diagnosis is a definitive statement of the patient's actual or potential difficulties that are amenable to nursing intervention.

   b. Development of nursing diagnosis using approved NANDA-I-approved nursing diagnosis (NANDA, 2003).

      (1) Excludes all non-nursing diagnoses.

      (2) Excludes all medical treatment.

      (3) Includes environmental stressors.

      (4) Includes data identified during assessment.

3. The diagnosis provides direction for care by directing specific interventions.

4. Use of nursing diagnoses provides criteria for quality improvement through review and evaluation.

5. Nursing diagnoses improve communication between health care professionals.

F. Nursing plan – Identifies specific nursing actions for achieving goals and desired outcomes that guide the implementation process. It is aimed at solving or alleviating the problems identified in the assessment process by setting realistic goals that are clear, concise, and established with the patient. The plan determines and identifies desired outcomes in timely and cost effective ways that are measurable and reflect the patient's response.

1. A plan of care (Alfaro-LeFevre, 2005):

   a. Promotes communication among caregivers to promote continuity of care.

   b. Directs care and documentation.

   c. Creates a record that can later be used for evaluation, research, and legal reasons.

   d. Previously identified nursing diagnoses are written on plan of care.

   e. Provides documentation of health care needs for insurance reimbursement purposes.

2. Clarification of outcomes and goals are guided by the use of:

   a. Protocols that:

      (1) Provide basis for consistency.

      (2) Describe steps/actions in exact order.

(3) Specify the procedures to be followed.

   b. Guidelines (see Chapter 13, Evidence-Based Practice).

      (1) Based on standards of care that guide nursing action.

      (2) Based on current best evidence.

      (3) Applied with clinical judgment (Hewitt-Taylor, 2003).

      (4) Aimed at achieving outcomes.

3. Patient outcomes are reflected in expected changes in the patient.

      (1) Must be objective, realistic, and measurable.

      (2) Provide standards of measure that can be used to determine if the goal of the patient and nurse have been achieved.

G. Implementation – Refers to the priority nursing actions performed to accomplish a specified goal. Implementation is the action component of the nursing process that involves giving direct care to the patient. The implementation phase of the nursing action must be appropriate and individualized for the patient (Smith, Duell, & Martin, 2000). Before implementing any nursing intervention, a review of the nursing plan ensures the nurse's understanding of the rationale of the action, the standard of care by use of protocols or guidelines, the principles for interventions, and the expected outcomes.

1. Nursing interventions – Actions performed to (Alfaro-LeFever, 2005):

   a. Monitor health status.

   b. Reduce risks.

   c. Resolve, prevent, or manage problems.

   d. Facilitate independence or assist with activities of daily living.

   e. Promote optimum sense of physical, psychological, and spiritual well being.

2. Nursing interventions include assessing patient for:

   a. Comfort including predisposition to alterations, and physical and emotional signs and symptoms of acute or chronic pain.

   b. Environmental conditions.

   c. Safety, including fall prevention, seizure precaution, and taking into account the patient's age and mobility.

3. Nursing Interventions Classifications (NIC) (Dochterman & Bulechek, 2004) describe the interventions and treatments nurses perform.
   a. Include independent and collaborative interventions.
   b. Are used by nurses, including advanced practice nurses, in all settings.
   c. Include illness treatment, illness prevention, and health promotion.
   d. The fourth edition (2004) includes 514 research-based interventions.
   e. Updated approximately every 4 years.
   f. Linked to NANDA nursing diagnoses.
4. Medically directed interventions include:
   a. Administrating oral, topical, and inhalant medications.
   b. Administering intradermal, subcutaneous, and intramuscular injections.
   c. Administering intravenous solutions and medications.
   d. Providing wound care.
   e. Following other orders as directed by a physician, advanced practice nurse, or physician's assistant.
5. Prior to performing a procedure, the nurse:
   a. Reviews the procedure, protocol, or guideline.
   b. Provides necessary information about the procedure to the patient.
   c. May include written instructions and/or teaching.
   d. Allows time for questions.
   e. Assures the safety of the patient.
H. Patient education and teaching – Communications to assist the patient in the prevention of illness or to promote wellness. The goals of *Healthy People 2010* are to increase the life span and quality of life and eliminate health disparities among different populations (deWit, 2005). Teaching is planned with specific learning objectives that aid the patient by increasing the knowledge needed to make informed decisions that enhance their quality of life. Learning objectives often describe what the patient will be able to do after successful teaching (refer to Chapter 19, *Patient Education and Counseling*). Goals of teaching:

1. Assist in gaining new knowledge of health or disease.
   a. Understanding or acquiring knowledge.
   b. Developing attitudes: Affective learning (such as, "What does the health problem mean to the individual?").
2. Assist in the management of a disorder or disease.
3. Facilitate the patient toward making decisions about his or her own care.
4. Assist in performing their activities of daily living.
5. Assist in identifying risks/problems with their health.
6. Assist in exploring all options regarding their care.
7. Decrease anxiety prior to procedure.
I. Evaluation – Assesses the patient's response to the plan of care by determining the effectiveness of the actions and the degree of goal attainment. Evaluation examines the appropriateness of nursing action and considers alternatives by re-assessing or revising the care plan. By comparing the outcome of care with the desired outcome, identification of problems solved, and those that need to be reassessed or re-planned are identified (Waltz & Jenkins, 2001). Identifying specific areas that need change in the evaluation process is based on the philosophy that the quality of heath care can always be improved by continuous quality improvement (Alfaro-LeFevre, 2005).
1. Identifying areas that may need change include:
   a. Outcome/goal achieved.
   b. Patient safety.
   c. Cost effective.
   d. Patient/family satisfaction.
   e. Completion in a time-efficient manner.
2. Outcomes – Specific statements of the goal the patient is expected to achieve as a result of nursing intervention (deWit, 2005). Outcomes are based on the established goals of care and are measured in the evaluation section of the nursing process.
   a. Derived directly from the problem.
   b. Time-specific, realistic, and attainable.
   c. Standards that contain measurable criteria to evaluate the plan's effectiveness.

d. Objectives aimed at reducing, eliminating, or alleviating the problem.

e. Require collaboration with the patient to assess patient satisfaction.

3. Nursing Outcomes Classifications (NOC) – Standardized classification for patient outcomes to evaluate the effects of nursing interventions.

   a. Developed for use in all settings and with all patient populations.

   b. Use a list of indicators to evaluate patient status in relation to outcomes.

   c. Yield more information than just whether a goal was met.

   d. Linked to NANDA international diagnosis and recognized by the ANA.

   e. The 3rd edition includes 330 NOC outcomes in the Nursing Outcome Classifications.

   f. Continually updated based on new research or user feedback, and is published on a 4-year cycle.

Invasive Procedures

An invasive procedure is one in which the normal protective barrier of the skin or mucus membrane is broken or compromised. When broken, there is an increased risk for pathogenic microorganisms to enter the body, causing a reaction to tissues and the toxins generated by them. When performing an invasive procedure, physical and chemical control of microorganisms is required. Medical or surgical asepsis makes the environment and objects free of microorganisms (deWit, 2005). For invasive procedures, the use of surgical asepsis is practiced for preparing and handling materials. This involves using sterile supplies and techniques for procedures that invade the body for care.

A. Venipuncture for diagnostic testing is used for the screening of early signs of alterations to the patient's health or the course of disease, or to monitor response to treatment.

   1. Assessment:

      a. Review purpose.

      b. Review orders.

      c. Determine if special conditions are needed; privacy for disrobing or restraint by adult for combative child.

      d. Assess patient for risks, fragile veins, or signs of infection.

      e. Assess patient cooperation.

      f. Assess contraindications that exclude certain sites: Site has signs of infection, infiltration, or thrombosis.

   2. Plan:

      a. Venipuncture procedure.

      b. Patient is free of discomfort.

      c. No complications.

      d. Document date, time, specimen collected, site, and patient response.

      e. Report abnormal findings.

   3. Implementation (Smith et al., 2000):

      a. Assemble equipment.

      b. Identify correct patient and explain procedure.

      c. Position patient and select site.

      d. Place protection pad under site.

      e. Wash hands.

      f. Apply tourniquet on upper arm at least 4 to 6 inches above site.

      g. Reassess site for suitability.

      h. Don gloves.

      i. Cleanse site according to agency policy.

      j. Stabilize the skin approximately 2 inches below insertion site.

      k. Perform venipuncture according to agency policy.

      l. Release tourniquet and withdraw needle.

      m. Assess site and patient response, apply dressing.

      n. Write date, time, and patient identifiers (such as name and date of birth or registration number) on tubes according to agency policy.

      o. Remove gloves and wash hands.

      p. Record procedure as stated by agency policy.

   4. Evaluation:

      a. Reinspect site for evidence of bleeding or hematoma.

      b. Patient response for pain or discomfort.

      c. Specimen collected and obtained properly according to agency guidelines.

   5. Teaching:

      a. Regarding procedure – Purpose and how obtained to decrease anxiety.

      b. Post procedure – Pressure at site,

report any discomfort, pain, or bruising at site.

B. Venipuncture for intravenous therapy – For medication or fluid administration to correct or prevent fluid and electrolyte disturbances.
  1. Assessment:
    a. Review purpose.
    b. Review orders.
    c. Determine if special conditions are needed; privacy for disrobing or restraint by adult for combative child.
    d. Assess patient for risks; fragile veins or signs of infection.
    e. Assess patient cooperation.
    f. Assess contraindications.
    g. Check intravenous (IV) bag for outdating, tears, and leaks by applying gentle pressure to bag.
    h. Hold bag up to dark and light background to examine for discoloration, cloudiness, or particulate matters.
    i. Determine if the patient is allergic to IV solution or medication.
  2. Plan:
    a. Venipuncture procedure.
    b. Patient free of discomfort.
    c. No complications.
    d. Documentation of date, time, IV solution, site, and patient response.
    e. Report abnormal findings.
  3. Implementation (Smith et al., 2000):
    a. Identify correct patient and explain procedure.
    b. Assemble equipment.
    c. Hang IV bag on IV pole.
    d. Prepare IV bag/tubing according to agency policy.
    e. Position patient and select site.
    f. Place protection pad under site.
    g. Wash hands.
    h. Apply tourniquet on upper arm at least 4 to 6 inches above site.
    i. Reassess site for suitability.
    j. Don gloves.
    k. Cleanse site according to agency policy.
    l. Stabilize the skin approximately 2 inches below insertion site.
    m. Perform venipuncture and begin IV according to agency policy.

    n. Reduce flow rate of IV to keep open until taped needle and tubing are in place.
    o. Apply occlusive transparent dressing over infusion site.
    p. Assess site and patient response while applying dressing.
    q. Write date, time, and nurse's initials on dressing/tape according to agency policy.
    r. Remove gloves and wash hands.
    s. Set drip rate according to order by pump or calculated gravity flow drips per minute.
    t. Immobilize infusion site in functional position.
    u. Clean up supplies and make the patient comfortable.
    v. Record procedure as stated by agency policy.
    w. Change cannula/tubing as stated by agency policy.
  4. Evaluation:
    a. Reinspect site for evidence of bleeding, infiltration, or hematoma.
    b. Patient response for pain or discomfort.
    c. Verify the solution is running at the correct rate into vein without pain and IV cannula is secure.
  5. Teaching:
    a. Regarding procedure – Purpose and how obtained to decrease anxiety.
    b. Post procedure – Report any discomfort, pain, or bruising at site; signs and symptoms of infiltration; and complications.

C. Tuberculin skin testing (TST) (U.S. Public Health Service, 1997) – Tuberculosis is an infection of the lungs caused by *Mycobacterium tuberculosis*, an acid-fast bacterium. Tubercle bacillus may be communicated to others by means of droplet formation (inhalation), ingestion, or inoculation. Testing determines the antibody response to tubercle bacillus.
  1. Predisposing factors to tuberculosis infection include:
    a. Alcoholism.
    b. Cardiovascular disease.
    c. HIV infection.
    d. Diabetes mellitus.

e. Cirrhosis.
f. End-stage renal disease.
g. Cancers of the upper gastrointestinal tract or oropharynx.
h. Poor nutrition.
i. Crowded living conditions.
j. Adverse social-economic conditions.
k. Persons known to inject illicit drugs.
l. Foreign-born individuals from countries with a high prevalence of tuberculosis.
m. Low income population who are medically underserved.
n. Patients who are non-compliant with appropriate drug therapy.
o. Close contact with persons who are known or suspected to have tuberculosis.
p. Residents and employees of high-risk congregate settings.
q. Health care workers who serve high-risk patients.

2. Assessment for disease:
a. Subjective: Malaise, pleuritic pain, easily fatigued.
b. Objective: Fever, night sweats, cough that progressively becomes worse, hemoptysis, and weight loss.

3. Assessment prior to testing.
a. Review purpose.
b. Review orders.
c. Determine if special conditions needed; disrobing, adult assistance with combative child.
d. Know expected reactions.
e. Check date of expiration of tuberculin Purified Protein Derivative (PPD).
f. Assess the patient's knowledge of procedure and its purpose.
g. Assess patient allergies.
h. Do not administer to patients who have a documented history of a positive Mantoux test; such testing has no diagnostic utility.
i. Review with the patient, as indicated, that potential cross reactions with antigens shared between Mycobacteria and prior vaccination with BCG may occur, but the test is still administered.

4. Plan:
a. Administration of test.
b. Normal reaction.
c. Patient knowledge of test and when/how to read test.
d. Safe and correct administration; no impaired skin integrity, no injury.
e. No transfer of microorganisms.
f. Follow Centers for Disease Control and Prevention (CDC) recommendations to prevent accidental exposure to blood and body fluids.
g. Document amount type of testing substance, date, time, site, appearance of skin and any undesirable effects from administration, patients response.
h. Live vaccines (such as measles-mumps-rubella [MMR], varicella, and polio vaccines) may interfere with the response to the Mantoux test. Give live vaccines with TB test concurrently or delay TB test for 4 to 6 weeks.

5. Implementation.
a. Verify order and properly identify patient.
b. Assemble supplies and select site inside forearm.
c. Check the patient's understanding of the test and when/how to read.
d. Position patient, wash hands, and don gloves.
e. Follow agency policy for administration of intradermal injection.
f. Mantoux test is the standard method of testing.
    (1) Administer 0.1 ml. of PPD containing 5 Tuberculin units (TU) on the ventral surface of the forearm.
    (2) Administer injection intradermally with the bevel of the needle facing upward. Injection should produce a pale, discrete 6-mm to 10-mm weal on the skin.
g. Interpret results as described in *Evaluation* (see next page).

6. Teaching.
a. Purpose of test.
b. How test is administered, low concentration of medication.

c. Positive test may indicate exposure but not active disease.

d. Return for reading within 48 to 72 hours (see *Reading Results* in *Evaluation* section C.7.j.)

e. Self reading by patient – Instruct patient according to agency policy.

7. Evaluation:

   a. Verify bleb remains.

   b. Patient experiences no discomfort.

   c. Safe and correct administration.

   d. Timely documentation.

   e. A positive skin test necessitates additional workup.

   f. Reactions may wane with age, but can be restored by repeated testing. The "booster" phenomenon may occur at any age, but frequency increases with age, highest among persons >55 years of age and/or among persons who have had prior BCG vaccination. This "booster" effect of patients who undergo repeat testing may be falsely considered a new conversion of the skin test from non-reactive to reactive if the second test is administered at some later interval, such as in health care workers getting a second test a year after employment. The CDC (1995) recommends a two-step procedure for the initial screening of residents and employees of long-term care facilities.

     (1) The two step procedure – If the first Mantoux test results is non-reactive, perform a second test 1 to 2 weeks later.

     (2) Reaction to the "booster" test usually indicates old, not new, TB infection.

   g. Absence of a tuberculin reaction does not exclude a diagnosis of TB infection, when symptoms suggest the presence of active disease.

   h. A small percentage of tuberculin reactions may be caused by errors in administering the test or reading the results.

   i. Reading the results (CDC, 2005):

     (1) Skin test should be read between 48 to 72 hours.

     (2) The patient who does not return within 72 hours will need to be retested.

     (3) Basis for the reading test is the presence or absence of induration.

     (4) Erythema should not be measured.

     (5) Reactions at injection site can range from no induration to a large, well-defined induration.

     (6) Induration is not always visible; palpate with fingertips for induration.

     (7) With a light gentle motion, sweep the surface of the forearm in a 2-inch diameter in all four directions to locate margins of induration.

     (8) Mark and measure, using the millimeter ruler, the longest diameter across the forearm.

     (9) Document the measurement and record any blistering. Do not record as positive or negative. Actual measurement is needed. If no induration, then record as "0 mm."

     (10) Positive reading: > 5mm with risk factors; > 10mm without risk factors but in high-incidence group; >15mm without risk factors and in low-incidence group.

     (11) Check agency policy regarding patient reading of TST.

     (12) The CDC (2005) offers educational materials for TST and provides directions for administering and reading the test (www.cdcnpin.org/Guides/tbguide.pdf).

Noninvasive Procedures

Noninvasive procedures are diagnostic or therapeutic techniques that do not require the skin to be broken or the body to be entered. Noninvasive procedures reduce discomfort to the patient and the spread of microorganisms. Medical asepsis, or the clean technique, is used for these procedures. Proper hand washing and disinfecting anything that may have been contaminated while performing a noninvasive procedure reduces the risk for transmission of organisms from person to person or to items in the environment (deWit, 2005).

A. Vital signs – The measurements of 5 vital signs provide important indications regarding the state of health of an individual. Vital signs provide baseline data that reflect the status of several body systems where any deviations or changes can be easily recognized. Vital signs are not assessed in isolation but in addition to assessing signs, symptoms, patient's medications, lab tests, history, and records.
    1. Factors that may influence vital signs:
        a. Age.
        b. Gender.
        c. Race and heredity.
        d. Medications.
        e. Pain.
        f. Time of day.
        g. Caffeine, nicotine.
        h. Exercise.
        i. Emotions.
        j. Pregnancy.
        k. Presence of disease.
        l. Blood loss.
        m. Degree of hydration.
        n. Environmental temperature.
    2. Blood pressure – Measuring arterial blood pressure provides important information about the overall health of the patient. The systolic pressure provides a database about the condition of the heart and great arteries. The diastolic pressure indicates arteriolar or peripheral vascular resistance. The difference between the systolic and diastolic pressure provides information about cardiac function and blood volume. A series of blood pressure readings should be taken to establish a baseline to provide adequate data about all these factors (Smith et al., 2000).
        a. Assessment.
            (1) Blood pressure reading initially and whenever patient status changes.
            (2) Size of cuff needed for accurate reading.
                (a) Bladder width should cover 40% of arm circumference at midpoint; bladder length should cover 80% to 100% of upper arm or thigh circumference. Bladder ends should not overlap.
                (b) Improper cuff size:
                    (i) Too small or narrow will result in falsely elevated measurements.
                    (ii) Too large or wide will result in falsely low measurements.
            (3) Presence of factors that can alter readings (such as smoking or ingesting caffeine within prior 30 minutes).
            (4) Any changes from prior readings.
        b. Planning.
            (1) Determine if reading is within normal range for the patient.
            (2) Establish a baseline for further evaluation.
            (3) Identify alternations in reading results from changes in the patient's condition.
            (4) Correlate readings with pulse and respirations.
            (5) Frequency of measurement is individualized.
            (6) Manage and minimize vascular complications.
            (7) Assess if contraindicated to taking blood pressure on either arm (such as mastectomy, serious injury, lymph node dissection).
            (8) Blood pressure is dependent on the position of body and arm.
            (9) A validated electronic device meeting the requirements of the American National Standard for Electronic Advancement of Medical Instruments may be used (U.S. Public Health Service, 1997).
        c. Implementation.
            (1) Identify the patient.
            (2) Provide privacy.
            (3) Provide a quiet environment. Have the patient sit and rest for 5 minutes.
            (4) Wash hands.
            (5) Expose upper part of patients arm and position palm up, arm slightly flexed and arm supported at heart level. Wrinkled clothing prevents correct placement of cuff.

(6) Wrap deflated cuff snugly and smoothly around arm (lower border of cuff 1 inch above antecubital space, center of cuff over brachial artery). Make sure pressure dial is at zero.

(7) Apply stethoscope lightly to the antecubital fossa. Close valve on sphygmomanometer pump.

(8) Inflate cuff rapidly to a level 30mm Hg above point where the radial pulse is no longer palpable.

(9) Deflate cuff gradually at a constant rate by opening valve on pump no more than 2 to 3 mm Hg per second until first Korotkoff's sound is heard (systolic pressure). Note reading. Continue to deflate cuff. Note the disappearance of Korotkoff's sound (diastolic pressure).

(10) Deflate cuff completely, remove from arm. Check that patient is comfortable.

(11) Document position, limb used, and cuff size for consistency.

  d. Teaching.

(1) Educate regarding expected or desired blood pressure.

(2) Risks of hypertension.

(3) Develop education plan for self measurement, if indicated.

(4) Describe signs and symptoms that must be reported to health care professionals.

(5) Importance for monitoring blood pressure.

  e. Evaluation.

(1) Blood pressure for adults 18 years or older within normal range <120 systolic and < 80 diastolic (U.S. Department of Health and Human Services, 2004).

(2) The normal range of blood pressure in children and adolescents is based on sex, age, and height, and is classified according to body size (National Institute of Health National Heart, Lung and Blood Institute [NHLBI], 2005).

(3) Alterations are identified early and appropriate treatment initiated.

(4) Severely altered readings are rechecked on another limb, different equipment used, or validated by another health care professional.

(5) Initial visit use the average of at least 2 readings. Permit the blood to be released from veins by waiting 1 to 2 minutes before repeated readings.

(6) Altered readings are reported to physician.

3. Pulse – The palpable bounding of blood flow noted at various points on the body. Each time the heart contracts to force blood into an already full aorta, the arterial walls in the vascular system must expand to accept the increased pressure. The pulse rate is determined by counting each pulsation of the arterial wall (deWit, 2005). The radial and apical pulses are the most common sites for assessment of vital signs.

  a. Assessment.

(1) Appropriate site, rate, rhythm, volume, and quality.

(2) Obtaining baseline.

(3) Any changes from prior readings.

(4) Consider factors that normally influence pulse character; age, exercise, postural changes.

  b. Plan.

(1) Determine if pulse rate is within the normal range.

(2) Monitor for health changes.

(3) Take apical rate before administration of cardiac medication.

(4) Apical pulse is used to assess if infant or child, or if there is question about radial pulse in adolescent or adult.

  c. Implementation (radial pulse).

(1) Assess radial pulse at rest to allow for comparison of values.

(2) Identify the patient.

(3) Wash hands.

(4) Patient sitting – Bend elbow 90 degrees and support lower arm on chair, slightly extending wrist with palm down.

(5) Place tips of first two fingers of your hand over groove along radial (thumb side) of patient's inner wrist.

(6) Lightly compress against radius so that pulse is easily palpable.

(7) Begin to count with zero. If pulse is regular, count rate for 30 seconds and multiply by 2. If pulse is irregular, count for 1 full minute.

(8) Determine strength of pulse.

(9) Palpate with two fingers along course of artery toward wrist to determine elasticity of arterial wall.

(10) If irregular or skipped beats, two people need to assess radial and apical pulse at the same time.

(11) Document pulse rate, rhythm, and intensity.

d. Teaching.
(1) Teach the patient to assess his or her own pulse if taking certain medications or if there is a need in response to exercise.
(2) Describe signs and symptoms to report to health care professional.
(3) Normal adult pulse range is 60 to 100 beats/minute.

e. Evaluation.
(1) Palpated pulse without difficulty.
(2) Pulse within normal range and easily detected.
(3) Response to activities of daily living or exercise.
(4) Cardiac status is stable; radial artery is patent.

4. Respirations – Involve the processes of ventilation, diffusion, and perfusion. Accurate assessment of respirations depends on recognizing normal thoracic and abdominal movements. Monitoring respirations assists in the detection of abnormal conditions or diseases in the pulmonary or metabolic system.

a. Assessment.
(1) Risk factors of disease or illness on respiratory functions.
(2) Alterations including fever, pain, anxiety, smoking, medications, postural changes, chest or abdominal dressings, or gastric distention.

(3) Signs and symptoms of respiratory alterations; cyanotic appearance, labored breathing, pain, or coughing.
(4) Presence of dyspnea.
(5) Use of accessory muscles.

b. Plan.
(1) Determine previous baseline rate, if available.
(2) Compare with other vital signs.
(3) Identify if difficulty sleeping, snoring, or shortness of breath.
(4) Note changes from previous readings.

c. Implementation.
(1) Assess after pulse measurement while patient is not aware.
(2) Observe complete respiratory cycle of one inspiration and one expiration.
(3) Count one with first full respiratory cycle.
(4) If rhythm is regular, count for 30 seconds and multiply by 2. If irregular, less than 12 or greater than 20, count for 1 full minute.
(5) Assess the three objective qualities of rate, depth, and rhythm.
(6) Document time, respiratory rate, and any abnormalities.

d. Teaching.
(1) Effective breathing techniques.
(2) Signs or symptoms to report to health care professional.
(3) Modifications of activities of daily living if indicated.

e. Evaluation.
(1) Compare with patient's baseline.
(2) Regular rate and effortless breathing.
(3) Respirations are effective, relaxed, and of normal depth.

5. Temperature – The balance of body temperature is regulated by physiological and behavioral mechanisms. Temperature control mechanisms keep the body's core temperature in a relatively constant range. The core body temperature is the temperature of the deep tissues of the body, not of the skin tempera-

ture. For the body to function on a cellular level, a core temperature between 36.5°C and 37.7°C (96.0°F and 99.9°F) must be maintained (Weber & Kelley, 2003). Variations of heat loss and gain in individuals are influenced by body surface, peripheral vasomotor tone, and quantity of subcutaneous tissue.

a. Assessment (deWit, 2005).
  (1) Most appropriate method of obtaining.
    (a) Oral – Glass thermometer (non-mercury) or electronic.
    (b) Electronic digital – For oral, rectal, axillary.
      (i) Readings appear in seconds.
    (c) Tympanic – Portable, electronic auditory canal probe.
      (i) Readings appear in seconds.
      (ii) Most accurate and good indicator of core body temperature.
      (iii) Measures heat radiated from infrared energy; same blood vessels that serve hypothalamus.
    (d) Disposal – Single use, disposable.
      (i) Thin plastic strips with chemically impregnated paper.
      (ii) Least reliable.
  (2) Determine physician orders and number of times to be taken.
  (3) Temperature in relationship to time of day and age of patient.
  (4) No single temperature is normal for all patients.

b. Plan.
  (1) Factors that influence site chosen.
    (a) Safety.
    (b) Accuracy.
    (c) Convenience.
    (d) Age.
    (e) Patient cooperation.
  (2) Reliability of temperature depends on:
    (a) Accurate temperature taking technique.

    (b) Minimization of variables that influence.
    (c) Site chosen.
  (3) Determine if patient has consumed hot or cold liquids or smoked within 15 to 30 minutes prior to taking orally.

c. Implementation.
  (1) Measurements of any site includes:
    (a) Most appropriate site chosen.
    (b) All equipment assembled prior to procedure.
    (c) Patient identified.
    (d) Patient positioned properly and privacy ensured.
    (e) Explanation of purpose and method.
    (f) Wash hands and don gloves.
    (g) After removing device, wipe from stem to bulb tip.
    (h) Assist the patient to a comfortable position.
    (i) Document temperature, time, and how obtained.
  (2) Oral – Electronic.
    (a) Check battery of electronic thermometer to ensure proper functioning.
    (b) Place probe with proper cover/sleeve under tongue, to the right or left of the frenulum.
    (c) Ask the patient to keep lips tightly closed around thermometer. Open mouth breathing will result in lower readings.
    (d) Remove probe when light or audible signal occurs.
    (e) Read temperature.
    (f) Push ejection button of probe, dispose of disposal cover/sleeve.
  (3) Axillary – Electronic.
    (a) Reliable for skin temperature.
    (b) Used if oral/rectal/tympanic contraindicated.
    (c) Check battery of electronic thermometer.
    (d) Hold under axilla firmly.
    (e) Remove when light or audible signal occurs.
    (f) Read temperature.

(g) Push ejection button of probe, dispose of disposal cover/sleeve.

(4) Rectal – Electronic.

    (a) Do not use if contraindicated (for example, severe coagulation disorders).

    (b) Switch to rectal probe attachment.

    (c) Used if other routes not practical.

        (i) If patient cannot cooperate.

        (ii) If patient cannot close mouth.

    (d) Use disposable sleeve/lubricate according to agency protocol.

    (e) Insert probe 1 inch into rectum; never force probe into rectum.

    (f) Remove when light or audible signal occurs.

    (g) Read temperature.

    (h) Push ejection button of probe; dispose of disposal cover/sleeve.

    (i) Assist patient by cleansing area, repositioning.

(5) Tympanic – Electronic auditory canal probe.

    (a) Do not use in infected or draining ear.

    (b) Place probe gently at opening of auditory canal.

    (c) Remove when light or audible signal occurs.

    (d) Read temperature.

    (e) Push ejection button of probe; dispose of disposal cover/sleeve.

d. Teaching.

(1) Need to monitor.

(2) Appropriate site.

(3) How to obtain and positioning.

(4) Glass thermometers should be disinfected in 70% to 90% isopropyl alcohol, then rinsed with clear water, dried, and stored in dry container.

e. Evaluation.

(1) Comparison to normal range.

(2) Normal ranges (deWit, 2005):

    (a) Oral 36.4°C to 37.5°C (97.5°F to 99.5°F).

    (b) Axillary 0.5°C (1°F) lower than oral temperature.

    (c) Rectal between 0.4°C and 0.5°C (0.7°F to 1°F) higher than oral.

    (d) Tympanic 0.8°C (1.4°F) higher than oral.

6. Pain – The feeling of distress, suffering, and/or discomfort that has long been regarded as a symptom of a condition to be diagnosed and treated (deWit, 2005). Today, it is often regarded as the "fifth" vital sign. It is subjective and individualized, and involves psychosocial and cultural factors. The Joint Commission on Accreditation of Healthcare Organizations (JCAHO) has established standards that state all patients have the right to appropriate assessment and management of pain. In outpatient settings, this standard is interpreted to mean assess "as appropriate to the reason the patient is presenting for care or services" (JCAHO, 2006, p. 1).

a. Assessment.

(1) Type of pain.

(2) Characteristics of pain:

    (a) Location – Diffuse or localized.

    (b) Quality – Description.

    (c) Intensity – Rating.

    (d) Precipitating factors – Fears, anxiety, trauma, disease state.

    (e) Aggravating factors – Position change, environment, fatigue, inadequate pain relief measures.

    (f) Frequency and duration.

(3) Nonverbal indication of pain.

(4) Patient's ability or reluctance to report pain.

(5) Patient's beliefs and fears.

(6) Cognitive status.

b. Plan.

(1) Review patient history.

    (a) Characteristics.

    (b) Management strategies.

    (c) Relevant medical and family history.

    (d) Psychosocial history.

    (e) Impact of pain on patient's daily life.

(f) Patient expectations and goals.

(2) Establish a positive relationship.

(3) Identify appropriate pain scale.

    (a) Numeric – 0 to 10 rating; 0 = no pain to 10 = worst pain.

    (b) Verbal – Word; no pain to worse pain.

    (c) Visual (visual analog scale); Categorical scale (such as the Faces Pain Scale).

    (d) Multidimensional pain assessment tools; Brief Pain Inventory; Initial Pain Assessment Inventory; McGill Pain Questionnaire.

(4) Set realistic goals with the patient for pain management.

(5) Use of time frames.

(6) Identify pharmacologic and non-pharmacologic therapies.

c. Implementation.

(1) Pain scale used.

(2) Physician orders, which may include pharmacologic treatment.

(3) Non-pharmacologic treatments for pain.

    (a) Patient education.

    (b) Psychological approaches.

    (c) Physical rehabilitative approaches.

    (d) Surgical approaches.

(4) Document the patient's preferred pain assessment tool and goals.

(5) Document using common language across the continuum of care.

d. Teaching.

(1) Educate about pain assessment, use of pain scales.

(2) Explore misconceptions of pain.

(3) Signs and symptoms to report to the health care professional.

(4) Physical and psychological consequences of unrelieved pain.

(5) Importance of following medication schedules and plan of care.

(6) Behavioral changes if medication prescribed.

(7) Provide written information and contact persons.

(8) Give patient permission to report pain.

e. Evaluation.

(1) Pain is controlled to patient's satisfaction.

(2) Patient report of deceased anxiety.

(3) Patient reaction, tolerance, and dependence.

(4) Activities of daily living are achieved to the patient's expectations.

(5) Patient reporting of unrelieved or new appearance of pain.

B. Physical assessment – Provides a complete picture of the physiologic functioning of the patient. It is conducted in a systematic way and begins with measuring the height, weight, and vital signs. A brief medical history and psychosocial history is also noted. A health database is formed by combining the above with the physical examination techniques of inspection, palpation, percussion, and auscultation (deWit, 2005).

1. Inspection and observation.

a. Involves sense of vision, smell, and hearing to detect normal and abnormal characteristics and findings.

b. General appearance, color, patterns, size, location, consistency, symmetry, movement, behavior, odors, and sounds.

2. Palpation.

a. Sense of touch to feel various parts of the body.

b. Texture, temperature, moisture, mobility, consistency, strength of pulses, size, shape, and degree of tenderness.

c. Light palpation for to determine areas of tenderness.

d. Deep palpation to examine condition of organs.

3. Percussion.

a. Light tapping on the body structures to produce sound waves.

b. Used to elicit pain, detect abnormal masses, elicit reflexes.

c. Location, size, and density of underlying structures are determined.

d. Type of tapping:

    (1) Direct – Using one or two fingertips to check tenderness.

(2) Indirect – One hand flat; with fist of other hand to strike back of hand or place the middle finger of non- dominant hand and strike with finger of dominant hand.

(3) Sounds produced – Tympany, resonance, hyperresonance, dullness, and flatness.

4. Auscultation.
   a. Listening to sounds produced in the body by use of a stethoscope.
   b. To listen to lungs, assess heart sounds, and detect presence of bowel sounds.
5. Abdominal examination.
   a. Differs slightly from other assessments because ausculating bowel sounds should be performed prior to palpation of bowel, which may stimulate sounds.
   b. Order of assessment of abdomen is inspection, auscultation, palpation and percussion.

C. Electrocardiogram (EKG/ECG) – A graphic representation of electrical impulses generated by the heart used to establish a baseline and as a diagnostic tool in the evaluation of heart failure.
   1. Assessment.
      a. Determine if preexisting cardiac disease.
      b. Rationale for obtaining EKG/ECG.
      c. Identify pharmacologic agents currently prescribed.
      d. Determine subjective complaints.
      e. Identify electrolyte abnormalities.
      f. Patient's knowledge of procedure.
      g. Baseline vitals.
   2. Plan.
      a. Obtain an accurate 12-lead EKG/ECG.
      b. Determine EKG/ECG changes.
      c. Identify electrolyte abnormalities.
      d. Determine cardiac irregularities.
      e. Identify and report potentially dangerous rhythms.
      f. Determine if relationship exists between subjective complaints and EKG/ECG changes.
   3. Implementation.
      a. Obtain tracing (Smith et al., 2000).
         (1) Follow the EKG/ECG machine's own set of operating instructions and agency protocol.

(2) Check the color coding on the manufacture's directions before placing electrodes to ensure they are placed on correct wires.

(3) Review order and identify patient.

(4) Provide privacy and determine if skin site care is necessary.

(5) Attach electrodes to wires before pressing on patient's chest.

(6) Wash hands.

(7) Place electrodes on fleshy areas avoiding bone and muscle.

(8) Place four limb leads on each limb according to color coding.

(9) Place the chest leads as follows:
   (a) V1 – Fourth intercostal space, right sternal border.
   (b) V2 – Fourth intercostal space, left sternal border.
   (c) V3 – Midway between V2 and V4.
   (d) V4 – Fifth intercostal space, left midclavicular line.
   (e) V5 – Fifth intercostal space, anterior axillary line.
   (f) V6 – Fifth intercostal space, left midaxillary line.

b. Monitor EKG/ECG.
c. Remove electrodes; assist the patient with cleansing ensuring privacy.
d. Assist the patient to a comfortable position.
e. Interpretation of EKG/ECG strip.
f. Document and record a 12-lead EKG/ECG, vital signs, date, time, and patient's response.
g. Monitor any patient complaint or discomfort.
h. Report any unexpected outcomes immediately.

4. Teaching.
   a. Purpose and steps of procedure.
   b. Electric current is from patient to machine; therefore, no danger of electric shock.
   c. Contact physician or health care provider regarding test results.

5. Evaluation.
    a. EKG/ECG performed accurately.
    b. Abnormal findings interpreted accurately.
    c. Patient's tolerance of procedure.
    d. Vital signs stable.
    e. Clear EKG/ECG strip obtained.
D. Body mass index (BMI) – Describes relative weight to height. It is used to assess overweight and obesity, and to monitor changes in body weight. The calculation and classification of BMI provides the most current evidence-based guidelines on the identification, evaluation, and treatment of adults who are overweight and obese (McInnis, Franklin, & Rippe, 2003).
    1. Assessment.
        a. Frequency of measurement in adults is based on clinical discretion.
        b. Formula for calculation: Weight (kg)/Height (m)^2
        c. BMI values (National Institutes of Health [NIH], 1998):
            (1) Overweight = 25-29.9.
            (2) Obesity = 30 or greater.
        d. Determine need for BMI measurements.
        e. Review disease conditions, cardiovascular risk factors, physical inactivity, and patient motivation.
    2. Plan.
        a. Establish baseline data.
        b. Identify excess or deficit fluid balance.
        c. Determine patient's expectations.
    3. Implementation.
        a. Obtain height, weight, and calculation of BMI.
        b. Document height, weight, BMI, vital signs, and general appearance.
    4. Teaching.
        a. Normal range of BMI.
        b. Weigh at same time each day.
        c. Diet.
        d. Exercise.
    5. Evaluation
        a. Indication of losses/gains.
        b. Assessment of nutritional status by presence/absence of body fat.
        c. Possible indication of growth disorder.
        d. Possible indication for referral to treatment program.

E. Visual acuity – The purpose of the eye and vision examination is to identify any changes in vision or signs of eye disorders (Weber & Kelley, 2003).
    1. Assessment.
        a. History of difficulty with vision.
        b. History of ocular disease, trauma, diabetes, hypertension, or eye surgery.
        c. Subjective complaints.
        d. Use of glasses or contacts.
        e. Medications used.
        f. Date of last eye examination.
    2. Plan.
        a. Determine visual acuity with or without correction.
        b. Patient denies discomfort during exam; identification of visual problems.
    3. Implementation.
        a. If glasses/contacts are worn at all times, they are to be used for test.
        b. Vision of each eye is tested individually and in both eyes.
        c. Identify patient, and explain purpose and procedure.
        d. Test visual acuity using appropriate chart (U.S. Public Health Service, 1997).
            (1) Snellen (letters or numbers) – The patient reads as many of the symbols as possible, reading each line and proceeding down from the top.
            (2) Tumbling E – Used if the patient not familiar with western alphabet.
            (3) HOTV.
            (4) Allen Figures.
            (5) LH (Leah Hyvarinen) Test.
        e. Test for visual acuity at 10, 15, or 20 feet using the appropriate chart.
        f. Document results and chart used.
    4. Teaching.
        a. Importance of regular eye exam.
        b. Signs and symptoms of eye disease.
        c. Safety precautions for visual deficits.
        d. Signs and symptoms to report to health care professional.
    5. Evaluation.
        a. Compare results to other findings if available and report abnormal results to health care provider.
        b. Patient safety and self care measures reviewed with patient.

c. Home environment assessment completed if indicated.

d. If visual acuity is at 20/40 or less with corrective lenses, refer to eye care specialist.

F. Peak flow meter – Designed for monitoring of airflow in patients with asthma, but it is not used as a diagnostic tool. The severity of asthma signs and symptoms must be classified for appropriate treatment and monitoring. "Initially and before treatment has been optimized, clinical signs, symptoms, and peak flow monitoring or spirometry are used to classify severity" (U.S. Department of Health and Human Services, 2003, p. 4).

1. Assessment.
   a. Obtain medical, social and family history.
   b. Review lifestyle and patient cooperation.
   c. Signs of airway obstruction.
   d. Respiratory assessment.
   e. Includes a review of aggravating factors and how they are managed.
   f. Functional status and quality of life.
   g. Pharmacotherapy.

2. Plan.
   a. Allow for individualized plan of action to address changes.
   b. Monitor for signs and symptoms of distress.
   c. Maintain near normal pulmonary function.
   d. Maintain normal activities.
   e. Prevent chronic and troublesome symptoms.
   f. Meet patient/family expectations.

3. Implementation.
   a. Review orders.
   b. Educate about the use of a peak flow meter and proper procedure.
   c. Observe the patient properly using peak flow meter (NIHLB, 2001).
      (1) Move the indicator to the bottom of the number scale.
      (2) Stand up.
      (3) Take a deep breath, filling lungs completely.
      (4) Place mouthpiece in mouth, close lips around it.
      (5) Blow out as hard and fast as possible.
      (6) Write down the number.
      (7) Repeat 2 more times.

(8) Write down the best (highest) number of 3 blows. Peak Flow Meter interpretation is based on personal best reading:
   (a) Green 80% to 100% – Indicates good control of asthma.
   (b) Yellow 50% to 80% – Signals caution, take quick relief medicine.
   (c) Red < 50% – Signals danger, take quick relief medicine, and seek medical care if not returned to yellow or green immediately.

(9) Assist patient with setting realistic goals with a written action plan.

(10) Document patient understanding, use, tolerance, time, and results.

4. Teaching.
   a. State signs and symptoms to report to health care professionals.
   b. Keep scheduled followup appointments.
   c. Maintain adequate hydration.
   d. Proper use of hand-held nebulizer, oxygen therapy, and inhalers, if prescribed.
   e. Disease process.
   f. Use peak flow meter as instructed by health care professional.

5. Evaluation.
   a. Vital signs stable and within normal range.
   b. Patient able to breath with normal inspiratory capacities.
   c. Realistic short and long-term goals set.
   d. Understanding of follow up care and medication plan as ordered.

Onsite Testing

Also referred to as *Point of Care Testing*. Listed are several of the most common tests that are performed in ambulatory care settings. Onsite testing may include other tests as directed by the agency.

A. Blood glucose testing – Is essential in the diagnosis and control of diabetes (deWit, 2005).
   1. Assessment.
      a. Understanding and purpose of test.
      b. Determine if specific conditions need to be met.

    c. Area of skin to be used.
    d. Note specific requirement for test (such as fasting).
    e. Check to see if test is routine or urgent.
2. Plan.
    a. Obtain an uncontaminated blood specimen.
    b. To obtain accurate blood glucose level.
    c. Review lab parameters.
    d. Obtain blood sample without complications.
3. Implementation.
    a. Review physicians order.
    b. Gather equipment.
    c. Identify patient and explain purpose of test and procedure.
    d. Plan which finger to use; have patient allow hand to hang downward. If hand is cold, have patient warm hand under warm water.
    e. Wash hands and don gloves.
    f. Cleanse chosen fingertip with an alcohol swab.
    g. Turn the machine on, place lancet in holder and remove lancet cover.
    h. Cock the lancet device.
    i Check the control number on the screen with the control number on test strips.
    j. Remove a test strip and insert the metal strip end into machine. Follow manufacturer's directions on machine.
    k. Place the finger stick device firmly on skin and push the release button allowing lancet to penetrate the skin.
    l. Lightly squeeze the finger, gently milking down toward the tip.
    m. Lightly apply the drop of blood to the test strip pad and apply a cotton ball to the puncture wound.
    n. Follow manufacturer's directions regarding timing for test. When complete, record the reading and turn machine off.
    o. Assess the patient's finger.
    p. Dispose of test strip, lancet, and supplies in appropriate waste receptacles.
    q. Remove gloves and wash hands.
    r. Document procedure and results.
    s. Report abnormal levels.
    t. Determine level of instruction needed.

4. Teaching.
    a. Review of disease process.
    b. Review and update goals.
    c. Review of risk factors.
    d. Management of hyperglycemia and hypoglycemia.
5. Evaluation.
    a. Uncontaminated specimen obtained.
    b. Sample obtained with complications.
    c. Patient's understanding of home monitoring, disease, nutrition, and physical activity.
B. Fecal occult blood – A guaiac test is a common laboratory test that can be done in the office following a rectal exam or at home. This test measures microscopic amounts of blood in the feces.
1. Assessment.
    a. Patient's ability to cooperate.
    b. Medical history for bleeding or gastrointestinal disorders.
    c. Medications; note drugs that can cause gastrointestinal bleeding.
    d. Diet.
    e. Use of laxatives.
    f. Exercise.
2. Plan.
    a. Monitor for signs and symptoms of gastrointestinal bleeding, anemia, pain.
    b. Patient instructed (if performed at home) to:
        (1) Do not collect if obvious hematuria, rectal bleeding, or menstruation.
        (2) Avoid aspirin and non-steroidal anti-inflammatory drugs (NSAIDs) 7 days prior to test.
        (3) Do not consume vitamin C in diet or supplemental, red meats, and raw fruits or vegetables.
        (4) Patient understanding of instructions, when and how to return samples.
        (5) Collect two separate samples from three separate bowel movements.
3. Implementation (in ambulatory care setting).
    a. Identify patient and explain procedure.
    b. Prepare necessary equipment.
    c. Check if dietary or medication restrictions were followed.
    d. Wash hands and don gloves.

e. Obtain uncontaminated stool specimen.

f. Use tip of applicator to obtain a small portion of feces.

g. Perform Hemoccult® slide test:

(1) Open flap of slide and apply thin smear of stool in first box.

(2) Obtain second feces specimen from different portion of stool and apply to second box.

(3) Close slide cover and turn over, opening flap.

(4) Apply 2 drops of Hemoccult® developing solution on each box of guaiac paper.

(5) Read results of test after 30 to 60 seconds, note color changes.

(6) Dispose of supplies, remove gloves, and wash hands.

(7) Document results.

4. Teaching.

a. Regarding effect of diet and medications on test result.

b. Importance of following instructions of test, if sending specimens from home.

c. Risk factors for colon cancer, warning signs, and screening tests.

5. Evaluation.

a. Test completed and returned as instructed.

b. Results recorded.

References

Alfaro-LeFevre, R. (2005). *Applying nursing process a tool for critical thinking* (6th ed.). Philadelphia: Lippincott Williams & Wilkins.

American Nurses' Association (ANA). (2004). *Nursing scope and standards of performance and standards of clinical practice.* Washington, DC: American Nurses Publishing.

Centers for Disease Control and Prevention (CDC). (1995). Screening for tuberculosis and tuberculosis infection in high-risk populations: Recommendations of the Advisory Committee for the elimination of tuberculosis. *Morbidity and Mortality Weekly Report, 44*(No. RR-11), 19-34.

Centers for Disease Control and Prevention (CDC). (2005). *Mantoux tuberculosis skin test facilitator guide.* Retrieved November 22, 2005, from http://www.cdc.gov/nchstp/tb/pubs/Mantoux/part2.htm

deWit, S. (2005). *Fundamental concepts and skills for nursing.* Philadelphia: Elsevier Saunders.

Dochterman, J., & Bulechek G. (Eds.). (2004). *Nursing interventions classification (NIC)* (4th ed.). St. Louis: Mosby.

Hewitt-Taylor, J. (2003). Developing and using clinical guidelines. *Nursing Standard, 18*(5), 41-44.

Joint Commission on Accreditation of Healthcare Organizations (JCAHO). (2006). *Nutritional functional, pain assessments and screens.* Retrieved from http://www.jointcommission.org/AccreditationPrograms/AmbulatoryCare/Standards/FAQs/Provision+of+Care/Assessment/Nutritional_Functional_Pain_Assessments_Screens.htm

McInnis, K.J., Franklin, B.A., & Rippe, J.M. (2003). Counseling for physical activity in overweight and obese patients. *American Family Physician, 67*(6), 1249-1256.

National Institutes of Health National Heart, Lung and Blood Institute (NIHLBI). (1998). *Obesity* (NIH Publication No. 98-4083). Bethesda, MD: U.S. Government Printing Office.

National Institutes of Health National Heart, Lung and Blood Institute (NIHLBI). (2001). *Controlling your asthma* (NIH Publication No. 01-2339). Bethesda, MD: U.S. Government Printing Office.

National Institutes of Health National Heart, Lung and Blood Institute (NIHLBI). (2005). *The fourth report on the diagnosis, evaluation, and treatment of high blood pressure in children and adolescents* (NIH Publication No. 05-5267). Bethesda: U.S. Government Printing Office.

North American Nursing Diagnosis Association (NANDA). (2003). *Nursing diagnoses: Definitions and classification 2003-2004.* Philadelphia: Author.

Smith, S., Duell, D., & Martin, B. (2000). *Clinical nursing skills: Basic to advanced skills* (5th ed.). Upper Saddle River, NJ: Prentice Hall Health.

U.S. Department of Health and Human Services. (2003). Key clinical activities for quality asthma care. *Morbidity and Mortality Weekly Report. 52*(RR-6), 1-6.

U.S. Department of Health and Human Services. (2004). *The seventh report of the joint national committee on prevention, detection, evaluation, and treatment of high blood pressure* (NIH Publication No. 04-5230). Bethesda, MD: U.S. Government Printing Office.

U.S. Public Health Service. (1997). *Put prevention into practice: Clinicians's handbook of preventive services* (2nd ed.). Germantown, PA: International Medical Publishers.

Waltz, C., & Jenkins, L. (2001). *Measurement of nursing outcomes.* New York: Springer.

Weber, J., & Kelley, J. (2003). *Health assessment in nursing.* Philadelphia: Lippincott Williams & Wilkins.

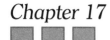
Application of the Nursing Process in Ambulatory Care

This test may be copied for use by others.

COMPLETE THE FOLLOWING:

Name: _____

Address: _____

City: _____ State: _____ Zip: _____

Preferred telephone: (Home)_____ (Work)_____

E-mail_____

AAACN Member Expiration Date: _____

Registration fee: AAACN Member: $12.00
                      Nonmember: $20.00

Answer Form:

1. If you applied what you have learned from this activity into your practice, what would be different?

_____

_____

_____

Evaluation	Strongly disagree				Strongly agree
2. By completing this activity, I was able to meet the following objectives:					
a. Outline the steps of the nursing process and how they promote critical thinking.	1	2	3	4	5
b. Describe the methods of assessment applicable in ambulatory care, including triage.	1	2	3	4	5
c. Identify knowledge necessary for technical skills applicable in the practice of ambulatory care nursing.	1	2	3	4	5
d. Explain how to determine if outcomes are achieved.	1	2	3	4	5
e. Describe the interaction of the components of the nursing process.	1	2	3	4	5
3. The content was current and relevant.	1	2	3	4	5
4. The objectives could be achieved using the content provided.	1	2	3	4	5
5. This was an effective method to learn this content.	1	2	3	4	5
6. I am more confident in my abilities since completing this material.	1	2	3	4	5

7. The material was (check one) ___new ___review for me.

8. Time required to read this chapter: _____minutes

I verify that I have completed this activity: _____
                                          Signature

Comments: _____

_____

_____

Objectives

This educational activity is designed for nurses and other health care professionals who practice in ambulatory care. For those wishing to obtain CE credit, an evaluation follows. After studying the information presented in this offering, you will be able to:

1. Outline the steps of the nursing process and how they promote critical thinking.
2. Describe the methods of assessment applicable in ambulatory care, including triage.
3. Identify knowledge necessary for technical skills applicable in the practice of ambulatory care nursing.
4. Explain how to determine if outcomes are achieved.
5. Describe the interaction of the components of the nursing process.

Posttest Instructions

1. To receive continuing education credit for individual study after reading the article, complete the answer/evaluation form to the left.

2. Detach and send the answer/evaluation form along with a check or money order payable to the *American Academy of Ambulatory Care Nursing (AAACN)*, East Holly Avenue Box 56, Pitman, NJ 08071–0056.

3. Test returns must be postmarked by August 1, 2011. Upon completion of the answer/evaluation form, a certificate for **1.4** contact hour(s) will be awarded and sent to you. Should the material contained in this chapter become outdated prior to the above expiration date, AAACN reserves the right to withdraw this CE test.

This activity is co-provided by the *American Academy of Ambulatory Care Nursing (AAACN)* and Anthony J. Jannetti, Inc. (AJJ). AJJ is accredited as a provider of continuing nursing education by the American Nurses' Credentialing Center's Commission on Accreditation (ANCC-COA). AAACN is a provider approved by the California Board of Registered Nurses, provider number CEP 05336.

This article was reviewed and formatted for contact hour credit by Sally S. Russell, MN, CMSRN, AAACN Education Director; and Candia Baker Laughlin MS, RN, C, Editor.

Multicultural Nursing Care
In the Ambulatory Care Setting

Barbara G. White, MS, RN

Objectives

Study of the information presented in this chapter will enable the learner to:

1. Describe the concept of multicultural care in the 21st century.
2. Discuss the application of culturally competent care in the ambulatory care environment.
3. Integrate cultural differences into ambulatory nursing care practice.
4. Consider cultural disparities in planning health care services.
5. Identify sources of regulations, guidelines, and information to guide culturally competent care.

Key Points

1. Culture affects a person's way of perceiving the world, and it serves as a guide for beliefs and practices related to health and illness.
2. Providing culturally competent health care is a professional and social mandate in modern health care.
3. In this increasingly multicultural environment, the ambulatory care nurse will encounter individuals from many cultures, and will need an understanding of cultural beliefs and practices to effectively plan and provide culturally competent care.
4. Racial and ethnic minorities experience a lower quality of health services and are less likely to receive even routine medical procedures than are Caucasian Americans, even when insurance status, income, age, co-morbid conditions, and symptom expression are taken into consideration.
5. There are increasing numbers of research studies that can assist the nurse to understand biological and other differences between and within cultural groups. Resources to find some of these studies are included in this chapter.

Human beings come together in groups and subgroups as they modify and organize their social and physical environments in ways that improve their quality of life. The resulting cultural patterns of behavior, beliefs, values, knowledge, morals, law, customs, and habits then guide their world view and decision-making. These patterns may be explicit or implicit, are primarily learned and transmitted within the family, are shared by most members of the culture, and change over time in response to various global phenomena. Culture affects a person's way of perceiving the world, and serves as a guide for beliefs and practices related to health and illness (Geiger &

Davidhizar, 1999; Purnell & Paulanka, 2003).

Providing culturally competent health care is a professional and social mandate in modern health care. In today's increasingly multicultural environment, it is essential that health care providers consider the potential impact of the culture of patients and their families, the health care system, and the health care providers themselves. Culture is complex and largely unconscious, and has been shown to have a significant impact on choices made by patients, their families, and health care providers. In the health care setting, it is vitally important that providers develop cultural expertise that will enhance relationships, processes, and outcomes for consumers and providers.

This chapter describes the importance of cultural competency in providing ambulatory care nursing services. With the increasingly diverse population in the U.S., the nurse must have a working understanding of cultural factors that can be involved in the nurse/patient encounter. Many reasons for current disparities in health for minority groups and potential causes for those differences and suggestions for improvement are addressed. In addition, this chapter describes regulations, guidelines, and resources for further exploration of pertinent information.

Increasing Diversity of the Population

A. Minority populations have been increasing in the U.S. in recent years. The percentages of select minority populations as reported in the 2000 census are as follows (U.S. Census Bureau, 2001):
1. Total Population in 2000 census = 281,421,906 (100.0%).
2. White (77.1%).
3. Black or African American (12.9%).
4. Hispanic or Latino of any race (12.5%).
5. Asian (4.2%).
6. American Indian and Alaska Native (1.5%).
7. Total Arab population (0.42%).
8. Native Hawaiian and Other Pacific Islander (0.3%).
B. In this increasingly multicultural environment, the ambulatory care nurse will encounter individuals from many cultures, and will need an understanding of cultural beliefs and practices to effectively plan and provide culturally competent care.

Cultural Competency of Health Care Professionals

A. Pew Health Professions Commission.
1. The Pew Health Professions Commission identified 21 competencies for health care professionals in the 21st century (O'Neil & Pew Health Professions Commission, 1998).
2. The competencies most closely related to cultural competence are (The Center for the Health Professions, 2001):
a. Improve access to health care for those with unmet health needs.

b. Practice relationship-centered care with individuals and families.
c. Provide culturally sensitive care to a diverse society.
d. Partner with communities in health care decisions.
e. Ensure care that balances individual, professional, system, and societal needs.
f. Take responsibility for quality of care and health outcomes at all levels.
g. Advocate for public policy that promotes and protects the health of the public.

Mandates, Regulations, and Guidelines Related to Culture and Health Care

A. *Healthy People 2010* (U.S. Department of Health and Human Services [DHHS], 2000).
1. Is an initiative designed to improve the health of each individual, the health of communities, and the health of the nation.
2. Builds on prior health initiatives, the Surgeon General's Reports of 1979 and 1980, and the *Healthy People 2000* movement as an instrument to improve health for the first decade of the 21st century.
3. Serves as a guide to promote health and to prevent illness, disability, and premature death.
4. Serves as a guide for policy makers and health care organizations including ambulatory care providers.
5. States, "*Healthy People 2010* is firmly dedicated to the principle that – regardless of age, gender, race or ethnicity, income, education, geographic location, disability, and sexual orientation – every person in every community across the nation deserves equal access to comprehensive, culturally competent, community-based health care systems that are committed to serving the needs of the individual and promoting community health" (DHHS, 2000).
6. Includes two goals and 467 objectives in 28 focus areas. The objectives include specific targets for improvement by 2010.
a. Goal 1: Increase Quality and Years of Healthy Life – To help individuals of all

ages increase life expectancy and improve their quality of life. Evaluation will include measuring changes in the following indicators:

(1) *Life expectancy* – Is the average number of years people born in a given year are expected to live based on a set of age-specific death rates. Differences in life expectancy between populations suggest a substantial need and opportunity for improvement.

(2) *Quality of life.*

    (a) *Health-related quality of life* – Subjective, personal sense of physical and mental health and the ability to react to factors in the physical and social environments.

    (b) *Global assessments* – Personal ratings of one's own health status.

    (c) *Healthy days* – Measure of health-related quality of life that estimates the number of days of poor or impaired physical and mental health in the past 30 days.

    (d) *Healthy life* – Difference between life expectancy and years of healthy life reflects the average amount of time spent in less than optimal health because of chronic or acute limitations.

  b. Goal 2: Eliminate Health Disparities – To eliminate health disparities among segments of the population, including differences that occur by gender, race or ethnicity, education or income, disability, geographic location, or sexual orientation.

B. Culturally and Linguistically Appropriate Services (CLAS).

  1. In 1997, the Office of Minority Health of the DHHS initiated a project to recommend national standards that would support a consistent and comprehensive approach to cultural and linguistic competence in health care (U.S. Department of Health and Human Services Office of Minority Health [OMH], 2001).

  2. A comprehensive final report on the project, *National Standards on Culturally and Linguistically Appropriate Services (CLAS) in Health Care: Final Report*, was completed in March 2001.

    a. Describes 14 individual standards and outlines the development, methodology, and analysis undertaken to create the national standards.

    b. Lists standards for culturally competent care, language access services, and organizational supports for cultural competence.

    c. Includes mandates, guidelines, and recommendations. CLAS mandates serve as current Federal requirements for all recipients of Federal funds.

C. Joint Commission on Accreditation of Healthcare Organizations (JCAHO).

  1. On May 12, 2005, JCAHO (2005b) posted the document *Joint Commission 2005 Requirements Related to the Provision of Culturally and Linguistically Appropriate Health Care* on its Web site:

    a. Indicates that JCAHO considers the provision of culturally and linguistically appropriate health care services as an important quality and safety issue.

    b. Has several standards that are related to providing care, treatment, and services in a manner that supports the cultural, language, literacy, and learning needs of individuals.

  2. JCAHO's standards are compared with the CLAS standards in the document *Office of Minority Health National Culturally and Linguistically Appropriate Services (CLAS) Standards Crosswalked to Joint Commission 2004 Standards for Hospitals, Ambulatory, Behavioral Health, Long-Term Care, and Home Care* (JCAHO, 2004).

Cultural Disparities in Health

A. The Institute of Medicine (IOM) reported in *Unequal Treatment: Confronting Racial and Ethnic Disparities in Health Care* (Smedley, Stith,

& Nelson, 2003). Findings from their extensive review of published research follow:

1. Sources of disparities include (Smedley et al., 2003, pp. 1-3):
   a. Historic and contemporary inequities.
   b. Health systems.
      (1) Administrative and bureaucratic processes.
      (2) Utilization managers.
      (3) Financial and institutional arrangements.
      (4) Health care professionals.
      (5) Patients.
   c. High time pressures.
   d. Cost containment.
   e. Language barriers.
   f. Geography.
   g. Stereotyping, biases, and discrimination at the individual (provider and patient), institutional, and health system levels (Smedley et al., 2003, pp. 2-6).

2. Racial and ethnic minorities experience a lower quality of health services and are less likely to receive even routine medical procedures than are White Americans, even when studies control for insurance status, income, age, co-morbid conditions, and symptom expression (Smedley et al., 2003).
   a. When compared with Whites, African Americans are less likely to receive:
      (1) Appropriate cardiac medications.
      (2) Cardiac bypass surgery.
      (3) Peritoneal dialysis.
      (4) Kidney transplantation.
      (5) Quality basic clinical services including intensive care.
   b. Racial differences have been found with:
      (1) Cancer diagnostic tests, treatments, and analgesics, and disparities in cancer care are associated with higher death rates among minorities.
      (2) HIV treatment and survival rates.
      (3) Diabetes care.
      (4) End-stage renal disease and kidney transplants.
      (5) Pediatric care.
      (6) Maternal and child health.
      (7) Mental health.
      (8) Rehabilitation and nursing home services.
      (9) Surgical procedures.
   c. Minorities have been found to be more likely to have procedures that are considered to be less desirable such as bilateral orchiectomy and amputation.

3. The IOM's review of research studies found that there are many reasons that minority patients have different care.
   a. Patient characteristics.
      (1) Minority patients have been found to be more likely to refuse recommended services, delay seeking care, and not follow prescribed treatment regimens. These can be the result of differences between the cultural backgrounds of the patient and provider, mistrust, misunderstanding of instructions, problems with previous interactions with the health care system, or lack of knowledge of how to access the health care system.
      (2) Patients also may present their symptoms/disease in different ways (Smedley et al., 2003, p. 7). The IOM determined that this does not fully explain the disparities.
   b. Health care system characteristics.
      (1) Language barriers may prevent patients from using a facility or negatively affect care because of lack of appropriate interpreter services.
      (2) Time pressures of the provider may hinder complete assessment that takes into account appropriate language and cultural aspects of the patient's situation.
      (3) Services may be geographically remote or may not be available to minorities.
      (4) Financial resources may be a barrier to care.
   c. Health care provider characteristics (Smedley et al., 2003, p. 9).
      (1) Bias or prejudice against minorities.
      (2) Clinical uncertainty when interacting with minority patients.
      (3) Beliefs or stereotypes about the behavior or health of minorities.
      (4) Misinterpretation of behaviors or

responses of patients to the provider.

(5) More research is needed in this area because little is known at this time.

(6) See the full report for descriptions of specific research findings and examples of the impact of provider effect on the disparities of health in minorities.

4. Suggestions from the IOM report:

a. Broader awareness of the scope, causes, and effective strategies to reduce health disparities.

b. Systems that insure financial incentives do not restrict minority patients' access to care.

c. Provision of interpretive services.

d. Financial incentives that reward appropriate screening, preventive services, and evidence-based care.

e. Increased numbers of minority health care professionals.

f. Culturally appropriate education of patients to improve access to care and participation in decision-making. Examples of successful strategies:

(1) Waiting room interventions have been shown to increase patients' participation in their interactions with providers, improve health, decrease physical limitations, and improve patients' health status and perceptions of their overall health. In one study, a research assistant "reviewed the medical record with the patient, helped the patient identify decisions to be made, rehearsed negotiation skills, encouraged the patient to ask questions, reviewed obstacles such as embarrassment and intimidation, and after the visit, gave the patient a copy of the medical record for that visit" (Smedley et al., 2003, p. 577).

(2) A booklet mailed to patients assisted them in preparing for their visit, and resulted in changes in their success of reporting and obtaining information, and improved self-reported

adherence to treatment plans (Smedley et al., 2003, p. 567).

g. Continuing education for health care providers that addresses current research on disparities in health, the role of unintentional bias and stereotyping, and clinical research related to differences in health responses related to ethnic and cultural factors.

5. Resources:

a. The IOM Report. The 780-page published report is available either as hard copy or in electronic format.

b. Collection and monitoring of patient care data. In association with JCAHO, a 30-month project funded by the California Endowment began in January 2004. The project was initiated to assess hospitals' capacity to address the issues of language and culture that impact the quality and safety of patient care (JCAHO, 2005a). The status of this project can be monitored by visiting the *Hospitals, Language, and Culture: A Snapshot of the Nation* Web site (http://www.jcaho.org/about+us/hlc/index.htm).

B. Agency for Healthcare Research and Quality (AHRQ) (2004).

1. AHRQ has been directed by Congress to produce an annual report that tracks disparities in health care delivery related to racial, ethnic, and socioeconomic factors for priority populations.

a. Examines differences in quality of and access to health care.

b. Priority populations include:

(1) Low-income groups.

(2) Minority groups.

(3) Women.

(4) Children.

(5) Older adults.

(6) Individuals with special health care needs, including individuals with disabilities and individuals who need chronic care or end-of-life health care.

2. The first *National Healthcare Disparities Report*, which was released in 2003, pro-

vides a comprehensive national overview of disparities in health care among racial, ethnic, and socioeconomic groups in the general U.S. population and among priority populations.

3. The second report (AHRQ, 2004) continues to examine disparities and adds a goal to track progress towards elimination of those disparities. It also examines differences within and across priority populations (for example, comparisons are made between black and white women, and between low-income and high-income women).

4. Details of the findings, including information about risk factors, screening, treatment, management, and mortality for high-priority diseases (breast cancer, diabetes, end-stage renal disease, heart disease, maternal and child health, etc.) of the priority population groups are included in the second report of the AHRQ (2004).

Cultural Competency

A. Developing cultural competence requires cultural awareness, cultural knowledge, cultural skill, and cultural encounter (Campinha-Bacote, 2003).
   1. Cultural awareness: Conscious learning process through which the individual becomes appreciative of and sensitive to the cultures of other people.
   2. Cultural knowledge: Process of understanding the key aspects of a group's culture, especially related to interpretations of health and illness, and health care practices.
   3. Cultural skill: Ability to collect relevant data regarding health histories and performing culturally specific assessments.
   4. Cultural encounter: Process that encourages individuals to engage directly in cross-cultural interactions with people from culturally diverse backgrounds.
B. Spector (2004) describes three components for professional health care that addresses the complex culture-bound health care needs of individuals, families, and communities. Care should be:
   1. Culturally sensitive: The provider possesses basic knowledge of health traditions of diverse cultural groups found in the practice setting.

2. Culturally appropriate: The provider applies cultural background knowledge to provide the patient with the best possible health care.
3. Culturally competent: The provider understands and attends to the total context of the patient's situation; includes a complex combination of knowledge, attitudes, and skills.
C. Purnell and Paulanka (2003) describe cultural competence as encompassing the following:
   1. Developing and appreciating an awareness of one's own existence, sensations, thoughts, and surroundings without letting it have an untoward influence on others.
   2. Demonstrating knowledge and understanding of the cultural preferences of others (patients, family, colleagues, etc.).
   3. Accepting and respecting the cultural differences of others.
   4. Avoiding ethnocentric responses.
   5. Being open to cultural encounters.
   6. Adapting professional practice so that it is congruent with the culture of others.
D. Cultural competence addresses differences among the health care team members as well as between providers and patients, families, and the community.
E. The health care encounter is affected by attributes of patients and their families, health care providers, and the health care system. Individuals make decisions based on their cultural beliefs and experiences. Each individual is culturally unique and brings with them "their personal characteristics, including their personalities, social attitudes and values, race, ethnicity, gender, sexual orientation, age, education, and physical and mental health" (Smedley et al., 2003, p. 557).
   1. Individuals are diverse in multiple dimensions including:
      a. Race.
      b. Gender.
      c. Religion.
      d. Age.
      e. Weight.
      f. Ethnicity (country/geographic area/culture of origin).
      g. Education.
      h. Physical and mental abilities and disabilities.

i.   Job-relevant abilities.
j.   Sexual orientation (heterosexual, homosexual, bisexual, asexual).
k.   Marital status (single, married, divorced, cohabitating, widow/widower).
l.   Family status (children, childless, single parent, two parent, single, grandparent).
m.   Appearance and clothing preferences (casual, formal, professional, business).
n.   Personality traits.
o.   Interest in technology (high-tech, low-tech, technophobe).
p.   Values and motivation.

F.   Developing cultural competence.
1.   Using guides to cultural assessment can facilitate the nursing process. Such guides can be used to explore the degree to which patients share or differ from commonalities with the cultural information generally attributed to their cultural group. Identifying potential similarities and differences can assist the nurse to deliver culturally relevant health care. One example of a guide is *Transcultural Communication in Nursing* (Munoz & Luckman, 2005).
2.   Increasingly, nurses are finding that approaching cultural knowledge from the viewpoint of a list of characteristics of a specific cultural group is inadequate for their practice and can lead to stereotyping.
3.   Fortunately, there is an increasing number of research studies that can assist the nurse to understand biological and other differences between and within cultural groups. Resources to find some of these studies are included later in this chapter.
4.   Strategies to improve cultural awareness.
a.   Explore one's own cultural background, values, and beliefs, especially related to health and health care.
b.   Examine one's own cultural biases toward people whose cultures differ from one's own culture.
5.   Strategies to improve cultural knowledge.
a.   Learn basic general information about predominant cultural groups in the geographic area of the ambulatory care setting.
b.   Explore Web sites and cultural pocket guides as a resource for general information.
c.   Read research studies that describe cultural differences.
d.   View documentaries about cultural groups who receive care in the ambulatory care facility.

6.   Strategies to improve cultural skill.
a.   Become aware of cultural differences in predominant ethnic groups.
b.   Be alert for unexpected responses with patients, especially as related to cultural issues. Individuals have their own explanatory model based on their belief system about what has caused their illness and what the illness does to them. This model also includes their beliefs about what will help cure them. For example, a Hispanic mother may believe that her child has *Mal d'ojo*, or has been cursed with the "evil eye." An Asian patient may believe she is having a difficult birth because of an imbalance between hot and cold in her body. As pregnancy is a "cold" condition, she may request a drink of hot water for balance (Pediatric Pulmonary Centers, 2005).
c.   Develop assessment skills to do a competent cultural assessment for any patient. To facilitate this, the health care provider in the ambulatory care setting can ask patients what they need, what they expect to receive, and whether they have received what they think will help them feel better (McKenna, 1999).
d.   Learn assessment skills for different cultural groups including cultural beliefs and practices.
7.   Strategies to improve cultural encounters.
a.   Create opportunities to interact with predominant cultural groups.
b.   Visit cultural events, such as religious ceremonies, significant life passage rituals, social events, and demonstrations of cultural practices.
c.   Visit markets and restaurants in ethnic neighborhoods.
d.   Explore ethnic neighborhoods, listen to

different types of ethnic music, and learn games of various ethnic groups.
- e. Visit or volunteer at health fairs in local ethnic neighborhoods.
- f. Learn about prominent cultural beliefs and practices, and incorporate this knowledge into planning nursing care.

G. Cultural competence benefits the individual and the organization in that it:
1. Fosters mutual trust and respect for differences among individuals and groups.
2. Acknowledges the contributions of each individual involved.
3. Values and utilizes cultural variations to the benefit of all.
4. Maintains a learning environment where cultural behavior is assessed and interpretations are pursued and valued as well as integrated into health care and nursing care delivery.

H. Attributes to consider when planning for culturally competent care:
1. Communication styles: Communication is the mechanism whereby individuals and groups connect.
   a. Assessing communication styles and patterns from the cultural perspective can include the following:
      (1) Visit areas where different ethnic communities gather, watching and listening to how they communicate, interact, and conduct business.
      (2) Observe how individuals interact with regard to dialect, volume of speech and silence, the context of speech including emotional tone, and kinesics (gestures, stance, eye behavior).
      (3) Determine from reliable resources the implications of the behaviors observed in different cultural groups.
   b. To develop and apply culturally competent communication skills that are central to positive working relationships, nurses, and other professionals would:
      (1) Modify communication patterns to adapt to the style of the individual or group addressed.
      (2) Identify and avoid using gestures

that individuals or groups might find threatening or insulting.
      (3) Use clarifying and validating techniques.
      (4) Utilize team members from different cultures as resources in learning about and using culturally sensitive behaviors.
      (5) Employ trained interpreters as appropriate. Avoid use of family, friends, or hospital workers who are not trained as professional interpreters.
2. Space, in terms of cultural behavior, is defined as the physical distance occurring in personal interactions and the intimacy techniques utilized when relating to others, both verbally and nonverbally.
   a. Assessing the relevance of space includes acknowledging that space has distinct zones for different interactions.
      (1) Intimate.
      (2) Personal.
      (3) Public.
   b. Acquire knowledge of the appropriate distances to maintain in different cultures. Comfort with space and distance has different meanings in different cultures.
   c. Integrating culturally competent space skills includes the ability to:
      (1) Honor space distances according to cultural and personal preference.
      (2) Communicate personal space comfort levels appropriately.
3. Social organization as a cultural dimension refers to the values that individuals place on important groups in their life (such as family, work group, etc.).
   a. Assess the importance and value individuals place on the different groups in their lives.
   b. Value, respect, and integrate individual differences for preferred social organization into professional interactions with individuals and groups. For example, ask who the primary decision maker of the family is for this patient. Among many traditional Chinese, it is the eldest

son. In some Muslim cultures, it may be the husband or father.

4. Time as a key element in culture is defined by the clock and the calendar but also includes a person's orientation to the past, present, and future.
   a. Past-oriented people have a tendency to value tradition and stability. In some Asian cultures, remedies of their ancestors are honored and may be in conflict with modern medical care.
   b. Present-oriented people tend to focus on activities that meet current demands, and may not see the importance of immunizations or for treatments of asymptomatic diseases, such as hypertension.
   c. Future-oriented people tend to conduct activities in light of their contributions to achieving goals, such as taking steps to promote health or use preventive care services.
   d. Assessing and integrating cultural competency regarding time includes evaluating an individual's or group's orientation to time (for example, are they prompt, on time, or late for scheduled appointments; how are they oriented to the past/present/future; and how do they define "late?").
   e. Using time in a culturally sensitive manner includes engaging in activities and interactions that utilize time orientation to the individual's and the group's benefit.

5. Environmental control refers to an individual's perceived ability to control external occurrences. These perceptions are a source of the individual's feelings of safety and security.
   a. Environmental control has two aspects.
      (1) An individual's attachment to a certain terrain, climate, or location (such as individual preferences or affinity with a particular country or section of a country, desert living, or locating by water).
      (2) An individual's belief about the degree to which they control

events. This belief has two general categories:
      (a) Internal locus of control: A person believes actions can evoke events.
      (b) External locus of control: A person believes that events occur by chance, luck, or fate, and they have little control over what happens to them.
   b. Cultural competency regarding environmental control includes:
      (1) Assessing the individual's or group's perceptions about the ability to control external events. The health care provider can explore the patient's explanatory model to determine beliefs about the cause of a health condition and the patient's perceived ability to influence outcomes by his or her own actions. If the patient believes that a condition is caused by fate or as a result of his or her own bad behavior, the prescribed treatment interventions may not be carried out.
      (2) Framing interventions and programs in a way that facilitates comfort levels of patients and leads to successful outcomes.

6. Biological variation, as a dimension in cultural competence, refers to the genetic differences among individuals.
   a. Genetic biological variations among specific ethnic, gender, or cultural groups is increasingly being associated with risk factors for specific diseases or responses to therapeutic pharmaceuticals or regimens (Kudzma, 1999; Munoz & Hilgenberg, 2005).
   b. Cultural competence regarding biological variations includes:
      (1) Developing knowledge about cultural differences.
      (2) Assessing for them.
      (3) Adapting interventions to maximize positive outcomes and minimize risk from disability and disease.

7. Ethnopharmacology.

a. Ethnopharmacology reflects an emerging field of research that is increasingly focusing on the effect of genetic and cultural factors on the absorption, metabolism, distribution, and elimination (pharmacokinetics) and the mechanism of action and effects (pharmacodynamics) of drugs. (Munoz & Hilgenberg, 2005).

b. Cultural competence includes understanding a person's response to treatment, including how genetic and cultural influences might affect a person's treatment choices and responses (Munoz & Hilgenberg, 2005).

c. Genetic variations in certain enzymes can cause different responses, with some ethnic groups having more variation than others. There are also significant differences between subcultures that have traditionally been grouped together, for example, Hispanics (Latino, Mexican, Latin American, etc.), Pakistani groups (Muhajir, Punjabi, Sindhi, Pashtun, and Baluchi), Asians (Korean, Chinese, Japanese, Indian, Pakistani, Vietnamese), and American Indians (Munoz & Hilgenberg, 2005).

  (1) Cytochrome P-450 (CYP) enzyme abnormalities are common and vary based on race or ethnic group. As a result, some people are "ultrarapid metabolizers" who metabolize a drug quickly, and others may be "poor metabolizers" who metabolize a drug more slowly and have higher serum levels at the same dose. Additionally, a person can be a rapid metabolizer of one medication and a slow metabolizer of another (Munoz & Hilgenberg, 2005).

  (2) Psychotropic drugs.

    (a) Haloperidol: "American-born Asian Americans" and "Foreign-born Asians" were found to have higher serum concentrations than the "Caucasians" in a study by Lin and Poland (Munoz & Hilgenberg, 2005). In a study of Asian and White patients diagnosed with schizophrenia, Asians required lower doses of haloperidol, and when given the same dose as White patients, they experienced more extrapyramidal symptoms. (Lin and Poland in Munoz & Hilgenberg, 2005).

    (b) Blacks were more at risk for tardive dyskinesia than Whites with traditional antipsychotics (haloperidol, fluphenazine, chlorpromazine, thioridazine).

    (c) Newer antipsychotic agents (risperidone, clozapine and olanzapine) may be less likely to cause extrapyramidal and other adverse effects in Asians, Hispanics, Blacks, and Whites (Munoz & Hilgenberg, 2005).

  (3) Some antihypertensive drugs (for example, captopril, losartan) may be less effective in Blacks than in Whites, while others (thiazide diuretics) may be more effective in Blacks.

d. Another source of difference in drug responses may be clinician biases and prescribing practices rather than to pharmacokinetic or pharmacodynamic variability (Munoz & Hilgenberg, 2005).

e. The culturally competent nurse will take into account the potential variations in effects of treatments, the potential effect of patients discontinuing their therapies based on side effects, and the effects of beliefs and previous experience in planning and delivering care for all patients, including those from diverse cultural backgrounds.

Cultural Differences in Disease Incidence and Management

A. Hepatitis.

  1. Effectiveness of Interferon treatment for chronic hepatitis C varies in racial and ethnic groups (Doctor's Guide, 1999) with African Americans

having the lowest effectiveness rates:
- a. Interferon treatment resulting in hepatitis C virus RNA negative status.
  - (1) Asian 40%.
  - (2) Caucasian 33%.
  - (3) Hispanic 28%.
  - (4) African American 5%.
2. Individuals with chronic hepatitis B are at high risk of developing liver cancer.
   - a. Immigrants from some countries have higher rates of hepatitis B, and screening programs should be in place to screen for liver cancer because studies indicate that early detection and treatment of cancer improves the survival rate. Screening programs in rural areas, such as the Alaska Native populations, have proven to be cost effective.
3. The reasons for the variations have not been fully explained; however, the health care provider can provide culturally relevant care by being observant and aware of the potential implications in minority patients.

B. Asthma and other lung diseases.
1. African Americans have the highest asthma prevalence of any racial/ethnic group in the US. The asthma prevalence rate in African Americans was almost 38% higher than that in Whites (American Lung Association, 2005).
2. Data from some studies indicate that American Indians/Native Americans may have equal if not greater rates of asthma than other racial groups.

C. Pain management.
1. Research has documented that as a group ethnic minorities' pain is consistently under-treated (Cleeland, Serlin, Nakamura, & Mendoza, 1996). The Intercultural Cancer Council (2003) summarized the effect of culture on pain management:
   - a. Increasingly, studies report that minorities are significantly less likely than White patients to receive prescriptions for analgesic agents, are at risk for inadequate pain control and under-treatment of pain, and that unrelieved pain among minority groups is highly prevalent.
   - b. Hispanics with isolated long-bone fractures are twice as likely as similar non-Hispanic Whites to receive no pain medication in the emergency department. Fifty-five percent of Hispanics receive no analgesic medication, as compared with 26% of non-Hispanic Whites.
   - c. African American and Hispanic patients are less likely to have their pain recorded compared to non-Hispanic Whites.
   - d. Metastatic cancer patients at centers that treat predominantly minorities are three times more likely than those treated elsewhere to have inadequate pain management.
   - e. White patients are significantly more likely than African American patients to receive analgesics (74% versus 57%), despite similar records of pain complaints.
2. Managing pain in culturally diverse populations can be a challenge as there are differences in beliefs about the causes of pain, ways to express or hide pain, and ways to treat pain (Intercultural Cancer Council, 2003).
   - a. African Americans with chronic illness use more pain-coping techniques that employ distraction, praying, or hoping, while Whites use more pain-coping techniques that involve ignoring pain.
   - b. Religion and faith are important ways with which Hispanic patients cope with cancer and pain.
   - c. Poor postoperative pain relief is often more prevalent when patients are passive in their relationship with health professionals.
   - d. Inadequate education of patients in pain and analgesia expectations may contribute to poor postoperative pain relief in the Asian population.
   - e. More than 80% of African American and Hispanic cancer patients wait until their pain severity is a 10 on a 10-point scale before calling their health care provider or oncology clinic for assistance with pain management.

f. Attitudes and cultural beliefs about coping with pain may explain why Asian patients are less likely to request an opioid or are likely to cease its use prematurely even when there is some pain relief.

g. The meaning of cancer-related pain differs somewhat between African American and Hispanic cancer patients. Hispanic patients are more likely to describe pain as "suffering," whereas African American patients describe it as "hurt." When defining what pain means to them, Hispanic patients tend to focus more on the emotional component of pain, whereas African American patients talk more about the sensory component.

3. While numeric rating scores for pain are widely used (rate pain from 0 to 10), some cultural groups would more readily describe the full nature of their pain as a constellation of feelings, symptoms, and consequences of the pain. Some cultures also respond to pain in stoic or very expressive ways, and these, too, do not fit readily on the standard scales (Douglas, 1999).

4. Assessment of pain in non-English-speaking or limited-English-speaking patients may require the nurse to learn key phrases in the patient's language. Collins, Gullette, and Schnepf (2004) found this an effective strategy among Hispanic patients.

D. Maternal and child health.

1. While Mexican American women may have risk factors during their pregnancy, there are cultural factors that have an impact on favorable birth outcomes. Cultural practices include protection of the mother and fetus by older Mexican American women, religious beliefs and practices, family obligations to provide aid and be with the childbearing mother, and respect for familial caring roles in relation to age and gender (Berry, 1999).

2. In some cultures, high fertility rates are desirable. In the Muslim population, irreversible forms of birth control, such as vasectomy or tubal ligation, would be forbidden, and abortion would be an option only when a pregnancy-induced disease is present or the mother's life is threatened (Purnell & Paulanka, 2003).

E. Cancer care.

1. The Intercultural Cancer Council (2001a & b) reports low screening rates for some cultural groups:

a. Hispanic women have lower breast cancer screening rates than non-Hispanic White women and tend to seek and attain health care services less than other ethnic groups. Only 38% of Hispanic women age 40 and older have regular screening mammograms (Intercultural Cancer Council, 2001b).

b. Age, income, education, health insurance coverage, language proficiency, physician referrals, and system barriers are some of the factors that influence Hispanic women in participating in screening services. Other factors include cultural beliefs about modesty and sexual behavior, fatalism, acculturation factors unrelated to language use, family-centered values, and existing social support networks. The degree to which each Hispanic population group in each locale holds onto beliefs about cancer may play an important role in levels of participation (Intercultural Cancer Council, 2001b).

c. According to the 1992 National Health Interview Survey Results, Hispanics are less likely than non-Hispanics to report having had a screening test for colorectal cancer. Low screening rates among Hispanics indicate a great need for providing education to Hispanics about the importance of early screening for and detection of colorectal cancer, and an equally great need for increasing Hispanics' access to these critical health services (Intercultural Cancer Council, 2001b).

2. Individuals from many cultural groups use home remedies for treatment of medical conditions such as cancer. For instance, a major problem in Chinese women is that approximately 22% often use herbal remedies when diagnosed with breast cancer (Intercultural Cancer Council, 2001a).

Resources for Cultural Competence and Knowledge about Disease Management In Various Cultural Groups

A. Alzheimer's disease: The Alzheimer's Association Web site includes information on cultural variations (www.alz.org/Resources/Diversity/general.asp).

B. Respiratory: American Lung Association provides information on incidence, causes and treatment of respiratory problems in cultural populations (http://www.lungusa.org/site/pp.asp?c=dvLUK9O0E&b=312474).

C. Cancer: The Office of Minority Health, Health Resources and Services Administration published a 84-page handbook to guide heath care providers who want to decrease cancer health disparities. The guide takes the professional along a cultural journey that moves from an assessment of the health care provider to essential information on the cancer experience for specific cultural groups. It is available through the Intercultural Cancer Council Web site (http://icc network.org). This Web site also includes other information on cancer and cultural variations.

D. Developing cultural competence: The "Cross Cultural Health Care-Case Studies" program is an online interactive self-study program consisting of a series of 5 tutorials in cultural competence. The tutorials include a home page to introduce the topic and define concepts, a case story to illustrate the topic, a multimedia lecture about the topic, and a series of learning activities to engage the learner in applying the concepts to the case story. The Cross Cultural Health Care Case Studies were developed collaboratively by seven Pediatric Pulmonary Centers. The tutorials are available at no charge (http://ppc.mchtrain ing.net/).

E. Working with minority patients and health care providers: The Minority Nurse Web Site and Journal – The Minority Nurse Web site (http://minority nurse.com) is a valuable resource for minority nurses and provides insight into working with nurses from various cultural backgrounds. Their journal, *Minority Nurse*, provides information that will help any nurse improve care for patients from different cultural backgrounds.

F. Transcultural nursing: The mission of the Transcultural Nursing Society is "to enhance the quality of culturally congruent, competent, and equitable care that results in improved health and well being for people worldwide" (http://www.tcns.org/). The journal of this society (*Journal of Transcultural Nursing: A Forum for Cultural Competence in Health Care*) publishes research that explores the influence of culture on nursing practice and the delivery of health care (http://www.sagepub.com/journal.aspx?pid=71).

References

Agency for Healthcare Research and Quality. (2004, December). *2004 National healthcare disparities report.* Retrieved December 23, 2005, from http://www.qualitytools.ahrq.gov/disparitiesreport/2004/browse/browse.aspx

American Lung Association. (2005). *Lung disease data at a glance: Asthma.* Retrieved December 23, 2005, from http://www.lungusa.org/site/pp.asp?c=dvLUK9O0E&b=312474

Berry, A.B. (1999). Mexican American women's expressions of the meaning of culturally competent prenatal care. *Journal of Transcultural Nursing, 10*(3), 201-211.

Campinha-Bacote, J. (2003, January 31). *Many faces: Addressing diversity in health care.* Retrieved April 24, 2006, from http://nursingworld.org/ojin/topic20/tpc20_2.htm

Cleeland, C.S., Serlin, R., Nakamura, Y., & Mendoza, T. (1996). Effects of culture and language on ratings of cancer pain and patterns of functional interferences. In T.S. Jenson, J.A. Turner & Z. Hallin-Weosnefeld (Eds.), *Proceedings of the 8th World Congress on Pain* (pp. 35-51). Seattle, WA: IASP Press.

Collins, A.S., Gullette, D. & Schnepf, M. (2004). Break through language barriers. *Nursing Management, 35*(8), 34-38.

Doctor's Guide. (1999). *AASLD meeting: For African Americans, Interferon much less effective against hepatitis C.* Retrieved December 23, 2005, from http://www.pslgroup.com/dg/C0186.htm

Douglas, M. (1999). Pain as the fifth vital sign: Will cultural variations be considered? *Journal of Transcultural Nursing, 10*(4), 285.

Geiger, J.N. & Davidhizar, R.E. (1999) *Transcultural nursing: Assessment and intervention* (3rd ed.). St Louis: Mosby.

Intercultural Cancer Council. (2001a). *Asian Americans & cancer.* Retrieved March 10, 2006, from http://www.iccnetwork.org/cancerfacts/ffs3.htm

Intercultural Cancer Council. (2001b). *Hispanics/Latinos & cancer.* Retrieved March 10, 2006, from http://www.iccnetwork.org/cancerfacts/cfs4.htm

Intercultural Cancer Council. (2003). *Pain & cancer.* Retrieved May 18, 2006, from http://www.iccnetwork.org/cancerfacts/cfs7.htm

Joint Commission on Accreditation of Healthcare Organizations (JCAHO). (2004) *Office of Minority Health national culturally and linguistically appropriate services (CLAS) standards crosswalked to Joint Commission 2004 standards for hospitals, ambulatory, behavioral health, long term care, and home care.* Retrieved December 23, 2005, from http://www.jcaho.org/about+us/hlc/hlc_omh_xwalk.pdf

Joint Commission on Accreditation of Healthcare Organizations (JCAHO). (2005a). *Hospitals, language, and culture: A snapshot of the nation.* Retrieved December 23, 2005, from http://www.jcaho.org/about+us/hlc/index.htm

Joint Commission on Accreditation of Healthcare Organizations (JCAHO). (2005b). *Joint Commission 2005 requirements related to the provision of culturally and linguistically appropriate health care.* Retrieved December 23, 2005, from http://www.jcaho.org/about+us/hlc/hlc_jc_stds.pdf

Kudzma E.C. (1999). Culturally competent drug administration. *American Journal of Nursing, 99*(8), 46-51.

McKenna, M. (1999). Let us try to keep culturally competent care in managed care. *Journal of Transcultural Nursing, 10*(3), 293-294.

Munoz, C., & Hilgenberg, C. (2005). Ethnopharmacology. *American Journal of Nursing, 105*(8), 40-49.

Munoz, C., & Luckman, J. (2005). *Transcultural communication in nursing* (2nd ed.). Clifton Park, NY: Delmar Learning.

O'Neil, E.H., & Pew Health Professions Commission. (1998). *Recreating health professional practice for a new century.* Retrieved December 23, 2005, from http://future health.ucsf.edu/pdf_files/recreate.pdf

Pediatric Pulmonary Centers. (2005). *Cross cultural health care.* Retrieved April 24, 2006, from http://ppc.mchtraining.net /custom_pages/national_ccce/case0/home.html#

Purnell, L.D. & Paulanka, B.J. (2003). *Transcultural health care.* Philadelphia: FA Davis.

Smedley, B.D., Stith, A.Y., & Nelson, A.R. (Eds.). (2003). *Unequal treatment: Confronting racial and ethnic disparities in health care.* Washington DC: The National Academies Press.

Spector, R.E. (2004). *Cultural diversity in health and illness* (6th ed.). Upper Saddle River, NJ: Pearson Education.

The Center for the Health Professions. (2001). *Twenty-one competencies for the twenty-first century.* Retrieved December 23, 2005, from http://futurehealth.ucsf.edu/pewcomm/ competen.html

U.S. Census Bureau. (2001). *Census 2000 briefs.* Retrieved November 27, 2005, from http://www.census.gov/population/www/cen2000/briefs.html

U.S. Department of Health and Human Services (DHHS). (2000). *Healthy people 2010.* Retrieved December 23, 2005, from http://www.healthypeople.gov/Document/html/uih/uih_2.h tm#obj

U.S. Department of Health and Human Services Office of Minority Health (OMH). (2001). *National standards for culturally and linguistically appropriate services (CLAS) in health care: Final report.* Retrieved December 23, 2005, from http://www.omhrc.gov/assets/pdf/checked/finalreport.pdf

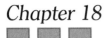

Multicultural Nursing Care in the Ambulatory Care Setting

This test may be copied for use by others.

COMPLETE THE FOLLOWING:

Name: _____

Address: _____

City: _____ State: _____ Zip: _____

Preferred telephone: (Home)_____ (Work)_____

E-mail_____

AAACN Member Expiration Date: _____

Registration fee: AAACN Member: $12.00
                    Nonmember: $20.00

Answer Form:

1. If you applied what you have learned from this activity into your practice, what would be different?

_____

_____

_____

Evaluation	Strongly disagree				Strongly agree
2. By completing this activity, I was able to meet the following objectives:					
a. Describe the concept of multicultural care in the 21st century.	1	2	3	4	5
b. Discuss the application of culturally competent care in the ambulatory care environment.	1	2	3	4	5
c. Integrate cultural differences into ambulatory nursing care practice.	1	2	3	4	5
d. Consider cultural disparities in planning health care services.	1	2	3	4	5
e. Identify sources of regulations, guidelines, and information to guide culturally competent care.	1	2	3	4	5
3. The content was current and relevant.	1	2	3	4	5
4. The objectives could be achieved using the content provided.	1	2	3	4	5
5. This was an effective method to learn this content.	1	2	3	4	5
6. I am more confident in my abilities since completing this material.	1	2	3	4	5

7. The material was (check one) ___new ___review for me.

8. Time required to read this chapter: _____minutes

I verify that I have completed this activity: _____
                                            Signature

Comments: _____

_____

_____

Objectives

This educational activity is designed for nurses and other health care professionals who practice in ambulatory care. For those wishing to obtain CE credit, an evaluation follows. After studying the information presented in this offering, you will be able to:

1. Describe the concept of multicultural care in the 21st century.
2. Discuss the application of culturally competent care in the ambulatory care environment.
3. Integrate cultural differences into ambulatory nursing care practice.
4. Consider cultural disparities in planning health care services.
5. Identify sources of regulations, guidelines, and information to guide culturally competent care.

Posttest Instructions

1. To receive continuing education credit for individual study after reading the article, complete the answer/evaluation form to the left.

2. Detach and send the answer/evaluation form along with a check or money order payable to the *American Academy of Ambulatory Care Nursing (AAACN)*, East Holly Avenue Box 56, Pitman, NJ 08071–0056.

3. Test returns must be postmarked by August 1, 2011. Upon completion of the answer/evaluation form, a certificate for **1.5** contact hour(s) will be awarded and sent to you. Should the material contained in this chapter become outdated prior to the above expiration date, AAACN reserves the right to withdraw this CE test.

This activity is co-provided by the *American Academy of Ambulatory Care Nursing (AAACN)* and Anthony J. Jannetti, Inc. (AJJ). AJJ is accredited as a provider of continuing nursing education by the American Nurses' Credentialing Center's Commission on Accreditation (ANCC-COA). AAACN is a provider approved by the California Board of Registered Nurses, provider number CEP 05336.

This article was reviewed and formatted for contact hour credit by Sally S. Russell, MN, CMSRN, AAACN Education Director; and Candia Baker Laughlin MS, RN, C, Editor.

Chapter 19

Patient Education and Counseling

Mary Anne Bord-Hoffman, MN, RN, C

Objectives

Study of the information presented in this chapter will enable the learner to:
1. Describe factors that influence the educational process in ambulatory care.
2. List the goals of education in ambulatory care.
3. Describe teaching strategies used for patient education and counseling in ambulatory care.
4. Discuss major health topics that are included in patient counseling to promote health behaviors in ambulatory care settings.

Key Points

1. Patient education and counseling in the ambulatory care nursing setting have long been identified as important by the American Nurses Association (ANA) and the International Council of Nurses.
2. Education in ambulatory care nursing draws on basic principles and theories of education and behavioral psychology.
3. In the ambulatory care setting, patients seek care and counseling for disease prevention and health promotion, as well as care for illnesses.
4. Health and wellness issues for children, adolescents, and adults, and specific issues to include in counseling are reviewed.

Patient Education in Ambulatory Care

A. Patient education in nursing practice.
   1. Historical foundations for nurses' teaching role (Bastable, 2003).
      a. Mid 1800s: Florence Nightingale educates those who deliver health care.
      b. Early 1900s: Public health nurses in the U.S. teach prevention of disease and maintenance of health.
      c. 1918: The National League of Nursing Education recognizes health education as a component of the scope of nursing practice.
      d. 1950: The National League of Nursing Education's course content aims to prepare nurses upon completion of their basic program to assume the teaching role.
      e. Both the American Nurses Association (ANA) and the International Council of Nurses have long identified the importance of the teaching component in nursing practice.
   2. Legal mandates:
      a. All state nurse practice acts include teaching within the scope of nursing practice.
      b. The *Patient Self Determination Act of 1990* defines informed consent (see Chapter 8, *Legal Aspects of Ambulatory Care Nursing*, for more details).
   3. Accreditation mandates:
      a. Joint Commission on Accreditation of Healthcare Organization (JCAHO) standards require evidence that patients have been taught, and that they understand what they have been taught (JCAHO, 2005).
      b. The American Hospital Association's (AHA) Patient's Bill of Rights establishes a patient's right to receive information about diagnosis, treatment, and prognosis in terms that can be reasonably understood (AHA, 1998).
   4. Professional mandates:
      a. As mentioned above, the ANA identifies teaching as a major component of the nurse's practice.

b. The American Academy of Ambulatory Care Nursing (AAACN) *Conceptual Framework for Ambulatory Care Nursing* lists patient education as the first element in the clinical nursing role (AAACN, 2004).

c. AAACN includes integration of patient and family education into the delivery of care in its *Ambulatory Care Nursing Administration and Practice Standards* (AAACN, 2004).

B. The education process (Bastable, 2003).

1. Definitions (Bastable, 2003).

a. *Education process* – A systematic, planned course of action consisting of two major interdependent operations: Teaching and learning.

b. *Teaching* – A deliberate intervention to meet intended learner outcomes.

c. *Learning* – An action by which knowledge, skills, and attitudes are consciously or unconsciously acquired so that behavior is altered in some way that can be observed or measured.

d. *Patient education* – A process of assisting people to learn health-related behaviors (knowledge, skills, attitudes, and values) so they can incorporate them into their everyday lives.

2. Learning theories: Learning theory is a framework that describes, explains, or predicts how people learn. There are several theories of learning, and each provides its own perspective. The testing of these theories has made significant contributions to understanding how people acquire knowledge and change their ways of thinking, behaving, and feeling. The major learning theories form the foundation, not only for education, but also for psychological counseling, from which many of the principles of behavioral change have been developed (Bastable, 2003). This has implications for nurses teaching patients because the principles of behavioral change are utilized in counseling patients regarding healthy lifestyle choices. Learning theories are useful in guiding an approach to education and are often combined to address specific situations.

a. Behaviorist learning theory:
(1) Examines learning as the product of a stimulus condition and the response it elicits.
(2) Is sometimes called the S-R model of learning.
(3) Focuses on external conditions and does not consider what goes on inside an individual.

b. Cognitive learning theory:
(1) Stresses the importance of what goes on inside the learner.
(2) Involves processing information based on what is already known and reorganizing it into new insights or understanding.

c. Social learning theory:
(1) Views learning as a social process.
(2) Emphasizes importance of significant others providing examples or role modeling for how to feel, think, or behave.

d. Psychodynamic learning theory:
(1) Utilizes constructs of theories based on Freud.
(2) Stresses the importance of conscious and unconscious forces in guiding behavior.

e. Humanistic learning theory:
(1) Assumes that each individual is unique.
(2) Assumes that all individuals desire to grow in a positive way.

3. Factors that influence the educational process.

a. Learner developmental stage.

b. Learner level of literacy.

c. Learner readiness to learn:
(1) Physical readiness: Physical ability, health status, gender, environment.
(2) Emotional readiness: Acceptance of need to learn, level of anxiety, support systems, motivation.
(3) Experiential readiness: Cultural background, past coping mechanisms, short and long-term goals.
(4) Knowledge readiness: What is already known, cognitive ability, learning style, presence or lack of learning disability.

d. Environment in which education takes place.
e. Time allotted for the education.
4. Teaching approaches related to developmental stage of the learner.
   a. Infant and toddler (0 to 3 years of age).
       (1) Focus instruction toward parents.
       (2) Allow older toddlers, if appropriate, to participate to some extent in the process (perform procedures on a teddy bear or doll first to help the child comprehend; keep teaching lessons brief; avoid analogies and explain in simple terms).
   b. Preschooler (3 to 6 years of age).
       (1) Instruct about health promotion and disease prevention, emphasizing importance of this to parents. Parents are strong role models for a variety of health habits.
       (2) Allow the child to handle equipment and play with dolls to learn about body parts. There are special kidney, ostomy, and stoma dolls, as well as those which can have splints and traction attached.
       (3) Use praise, approval, and tangible rewards, such as stickers and badges as reinforcement for a successful learning experience.
   c. Adolescent (12 to 18 years of age).
       (1) Recognize that adolescents' language skills and ability to conceptualize mean a wide variety of teaching methods and instructional tools may be used.
       (2) Assure confidentiality by using one-on-one instruction about sensitive information.
       (3) Provide for control by sharing decision-making whenever possible, and suggest options to help provide choices. Including the adolescent in determining the best way to master information helps to support his or her sense of autonomy.

(4) Anticipate negative responses when adolescent self-image/self-integrity is threatened. Approach with respect, flexibility, and openness to encourage responsiveness to teaching-learning situations.
   d. Adult (18 years of age and older). Malcom Knowles pioneered the field of adult leaning (Lieb, 1991). Adult learning principles suggest that the adult learner is the center of the activity, not the end point at which teaching is directed. Teaching strategies should be based on principles that guide adult learning (Bastable, 2003).
       (1) What is to be learned must be related to an immediate need.
       (2) Learning is voluntary, self-initiated, person-centered, and problem-centered.
       (3) Learning is self-directed.
       (4) The role of the teacher is that of facilitator.
       (5) Learning new material draws on past experience and is related to something the learner already knows.
       (6) Information and assignments must be relevant.
       (7) Learning is reinforced by application and prompt feedback.
C. Goals of education in ambulatory care.
   1. Self management.
   2. Health promotion.
   3. Disease prevention.
   4. Appropriate patient/significant other involvement in treatment, care, and service decisions.
D. Specific topics for patient education in ambulatory care.
   1. JCAHO standards define what is required for patient education in ambulatory care. The patient and his or her needs are assessed and as appropriate to the patient's condition and the specific setting, the patient is educated about:
       a. The plan of care, including treatments and services.
       b. Basic health practices.
       c. Basic safety.

d. Safe and effective use of medications.
e. Nutrition, modified diets, oral health.
f. Safe and effective use of medical equipment or supplies.
g. Pain, including:
(1) What it is.
(2) The risk for pain.
(3) Importance of pain management.
(4) How to evaluate for pain and measure it.
(5) Methods for pain management.
E. Unique challenges for educating patients in ambulatory care:
1. Episodic nature of visits.
2. Time constraints.
3. Wide geographic catchments areas, making it difficult to get patients back for structured classes.
4. Wide variety of cultural and age grouped patients.
F. Teaching strategies encompass a wide range and are chosen based on patient factors, setting, skill of the educator, and available resources.
1. Lecture.
2. Group discussion.
3. Simulation and learning exercises.
4. Printed materials.
5. Web sites and on-line information.
6. Computer-assisted instruction (CAI).
7. Video and CD.
8. Interactive video programming.
9. Virtual reality.
G. Documentation of education and patient response is part of the process for nurses in ambulatory care.

Patient Counseling for Health Promotion and Disease Prevention

Primary Care is such a strong collaboration between provider and nursing staff that the role of nurse as educator in primary care cannot be divorced from the overall goals of that discipline. While the physician or nurse practitioner may be the "provider" of record and the one held accountable for meeting practice guidelines, the nurse is, more often than not, the one who provides the education or counseling for preventative health behaviors.

A number of factors that contribute to premature death in the U.S. have been identified. These include smoking tobacco, poor diet, physical activity patterns, alcohol consumption, toxic agents, firearms, sexual behavior, motor vehicles, and illicit use of drugs. Behavioral choices determine the effect these have on an individual's health. Often, patients in ambulatory care are not ill but are seeking preventative care or followup for chronic conditions. Therefore, it is important to place strong emphasis on counseling that leads to improved personal health practices.

The following section identifies specific content in counseling patients. It has been divided into *Providing Counseling for Infants, Children, and Adolescent Health*; and *Providing Counseling for Adult and Older Adult Health*. Counseling topics and many of the specific counseling strategies parallel those described in *Put Prevention into Practice: Clinician's Handbook of Preventive Services, 2nd Edition* (U.S Public Health Services [USPHS], 1998), and updates found on the Agency for Healthcare Research and Quality (AHRQ) Web site (www.ahrq.gov). In the section on *Infants, Children, and Adolescent Health*, counseling would be directed at parents as appropriate.
A. Counseling for infants, children, and adolescent health.
1. Alcohol and other drug abuse.
a. *Scope of the problem*: Abuse of alcohol and other drugs is a major health problem for older children and adolescents. Accidental injury is the leading cause of death for adolescents, and 40% of such injuries are related to alcohol use (USPHS, 1998). Alcohol has also been implicated in a significant percentage of homicides and suicides, the second and third leading causes of death in this age group.
b. Cocaine use leads to increased cardiovascular morbidity and mortality, and is indirectly a contributor to deaths related to illegal drug activities. Use of illegal drugs is also related to academic and occupational problems and illegal behavior (Centers for Disease Control and Prevention [CDC], 2005a). Steroid use to enhance physical performance has

been demonstrated to have severe and long-term effects on multiple body systems.

c. Topics to include in counseling.
(1) Physical effects of drug and/or alcohol use.
(2) Psychosocial effects of drug and/or alcohol use.
(3) Dangers of drinking alcohol and driving.
(4) Parental role in educating about the dangers of drug and alcohol use.
(5) Dangers of using performance enhancing drugs, such as anabolic steroids.
(6) Resources for parents and children.

2. Dental and oral health.
a. *Scope of the problem*: Dental caries (tooth decay) and periodontal diseases are the most common dental and oral health problems in children. It is estimated that about 80% of those in late adolescence have acquired dental caries, a preventable infectious disease (AHRQ, 2001). The dental health of adults is in great part determined by the quality of preventative treatment and services received during childhood.
b. Topics to include in counseling.
(1) Proper dosage and technique of application of fluoride supplements, if needed.
(2) Techniques parents can use to sooth irritability caused by teething.
(3) Strategies to prevent tooth decay.
(4) Proper technique for brushing children's teeth.
(5) Importance of consulting a dentist or hygienist regarding a child's use of dental floss and need for dental sealants on permanent molars.
(6) The impact of dietary habits on oral health: Importance of avoiding foods that are high in simple sugars or starches, and encouraging the consumption of raw fruits and vegetables.
(7) Correct technique for replacing a permanent tooth that has been

knocked out and is intact, and the action to take if this is not possible.
(8) Importance of wearing helmets, wearing appropriate mouth protectors, and avoiding the use of chewing tobacco.

3. Nutrition.
a. *Scope of the problem*: Inadequate nutrition during infancy and childhood prevents proper growth and development. Calcium and iron are the most common nutrients deficient in children's diets, but excessive caloric intake is a much greater problem for children in the U.S. Many children have a high intake of dietary total and saturated fat, are physically inactive, and are substantially overweight. These factors may lead to obesity and poor nutritional habits in adulthood, resulting in a higher risk of heart disease, type 2 diabetes, and other health problems.
b. Topics to include in counseling.
(1) Benefits of breastfeeding infants for the first 6 to 12 months of life.
(2) New food introduction: One food at a time at 3 to 5-day intervals.
(3) Use of iron-rich foods, such as iron-fortified cereal and infant formula.
(4) Need for a balanced diet for children over the age of 2 years.
(5) How to choose a diet low in fat, saturated fat, and cholesterol.
(6) The importance of using sugar and salt in moderation.
(7) Sugar and salt content of prepared and packaged food.
(8) Importance of maintaining a healthy weight.
(9) Importance of adolescent females consuming adequate folic acid and dietary options for doing this.

4. Physical activity.
a. *Scope of the problem*: Despite all the well-demonstrated benefits of physical activity, most American children and adolescents are not physically active. In 1996, the Surgeon General reported that only about half of young people,

aged 12 to 21, engaged in regular and vigorous physical activity (U.S. Department of Health and Human Services [DHHS], 1996). Obesity among young children and adolescents is felt to be associated with this lack of activity. In a highly cited work that controlled for adult weight, it was found that being overweight in adolescence was a more powerful predictor of premature mortality than was being overweight as an adult (USPHS, 1998).

   b. Topics to include in counseling.

     (1) Importance of choosing a physical activity for enjoyment (sometimes children's experience with physical activity is only in the form of competition and is not positive).

     (2) Importance of engaging in a variety of activities to help with the development of a range of abilities.

     (3) Importance of safety equipment, such as helmets, guards, and pads, and protection against sunburn for outdoor activities with use of sunscreens, lip balm, and protective clothing.

     (4) The effect of drugs, cigarettes, and alcohol on performance and increasing the chance of injury.

     (5) The reduction of the risk of injury with proper training and gradual increase in intensity of exercise.

     (6) Dangers of performance-enhancing drugs, such as anabolic steroids.

5. Safety.

   a. *Scope of the problem*: Injuries are the leading cause of death for children in the U.S. (CDC, 2003). Approximately one-half of injury-related deaths of children involve motor vehicles (USPHS, 1998). Additional causes include burns, drowning, scalds, choking, firearms, falls, poisoning, and sports. The majority of unintentional injuries are preventable, and among adolescents, the use of alcohol and drugs presents a significant risk. Among adolescents, violence within the dating context can also present a safety risk. Dating violence includes verbal or emotional abuse, physical violence, and sexual assault (CDC, 2004).

   b. Topics to include in counseling.

     (1) Importance of parents learning life-saving skills, such as cardiopulmonary resuscitation (CPR) and the Heimlich maneuver.

     (2) Importance of using appropriate child safety seats/seatbelts in automobiles.

     (3) Importance of teaching children to use the community emergency response system (for example, 911 or other emergency numbers).

     (4) Importance of parents' role in modeling safety (for example, wearing seat belts and bike helmets; not driving after drinking alcohol).

     (5) How to avoid and protect children from choking and suffocation, drowning, electrocution, falls, burns, firearms, motor vehicle accidents, poison ingestion, pedestrian injuries, recreational injuries, and sudden infant death syndrome (SIDS).

     (6) Importance of having a dating safety plan (Alabama Coalition Against Domestic Violence [ACADV], n.d.).

6. Sexually transmitted diseases and HIV infection.

   a. *Scope of the problem*: Sexually active young people are at high risk of getting a sexually transmitted disease (STD) including infection with the human immunodeficiency virus (HIV). In 2003, 47% of high school students reported ever having had sexual intercourse (CDC, 2005b), and among those who did report that they had ever had sexual intercourse, only 63% reported having used a condom the last time they had intercourse (Klein & the American Academy of Pediatrics Committee on Adolescence, 2005). The consequences of sexually transmitted diseases can be very serious for teenagers. Because of the histology of their cervix, female adolescents are more susceptible to certain

STDs than are older women; pelvic inflammatory disease and sterility can result from gonorrhea and chlamydia infections; human papilloma virus, which may be the most prevalent STD in adolescents, can lead to cervical cancer; the presence of other STDs may increase susceptibility to the HIV virus; and untreated STDs during pregnancy can lead to serious consequences for the fetus or newborn child (USPHS, 1998).

  b. Topics to include in counseling.
    (1) Risk of STDs and HIV infections.
    (2) Routes of transmission of STDs and HIV infections.
    (3) Importance of communication between parents and their adolescents regarding responsible, safe, sexual behavior.
    (4) Abstinence as the most effective way to prevent STDs and HIV infection.
    (5) Importance of using condoms to prevent STDs and HIV infection.
    (6) The proper way to use condoms.
    (7) How to access resources about specific topics related to sexual activity and STDs/HIV infection.

7. Tobacco use.
  a. *Scope of the problem*: Passive exposure to tobacco smoke is a potential health hazard for infants and children, exacerbating the symptoms of asthma and allergies, and decreasing pulmonary function. Additionally parental smoking is a risk factor for beginning to smoke in adolescence. Health consequences of smoking include increased risk for multiple types of cancer, heart disease, and respiratory disease. Also of concern is the use of smokeless, or chewing, tobacco.
  b. Topics to include in counseling.
    (1) Importance of a smoke-free home environment.
    (2) Parental role modeling and its effect on children and adolescents.
    (3) Negative health consequences on the child of parental smoking.
    (4) Importance of beginning to discuss tobacco use and its negative effects when children are early elementary school age.
    (5) Negative cosmetic and athletic effects of smoking (in discussions with children and adolescents).

8. Unintended pregnancy.
  a. *Scope of the problem*: Approximately 900,000 teenagers become pregnant each year in the U.S., and despite decreasing rates, more than 4 in 10 adolescent girls have been pregnant at least once before 20 years of age. Greater than 90% of 15 to 19-year-olds, as compared with half of all adults, describe their pregnancies as being unintended. Adolescent pregnancy has a higher incidence of low birth weight, prematurity, and neonatal death than for adult pregnant women. Psychosocial complications of adolescent pregnancy include school interruption and/or lack of completion of education. This can have longer term effects in terms of socioeconomic future for both parent and child (Klein & the American Academy of Pediatrics Committee on Adolescence, 2005).
  b. Topics to include in counseling.
    (1) Options for contraception for a sexually active adolescent.
    (2) How to support an adolescent's decision of abstinence (for parents).
    (3) Importance of using condoms as a means of preventing STDs and HIV infection, even if another form of contraception is being used.
    (4) Importance of sexually active adolescents talking freely with their partners about STDs, HIV, and hepatitis B infection, as well as the use of contraceptives.
    (5) Importance of adolescents being assertive with their partners about using contraception and protective measures against STDs.
    (6) Importance of close followup with

their health care provider after initiating use of contraceptives. This provides opportunity to clarify any misconceptions and address any concerns, thus promoting continued use.

9. Violent behavior and firearms.
   a. *Scope of the problem*: Violence is a major health problem for children and adolescents in the U.S. Homicide is the second leading cause of death among 15 to 24-year-old individuals, and for African American males and females and Hispanic males in this age group, it is the leading cause of death. Violence to females, in the form of dating violence, sexual assault, and rape, is also a concern (USPHS, 1998).
   b. Topics to include in counseling.
      (1) Risk factors for violent injury (history of violent injury to the child or other family members, history of alcohol or other drug abuse by the child or other family members, guns or other weapons kept in the house, prevalence of violence-related injury in the community).
      (2) Dangers of keeping a gun in the home.
      (3) For those who do have a gun in the home, review the specifics of gun safety.
      (4) Availability of guns in places where children spend time, such as school, friends' homes, and recreational facilities.
      (5) Ways of dealing with anger.
      (6) Importance of having a dating safety plan (ACADV, n.d.).
      (7) Resources for information about prevention of violence.

B. Counseling for adult and older adult health.
   1. Alcohol and other drug abuse.
      a. *Scope of the problem*: Alcohol and drug abuse are physically damaging and are associated with other major causes of death including suicide, traffic accidents, homicide, and HIV infection (USPHS, 1998). Consumption of alcohol

during pregnancy can lead to the development of fetal alcohol syndrome, which can produce a wide variety and severity of physical and mental problems in infants.
      b. Topics to include in counseling.
         (1) Importance of discontinuing alcohol/substance abuse.
         (2) Information about the negative impact on health of alcohol/substance abuse.
         (3) Risks of HIV infection, hepatitis B or hepatitis C infection, and other disorders associated with shared needle use.
         (4) Resources to assist with discontinuing alcohol/substance abuse.
   2. Dental and oral health.
      a. *Scope of the problem*: Most adults have dental or oral problems at some time in their lives. The most common are dental caries (tooth decay) and periodontal diseases, both of which are preventable. Clinical trials have demonstrated that personal oral hygiene measures can help control plaque and gingivitis in most individuals. The progression of periodontal disease can be retarded by a combination of meticulous personal oral hygiene practices and professional care. Oral cancer is also a major concern among adults, with 30,000 cases diagnosed each year (American Cancer Society [ACS], 2005). Use of tobacco in all forms and heavy consumption of alcohol are major contributing factors.
      b. Topics to include in counseling.
         (1) Importance of regular preventative health care with an oral care professional.
         (2) Importance of brushing and flossing daily.
         (3) Importance of limiting intake of refined sugars, especially for those patients with a history of dental carries.
         (4) Risks associated with tobacco and alcohol use.
         (5) Importance, especially for those who use alcohol or tobacco, of see-

ing a dentist or physician for any irregularities of the oral cavity (such as color changes, ulcers, bleeding, swelling or thickening in lips, cheeks, tongue, gums, or roof of the mouth) that lasts for more than two weeks.

(6) Importance of using protective equipment, including headgear and mouth guards, when engaging in sports or other activities that have a potential for oral/dental trauma.

(7) The need for endocarditis prophylaxis for dental or operative procedures in the oral cavity (for those patients for whom this is applicable).

(8) Oral effects and complications of medication and other treatments.

3. Injury and domestic violence.

a. *Scope of the problem*: The fifth leading cause of death in the U.S. is unintentional injuries, with motor vehicle crashes accounting for over half of these, and alcohol being a factor in both fatal and non-fatal crashes. While nation-wide seat belt use is estimated to be 68%, in fatal crashes, seat belt use is lower than 50%. Falls, especially in older adults, are a leading cause of injury death, with hip fractures being the most common fall-related injury leading to hospitalization. Roughly half of all persons sustaining hip fractures never regain full function. Domestic violence is a health risk especially for women and older adults (USPHS, 1998). The amount of death and disability caused by preventable injuries and violence warrant a discussion of these topics with every patient.

b. Topics to include in counseling.

(1) Questions about safety including seatbelt and helmet use.

(2) Importance of not consuming alcohol prior to driving or operating equipment.

(3) Importance of installing and maintaining smoke detectors in homes.

(4) Dangers of hazards and importance of safety rules at worksites.

(5) Importance of safety in the home.

This can be facilitated with the use of home safely check lists. This list reviews such things as adequate lighting, conditions that may result in falls, and presence of handrails and traction strips on stairs and in bathtubs.

(6) Unacceptability of violence when abuse is disclosed.

(7) Information on community, social, and legal resources available to abuse victims.

4. Nutrition.

a. *Scope of the problem*: Obesity among adults has increased significantly over the last 20 years. Over 30 percent of U.S. adults are obese. This increasing rate is of concern because being overweight or obese increases the risk of many diseases and health concerns (CDC, 2005c). Obesity has become a major health problem in the U.S. and is attributed to over consumption of calories and low levels of physical activity. Good nutrition is essential to good health throughout the lifespan, and it is also a component in the prevention and treatment of many diseases. Many patients look to their primary care providers to give them basic information that they can follow to assure adequate and appropriate nutrition (USPHS, 1998).

b. Topics to include in counseling.

(1) Dietary habits.

(2) Basic information about maintaining a healthy diet. *Dietary Guidelines for Americans* published by DHHS (2005) contains specific recommendations.

(3) Importance of women consuming adequate amounts of calcium and folic acid, including options for assuring adequate intake.

(4) Dietary strategies for weight reduction (fewer total calories, increase fruits and vegetables, decrease fat intake), for overweight patients.

(5) Low cholesterol diet for patients

with borderline or high cholesterol.

(6) Resources to assist with weight reduction for patients who wish to lose weight.

5. Physical activity.

a. *Scope of the problem*: Regular exercise has been shown to reduce the risk of cardiovascular disease, the leading cause of death in the U.S. In addition, it helps prevent diabetes, control weight, improve musculoskeletal functioning, and decrease stress; it may also help prevent bone loss associated with aging. Despite the many benefits of exercise, according to the 1996 *Surgeon General's Report on Physical Activity and Health* (DHHS, 1996), more than 60% of adults are not regularly exercising, and 25% report no physical activity at all. When all the benefits of regular exercise are taken into consideration, counseling patients on this one behavior may have the greatest positive effect on the health of American adults. Patients who are unable or unwilling to engage in regular exercise should be encouraged to increase physical activity in their usual routine by such things as parking farther away from a destination, walking to the supermarket, and taking the stairs rather than the elevator.

b. Topics to include in counseling.

(1) Importance of moderate intensity exercise for 30 minutes or longer daily.

(2) That exercise programs should include the following characteristics: Medically safe, enjoyable, convenient, structured, and realistic.

(3) Examples of daily exercise regimens.

(4) Importance of developing a routine which gradually increases in intensity and/or is modified to meet physical limitations.

(5) Importance of followup for ongoing support and reinforcement for patients who are beginning a new regimen.

6. Sexually transmitted diseases (STD) and HIV infection.

a. *Scope of the problem*: While substantial progress has been made in preventing, diagnosing, and treating certain STDs in recent years, sexually transmitted diseases remain a major public health challenge in the U.S. The CDC (2004) estimates that 19 million new infections occur each year, almost half of them among young people ages 15 to 24. In addition to the physical and psychological effects of these diseases, a tremendous economic toll exists; it is estimated that direct medical costs associated with STDs in the U.S. are approximately $13 billion per year (CDC, 2005d).

b. Topics to include in counseling.

(1) Information about STD and/or HIV transmission.

(2) Information about how to prevent STD and/or HIV infection.

(3) Risks of having sex with partners who use injected drugs, have multiple or anonymous sex partners, or have had any STD within the last 10 years, even if they are symptom-free.

(4) Health consequences of injection drug use, if indicated.

7. Smoking cessation.

a. *Scope of the problem*: The 2004 Surgeon General's report on health consequences of smoking concluded that smoking harms nearly every organ in the body, causing diseases and reducing the health of smokers in general; smoking cigarettes with lower machine measured yields of tar and nicotine provide no clear health benefit (DHHS, 2004). The list of diseases caused by smoking has been expanded to include abdominal aortic aneurysm; acute myeloid leukemia; cataract, cervical, kidney, pancreatic, and stomach cancers; pneumonia; and periodontitis. Quitting smoking has immediate as well as long-term benefits, reducing risks of diseases caused by smoking and improving health in general. This last finding gives added importance to counseling patients on smoking cessation.

 b. Counseling strategies.

  (1) AHRQ (2005) has developed a pocket guide for nurses to help their patients quit smoking. The following counseling strategies are taken from that guide, and are based on the "5 As" approach to cessation intervention.

   (a) **Ask** about tobacco use at every visit. This might be accomplished by considering tobacco use assessment as part of the vital signs assessment.

   (b) **Advise** tobacco users to quit. Tell patients, "Quitting smoking is the most important thing you can do to protect your health."

   (c) **Assess** readiness to quit. If the patient is ready to quit, provide resources and assistance. If the patient is unwilling to quit, provide resources and help the patient identify barriers to quitting.

   (d) **Assist** tobacco users with a quit plan. This should include specific goals of setting a quit date; getting support from family, friends, and coworkers; and using past experiences to identify what worked and what did not. Also, give advice on successful quitting, encourage the use of pharmacotherapy if not contraindicated, and provide resources.

   (e) **Arrange** for followup visits and provide the patient with information about these appointments. If the patient relapses, encourage a repeat quit attempt; tell the patient that relapse is part of the quitting process.

8. Unintended pregnancy.

 a. *Scope of the problem*: Unintended pregnancy is a pregnancy that is either mistimed or unwanted at the time of concep-

tion (CDC, 2005e). Half of all pregnancies in the U.S. are unintended. The two groups of women with the highest percentages of unintended pregnancies were those younger than 18, and those aged 40 or over (Henshaw, 1998). The consequences of these pregnancies include approximately 1.5 million abortions annually, children who are at increased risk of health and behavior problems in childhood and later life, and pregnancies that have not benefitted from preconception risk identification and management (USPHS, 1998). The main goal of counseling is to make sure family planning is a part of primary care for all sexually active patients.

 b. Topics to include in counseling.

  (1) Family planning that is culturally and ethnically specific.

  (2) Family planning topics specific to men's needs.

  (3) Varying forms of contraception and important characteristics of each.

  (4) Ability of different contraceptive methods to protect against STDs and HIV infection. Stress that even if the patient uses another form of birth control, condoms must be used if he or she is not involved in a mutually monogamous relationship with a person know to be infection-free.

  (5) Specific, in-depth information about the contraception method chosen including how it works, theoretical vs. actual effectiveness, advantages, disadvantages, how to use the method, side effects, warning signs, and backup methods.

  (6) Importance of early followup to evaluate the use of the method and to deal with any difficulties, misinformation and/or impediments to proper use.

9. Osteoporosis.

 a. *Scope of the problem*: Osteoporosis is the most common bone disease in humans (National Osteoporosis Foundation [NOF], 2003), and one-half of all post-menopausal women will have an osteoporosis-related fracture during their lives. Although osteoporosis is well-recognized and more common in women than in men, osteoporosis does affect men. One in five men over the age of 50 will experience an osteoporotic fracture, and hip fractures in men result in almost twice the mortality at one year post fracture as they do in women (Bord-Hoffman & Donius, 2005). Osteoporosis is largely preventable and prevention is important because while there are treatments for osteoporosis, there is no cure.

  b. Topics to include in counseling.

    (1) Daily recommended amounts of calcium and Vitamin D, including foods rich in these nutrients.

    (2) Impact of smoking and excessive amounts of alcohol on bone health.

    (3) Importance of regular weight bearing exercise.

    (4) Benefits and risks of hormone replacement therapy in menopausal women.

    (5) Home safety for the prevention of falls.

    (6) Medications prescribed for the prevention/treatment of osteoporosis, as indicated.

References

Agency for Healthcare Research and Quality (AHRQ). (2001). *Preventive oral care in primary pediatric care can help reduce disparities in children's oral health.* Retrieved December 23, 2005, from http://www.ahrq.gov/research/feb01/201RS22.htm

Agency for Healthcare Research and Quality (AHRQ). (2005). *Helping smokers quit: A guide for nurses.* Retrieved December 12, 2005, from http://www.ahrq.gov/about/nurisng/hlpsmksqt.htm

Alabama Coalition Against Domestic Violence (ACADV). (n.d). *Dating violence.* Retrieved December 29, 2005, from http://www.acadv.org/dating.html#safety

American Academy of Ambulatory Care Nursing (AAACN). (2004). *Ambulatory care nursing administration and practice standards* (6th ed.). Pitman, NJ: Author.

American Cancer Society (ACS). (2005). *What are the key statistics about oral cavity and oropharyngeal cancer?* Retrieved December 29, 2005, from http://www.cancer.org

American Hospital Association (AHA). (1998). *Management advisory: A patient's Bill of Rights.* Retrieved February 16, 2006, from www.injuredworker.org/Library/Patient_Bill_of_Rights.htm

Bastable, S.B. (2003). *Nurse as educator.* Boston: Jones and Bartlett.

Bord-Hoffman, M.A., & Donius, M. (2005). Loss in height: When is it a problem? *AAACN Viewpoint, 27*(5), 1, 14-15.

Centers for Disease Control and Prevention (CDC). (2003). *National center for injury prevention and control (NCIPC): Leading cause of deaths, United States.* Retrieved May 19, 2006, from http://www.cdc.gov./ncipc/wisquars/default.htm

Centers for Disease Control and Prevention (CDC). (2004). *National center for injury prevention and control (NCIPC): Youth violence: Overview.* Retrieved December 29, 2005, from http://www.cdc.gov/ncipc/factsheets/yvoverview.htm

Centers for Disease Control and Prevention (CDC). (2005a). *Healthy youth!: Alcohol and drug use.* Retrieved December 20, 2005, from http://www.cdc.gov/HealthyYouth/alcoholdrug/index.htm

Centers for Disease Control and Prevention (CDC). (2005b). *Healthy youth!: Sexual behaviors.* Retrieved December 28, 2005, from http://www.cdc.gov/HealthYouth/sexualbehaviors/index.htm

Centers for Disease Control and Prevention (CDC). (2005c). *Overweight and obesity: Home.* Retrieved December 29, 2005, from http://www.cdc.gov/nccdphp/dnpa/obesity/index.htm

Centers for Disease Control and Prevention (CDC). (2005d). *Trends in reportable sexually transmitted diseases in the United States, 2004.* Retrieved December 12, 2005, from http://www.cdc.gov/std/stats/trends2004.htm

Centers for Disease Control and Prevention (CDC). (2005e). *Unintended and teen pregnancy prevention: Home.* Retrieved December 20, 2005, from http://www.cdc.gov/reproductive health/UnintendedPregnancy/

Henshaw, S.K. (1998). Unintended pregnancy in the United States. *Family Planning Perspectives, 30*(1), 24- 29, 46.

Joint Commission on Accreditation of Healthcare Organizations (JCAHO). (2005). *Comprehensive accreditation manual for hospitals.* Oakbrook Terrace, IL: Author.

Klein, J.D., & the American Academy of Pediatrics Committee on Adolescence. (2005). Adolescent pregnancy: Current trends and issues. *Pediatrics, 116*(1), 281-286.

Lieb, S. (1991). *Principles of adult learning.* Retrieved February 13, 2006, from http://honolulu.hawaii.edu/intranet/committees/FacDevCom/guidebk/teachtip/adults-2.htm

National Osteoporosis Foundation (NOF). (2003). *NOF physician's guide: Impact and overview.* Retrieved December 20, 2005, from http://www.nof.org/physguide/impact and overview.htm

U.S. Department of Agriculture and Department of Health and Human Services (DHHS). (2005). *Nutrition and your health: Dietary guidelines for Americans.* Retrieved December 21, 2005, from http://www.health.gov/dietaryguidelines/dga2005/report/HTML?A_Exec.summary.htm

U.S. Department of Health and Human Services (DHHS). (1996). *Physical activity and health: a report of the Surgeon General.* Atlanta, GA: Author.

U.S. Department of Health and Human Services (DHHS). (2004). *Health consequences of smoking. A report of the Surgeon General.* Retrieved December 29, 2005, from http://www.cdc.gov/tobacco/sgr/sgr_2004/pdf/executivesummary.pdf

U.S. Public Health Services (USPHS). (1998). *Putting prevention into practice: Clinician's handbook of preventative services* (2nd ed.). McLean, VA: International Medical Publishers.

Patient Education and Counseling

This test may be copied for use by others.

COMPLETE THE FOLLOWING:

Name: _____

Address: _____

City: _____ State: _____ Zip: _____

Preferred telephone: (Home)_____ (Work)_____

E-mail_____

AAACN Member Expiration Date: _____

Registration fee: AAACN Member: $12.00
                   Nonmember: $20.00

Answer Form:

1. If you applied what you have learned from this activity into your practice, what would be different?

_____

_____

_____

Evaluation	Strongly disagree				Strongly agree
2. By completing this activity, I was able to meet the following objectives:					
a. Describe factors that influence the educational process in ambulatory care.	1	2	3	4	5
b. List the goals of education in ambulatory care.	1	2	3	4	5
c. Describe teaching strategies used for patient education and counseling in abmulatory care.	1	2	3	4	5
d. Discuss major health topics that are included in patient counseling to promote health behaviors in ambulatory care settings.	1	2	3	4	5
3. The content was current and relevant.	1	2	3	4	5
4. The objectives could be achieved using the content provided.	1	2	3	4	5
5. This was an effective method to learn this content.	1	2	3	4	5
6. I am more confident in my abilities since completing this material.	1	2	3	4	5

7. The material was (check one) ___new ___review for me.
8. Time required to read this chapter: _____minutes

I verify that I have completed this activity: _____
                                                    Signature

Comments: _____

_____

_____

Objectives

This educational activity is designed for nurses and other health care professionals who practice in ambulatory care. For those wishing to obtain CE credit, an evaluation follows. After studying the information presented in this offering, you will be able to:

1. Describe factors that influence the educational process in ambulatory care.
2. List the goals of education in ambulatory care.
3. Describe teaching strategies used for patient education and counseling in ambulatory care.
4. Discuss major health topics that are included in patient counseling to promote health behaviors in ambulatory care settings.

Posttest Instructions

1. To receive continuing education credit for individual study after reading the article, complete the answer/evaluation form to the left.

2. Detach and send the answer/evaluation form along with a check or money order payable to the *American Academy of Ambulatory Care Nursing* (AAACN), East Holly Avenue Box 56, Pitman, NJ 08071–0056.

3. Test returns must be postmarked by August 1, 2011. Upon completion of the answer/evaluation form, a certificate for **1.3** contact hour(s) will be awarded and sent to you. Should the material contained in this chapter become outdated prior to the above expiration date, AAACN reserves the right to withdraw this CE test.

This activity is co-provided by the *American Academy of Ambulatory Care Nursing* (AAACN) and Anthony J. Jannetti, Inc. (AJJ). AJJ is accredited as a provider of continuing nursing education by the American Nurses' Credentialing Center's Commission on Accreditation (ANCC-COA). AAACN is a provider approved by the California Board of Registered Nurses, provider number CEP 05336.

This article was reviewed and formatted for contact hour credit by Sally S. Russell, MN, CMSRN, AAACN Education Director; and Candia Baker Laughlin MS, RN, C, Editor.

■ ■ ■

Chapter 20

Care of the Well Patient:
Screening and Preventive Care

Carol Jo Wilson, PhD, RN, CS, FNP

Gail De Luca, MS, RN, CS, FNP

Objectives

Study of the information presented in this chapter will enable the learner to:
1. Describe primary, secondary, and tertiary prevention.
2. Identify clinical guidelines for routine health screening.
3. Identify resources for healthy diet and exercise guidelines.
4. Identify resources for immunization education.
5. Describe methods of contraception, sexually transmitted disease (STD) prevention and treatment, and abnormal pap guidelines.

Key Points

1. Health care in the 21st century will be focused on prevention and health promotion within communities and home care.
2. Primary prevention includes health promotion and specific measures to keep people free from disease and injury.
3. Secondary prevention consists of early detection, diagnosis, and treatment.
4. Tertiary prevention includes recovery and rehabilitation, and specific measures to minimize disability and increase functioning.

Health care in the U.S. is undergoing revolutionary changes at an increasingly accelerated pace. In the 19th century, health care focused on illnesses caused by unsanitary conditions and epidemics. As our agrarian culture became industrialized in the 20th century, the populace looked to employers and then to the government to provide basic necessities, such as health care. Following World War II, acute illness care moved from the home into the hospital. The 1960s saw the federal government addressing inequities in health care with the implementation of Medicare and Medicaid. Today, our country is still struggling with many of the same societal ills, such as poverty, lack of education, and class differences that have historically plagued the world.

Health care in the 21st century will be focused on prevention and health promotion within communities and home care. Indeed, the comprehensive plan for U.S. health care, *Healthy People 2010*, is aimed at increasing life span and access to preventive services while decreasing disparities in health (U.S. Department of Health and Human Services [DHHS], 2000). This chapter will present care of the well client and address current issues regarding primary, secondary, and tertiary prevention; child, adolescent, and adult screening; immunizations; prevention of pregnancy and STDs; and protocols for the abnormal pap.

Wellness, Health Promotion, and Disease Prevention

A. Consumers are increasingly knowledgeable and interested in health promotion. The relationship between stress and illness, the importance of wellness care (rather than disease-focused care), and the need to treat the whole person are increasingly recognized as essential elements in society today.
B. The family unit teaches health/illness beliefs, values, and behaviors, and serves as the focal point for the individual, client, system, or component of society. It is known that family functioning affects an individual's health while an individual's lifestyle, practices, and health affect the family. Nurses in ambulatory care settings can influence the family's

quality of life with health promotion.
C. Life-lengthening habits include:
1. Abstaining from tobacco use.
2. Limited or no alcohol.
3. Seven to eight hours of sleep nightly.
4. Regular, frequent, nutritionally dense small meals.
5. Daily breakfast.
6. Maintaining a normal weight.

Primary, Secondary, and Tertiary Prevention

A. Primary prevention includes health promotion and specific measures to keep people free from disease and injury.
B. Secondary prevention consists of early detection, diagnosis, and treatment.
C. Tertiary prevention includes recovery and rehabilitation, and specific measures to minimize disability and increase functioning.
D. The following example of smoking and lung cancer illustrates the three forms of prevention. Primary prevention would be patient education about not using tobacco products; secondary prevention would be patient education about signs and symptoms of lung cancer, smoking cessation information, and using cessation products/methods resulting in early diagnosis of lung cancer; and tertiary prevention would be smoking cessation and pulmonary rehabilitation.

U.S. Preventive Services Task Force Recommendations

The Agency for Healthcare Research and Quality (AHRQ, 2005) publishes recommendations for screenings and clinical preventive services, as well as the strength of these recommendations as guided by research. The categories of recommendation strength are classified as A, B, C, D, or I, incorporating research strength, as well as evaluation of risk vs. benefit.
A. Category A strongly recommends the service or screening because beneficial health outcomes from screening is evident.
B. Category B recommends that the service or screening be provided and has fair evidence of improved health outcomes. In both categories A and B, benefit of the screening outweighs the risk incurred.

C. Category C also demonstrates fair evidence of benefit, but the risk involved in the screening vs. the benefit is increased. Therefore, recommendation for general screening is not justified. Some targeted patients, however, may benefit from the screening.
D. Category D finds that the service or screening is either ineffective or that the harm exceeds any benefits; therefore, it recommends against the routine screening of asymptomatic patients.
E. Finally, category I is inconclusive; that is, either the strength of the recommendation is poor or conflicting data exist, and making a decision of benefit to harm is undeterminable (AHRQ, 2005).

Adult Screening: Blood Pressure and Lipids

A. Overview of blood pressure and lipid screening.
1. Because poor control of blood pressure and dyslipidemia both have interrelated adverse effects on the cardiovascular system, screening and treatment of these conditions will be discussed together.
   a. Normal blood pressure in adults is defined as systolic measurements of less than 120 mmHg with diastolic measurements of less than 80 mmHg (National Heart, Lung and Blood Institute [NHLBI], 2003b).
   b. Currently in the U.S., of the 25% of adults with hypertension, only 25% of them are at or below this goal.
   c. As blood pressure increases, risk for cardiovascular, renal, and cerebral disease increases (Uphold & Graham, 2003).
   d. Benefits of lowering blood pressure include reductions of stroke incidence by up to 40%, and heart failure by greater than 50% (AHRQ, 2005).
   e. Lifestyle and genetic predisposition are risk factors for hypertension.
B. Lipid and blood pressure screening.
1. Hyperlipidemia or dyslipidemia refers to an elevation of any lipid in blood plasma. The association between hyperlipidemia, hypertension, and cardiovascular disease is well documented.
   a. Blood lipids can be fractionated into:

(1) Triglycerides.
(2) Total cholesterol (TC).
(3) High density lipoproteins (HDL).
(4) Low density lipoproteins (LDL).
(5) Very low density lipoproteins (VLDL).

b. HDLs are cardio-protective, and low levels are an independent cardiac risk factor.

c. The Framingham Heart Study has documented that patients are three times more likely to develop coronary artery disease when TC exceeds 259 mg/dl (Dunphy & Winland-Brown, 2001).

d. Control of TC, as well as a reduction in LDL, has led to significant reductions in cardiovascular disease.

e. Family history is a significant risk factor in both hypertension and dyslipidemia. Other risk groups include people who:
(1) Smoke.
(2) Are sedentary.
(3) Drink alcohol excessively.
(4) Are overweight.
(5) Have diabetes.

f. Diets rich in saturated fats play a role in the genesis of both disorders, with excess sodium intake key in hypertension.

g. Because the higher the number of cardiovascular risk factors, the greater the probability of future disease, normalizing risk indicators (such as hypertension and abnormal lipid profiles) contribute to the overall reduction of cardiovascular disease (Neiderhauser & Arnond, 2004).

C. Anatomy and physiology.
1. Stroke volume, heart rate, and peripheral vascular resistance all affect blood pressure.
2. The body's baroreceptors, chemoreceptors, fluid status, renin-angiotensin system, and vascular autoregulation are control mechanisms of arterial blood pressure.
3. Over time, there is a loss of control in these regulating mechanisms resulting in increased peripheral vascular resistance (Uphold & Graham, 2003).
4. Over time, the elevated peripheral vascular resistance of high blood pressure results in the loss of vascular elasticity and a remodel-

ing of the blood vessel.
5. The left ventricle hypertrophies as a compensatory mechanism.
6. The stiffening of the arterial walls occurs in all areas of the body, compromising blood flow and damaging the tissues over time. This effect can be seen especially in:
a. Heart (hypertensive cardiomyopathy, congestive heart failure).
b. Brain (stroke, vascular dementia).
c. Kidneys (chronic renal insufficiency to end-stage renal disease).
7. While much of dyslipidemia is lifestyle-induced, other factors can contribute to its origin. Known potential causes of dyslipidemia include:
a. Diabetes.
b. Alcohol abuse.
c. Hypothyroidism.
d. Chronic renal insufficiency.
e. Genetic factors.
f. Some medications.
8. In dyslipidemia, increased levels of LDL incorporate themselves into fatty plaque developments on the intima wall of the blood vessel causing atherosclerotic changes, stiffening of the arteries, and reducing blood flow to vital organs, similar to the vessel and organ damage of hypertension.

D. Nursing assessment/screening recommendations.
1. Blood pressure (AHRQ, 2005).
a. Recommendation strength – A.
b. Normotensive individuals – Every two years.
c. Individuals with systolic blood pressure greater than 120 – At more frequent intervals.
2. Lipid screening (AHRQ, 2005).
a. Recommendation strength – A.
b. Optimal screening interval – Every five years, beginning at age 20 years (Grundy et al., 2004).
c. Individuals whose lipid levels are elevated may be screened at closer intervals.
3. Nursing history.
a. Duration of hypertension and/or dyslipidemia.
b. Co-morbid conditions.

(1) Diabetes.
(2) Gout.
(3) Peripheral vascular disease.
(4) Renal disease.
(5) Sexual dysfunction.

c. Nutritional history.
(1) Intake of caffeine.
(2) Sodium.
(3) Alcohol.
(4) Fats.
(5) Fiber.

d. Family history.
(1) Hypertension.
(2) Cardiovascular disease.
(3) Dyslipidemia.
(4) Stroke.
(5) Diabetes.
(6) Kidney disease.

e. Lifestyle questions.
(1) Smoking, including amount and number of years.
(2) Alcohol consumption as number of drinks per week/month.
(3) Patterns of exercise.
(4) Weight gain.

f. Medication.
(1) Prescription.
(2) Over-the-counter.
(3) Herbal preparations.

g. Psychosocial.
(1) Stress from work or family.
(2) Coping mechanisms.

4. Physical assessment.
a. Height, weight, body mass index, waist circumference.
(1) Abdominal fat is correlated with increased risk of cardiovascular disease.
(2) Body mass index higher than 27 kg/m2 is associated with elevations in blood pressure.

b. Blood pressure measurement.
(1) Taken with the patient seated in a chair after resting for 5 minutes.
(2) Cuff bladder size encircling at least 80% of the arm to avoid false low or high readings.
(3) Patient arm at heart level.
(4) Verification of blood pressure in the opposite arm.
(5) Ambulatory blood pressure monitoring.
(a) Necessary for evaluation of 'white-coat' hypertension.
(b) Provides 24-hour information about blood pressure and variances.
(6) Self-measurement of blood pressure.

c. Heart.
(1) Rhythm, rate, and regularity.
(2) Abnormal sounds.
(a) Murmurs.
(b) Extra heart sounds (S3, S4).

d. Lungs: Auscultate for rales or wheezing.
e. Neurological.
f. Abdomen.
(1) Masses.
(2) Abnormal pulsations.

g. Peripheral vascular.
(1) Carotid, abdominal, or femoral bruits.
(2) Edema of the lower extremities.
(3) Temperature or color changes of the lower extremities.

5. Diagnostic studies.
a. Laboratory evaluation.
(1) Urinalysis.
(2) Blood glucose.
(3) Electrolytes.
(4) Lipid profile.
(5) Liver function tests if on lipid lowering medication.

b. Optional laboratory tests.
(1) Urine protein.
(2) Urine albumin/creatinine ratio.

E. Physiologic alterations.
1. Clinical manifestations.
a. Most patients are asymptomatic.
b. May have morning occipital headache with hypertension.
c. May have evidence of target organ damage.

2. Common therapeutic modalities.
a. Lifestyle modifications.
(1) Weight reduction.
(2) Regular aerobic physical activity 30 to 45 minutes most days of the week.

(3) Alcohol intake less than two drinks per day.

(4) Tobacco cessation.

b. Nutritional recommendations.

(1) Sodium restriction to less than 2.4 grams per day.

(2) DASH diet (Dietary Approaches to Stop Hypertension) (National Heart, Lung, and Blood Institute [NHLBI], 2003a).

(a) Seven to 8 servings of grains or grain products daily.

(b) Four to 5 servings of fruits and vegetables daily.

(c) Two to 3 servings of low fat dairy foods daily.

(d) Two or fewer servings of lean meats, poultry, or fish daily.

(e) Four to 5 servings per week of nuts, seeds, and legumes.

(3) Low fat, low cholesterol diet (NHLBI, 2001).

(a) Saturated fat less than 7% of calories.

(b) Cholesterol intake less than 200 mg/day.

(c) Soluble fiber (10 to 25 grams/day).

(d) Plant stanols/sterols (2grams/day).

Adult Screening: Cancer, Hearing, and Vision

A. Overview.

1. To enjoy a high level of wellness into advanced adult years, both health care providers and individuals should ideally strive to identify disease risk factors through family history and lifestyle habit assessment, and incorporate preventive measures into current health practices. While primary prevention (health promotion through advocacy of healthy lifestyles and disease prevention) can prevent or minimize some disease, it does not eliminate it. Secondary levels of prevention provide an opportunity for early diagnosis and treatment, and limiting disease burden is assisted by screenings and immunizations (Dunphy & Winland-Brown, 2001).

B. Physiology and epidemiology.

1. Certain cancers have a hereditary predisposition and increasing incidence with age. Consideration must be given to the age at which certain cancers become more prevalent, and screening should be tailored appropriately.

a. In the age group 25 to 64 years, malignant neoplasms rank first in the leading causes of death followed by heart disease.

b. In the age group older than 65 years, heart disease is the leading cause of death followed by malignant neoplasms (Uphold & Graham, 2003).

2. In the aging adult, both central acuity and peripheral vision may be diminished.

a. Presbyopia, or difficulty with near vision, occurs as early as 40 years old. As individuals age, more light is necessary to see due to poorer adaptation to darkness.

b. The incidence of cataracts, glaucoma, and macular degeneration increases.

c. Glaucoma affects more men (incidence of 7.2% at age 75) than women, and without treatment, it can gradually reduce peripheral visual fields.

d. Macular degeneration is a loss of central vision and is the most common cause of blindness. Women (up to 28%) are affected more than men (Jarvis, 2003).

3. Hearing loss commonly occurs in the aging population because of reduced sound wave transmission due to increasing stiffening of cilia motion in the ear canal or by gradual nerve degeneration in the inner ear. Individuals may begin to notice these changes in their 5th decade. Previous lifestyle or environmental factors, such as chronic exposure to noise pollution or previous ear infections, can also contribute to hearing loss in older adults (Jarvis, 2003).

C. Nursing assessment/monitoring.

1. Nursing history.

a. Cancer.

(1) Any past medical history of cancer.

(2) Any family history of cancer.

(3) Lifestyle risk assessment.

(a) Blood pressure.
(b) Lipids.
(c) Exercise.
(d) Diet.
(4) Current chronic conditions.
(5) Any unintended weight loss.
(6) Fever, fatigue.
(7) Pain.
(8) Skin changes.
(9) Changes in bowel or bladder function.
(10) Lesions that change or do not heal.
(11) Thickening or a lump in the breast.
(12) Indigestion or change in swallowing.
(13) Nagging cough or hoarseness (5 through 13 from the American Cancer Society [ACS], 2005).

b. Vision (Jarvis, 2003).
(1) Eye pain.
(2) Double vision.
(3) Redness, swelling, or watering.
(4) Vision difficulty.
  (a) Visual acuity, blurred vision.
  (b) Halos or blind spots.
  (c) Right blindness.
  (d) Unilateral or bilateral.
  (e) Gradual or sudden.
(5) Past history of:
  (a) Ocular problems.
  (b) Cataracts.
  (c) Glaucoma.
  (d) Macular degeneration.
  (e) Hypertension.
  (f) Diabetes.
  (g) Trauma to the eye.
(6) Use of corrective lenses or contacts.
(7) Last eye examination.

c. Hearing (Jarvis, 2003).
(1) Ear pain.
(2) Ringing.
(3) Past ear infections.
(4) Discharge.
(5) Hearing loss.
  (a) Onset.
  (b) Ask if it is worse with background noise.
(6) Environmental noise exposure.
(7) Vertigo.
(8) Last hearing examination.

2. Physical assessment (Jarvis, 2003).
a. Vision.
(1) Snellen chart or Snellen E chart.
  (a) Provides assessment of visual acuity.
  (b) Vision may be examined with corrective lenses or contacts.
  (c) Each eye is tested individually at a distance of 20 feet.
(2) Jaeger card.
  (a) Tests for near vision.
  (b) Each eye is tested individually at a distance of 14 inches.
  (c) Vision may be examined with corrective lenses or contacts.
(3) Amsler grid.
  (a) Tests for macular degeneration.
  (b) Vision may be examined with corrective lenses or contacts.
  (c) Each eye is tested individually.
  (d) While looking at the center dot, surrounding lines should appear straight.
  (e) Amsler Web site (http://www.diabetesnet.com/diabetes_co mplications/diabetes_eye_ams ler.php).

b. Hearing.
(1) Note if the individual is lip reading, asks to repeat, misunderstands questions, and/or turns a favored ear to hear.
(2) Whispered hearing test.
  (a) Have the person occlude one ear.
  (b) Whisper a two-syllable word standing 3 feet behind the person on the unoccluded side.
(3) Otoscopic examination for cerumen occlusion.

3. Screening recommendations. While not all U.S. Preventive Services Task Force (USP-STF) recommendations (AHRQ, 2005) merit a strong level-A recommendation, targeted screening may reduce morbidity and improve quality of life for some individuals.
a. Cancer (AHRQ, 2005).
(1) Bladder cancer.

(a) Increased incidence among smokers.

(b) USPSTF recommends against routine screening.

(c) Strength of recommendation: D.

(2) Breast cancer.

(a) USPSTF recommends mammography every 1 to 2 years for women 40 years old or greater.

(b) Strength of recommendation: B.

(3) Cervical cancer.

(a) USPSTF strongly recommends cervical cancer screening in women with a cervix who have been sexually active beginning 3 years after becoming sexually active or at age 21.

(b) Annual Pap smears are recommended until 2 or 3 consecutive smears are cytologically normal, then the interval may be lengthened to every 3 years.

(c) Strength of recommendation : A.

(d) Recommendation against routine Pap screening in women older than 65 years if previous Pap screens were normal and in women who have had a hysterectomy for benign disease.

(4) Colorectal cancer.

(a) USPSTF strongly recommends screening of both men and women over 50 years of age.

(b) Strength of recommendation: A.

(c) Screening options.

(i) Fecal occult blood testing annually.

(ii) Flexible sigmoidoscopy every 5 years.

(iii) Colonoscopy every 10 years.

(iv) Double contrast barium enema every 5 years.

(d) Screening earlier than 50 years may be reasonable in persons with greater risk.

(5) Lung cancer.

(a) USPSTF has insufficient evidence to recommend screening for asymptomatic persons for lung cancer.

(b) Strength of recommendation: I.

(6) Ovarian cancer.

(a) USPSTF recommends against routine screening.

(b) Strength of recommendation: D.

(c) No evidence exists that earlier diagnosis reduces mortality.

(7) Pancreatic cancer.

(a) USPSTF recommends against routine screening in asymptomatic adults.

(b) Strength of recommendation: D.

(8) Prostate cancer.

(a) USPSTF finds evidence insufficient to recommend for or against routine prostate specific antigen (PSA) or digital rectal examination.

(b) Strength of recommendation: I.

(c) Benefit-to-harm ratio is uncertain.

(d) If screening is desired, screening should target men 50 to 70 years of age with average risk or men 45 years with increased risk.

(e) Older men or those with a life expectancy of less than 10 years of age may not benefit from screening.

(9) Skin cancer.

(a) USPSTF finds evidence insufficient to recommend for or against routine counseling to prevent skin cancer.

(b) USPSTF finds evidence insufficient to recommend for or against routine skin cancer screening utilizing a total body skin examination.

(c) Strength of recommendation: I.

(10) Testicular cancer.

(a) USPSTF does not recommend routine screening in asymptomatic adolescent or adult

males.
(b) Strength of recommendation: D.
(c) No evidence exists to confirm that teaching testicular self exam improves health outcomes.
b. Hearing.
(1) Routine screening for asymptomatic adults is not recommended.
(2) Screening of older adults for hearing impairment is recommended by:
(a) Asking them about their hearing.
(b) Educating about hearing aid devices.
(c) Referrals as needed.
c. Vision.
(1) USPSTF finds evidence insufficient for or against screening for glaucoma in adults.
(2) Strength of recommendation: I.

Adult Body Measurement

A. Overview.
1. Body measurements yield some objective measures of nutritional status. Nutritional screening can be done quickly and easily by evaluating an individual's:
a. Height.
b. Weight.
c. Weight history.
d. Diet history.
e. Food preferences.
f. Identification of nutritional risk factors identifying patterns for under-nutrition or over-nutrition.
2. If nutritional risk is identified through screening, obtain a full nutritional assessment including:
a. History.
b. Physical exam including body measurements.
c. Examination for any clinical signs of adequate or altered nutrition.
d. Laboratory evaluation may be warranted (Jarvis, 2003).
3. Nutritional status reflects the balance between the intake of essential nutrients and the body's metabolic requirements for basic needs, plus activity and growth or healing.
4. Under-nutrition occurs when the nutrient intake does not meet these needs; thus, nutritional stores are exhausted over time.
5. Over-nutrition, a condition far more prevalent in the U.S., is an imbalance in nutrients where nutrient requirements are exceeded by an excess of food intake. Frequently, this excess consists of calories dense in fats, sugars, and sodium, but not dense in nutrients.
6. Obesity affects approximately one-third of the American population and is a growing epidemic.
7. Simply, obesity is body fat in excess of that needed for metabolic function.
8. Obesity affects:
a. Both genders.
b. All age groups (though incidence increases with age).
c. All socioeconomic statuses, though it has a disproportionate prevalence among certain ethnic groups.
9. Obesity is a chronic disorder with multifactorial etiologies and is a risk factor for other disorders including:
a. Degenerative joint disease.
b. Hypercholesterolemia.
c. Type 2 diabetes.
d. Hypertension.
e. Heart disease.
10. Measurements defining obesity include:
a. Body weight 120% of ideal or:
b. Body mass index (BMI) equal to or greater than 27 (Uphold & Graham, 2003).
c. Adipose deposition patterns.
11. Persons with greater than 100% excess body weight are considered morbidly obese.
12. Of the 10 leading causes of death, 5 are related to poor diet. Adequate nutrition is crucial to the maintenance of health and prevention of major chronic diseases. This is achieved by intake of the 5 basic food groups, as well as regular exercise.
13. Optimal health benefits occur from regular exercise most days per week completed in either 30 minutes of continuous activity or an accumulation of 30 minutes daily in divided

activity. Both aerobic weight-bearing exercises as well as strengthening resistance exercises contribute to cardiovascular health, maintenance of ideal body weight, and prevention of bone demineralization with resultant osteoporosis. Endurance for aerobic types of activities can be increased gradually over time and provide excellent benefits (Uphold & Graham, 2003).

14. The U.S. Department of Agriculture (USDA) Food Guide Pyramid (2005) provides a visual key to the proper dietary balance of the 5 food groups. Proper adaptation of the pyramid into eating habits necessitates understanding of portion or serving size. In order for patients to familiarize themselves with proper portion size, food measurement may be utilized until visual inspection of portion size can be estimated.

15. The USDA (2005) recommends minimum daily consumption of the following:
   a. Three or more ounce-equivalents of whole-grain products per day, with the rest of the recommended grains coming from enriched or whole-grain products.
   b. Two cups of fruit and 2 cups of vegetables.
   c. Three cups per day of fat-free or low-fat milk or milk products, especially for adolescents, and pregnant or post-menopausal women.

16. The following is generally recommended:
   a. Maintenance of ideal body weight (IBW).
   b. Accurate interpretation of food label content.
   c. Balanced dietary intake following the Food Guide Pyramid.
   d. Regular exercise to increase caloric demand, lessen bone demineralization, and prevent lean tissue loss.

17. General dietary guidelines include:
   a. Increasing nutrient-dense, low-calorie, high-fiber foods.
   b. Increasing water consumption to 8 glasses per day.
   c. Increasing sources of complex carbohydrates (without added sugar or fat).
   d. Slowly increasing fiber between 25 to 40 grams per day.
   e. Limiting sources of concentrated sugars.
   f. Limiting fat intake to less than 30% of the total calories.
   g. Limiting after-dinner snacking.

18. Refer to www.mypyramid.gov for individualized diet and exercise plans.

B. Nursing assessment/monitoring.
   1. Nursing history.
      a. Weight milestones, including weight in late childhood, high school and college graduation, marriage, and pre- and post-pregnancies.
      b. Diet history including 24-hour food recall.
      c. Past dieting history and results.
      d. Family history of obesity, diabetes, cardiovascular disease, and sudden death.
      e. Amount and type of physical activity weekly.
      f. Psychosocial history including stressors and coping mechanisms.
         (1) Identification of maladaptive behaviors contributing to over or under-nutrition.
            (a) Food as a coping mechanism.
            (b) Food as a reward.
         (2) Identification of environmental cues to eat.
      g. Sleep apnea and snoring.
      h. Medications, tobacco, and alcohol use.
   2. Physical assessment.
      a. Height and weight. Review the record for weight history over the past 6 months and past year, noting any patterns/trends.
      b. Ideal body weight is based on the 1983 Metropolitan Life Insurance Tables, 1983 (Health Check Systems, 1997).
      c. Percent ideal body weight = Current weight ÷ Ideal weight X 100.
         (1) Eighty percent to 90% of ideal body weight indicates mild malnutrition.
         (2) Greater than 120% ideal body weight is obesity.
      d. Percent usual body weight = Current weight ÷ Usual weight X 100. Significant weight loss is unintentional weight loss of more than 5% over 1 month, 7.5%

over 3 months, or more than 10% over 6 months (Jarvis, 2003).

e. Body mass index (BMI). BMI: Weight (kilograms) ÷ Height (meters)^2 or Weight (pounds) ÷ Height (inches)^2 X 703.
   (1) BMI less than 18.5 is underweight, 18.5 to 24.9 is normal weight, 25.0 to 29.9 is overweight, 30.0 to 39.9 is obesity, greater than 40 is extreme obesity (NHLBI, 1991).
   (2) BMI may overestimate body fat in people with muscular builds.
   (3) BMI may underestimate body fat in people who have diminished muscle mass or older persons.

f. Waist-hip ratio (WHR). WHR = Abdominal girth ÷ Hip circumference.
   (1) Values greater than 1.0 for men or 0.8 for women indicates upper body obesity.
   (2) Upper body obesity predicts future risk of diabetes, hypertension, heart disease, and stroke.

g. Waist circumference.

h. Relative weights.
   (1) Men: 106 pounds plus 6 pounds for each inch of height over 5 feet.
   (2) Women: 100 pounds plus 5 pounds for each inch of height over 5 feet.

i. Bioelectric impedance analysis measures both fat and lean body mass.

3. Diagnostic studies.
   a. Fasting lipid profile.
   b. Fasting glucose.
   c. Comprehensive metabolic profile.
   d. Thyroid studies.

C. Physiologic alterations.
1. Clinical manifestations.
   a. Fatigue.
   b. Decreased energy.
   c. Weakness.
   d. Joint pain.
   e. Depression.
   f. Weight gain.
2. Common therapeutic modalities.
   a. Nursing interventions.
      (1) Identification of at-risk individuals.
      (2) Obesity prevention counseling for non-obese family members.
      (3) Nutritional and weight trend screening.
      (4) Encouragement of lifestyle changes including physical activity.
      (5) Follow general dietary guidelines.
      (6) Create a partnership with the individual.
         (a) Mutually set achievable goals.
         (b) Help the individual modify problem behaviors.
      (7) Referral to appropriate support groups.

3. Continued care and rehabilitation.
   a. Emphasize that proper body composition results from daily strategies.
   b. Emphasize the pitfalls of perfectionism.

D. Pharmacologic interventions. In addition to the following interventions, behavioral change is paramount for permanent results.
1. Weight loss.
   a. Antidepressants (partial list).
      (1) Selective serotonin reuptake inhibitors (SSRI) (most common).
         (a) Sertraline (Zoloft®).
         (b) Paroxetine (Paxil®).
         (c) Fluoxetine (Prozac®).
         (d) Citalopram (Celexa®).
         (e) Escitalopram (Lexapro®).
      (2) Serotonin norepinephrine reuptake inhibitors (SNRI).
         (a) Venlafaxine (Effexor®).
         (b) Duloxetine (Cymbalta®).
      (3) Side effects (partial list) include nausea, nervousness, fatigue, and orgasmic dysfunction.
      (4) Contraindicated within 14 days of MAO inhibitor.
      (5) Bupropion (Wellbutrin®).
         (a) Atypical antidepressant.
         (b) May be used with SSRI or SNRI.
         (c) Side effects (partial list) include insomnia, dry mouth, headache, and seizures.
   b. Anti-obesity drugs.
      (1) Sibutramine (Meridia®).
         (a) Inhibits the uptake of norepinephrine, dopamaine, and serotonin.

  (b) May cause increase in heart rate and blood pressure (partial list).

  (c) Contraindicated in patients already on SSRI or MAO inhibitor within 14 days.

 c. Surgical interventions.

2. Weight gain.

 a. Antidepressants.

  (1) SSRI.

  (2) SNRI.

 b. Other medications, such as mirtazapine (Remeron®), are sometimes used because weight gain is a common side effect of these drugs.

Adult Immunization

A. Overview.

1. In contrast to childhood immunizations, which are required by law, immunization of adults is voluntary. Thus, to prevent the 50,000 to 70,000 deaths occurring every year from influenza, pneumococcal, and hepatitis B infection, health professionals should routinely review each adult's immunization status annually in the fall to reduce these communicable diseases. Consideration and review of other vaccines should occur; including tetanus, varicella, and hepatitis A for individuals at risk who could benefit from these vaccines (Dunphy & Winland-Brown, 2001). Many middle-aged and older adults have had actual diseases, such as varicella. With this understanding, the health care provider during routine history should inquire about both immunization status and past occurrence of actual disease.

B. Nursing assessment/monitoring.

1. Nursing history: Immunization. Refer to the Centers for Disease Control (2005b) for most recent guidelines and updates.

 a. Influenza: Date of last immunization.

  (1) Nineteen to 49 years old.

   (a) Annually for persons with medical or occupational indications.

   (b) Annually for household contacts of persons with indications.

  (2) Fifty years and older: Annually.

 b. Pneumococcal: Date of last immunization.

  (1) Recommended for those 19 to 64 years of age. One dose with 1 revaccination dose in 5 years for those at risk:

   (a) Persons with medical or occupational indications.

   (b) Household contacts of persons with indications.

   (c) Those aged 65 years and older.

   (d) Those who have a serious long-term health problem, such as heart disease, sickle cell disease, alcoholism, leaks of cerebrospinal fluid, lung disease (not including asthma), diabetes, or liver cirrhosis.

   (e) Those whose resistance to infection is lowered due to Hodgkin's disease, multiple myeloma, cancer treatment with X-rays or drugs, treatment with long-term steroids, bone marrow or organ transplant, kidney failure, HIV/AIDS, nephrotic syndrome, damaged spleen or no spleen, and lymphoma, leukemia, or other cancers.

   (f) Alaskan Natives or from certain Native American populations.

 c. Tetanus/diphtheria (Td): Date of last immunization – 1 booster dose every 10 years for ages 19 and older. (Editor's note: The Advisory Committee on Immunization Practices [ACIP] made a provisional recommendation in March 2006 for a single dose of Tetanus Toxoid, Reduced Diphtheria Toxoid, and Acellular Pertussis Vaccine [Tdap] for adults to replace a single dose of Td [see http://www.cdc.gov/nip/recs/provisional_recs/default.htm].)

 d. Hepatitis B (series of 3 doses: initial, 1 to 2 months later, 4 to 6 months after second dose).

  (1) Date of last immunization.

(2) Completion of the series.

(3) Any past blood titers drawn.

(4) Nineteen years and older: Indicated for persons with medical, behavioral, occupational, or other indications.

e. Hepatitis A: Series of 2 doses – One at initial and the second after 6 to 12 months.

(1) Date of last immunization.

(2) Completion of the series.

(3) Nineteen years and older: Indicated for persons with medical, behavioral, occupational, or other indications.

f. Measles, Mumps, Rubella (MMR).

(1) Any past history of these diseases.

(2) Date of last immunization if applicable.

(3) Any past blood titers drawn.

(4) Age 19 to 49 years: 1 to 2 doses if:

(a) Lacks documentation of vaccination.

(b) Has no prior history of disease.

(5) Age 50 or older: 1 dose if other risk factors are present.

(6) Contraindicated in pregnant women or women planning to become pregnant in the next 4 weeks.

(7) Contraindicated in long-term immunosuppressive therapy or people who are severely immunosuppressed.

g. Varicella.

(1) Any past history of disease.

(2) Date of last immunization if applicable.

(3) Any past blood titers drawn.

(4) Nineteen years and older: 2 doses – Initial and at 4 to 8 weeks, if:

(a) Lacks documentation of vaccination.

(b) Has no prior history of disease.

(5) Fifty years and older; 19 years and older: 2 doses – Initial and at 4 to 8 weeks, if some other risk factor is present.

(6) Contraindicated in pregnant women or women planning to become pregnant in the next 4 weeks, and in persons with severely depressed immune systems.

h. Meningococcal conjugate vaccine (MCV4).

(1) One dose for persons with medical or other indications.

(2) All college freshmen living in dorms (MCV4 or MPSV4, meningococcal polysaccharide vaccine).

2. Nursing interventions.

a. Monitor for any adverse reactions.

b. Report vaccine reactions.

Adult Aspirin Prophylaxis

A. Overview.

1. Aspirin therapy has been used for some time in persons with known coronary heart disease, but only recently has been approved for primary prevention of cardiovascular events. Cardiovascular disease, including stroke, coronary artery disease, and peripheral vascular disease, is a leading cause of morbidity and mortality in the U.S., claiming 194 lives per 100,000 people with an estimated cost in excess of 145 billion dollars annually (Hayden, Pignone, Phillips, & Mulrow, 2002). Based on the evidence review of Hayden et al. (2002), the USPSTF concluded that aspirin chemoprophylaxis decreases incidence rates of coronary heart disease in adults at risk and should be offered as the primary prevention of cardiovascular events. Because aspirin is known to increase risk of gastrointestinal bleed and hemorrhagic stroke, the benefit-to-risk ratio is too low to recommend to all adults.

B. Screening.

1. USPSTF strongly recommends that clinicians discuss both potential benefits and harms of aspirin chemoprophylaxis with adults who are at increased risk for coronary heart disease.

2. Strength of recommendation: A.

3. Persons to consider aspirin therapy.

a. Men over 40 years old.

b. Post-menopausal women.

c. Younger adults with risk factors for coronary heart disease.

(1) Diabetes.
(2) Hypertension.
(3) Smoking.
C. Nursing history.
   1. Ask about past medical history of:
      a. Heart disease.
      b. Stroke.
      c. Peripheral vascular disease.
      d. Dyslipidemia.
      e. Hypertension.
      f. Diabetes.
      g. Rectal bleeding.
      h. Gastric bleeding.
      i. Smoking history.
   2. Family history of heart disease, stroke, peripheral vascular disease, dyslipidemia, hypertension, and diabetes.
   3. Nutritional history.
      a. Intake of caffeine.
      b. Sodium.
      c. Alcohol.
      d. Fats.
      e. Fiber.
   4. Lifestyle questions.
      a. Smoking including amount and number of years.
      b. Alcohol consumption as number of drinks per week/month.
      c. Patterns of exercise.
      d. Weight gain.
   5. Medication.
      a. Prescription.
      b. Over-the-counter.
      c. Herbal preparations.
   6. Psychosocial.
      a. Stress from work or family.
      b. Coping mechanisms.
D. Physical assessment.
   1. Height, weight, BMI, waist circumference.
      a. Abdominal fat is correlated with increased risk of cardiovascular disease.
      b. BMI higher than 27 kg/m2 is associated with elevations in blood pressure.
   2. Blood pressure measurement: See "Blood pressure and lipid screening" in the Adult Screening section of this chapter.
   3. Heart.
      a. Rhythm, rate, and regularity.
      b. Abnormal sounds.

(1) Murmurs.
(2) Extra heart sounds (S3, S4).
   4. Lungs: Auscultate for rales or wheezing.
   5. Neurological exam.
   6. Abdomen.
      a. Masses, abnormal pulsations.
      b. Stool hemoccult for occult bleeding.
   7. Peripheral vascular: Carotid, abdominal, or femoral bruits.
E. Diagnostic studies.
   1. Stool hemoccult for gastrointestinal bleeding.
   2. Complete blood count may be indicated.
F. Physiologic alterations.
   1. Clinical manifestations.
      a. Most are asymptomatic.
      b. Some may complain of gastric upset.
   2. Common therapeutic modalities.
      a. Optimum chemoprevention dose of aspirin is unknown (USPSTF).
      b. Doses of 75 mg seem to be as effective as higher doses (USPSTF).
      c. Incidence of gastrointestinal bleeding is higher in older adults.
      d. Some clinicians may add a proton pump inhibitor to the medication regime for gastric protection.
G. Pharmacotherapeutics: Aspirin.
   1. Classification: Nonsteroidal anti-inflammatory drug (NSAID).
   2. Route of administration: Usually by mouth. Rectal suppositories are available.
   3. Adverse effects: Gastrointestinal bleed, ulcer, or perforation; angioedema; anaphylaxis; prolonged bleeding time; gastric upset; nausea; dyspepsia; abdominal pain (partial list).
   4. Contraindicated with MMR vaccine, varicella vaccine; and use with other NSAIDS. Causes gastrointestinal bleed (partial list).

Adult and Adolescent Screening: Pap Smears, Sexually Transmitted Diseases, Pregnancy Prevention

A. Overview.
   1. The scope of ambulatory women's health care offers opportunities to provide individualized, comprehensive nursing care to women of all ages from the onset of menses

through the completion of menopause. Many women see only their obstetrics and gynecology provider for health care during their childbearing years. However, women also need information about cancer warning signs, adult immunizations, Papanicolaou (Pap) smears, blood pressure, sexually transmitted disease (STD) prevention, and additional health promotion information (Rawlings, 2004). Professional nurses in women's health care provide many facets of nursing care, including patient assessment, education, counseling, prevention of diseases and complications, diagnosis, treatment, and evaluation of care.

B. Pap smears:
1. The goal of screening with the Pap smear is to detect cancerous or precancerous lesions, and to detect the earliest changes in the cervix where treatment modalities are less invasive.
2. Fifty million Pap smears are completed annually in the U.S. and have reduced death rates from cervical cancer to 5 in 10,000 women.
3. The Bethesda system (Dunphy & Winland-Brown, 2001) is used for the categorization of Pap smears for standardized reporting on individual specimens.
4. Human papilloma virus infection (HPV) is associated with cervical cancer. While many strains of HPV exist, subtypes HPV 16 or 18 are frequently present in diagnoses of cancer of the cervix.
5. Other risk factors for abnormal Pap include sexual activity prior to age 18, multiple sexual partners, a sex partner who has had multiple sex partners, other STD(s), smoking, and increasing age.

C. Sexually transmitted diseases (STDs).
1. STDs are very common, affecting 1 in 4 adults of all socioeconomic levels in the U.S.
2. Women of all age groups have more risk than men, and young women have a greater risk than older women.
3. Untreated, STDs may lead to pelvic inflammatory disease (PID) resulting in potential infertility and increased risk for ectopic pregnancy.
4. Encouraging communication about sexual history between sexual partners, counseling

for STDs including HIV, and providing assurance of the confidentiality of the patient's treatment and testing is critical to meet the patient's health care needs (Nelson, Hough, & Paskiewicz, 2001).

D. Pregnancy prevention.
1. It is estimated that 6 of every 10 pregnancies is unplanned.
2. For women to make informed choices about their reproductive care, they must be informed and understand each type of contraceptive; the safety, efficacy, and risk profile of each is also necessary.
3. Individual birth control choices are made based on many factors, including a person's health, religious beliefs, desire for children currently or in the future, current health, number of sexual partners, frequency of sexual activity, and the safety and efficacy of the contraceptive option.
4. The U.S. Food and Drug Administration (FDA) (2003) cites that abstinence is the most effective means to avoid unintended pregnancy and STDs.

E. Screening recommendations.
1. USPSTF (AHRQ, 2005) recommends Pap smears every 1 to 3 years beginning with the onset of sexual activity or age 21.
2. May discontinue at age 65 if previous smears have been normal.
3. Strength of recommendation : A.

F. Nursing assessment/monitoring.
1. Nursing history.
   a. Sexual and gynecological history.
      (1) Number of lifetime sexual partners.
      (2) Past history of STDs, abnormal Pap.
      (3) Any partner history of STDs, intravenous drug use.
      (4) Number of total pregnancies.
      (5) Number of abortions (spontaneous or elective).
      (6) Age at first intercourse.
      (7) Condom use and consistency of use.
      (8) Contraceptive methods.
      (9) Last Pap date and results.
      (10) Any history of abnormal Pap.
         (a) Number.

(b) Treatment.
(c) Followup.
(11) Abnormal vaginal discharge.
    (a) Amount.
    (b) Character.
    (c) Color, odor.
(12) Pelvic pain.
(13) Back pain.
(14) Genital lesions.
(15) Vaginal burning, itching.

b. Menstrual history.
  (1) First day of last normal menstrual period.
  (2) Cycle length.
  (3) Number of days of flow.
  (4) Character of flow.
  (5) Cramping/pelvic pain.

c. Lifestyle history.
  (1) Tobacco use.
  (2) Caffeine, alcohol, illicit drug use.

d. Pregnancy history: The entire sexual, gynecological, menstrual history, plus:
  (1) Fatigue.
  (2) Breast tenderness.
  (3) Change in menses.
    (a) Ask about implantational bleeding: Light bleeding with mild cramping that may appear 12 to 15 days after fertilization.
    (b) Ask about amenorrhea.
  (4) Results of any home pregnancy testing.
  (5) Urinary frequency (occurs at 6 to 8 weeks).
  (6) Nausea or morning sickness.
  (7) Headache.

2. Physical assessment.
  a. Vital signs.
  b. Height, weight, general appearance.
  c. Nutritional status, BMI.
  d. Thyroid enlargement.
  e. Heart.
    (1) Rhythm, rate.
    (2) Murmurs, extra sounds.
  f. Breast exam.
    (1) Abnormal skin changes.
    (2) Nipple discharge.
    (3) Lymph node enlargement.
  g. Abdomen.

    (1) Enlargement.
    (2) Tenderness.
  h. Gynecological exam.
    (1) Private setting.
    (2) Proper draping of the patient.
    (3) Patient education.
    (4) Tray set up for provider.

3. Diagnostic studies.
  a. Urine chorionic gonadotropin.
  b. Serum human chorionic gonadotropin.
  c. Gonorrhea/Chlamydia cultures.
  d. Potassium hydroxide and normal saline wet preps of vaginal secretions.
  e. Pap smear.
  f. HPV testing.
  g. HIV testing (based on risk assessment).
  h. Other testing (based on indications).
    (1) Culture of genital lesions.
    (2) Herpes simplex virus IGG, IGM.
    (3) Rapid plasma reagin (RPR) for syphilis testing.

G. Physiologic alterations.
1. Clinical manifestations: The patient may be asymptomatic or present with any of the following:
  a. STD and/or abnormal Pap.
    (1) Abnormal vaginal discharge.
    (2) Post coital bleeding or irregular vaginal bleeding.
    (3) Pelvic pain, back pain (may indicate extensive disease).
    (4) Weight loss (may indicate extensive disease).
  b. Pregnancy.
    (1) Fatigue.
    (2) Breast tenderness.
    (3) Change in menses.
      (a) Implantational bleeding.
      (b) Amenorrhea.
    (4) Results of any home pregnancy testing.
    (5) Urinary frequency (occurs at 6 to 8 weeks).
    (6) Nausea or morning sickness.
    (7) Headache.

2. Common therapeutic modalities.
  a. Medical interventions.
    (1) Gonorrhea, chlamydia, syphilis.
      (a) Culture or blood testing.
      (b) Antibiotic treatment.

(c) Education to complete full treatment spectrum.
(2) Genital herpes.
  (a) Genital culture or HSV IGG, IGM blood tests.
  (b) Antiviral therapy.
  (c) Possibly give at each outbreak or continuous suppressive therapy.
(3) HIV.
  (a) Laboratory studies.
  (b) Antiviral therapy.
  (c) Teach importance of adherence to therapy.
(4) Abnormal Pap.
  (a) May be referred for colposcopy.
  (b) Teach importance of follow up.

b. Nursing interventions: Education.
(1) Encourage regular health checks.
(2) Patient education (Nelson et al., 2001).
  (a) Communication with present and past sexual partner if indicated.
  (b) Pregnancy prevention.
    (i) Abstinence.
    (ii) Choice of contraceptive method.
  (c) Condoms for STI reduction.
  (d) Signs and symptoms of infection.
  (e) Signs and symptoms of pregnancy.
(3) Education about the need for evaluation, testing, and treatment of sexual partners.

c. Nursing interventions: Screening.
(1) Encourage sexually active asymptomatic persons for screening.
(2) Encourage partner screening.
(3) Reporting requirements.
  (a) Report according to individual state law.
  (b) Assure confidentiality.

d. Nursing interventions: Advocacy.
(1) Resources and referrals as needed.
(2) Social and community resources.
(3) Nurse as the informational resource.

Newborn Screening and Measurement

A. Screening tests.
1. Requirements vary by state.
2. All states require screening for:
  a. Phenylketonuria (PKU).
  b. Hypothyroidism.
3. Many also recommend screening for galactosemia and hemoglobinopathies.
4. Others, as indicated.
5. Vision testing consists of coordinated eye movements, tracking, and presence of red light reflex.
6. Hearing screening before discharge mandatory in about half the states.

B. Measurements: Measure and plot on age and sex appropriate standardized growth charts. Growth indicates nutritional status and overall health.
1. Length.
  a. Measure on flat surface with infant on back.
  b. Length generally increases by 50% by age 1 year.
2. Weight.
  a. Measure on infant scale. Adjust for any additional materials like a blanket.
  b. Initial weight loss of 10 %. Weight generally doubles by age 6 months, triples by age 1 year.
3. Head circumference.
  a. Measure broadest part across forehead and occiput.
  b. Average growth is 1 cm/month for first year.

Child and Adolescent Screening

A. Overview – See "Anatomy and Physiology," "Nursing History," "Physical Examination," "Diagnostic Studies," and "Physiologic Alterations" under the Adult Screening section of this chapter.
1. Hypertension is defined for children and adolescents as an average systolic and/or diastolic blood pressure that is over or equal to the 95th percentile for gender, age, and height on 3 or more separate occasions.
2. Approximately one million children in the U.S. have elevated lead levels in their blood (CDC, 2005a). Lead can cause anemia, hearing loss, kidney problems, physical and develop-

mental delays, seizures, and death.
3. Approximately 5% to 10% of children have vision problems.
   a. Three percent of children under the age of 6 have strabismus (misalignment of the visual axis) (Broderick, 1998).
   b. Strabismus is the most common cause of amblyopia. Ideally, both eyes move together in unison, focusing the retinal image on the macula.
   c. If the retinal image is distorted due to strabismus or other condition, such as cataracts or refractive differences between the eyes, over time the brain learns to suppress the poorer image leading to permanent visual impairment (amblyopia). The earlier this condition is treated, the more likely a full recovery will occur.
4. Hearing loss can result in speech delays and school performance issues. There currently is a movement to screen newborns before they leave the hospital to increase the early detection of hearing loss. Indicators for hearing loss include:
   a. Caregiver concern regarding hearing, speech, language, and/or developmental delay.
   b. Family history of childhood hearing loss.
   c. Syndromes associated with hearing loss.
   d. Postnatal infections and hyperbilirubinemia.
   e. In-utero infections.
   f. Neurodegenerative disorders.
   g. Head trauma.
   h. Recurrent otitis media.
B. Nursing assessment/screening recommendations.
   1. Blood pressure: Blood pressure screening is recommended for children ages 3 years and older at every health care encounter (Falkner & Daniels, 2004).
   2. Vision screening. Ocular history, vision assessment, external inspection, ocular motility assessment, pupil exam, and red reflex exam recommended at all well child visits from newborn to age 3. For ages 3 to 5, above plus-visual acuity measurement and ophthalmoscopy (AHRQ, 2005).

3. Hearing screening.
   a. All ages should be screened for hearing loss as needed, requested, mandated, or when conditions place them at risk for hearing disability.
   b. Infants not tested as newborns should be screened before 3 months of age.
   c. Preschoolers need to be screened for hearing impairment, especially for common middle ear disease at this age.
   d. School-aged children should be screened on first entry into school. Every year from kindergarten through the 3rd grade, in 7th grade, in 11th grade, upon entrance into special education, and upon grade repetition (American Speech-Language-Hearing Association [ASHA], 2005).
4. Lead screening. Specific lead screening guidelines are set by county health departments; however, the CDC (2005a) recommends screening all children between the ages of 1 to 2, and screening children between the ages of 36 to 72 months of age if never screened before. In addition, the following could warrant more frequent testing:
   a. Residence in a particular geographic area (usually defined by zip code).
   b. Membership in a high risk group.
   c. Positive answers to a personal risk questionnaire.

Childhood Immunizations

See CDC (2005c) for current immunization schedules.
A. Hepatitis B (HepB): First dose is given to all infants soon after birth. Second dose is given at least 4 weeks after the first dose; third dose is given at least 16 weeks after the first dose and at least 8 weeks after the second dose. The last dose should not be administered before age 24 weeks.
B. Diphtheria, tetanus, and acellular pertussis (DTaP): Doses at 2, 4, 6, and 15-18 months, and at 4 years of age. The adolescent preparation Tdap is recommended for adolescents aged 11 to 12 years who have completed the recommended childhood diphtheria and tetanus toxoids and acellular pertussis/diphtheria (DTP/DTaP)

vaccination series and have not received a tetanus and diphtheria toxoids (Td) booster dose. Adolescents aged 13 to 18 years who missed the age 11 to 12-year Td/Tdap booster dose should also receive a single dose of Tdap if they have completed the recommended childhood DTP/DTaP vaccination series.

C. Haemophilus influenzae type b (Hib) conjugate vaccine: Given at 2, 4, 6, and over 12 months of age.

D. Measles, Mumps, Rubella (MMR): Given at or after 12 months of age and between 4 to 6 years of age.

E. Varicella: Given at or after 12 months of age.

F. Pneumococcal conjugate: Given at 2, 4, 6, and after 12 months of age.

G. Meningococcal: All children ages 11 to 12 years, as well as unvaccinated adolescents at high school entry (15 years) and all college freshmen living in dorms (MCV4 or MPSV4, meningococcal polysaccharide vaccine).

H. Influenza.

1. Recommended annually to healthy children aged 6 to 59 months (new recommendation in 2006). Also given to children over 6 months of age with certain risk factors including asthma, sickle cell disease, cardiac disease, HIV, and diabetes.

2. Live, attenuated influenza vaccine (LAIV) is an intranasal alternative to the intramuscular trivalent inactivated influenza (TIV) vaccine for healthy people aged 5 to 49 years. Children under the age of 8 years receiving the vaccine for the first time should receive 2 doses separated by at least 4 weeks for TIV and 6 weeks for LAIV.

I. Hepatitis A: Recommended for children and adolescents in certain states and certain high-risk groups. Given in 2 doses separated by at least 6 months. (Editor's note: Proposed to be recommended for all children soon after this publication deadline. Please refer to the CDC web site http://www.cdc.gov/nip/default.htm).

J. Poliovirus, inactivated: 4 doses at 2, 4, 6 to 18 months, and at 4 to 6 years.

References

Agency for Healthcare Research and Quality (AHRQ). (2005). *The guide to clinical preventive services 2005: Recommendations of the U.S. Preventive Services Task Force.* Retrieved April 21, 2005, from http://www.ahrq.gov/clinic/pocketgd.pdf

American Cancer Society (ACS). (2005). *Cancer facts and figures 2005.* Atlanta, GA: Author.

American Speech-Language-Hearing Association (ASHA). (2005). *Hearing screening.* Retrieved November 11, 2005, from http://www.asha.org/public/hearing/testing

Broderick, P. (1998). *Pediatric vision screening for the family physician.* Retrieved November 11, 2005, from http://www.aafp.org/afp/980901ap/broderic.html

Centers for Disease Control (CDC). (2005a). *Lead guidelines.* Retrieved November 12, 2005, from http://www.cdc.gov/nceh/lead/guide/chapter 4.pdf

Centers for Disease Control (CDC). (2005b). *Adult immunization schedule.* Retrieved November 2, 2005, from http://www.cdc.gov/nip/recs/adult-schedule.htm#chgs

Centers for Disease Control (CDC). (2005c). *Recommended childhood and adolescent immunization schedule.* Retrieved November 12, 2005, from http://www.cdc.gov/nip/recs/

Dunphy, L.M., & Winland-Brown, J.E. (2001). *Primary care: The art and science of advanced practice nursing.* Philadelphia: Davis.

Falkner, B., & Daniels, S.R. (2004). Summary of the Fourth Report on the diagnosis, evaluation, and treatment of high blood pressure in children and adolescents. *Hypertension, 44,* 387-388.

Grundy, S.M., Cleeman, J.I., Merz, C.N., Brewer, H.B., Jr., Clark, L.T., Hunninghake, D.B., et al. (2004). Implications of recent clinical trials for the National Cholesterol Education Program Adult Treatment Panel III Guidelines. *Circulation, 110*(2), 227-239.

Hayden, M., Pignone, M., Phillips, C., & Mulrow, C. (2002). Aspirin for the primary prevention of cardiovascular events: A summary of the evidence for the U.S. Preventive Services Task Force. *Annals of Internal Medicine, 136*(2), 161-172.

Health Check Systems. (1997). *Height and weight charts.* Retrieved April 26, 2006, from http://www.healthchecksystems.com/heightweightchart.htm

Jarvis, C. (2003). *Physical examination and health assessment* (4th ed.). Philadelphia: W.B. Saunders.

National Heart, Lung, and Blood Institute (NHLBI). (1991). *Obesity education initiative.* Retrieved November 1, 2005, from http://www.nhlbi.nih.gov/health/public/heart/obesity/lose_wt/risk.htm

National Heart, Lung, and Blood Institute (NHLBI). (2001). *Third report of the national cholesterol education program expert panel on detection, evaluation, and treatment of high blood cholesterol in adults (Adult Treatment Panel III) executive summary.* Retrieved April 18, 2006, from http://www.nhlbi.nih.gov/guidelines/cholesterol/atp3xsum.pdf

National Heart, Lung, and Blood Institute (NHLBI). (2003a). *The DASH eating plan.* Retrieved October 31, 2005 from http://www.nhlbi.nih.gov/health/public/heart/hbp/dash/new_dash.pdf

National Heart, Lung, and Blood Institute (NHLBI). (2003b). *JNC 7 express. The seventh report of the joint national committee on prevention, detection, evaluation and treatment of high blood pressure.* Retrieved October 31, 2005 from http://www.nhlbi.nih.gov/guidelines/hypertension/express.pdf

Neiderhauser, V., & Arnold, M. (2004). Assess health risk status for intervention and risk reduction. *Nurse Practitioner, 29*(2), 35-42.

Nelson, S., Hough, M.B., & Paskiewicz, L.S. (2001). Women's health/gynecology. In J. Robinson (Ed.), *Core curriculum for ambulatory care nursing* (pp. 216-238). Philadelphia: W.B. Saunders.

Rawlins, S. (2004). Evolving standards in contraceptive wellness: The annual visit and personalized contraceptive care. An update on the periodic well-woman visit. *Women's Health Care, 3*(1), 7-14.

United States Department of Agriculture (USDA). (2005). *Dietary guidelines for Americans 2005*. Retrieved April 26, 2006, from http://www.mypyramid.gov

United States Department of Health and Human Services (DHHS). (2000). *Healthy people 2010: Understanding and improving health* (2nd ed.). Washington, DC: U.S. Government Printing Office.

United States Food and Drug Administration (FDA). (2003). *Birth control guide*. Retrieved November 4, 2005, from http://www.fda.gov/fdac/features/1997/babytabl.html

Uphold, C.R., & Graham, M.V. (2003). *Clinical guidelines in family practice* (3rd ed.). Gainesville, FL.: Barmarrae Books.

Additional Readings

Hill, N.H., & Sullivan, L.M. (2004). *Management guidelines for nurse practitioners working with children and adolescents* (2nd ed.). Philadelphia: F.A. Davis.

National Heart, Lung, and Blood Institute (NHLBI). (2000). *The practical guide: Identification, evaluation and treatment of overweight and obesity in adults*. Bethesda, MD: Author.

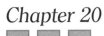
Care of the Well Patient: Screening and Preventive Care

This test may be copied for use by others.

COMPLETE THE FOLLOWING:

Name: _____

Address: _____

City: _____ State: _____ Zip: _____

Preferred telephone: (Home)_____ (Work)_____

E-mail_____

AAACN Member Expiration Date: _____

Registration fee: AAACN Member: $12.00
                    Nonmember: $20.00

Objectives

This educational activity is designed for nurses and other health care professionals who practice in ambulatory care. For those wishing to obtain CE credit, an evaluation follows. After studying the information presented in this offering, you will be able to:

1. Describe primary, secondary, and tertiary prevention.
2. Identify clinical guidelines for routine health screening.
3. Identify resources for healthy diet and exercise guidelines.
4. Identify resources for immunization education.
5. Describe methods of contraception, sexually transmitted disease (STD) prevention and treatment, and abnormal pap guidelines.

Answer Form:

1. If you applied what you have learned from this activity into your practice, what would be different?

_____

_____

_____

Evaluation	Strongly disagree			Strongly agree	
2. By completing this activity, I was able to meet the following objectives:					
a. Describe primary, secondary, and tertiary prevention.	1	2	3	4	5
b. Identify clinical guidelines for routine health screening.	1	2	3	4	5
c. Identify resources for healthy diet and exercise guidelines.	1	2	3	4	5
d. Identify resources for immunization education.					
e. Describe methods of contraception, sexually transmitted disease (STD) prevention and treatment, and abnormal pap guidelines.	1	2	3	4	5
3. The content was current and relevant.	1	2	3	4	5
4. The objectives could be achieved using the content provided.	1	2	3	4	5
5. This was an effective method to learn this content.	1	2	3	4	5
6. I am more confident in my abilities since completing this material.	1	2	3	4	5

7. The material was (check one) ___new ___review for me.
8. Time required to read this chapter: _____minutes

I verify that I have completed this activity: _____
                                                        Signature

Comments: _____

_____

_____

Posttest Instructions

1. To receive continuing education credit for individual study after reading the article, complete the answer/evaluation form to the left.

2. Detach and send the answer/evaluation form along with a check or money order payable to the *American Academy of Ambulatory Care Nursing (AAACN)*, East Holly Avenue Box 56, Pitman, NJ 08071–0056.

3. Test returns must be postmarked by August 1, 2011. Upon completion of the answer/evaluation form, a certificate for **1.3** contact hour(s) will be awarded and sent to you. Should the material contained in this chapter become outdated prior to the above expiration date, AAACN reserves the right to withdraw this CE test.

This activity is co-provided by the *American Academy of Ambulatory Care Nursing (AAACN)* and Anthony J. Jannetti, Inc. (AJJ). AJJ is accredited as a provider of continuing nursing education by the American Nurses' Credentialing Center's Commission on Accreditation (ANCC-COA). AAACN is a provider approved by the California Board of Registered Nurses, provider number CEP 05336.

This article was reviewed and formatted for contact hour credit by Sally S. Russell, MN, CMSRN, AAACN Education Director; and Candia Baker Laughlin MS, RN, C, Editor.

Chapter 21

Care of the Acutely Ill Patient

Lois J. Iiams, MSHCA, RN, HEM

Carolyn Pritchyk, MSN, RN, CNOR • Moderate Sedation

Patient Prototypes

Medical Emergencies
Loss of Consciousness • Cardiac Arrest • Respiratory Arrest • Seizure • Hypoglycemic Shock • Anaphylaxis
Moderate Sedation; Tuberculin Skin Test Conversion; Depression and Suicide
Children and Adolescents
Fever • Ear Pain • Upper Respiratory Infection • Nausea, Vomiting and Diarrhea
Adults
Headache • Back Pain • Sinusitis • Sexually Transmitted Diseases

Objectives

Study of the information presented in this chapter will enable the learner to:
1. Describe the assessment and care for life-threatening situations in ambulatory care.
2. Identify critical factors and care implications in the provision of ambulatory moderate sedation.
3. Identify the assessment and care for patients with acute illnesses commonly seen in ambulatory care settings.
4. Discuss patient and family education for acutely ill patients.

Key Points

1. It is important in ambulatory care to maintain one's knowledge base of emergency procedures through review of evidence-based guidelines.
2. Patients being sedated for outpatient procedures require special considerations related to education, safety measures, monitoring, and discharge care.
3. Patients with common acute illnesses may present at almost any ambulatory care setting or telehealth encounter, requiring timely and knowledgeable assessment and care.

Ambulatory health care has seen a paradigm shift in the last decade. Procedures once requiring hospital stays are now being performed in outpatient settings. The general population is aging as the "baby boomers" reach retirement age. Technology has aided our population to live longer and manage chronic disease better than ever before. A shift to outpatient status has also been fueled by rising health care costs to both patients and health care institutions. For the nurse in ambulatory care, not only providing care to patients but also managing employees, delegating nursing tasks within scope of practice, and triaging by telephone or other telehealth means require astute assessment skills and anticipation of the unexpected. It is important in ambulatory care to maintain one's knowledge base of emergency procedure through review of evidence-based guidelines. Written policies and protocols that are routinely updated according to facility guidelines will help the nurse remain current on developing technology and the nursing practice. Figure 21-1 provides a listing of Internet resources that offer updated guidelines and protocols for various procedures. Such measures will allow the nurse to implement condition-specific care in a timely and confident manner.

Medical Emergencies

Emergency conditions are an ever-present risk in ambulatory care. However, since they do not routinely occur, it is imperative that health care workers routinely practice emergency procedures to remain comfortable with processes and able to respond in a timely manner.

Figure 21-1.

Internet Resources

Asthma and Allergy Foundation of America – www.aafa.org
American College of Obstetricians and Gynecologists – www.acog.org
eMedicine – www.emedicine.com
Healthfinder – www.healthfinder.gov
National Mental Health Association – www.nmha.org
Centers for Disease Control – www.cdc.org
National Cancer Institute – www.cancernet.nci.nih.gov
National Domestic Violence Hotline – www.ndvh.org
National Institute for Allergy and Infectious Diseases – www.niaid.nih.gov
National Institutes of Health – www.nih.gov
National Osteoporosis Foundation – www.nof.gov
National Women's Health Information Center – www.4woman.gov
Office of Consumer Affairs, Food and Drug Administration – www.4woman.gov
Planned Parenthood – www.plannedparenthood.org
Smart Moms, Healthy Babies – www.smartmoms.org
Resolve, Inc (Impaired fertility) – www.resolve.org
La Leche League – www.lalecheleague.org
Special Supplemental Nutrition Program for Women, Infants, and Children (WIC) – www.usda.gov/fns/wic.html

Loss of Consciousness

Patient Population: Adult and Pediatric

Management of a patient who has lost consciousness requires careful and rapid assessment, both to determine the probable etiology and to provide supportive care. The most common causes for sustained loss of consciousness are uncontrolled diabetes (hyper or hypoglycemia), stroke, head injury, alcohol or drug overdose, bleeding, myocardial infarction (MI), or cardiac dysrhythmias. While head trauma and drug or alcohol overdoses are not usually experienced in the ambulatory care settings, other chronic illnesses are inherent to the primary and specialty care areas. Knowledge of the disease process and patient education may decrease the risk for loss of consciousness. Other conditions leading unconsciousness in ambulatory care include to vasovagal

response (such as fainting when receiving an injection) or dehydration (hypovolemia). Each situation requires a keen assessment by the nurse and timely action by protocol or in conjunction with a physician.

A. Assess/screen/triage.
  1. Assess airway, breathing, and circulation: Gently shake and call "Are you okay?" If unresponsive, call for help and activate the Emergency Management System (EMS), such as by calling 9-1-1.
     a. Assess airway: Head tilt, chin lift.
     b. Look, listen, and feel for respirations.
     c. If breathing is not present, refer to respiratory arrest guidelines later in this chapter.
     d. Assess vital signs.
     e. Initiate telemetry monitoring, if available.
     f. Assess blood glucose level.
     g. If possible, obtain history from accompanying family/friends.
        (1) Onset of symptoms.
        (2) Activity before onset of symptoms.
        (3) Recent complaints.
        (4) Recent injuries.
        (5) Medication and medical history.
        (6) Alcohol and/or recreational drug consumption.
  2. Nursing interventions.
     a. Notify provider immediately. In some settings or situations, it may be necessary to activate EMS, such as by calling 9-1-1.
     b. Protect the airway.
     c. Obtain IV access.
     d. Assess for bleeding or signs of trauma.
     e. Assess neurological function.
B. Primary/secondary/tertiary prevention.
  1. Decreasing risk for an unconscious episode due to diabetes:
     a. Perform regular blood glucose checks.
     b. Follow the prescribed diabetes diet plan.
     c. Follow prescribed medication regimen.
     d. Follow prescribed exercise plan.
     e. Abstain from smoking.
     f. Perform foot inspections daily for signs of open wounds or infection.
  2. Preventing hypoglycemic shock by good glycemic control (discussed later in this chapter).

3. Decreasing risk of stroke.
   a. Regularly check blood pressure readings, even if feeling well.
   b. Follow prescribed diet, such as a low-salt, low-fat diet.
   c. Follow prescribed medication regimen.
   d. Follow prescribed exercise plan.
   e. Abstaining from smoking.
4. Decreasing risk of seizure (discussed later in this chapter).

C. Clinical procedures:
1. Monitor blood pressure and heart rate at least every 15 minutes.
2. Obtain laboratory specimens per protocol or provider's order.
3. Obtain an electrocardiogram, as ordered.
4. Establish IV access.

D. Collaboration/resource identification and referral.
1. Convey assessment information to a provider.
2. Refer for tertiary care, as indicated.

E. Care management.
1. Support the family utilizing therapeutic communication skills.
2. Coordinate care with EMS and tertiary care.
3. Refer to social services or chaplain services, as indicated.

F. Patient education.
1. Client discharge teaching on chronic disease management, if applicable.
2. Client instruction on medication management, if applicable.

G. Telehealth practice.
1. Recognize emergency situations. Avoid delay in assessing and directing patients in emergencies. Procedure and protocols need to assure that office staff do not take messages but keep the patient with a potentially life-threatening emergency on the line until a nurse or other health professional can assess and determine the appropriate course of action.
2. Refer to EMS, such as calling 9-1-1.

H. Communication/documentation.
1. Time of onset.
2. Course of treatment.
3. Response to treatment including vital signs.
4. Report to EMS/tertiary health care workers.

I. Outcomes management.
1. Client regained consciousness.
2. Client safely transferred to tertiary care.
3. Family accepting of situation.
4. Coordination of care was accomplished.

J. Protocol development/usage.
1. Emergency care protocols should reflect latest evidence-based and expert agency guidelines (such as, the American Heart Association [AHA]).
2. Documentation tools.

Cardiac and Respiratory Arrest

Patient Population: Adult and Pediatric

In the U.S., approximately 400,000 deaths occur each year from sudden cardiac arrest. Without initiation of life-saving techniques, permanent cellular damage occurs within 4 to 6 minutes. Survival is less than 10% after 9 minutes. The AHA has developed the chain of survival in basic life support (BLS) training to increase survival rates from sudden cardiac arrest. The chain of survival consists of rapid EMS activation, initiation of cardiopulmonary resuscitation (CPR), early defibrillation, and fast access to advanced cardiac life support (ACLS) or pediatric advanced life support (PALS) protocols. The key to successful outcomes for sudden cardiac arrest due to ventricular tachycardia is timely defibrillation. In the ambulatory care setting, this step is most efficiently reached by use of the automated external defibrillator (AED). In the pediatric population, cardiac arrest is usually secondary to respiratory arrest, such as those caused by infectious processes (for example, croup), foreign body blockage of the airway, or drowning.

In November 2005, the AHA released recommendations for changes in BLS designed to simplify the guidelines, with more similarities across age groups (AHA, 2005). Other changes increase the number and improve the quality of chest compressions delivered, and decrease the interruptions in chest compressions. Priorities for health care providers are reflected in Table 21-1.

A. Definitions.
1. *Advanced cardiac life support (ACLS)* – Protocols and algorithms created through the AHA to provide guidelines for medical management of cardiac arrest and/or arrhythmia,

Table 21-1.

CPR Priorities for the Health Care Provider

> 1. **CALL FIRST** (activate the emergency response system) *except if* you are a lone rescuer with a victim of likely asphyxial cardiac arrest. Such victims will include all infants and children who do not have a sudden, witnessed collapse.
>
> 2. Use an **AED** as soon as it is available *except* if you are in the out-of-hospital setting with:
>   - An unresponsive child who did not have a sudden witnessed arrest. With such children you should perform 5 cycles (or 2 minutes) of CPR prior to using an AED.
>   - An adult with unwitnessed arrest (the adult is already unresponsive when you arrive) and you are an EMS responder with a call-to-arrival interval greater than 4 to 5 minutes. Then you may perform 5 cycles or about 2 minutes of CPR before using the AED.

Reproduced with permission. *Currents in Emergency Cardiovascular Care*, Volume 16, Number 4, Winter 2005-2006. © 2005, American Heart Association.

respiratory arrest and/or respiratory support, and stroke.

2. *Automated external defibrillator (AED)* – Device delivering electrical joules in response to shockable cardiac arrhythmias utilizing ACLS protocol.

3. *Basic life support (BLS)* – Process of providing circulation and respiration through artificial means (such as chest compressions and rescue breathing) in an organized, scientifically proven way in an effort to sustain life until advanced care can be provided.

4. *Pediatric advanced life support (PALS)* – Protocols and algorithms created through the AHA to provide guidelines for medical management of potentially fatal health conditions in the pediatric population, as well as to provide guidelines for medical management of cardiac arrest and/or arrhythmia, and respiratory arrest and/or respiratory support.

5. *Perfusion* – Tissues in the body exchanging metabolic waste (carbon dioxide) and receiving oxygen through arterial/venous circulation.

6. *Respiratory arrest* – Lung tissue is not able

to receive carbon dioxide or give oxygen to circulating blood.

7. *Ventilation* – Mechanism by which the blood gives off carbon dioxide and takes on oxygen in the lungs.

8. *Ventricular tachycardia* – Fatal heart arrhythmia with wide QRS complexes. Not necessarily resulting in pulselessness initially. The rapid rate of ventricular contraction inhibits adequate blood filling and decreased cardiac output.

9. *Ventricular fibrillation* – Fatal heart arrhythmia that results in pulselessness. The ventricles contract in an unorganized manner resembling a quiver and produce no cardiac output.

B. Assess/screen/triage.
1. Assess ABCDs of BLS (see Table 21-2).
   a. Gently shake and call "Are you OK?"
   b. If unresponsive, call for help and activate EMS according to facility's protocols (for example, call 9-1-1).
   c. Check airway: Use head tilt, chin lift to open airway.
   d. Breathing: Look, listen, and feel for respirations.
   e. If no respirations are present, reopen airway utilizing head tilt, chin lift.
   f. If no respirations, give two breaths utilizing BLS protocol.
   g. If unable to ventilate, check inside mouth for foreign object. Remove object if visible.
   h. If unable to visualize object, unblock airway utilizing BLS protocol for foreign body airway obstruction.
   i. Once airway is unblocked, begin supportive breathing.
   j. If no circulation, begin compressions utilizing BLS protocol.
2. When EMS providers arrive, direct them to the location of the emergency.
3. An AED should be available beside the patient within 3 to 4 minutes. Studies have shown increased survivability with fast intervention of cardiac arrhythmia with external defibrillation (AHA, 2005). Use of AEDs in the pediatric population requires adaptive pads to decrease the number of joules delivered.

Table 21-2.

Summary of BLS ABCD Maneuvers for Infants, Children, and Adults

Maneuver	Adult Lay rescuer: ≥ 8 years **HCP:** adolescent and older	Child Lay rescuers: 1 to 8 years **HCP:** 1 year to adolescent	Infant Under 1 year of age
Activate Emergency Response Number (lone rescuer)	Activate when victim found unresponsive. **HCP:** if asphyxial arrest likely, call after 5 cycles (2 minutes) of CPR	Activate after performing 5 cycles of CPR For sudden, witnessed collapse, activate after verifying that victim unresponsive	
Airway	Head tilt–chin lift (HCP: suspected trauma, use jaw thrust)		
Breaths: Initial	2 breaths at 1 second/breath	2 effective breaths at 1 second/breath	
HCP: Rescue breathing without chest compressions	10 to 12 breaths/min (approximately 1 breath every 5 to 6 seconds)	12 to 20 breaths/min (approximately 1 breath every 3 to 5 seconds)	
HCP: Rescue breaths for CPR with advanced airway	8 to 10 breaths/min (approximately 1 breath every 6 to 8 seconds)		
Foreign-body airway obstruction	Abdominal thrusts		Back slaps and chest thrusts
Circulation **HCP:** Pulse check (≤ 10 sec.)	Carotid (HCP can use femoral in child)		Brachial or femoral
Compression landmarks	Center of chest, between nipples		Just below nipple line
Compression method: Push hard and fast; Allow complete recoil	**2 Hands:** Heel of 1 hand, other hand on top	**2 Hands:** Heel of 1 hand with second on top; or **1 Hand:** Heel of 1 hand only	1 rescuer: 2 fingers **HCP,** 2 rescuers: 2 thumb–encircling hands
Compression depth	1½ to 2 inches	Approximately 1/3 to 1/2 the depth of the chest	
Compression rate	Approximately 100/min		
Compression-ventilation ratio	30:2 (1 or 2 rescuers)	30:2 (single rescuer) **HCP:** 15:2 (2 rescuers)	
Defibrillation			
AED	Use adult pads. Do not use child pads/child system. **HCP:** For out-of-hospital response may provide 5 cycles/2 minutes of CPR before shock if response > 4 to 5 minutes and arrest not witnessed.	**HCP:** Use AED as soon as available for sudden collapse and in-hospital. **All:** After 5 cycles of CPR (out-of-hospital). Use child pads/child system for child 1 to 8 years if available. If child pads/system not available, use adult AED and pads.	No recommendation for infants <1 year of age

Note: Newborn/Neonatal Information Not Included. Maneuvers used only by health care providers are indicated by "HCP."

Reproduced with permission. *Currents in Emergency Cardiovascular Care,* Volume 16, Number 4, Winter 2005-2006. ©2005, American Heart Association.

The user of the AED must be familiar with pediatric protocols and equipment before use.
   a. Turn AED on.
   b. Place external pads on upper right sub-clavicular region and left side mid-axillary region. Illustrations on the pads will aid in placement.
   c. Follow AED prompts. The nurse should be familiar with how to operate the model of AED in use.
   d. Announce "clear" loudly so no individual is touching the patient before delivering the shock.
   e. Follow AED prompts for discharging joules.
   5. In the ambulatory setting, sustained critical care is often not available in the same facility. Initiate EMS and transport to tertiary care.
C. Clinical procedures.
   1. All staff involved in direct patient care should be BLS certified. High-risk areas may have protocols for ACLS/PALS certification. Follow facility guidelines.
      a. Appropriate equipment is available to meet the requirements of the patient population (for example, bag- valve-mask, airways, etc.).
      b. One-way valve/masks should be available throughout the facility to provide mouth protection of the rescuer while waiting for AED and bag-valve-mask to arrive.
      c. Emergency carts or kits should be checked and ready at all times.
   2. Ensure AED equipment is available.
      a. Functioning equipment is critical to a successful outcome in cardiac arrest situations.
      b. Quality checks should be performed weekly to ensure battery is functional, and that pads are present and have not reached their expiration date.
   3. Cardiac arrest is not a frequent scenario in most ambulatory care areas, and periodic review of protocol and practice with peers is highly recommended.
D. Primary prevention.
   1. Teach parents about the importance of toddler-proofing the home.

   a. Small objects can become lodged in pediatric airways and cause respiratory arrest leading to death.
   b. Household cleaners and other poisons should be stored above child level.
   c. The poison control number should be posted near a telephone for easy access.
   2. Coronary risk factors should be controlled or eliminated, including smoking, hypertension, hyperlipidemia, diabetes, and a sedentary lifestyle.
   3. Patients and families should recognize early warning signs of cardiac or respiratory distress and seek immediate care.
E. Education.
   1. Once acute respiratory distress is resolved, educate the patient/parent regarding early signs and management of respiratory distress.
   2. Teach parents the signs of increased work of breathing in the pediatric population.
      a. Sternal notch sinking.
      b. Intercostal retractions.
      c. Audible wheezing.
   3. Teach clients how to best control active airway disease including:
      a. Use of metered dose inhalers.
      b. Medication management.
      c. Peak flow meters (see Chapter 17, *Application of the Nursing Process in Ambulatory Care*).
      d. Pursed-lip breathing.
      e. Postural drainage.
      f. Disease process and progression.
      g. Triggers for exacerbation of symptoms.
      h. Smoking cessation.
F. Care management.
   1. During the incident, crowds may gather, especially if it occurs in a public area. Assign a staff member to crowd control.
   2. Protect the patient's privacy as much as possible.
   3. Support for family/friends is essential. Utilize social services or chaplain services, if available.
   4. Provide assessment and treatment course information to EMS personnel as care is transferred.

5. Coordinate transfer to tertiary care.
G. Telehealth practice.
   1. Recognize emergency situations. Avoid delay in assessing and directing patients in emergencies. Procedure and protocols need to assure that office staff do not take messages but keep the patient with a potentially life-threatening emergency on the line.
   2. Refer to EMS, such as calling 9-1-1.
H. Communication/documentation.
   1. Careful documentation of event.
      a. Time of onset.
      b. Treatment course including tracings or memory disc from AED.
      c. Responses from treatment.
   2. Communication.
      a. Report of sequencing of events, assessment data and interventions to EMS personnel.
      b. Report of incident to receiving tertiary care unit, if possible.
      c. Use effective communication skills in conveying information to family.
      d. Coordinate with social services or chaplain services, as available.
I. Outcome management.
   1. Successful resuscitation efforts.
   2. Coordination of care to appropriate tertiary care setting.
   3. Family members' understanding of cardiac arrest incident.
J. Protocol development/usage.
   1. Facility specific code announcements and ACLS/BLS guidelines.
   2. Documentation tool.
   3. Post incident guidelines.

Seizure

Patient Population: Adult and Pediatric

A. Definitions
   1. *Absence seizure* – Type of seizure resulting in brief loss of consciousness, usually 10 seconds or less, with the absence of hypertonicity or muscular contracture. Presentation is predominantly in children.
   2. *Aura* – Subjective indication of oncoming seizure. Clients may describe a change in vision, taste, or smell pursuant to the onset of seizure activity.
   3. *Focal seizure* – Seizure activity initiating from one side of the brain. Presentation of seizure activity is seen on the opposite side of the body. The seizure may or may not generalize to include both sides of the body.
   4. *Epilepsy* – Diagnosis for congenital or acquired brain disease resulting in seizure activity.
   5. *Grand mal seizure (Tonic-clonic Seizure)* – Increased neuronal activity in the brain with presenting loss of consciousness, muscle rigidity, involuntary muscular twitching, and incontinence.
   6. *Post-ictal period* – Time after a seizure during which the patient may present with confusion and lethargy.
   7. *Seizure* – Increased neuronal activity in the brain caused by disease process or trauma leading to hypertonicity and muscular contracture.
   8. *Status epilepticus* – Increased neuronal activity in the brain resulting in seizure activity that continues for more than 10 minutes. Status Epilepticus is considered a medical emergency.
B. Assess/screen/triage.
   1. Active seizure activity.
      a. Ensure patient safety from injury.
         (1) If the patient is sitting or standing at onset, lay client on floor.
         (2) If the patient is lying on a bed, protect client from fall.
         (3) Protect airway by rolling onto side.
         (4) Protect the patient's head by cradling in lap or placing head on a pillow.
         (5) Loosen clothing.
         (6) Do not place a bite stick or other object in the patient's mouth.
      b. Objective assessment.
         (1) Time of onset.
         (2) Location(s) of initial muscle activity.
         (3) Progression of muscle activity, if any.
         (4) Monitor closely for patent airway.
         (5) Time of resolution.
      c. Nursing intervention.
         (1) Obtain suction equipment.

(2) Obtain IV access.

(3) Monitor heart rate and respirations.

(4) Monitor for subsequent seizure activity.

(5) Activate EMS, if appropriate, according to facility's protocol.

d. Determine history of seizure or recent head injury.

2. History of seizure without current seizure activity.

a. Type of seizure.

b. Sequence of events, if known.

c. Type of aura, if present.

d. Frequency and length of seizures, including time of last seizure.

e. Medications taken and consistency of use.

C. Clinical procedures.

1. Neurological assessment.

2. Blood tests, such as medication levels.

3. Lumbar puncture.

4. Electroencephalogram (EEG).

D. Primary/secondary/tertiary prevention.

1. Protect against head injury.

a. Wear head gear during contact sports or bike riding.

b. Wear seat belts while riding in automobiles.

2. Community resources and education.

a. Epilepsy Foundation of America (EFA).

b. National Institutes of Health (NIH).

E. Collaboration/resource identification and referral.

1. Neurology or neurosurgery consult.

2. Electrode implant.

F. Patient education.

1. Identify barriers to communication.

2. Use effective communication skills.

3. Discuss the disease process including stages of seizure activity (aura, unconsciousness, seizure activity, post-ictal phase, possible incontinence).

4. Identify learning needs related to seizure activity and safety measures.

a. If the patient experiences aura, lay down flat and make sure no objects are close by.

b. Instruct family/friends not to place anything in the patient's mouth and to pro-

tect the patient's head.

c. The patient should not drive a car.

d. Seizure disorder support groups.

e. Library and Internet information resources.

G. Care management.

1. Provide for patient privacy.

2. Discuss the episode and answer any questions.

H. Advocacy.

1. American Epilepsy Foundation (AEF) (www. aesnet.org).

2. National Society for Epilepsy (www.epilepsynse.org.uk).

3. Epilepsy Foundation (www.epilepsyfoundation. org).

I. Telehealth practice.

1. Information resource.

2. Triage/referrals.

3. Provide instruction for seizure management when necessary.

4. Support timely prescription renewals for anticonvulsants.

J. Communication/documentation.

1. Patient record.

2. Telephone advice documentation.

K. Outcome measurement.

1. The patient remains injury-free.

2. Seizure activity controlled.

3. Return demonstration and verbalization of safety measures to use during seizure activity.

4. Self-esteem intact.

L. Protocol development.

1. Emergent treatment guidelines or care maps.

2. Increase understanding of interventions and outcomes.

3. Decrease anxiety of the patient and family in home management of seizure disorder.

Acute Hypoglycemia and Hypoglycemic Shock

Patient Population: Adult and Pediatric

Hypoglycemia occurs when there is a significant decrease in circulating blood glucose. For diabetics, the most common cause is injection of insulin followed by inadequate intake of calories. Hypoglycemic shock is an emergent situation that requires fast response. Symptoms rapidly progress from confusion and lethargy to unconsciousness and possible death.

A. Assess/screen/triage.
  1. Blood glucose level.
  2. Vital signs.
  3. Level of consciousness.

B. Primary/secondary/tertiary prevention.
  1. Diabetic education and good glycemic control.
  2. Nutritional counseling.
  3. Insulin or oral hypoglycemic agent administration, as ordered.
  4. Jewelry identifying patient as a diabetic.
  5. Foot care.
  6. Medication management.
  7. Factors that affect blood glucose levels:
    a. Illness.
    b. Exercise.
    c. Fasting for procedures.

C. Clinical procedures.
  1. Blood glucose level measurement.
  2. Rapid glucose replacement.
    a. If responsive and able to eat, oral carbohydrates should be consumed, such as $1/2$ cup of fruit juice or skim milk, hard candies (3 to 5 pieces), glucose tablets, or a tablespoon of sugar, jelly, or honey.
    b. If unresponsive and/or unable to eat:
      (1) Obtain IV access and an order to administer dextrose, 50%. IV push.
      (2) If no IV access, obtain order and administer Glucagon 1 mg. IM or SQ.
    c. Recheck capillary blood glucose 15 minutes after glucose replacement.

D. Collaboration/resource identification and referral.
  1. Tertiary care if needed.
  2. Nutritional counseling.
  3. Group training classes.
  4. Podiatry.
  5. Community support groups.

E. Care management.
  1. Primary care provider for routine care.
  2. Nutritionists for ongoing meal planning.
  3. Telephone triage for health concerns.

F. Patient education.
  1. Self administration of insulin injection.
  2. Initial signs and symptoms of low blood glucose levels.
    a. Mild symptoms: Dizziness, irritability, hunger but no thirst, clumsiness, shakiness, diaphoresis, tachycardia.
    b. Moderate symptoms: Confusion, headache, poor coordination.
    c. Severe symptoms: Unconsciousness, seizures, coma.
  3. Treatment measures for self or family members to manage low blood glucose levels.
    a. Do not drive when blood sugar is low.
    b. Drink or eat some form of carbohydrate as soon as possible.
    c. If severe, call for EMS support, such as by calling 9-1-1.
  4. Self monitoring of capillary blood glucose.
  5. Self inspections of lower extremities.

G. Advocacy (See Chapter 22, *Care of the Chronically Ill Patient*)
  1. Family/community services.
  2. Library and Internet information resources.
    a. National Institute of Diabetes and Digestive and Kidney Disease (www.niddk.nih.gov).
    b. American Diabetes Association (www.diabetes.org).
  3. Specialty groups.

H. Telehealth practice.
  1. Information resource.
  2. Recognize emergent situations.
  3. Refer when necessary.

I. Communication/documentation.
  1. Patient record.
  2. Telephone advice documentation.

J. Outcome management.
  1. Hypoglycemic episode resolved.
  2. Patient free from injury.
  3. Patient verbalizes understanding of causes and prevention of hypoglycemia.

Anaphylactic Shock

Patient Population: Adult and Pediatric

Anaphylaxis is a rare but severe systemic allergic reaction. Roughly 30 out of 100,000 people will experience anaphylaxis in their lifetime. As the tissues of the body release histamine and other substances, the airways constrict. Blood vessels dilate, lowering blood pressure severely and causing lightheadedness. Fluid leaks from the bloodstream into the tissues, including the bronchioles, resulting pulmonary edema, lowering blood pressure, and if left unchecked, shock and cardiovascular collapse.

A. Definitions.
   1. *Anaphylactoid reaction* – An allergic reaction induced by drug infusion. Anaphylactoid reactions are not caused by immune globulins (IgE).
   2. *Anaphylaxis* – An allergic reaction caused by IgE that affects whole body systems. Can be fatal if not immediately treated.

B. Assess/screen/triage.
   1. Objective assessment.
      a. Airway, breathing and circulation.
      b. Lung sounds for air movement, wheezes.
      c. Skin rash.
      d. Swelling of eyes, lips, tongue.
      e. Blood pressure, including orthostatics, if possible.
      f. Pulse rate and quality.
      g. Pulse oximetry.
   2. Subjective assessment.
      a. Related symptoms, such as abdominal pain, vomiting, or diarrhea.
      b. Assess for insect bites.
      c. Assess for history of allergies. Allergies to food items such as nuts and fish have a high risk of anaphylactic-type reactions (Krause, 2005).

C. Primary/secondary/tertiary prevention.
   1. Patient education on allergy condition.
   2. Insect or allergen control measures in the home.
   3. Medication administration.

D. Clinical procedures.
   1. ABCDs of BLS, as indicated.
   2. Notify physician immediately. Symptoms not immediately life-threatening might progress rapidly unless treated promptly. Treatment recommendations are subject to physician discretion, and variations in sequence and performance rely on physician judgment.
   3. Nebulizer treatments.
   4. Oxygen administration.
   3. Intravenous access.
   4. Cardiac and blood pressure monitoring.
   5. Medication administration per protocol or provider's order.
      a. Aqueous epinephrine 1:1000 dilution (1 mg/mL), 0.2 to 0.5 mL (0.01 mg/kg in children, maximum 0.3-mg dosage) intramuscularly or subcutaneously every 5 minutes, as necessary, should be used to control symptoms and increase blood pressure.
      b. Other medications and fluids per provider order in response to assessed needs, such as bronchodialtors, Dopamine, corticosteroids, diphenhydramine, or ranitidine (Note: Diphenhydramine and other H1 antihistamines are considered secondary, and should never be administered alone in anaphylaxis) (Joint Council on Allergy, Asthma, and Immunology [JCAAI], 2005).

E. Collaboration/resource identification and referral.
   1. Allergist for screening and possible desensitization therapy.
   2. Refer to tertiary care, as indicated.

F. Patient education.
   1. Information on allergen and how to protect against exposure.
   2. Self injections with epinephrine (such as "Epipen") as indicated.
   3. Signs and symptoms that indicate an emergency situation.
   4. Family and patient aware of how to activate EMS and when to call.

G. Telehealth practice.
   1. Identify emergent situations and refer to EMS (9-1-1).
   2. Stay on the phone with the patient until EMS personnel arrive.

H. Communication/documentation.
   1. Patient record.
   2. EMS personnel, as indicated.
   3. Collaboration with allergist, as indicated.

I. Outcome measurement.
   1. Patient's airway is patent, and respirations are even and non-labored.
   2. Patient understands triggers that caused anaphylaxis.
   3. Patient recognizes and can verbalize symptoms of emergent disease process.
   4. Patient verbalizes and demonstrates correct technique for medication administration.

Moderate Sedation (Conscious Sedation)

Patient Population: Pediatric, Adult, Elderly
Carolyn Pritchyk, MSN, RN, CNOR

Moderate sedation is the use of medication resulting in amnesia and/or analgesia to sufficiently blunt but not remove a patient's protective reflexes to allow the performance of a procedure or test. The patient should exhibit a state of reduced consciousness that allows the patient to tolerate unpleasant procedures while retaining the ability to independently and continuously maintain cardiorespiratory function and appropriately respond to physical stimulation and/or verbal commands (American Society of Anesthesiologists [ASA], 1996).

A. Assess/screen/triage.
   1. The assessment and screening of ambulatory patients receiving moderate sedation is essential for a safe and uneventful experience.

Table 21-3.

American Society of Anesthesiology (ASA) Classification System

Classification	Description
ASA-1	Normal healthy patient
ASA-2	Patient with mild systemic disease (mild diabetes, controlled hypertension, anemia, chronic bronchitis)
ASA-3	Patient with severe systemic disease that limits activity but is not incapacitating (angina, obstructive pulmonary disease, prior myocardial infarction)
ASA-4	Patient with severe systemic disease that is a constant threat to life (heart failure, renal failure, acute myocardial infarction)
ASA-5	Moribund patient not expected to survive (ruptured aneurysm, head trauma with increasing ICP, shock caused by myocardial ischemia)
E	Emergency

Source: Somerson, Husted, & Sicilia, 1995.

   a. The Physical Status Classification of the ASA is a widely used screening tool (see Table 21-3).
   b. Accurate patient classification identifies patients with disease processes that may require hospitalization and management by anesthesiology. Typically, P3 and P4 patients are not candidates for ambulatory care nursing management.

2. The age range and developmental level of patient populations receiving moderate sedation must be considered.
   a. Adult and pediatric patients differ in:
      (1) Physical and psychological needs.
      (2) Type of medications and dosages.
      (3) Emergency resuscitation measures and equipment sizes.
      (4) Staff training requirements.
   b. Disabled and psychologically immature patients may require deep sedation or general anesthesia for safety and compliance.

3. Thorough medical record review and patient interview are essential and should include:
   a. Patient diagnosis.
   b. Medical history, including a review of previous use of alcohol and tobacco, and drug allergies.
   c. Last oral intake and a focused physical examination including cardiac, respiratory, and airway.
   d. History of sleep apnea.
   e. Prior surgical procedures: Previous uncomplicated procedures cannot be taken as a guarantee of a problem-free course.
   f. Specialty consultations to ascertain that other medical conditions are optimally treated.
   g. Use of prescription, over-the-counter (OTC) medications, or dietary supplements.
   h. History of prior anesthesia or moderate sedation.
      (1) Medications and dosages used.
      (2) Airway management used.
      (3) Drug reactions including latex products and anesthetic complications.

        i.   Determination of availability of post-procedure transportation. Assessment and monitoring intra-procedure includes oxygenation, ventilation, and circulation. Assessment immediately following the procedure and/or sedation includes level of consciousness, physiologic metrics, and pain level (Joint Commission on Accreditation of Healthcare Organizations [JCAHO], 2005b).

B.   Primary/secondary/tertiary prevention.
   1.   Primary prevention.
      a.   Early detection of potential complications can decrease the likelihood of adverse outcomes (ASA, 1996).
      b.   Continuous monitoring of the patient's physiological and psychological status is required.
      c.   Documentation of intra-operative monitoring at 5-minute intervals (may increase to 15-minute intervals as the patient progresses through the recovery process).
      d.   The most important monitor is the person designated to do the monitoring. The person assigned to monitor the patient should not be directly involved in the procedure.
   2.   Secondary prevention.
      a.   Appropriate training and competencies in operation of emergency equipment.
      b.   Knowledge of and immediate access to emergency resuscitative drugs.
   3.   Tertiary prevention – Immediate access to a higher level of care should the patient's condition warrant.

C.   Clinical procedures.
   1.   Sufficient number of qualified staff in addition to the person performing the procedure (JCAHO, 2005)
      a.   A registered nurse supervises periprocedural nursing care.
      b.   Individuals trained to manage patients in the event of any distress.
   2.   Prior to the procedure to ensure patient safety, the Universal Protocol is exercised: All documents and studies are available and have been reviewed, and the patient's expectations and team's understanding of the intended procedure are in concert (JCAHO, 2005b).

      a.   Verify the correct person, procedure, and site.
         (1) When the procedure is scheduled.
         (2) On entry into the facility.
         (3) At points in which care responsibility is transferred to another caregiver.
         (4) With the patient's involvement, if possible.
         (5) When the patient is transferred from the pre-procedure area to the procedure room.
         (6) Relevant documentation (such as consent, H & P), images, and implants or special equipment is available.
      b.   The operative site is marked.
         (1) Mark is unambiguous. No marks are used to indicate the non-operative site.
         (2) Mark is visible after the patient is positioned and draped.
         (3) Marking methodology is consistent throughout the institution.
         (4) Marking involved the patient, awake and aware.
         (5) Marking is performed in all cases involving laterality, multiple structures (for example, fingers), or multiple levels (for example, spine).
         (6) Marking is performed by the person performing the procedure.
      c.   A "time out" is performed immediately before starting the procedure.
         (1) Entire team in the procedure room use active communication and document on the patient record.
         (2) Team agrees to correct patient, correct side/site, correct procedure, correct position, and implants or special equipment are available.
   3.   Monitoring consists of vital signs, including heart rates and oxygenation using pulse oximetry, respiratory rate, and adequacy of ventilation, blood pressure checked at regular intervals, and cardiac monitoring in patients with cardiovascular disease or when dysrhythmias are anticipated (JCAHO, 2005).
   4.   Essential monitoring and support equipment and supplies.
      a.   Intravenous fluid and drug administration equipment and supplies, with capa-

bility of administering blood or blood products.
  b. Functional source of oxygen (and a back-up source).
  c. Positive-pressure ventilation (bag valve mask).
  d. Suction equipment and appropriate-sized suction catheters.
  e. Sufficient electrical outlets and clearly labeled emergency power supply.
  f. Adequate illumination with backup battery-powered equipment.
  g. Emergency cart with equipment appropriate for the patient's age and size (defibrillator, emergency drugs, airway equipment, and IV solutions and supplies).
  h. Equipment to monitor cardiac rate and rhythm, blood pressure, pulse rate, respiratory rate, oxygen saturation (pulse oximetry).
  i. Reliable means of two-way communication to summon help (Janikowski & Rockefeller, 1998).
D. Collaboration/resource identification and referral – Statements and standards for the provision of moderate sedation in the ambulatory setting.
  1. American Nurses' Association (ANA).
  2. Association of PeriOperative Registered Nurses (AORN).
  3. Association of PeriAnesthesia Nurses (ASPAN).
  4. Emergency Nurses Association (ENA) (Odom, 1997).
  5. Local standards per medical policy and procedure committees.
  6. American Society of Anesthesiology Guidelines on Sedation and Analgesia by Non-Anesthesiologists.
E. Care management.
  1. If any reversal agents are used, the patient must be observed for at least 2 hours post procedure to ensure that respiratory depression does not reoccur.
  2. Patients receiving moderate sedation should not drive or take public transportation within 24 hours after surgery or discharge from the facility.

3. Patient evaluation is ongoing until recovery and independence are achieved or chronic care is required.
F. Patient education.
  1. Verbal and written pre-procedure instructions.
    a. Dietary restrictions, NPO status, and preparation (such as bowl cleansing protocol).
    b. Skin care for operative site as indicated.
    c. Exercises required postoperatively.
    d. Medication instructions.
    e. Need for transportation following procedure.
  2. Verbal and written discharge instructions.
    a. Provide to patient and responsible adult caregiver/escort.
    b. Document in medical record.
  3. Discharge instructions.
    a. Self-care of operative site(s).
    b. Activity level and limitations.
    c. Symptoms to expect following procedure.
    d. Symptoms that need to be brought to the health care professional's attention.
    e. Signs and symptoms of infection or bleeding.
    f. Dietary restrictions.
    g. Medication instructions.
    h. Avoidance of operating motor vehicles, electric equipment, or heavy equipment as advised by the health care provider.
    i. Avoidance of alcohol consumption, tobacco, and making important decisions for 24 hours post-procedure.
    j. Followup care (time, place, and date).
    k. Phone number(s) for assistance in the event of post-procedure problems (Janikowski & Rockefeller, 1998; Odom, 1997).
G. Advocacy.
  1. JCAHO Standards for Moderate Sedation (2005b).
    a. Operative or other procedures and/or the administration of moderate or deep sedation or anesthesia are planned.
    b. Patients are monitored during the procedure and/or administration of moderate or deep sedation or anesthesia.

c. Patients are monitored immediately after the procedure and/or administration of moderate or deep sedation or anesthesia.

H. Telehealth practice.
   1. Pre-operative phone calls.
      a. Patient convenience.
      b. Provide and reinforce preoperative instructions.
      c. Obtain medical information.
   2. Post-operative phone calls.
      a. Evaluate progress and obtain medical information.
      b. Comfort level.
      c. Provide reassurance and positive reinforcement.

I. Communication/documentation.
   1. Terminology to describe the spectrum of consciousness.
      a. Alert and awake.
      b. Sedated and cooperative.
      c. Asleep and easily arousable.
      d. Asleep but slow to arouse to name.
      e. Arousable only to pain.
      f. Un-arousable (AORN, 1996; JCAHO, 2005b).
   2. Documentation of monitoring data on a time-based record.
      a. Cardiac rate and rhythm (continuous for patients with underlying cardiovascular disease because of increased risk for dysrhythmias).
      b. Blood pressure, pulse rate, respiratory rate (taken every 1 to 2 minutes during onset of sedation and every 5 to 10 minutes during the procedure).
      c. Oxygen delivery route (nasal cannula, face mask) and flow rate, oxygen saturation.
      d. Level of consciousness.
      e. Verbal response.
      f. Medication administered – Dosage, time, route, patient response, name of ordering physician or anesthesia provider.
      g. Type and amounts of IV fluids and blood components administered.
      h. Pre- and post-procedural temperatures on patients less than 16 years of age.
      i. Any interventions and the patient's response.
      j. Any significant events or untoward reactions and their resolution (AORN, 1996).
   3. Practical objective criteria, note time frames, ensure uniform, safe recovery, and discharge (Chung, 1995).
      a. The post-anesthetic recovery (PAR) score is an effective, reliable, and safe assessment and documentation tool but only addresses the early phases of recovery.
      b. The modified post-anesthetic recovery (PAR) score additionally determines street fitness and home readiness. Nine items are assessed:
         (1) Activity: Ability/inability to move extremities.
         (2) Respiration: Ability/inability to breathe and cough.
         (3) Circulation: Blood pressure readings within pre-anesthetic level.
         (4) Consciousness: Awake or arousable.
         (5) O_2 saturation: On room air or with oxygen supplement.
         (6) Pain: None, mild, or severe.
         (7) Ambulation: Dizziness/vertigo, able to walk.
         (8) Feeding: Nauseated/vomiting, able to drink.
         (9) Urine output: Voiding/unable to void (Janikowski & Rockefeller, 1998).
      c. The post-anesthesia discharge scoring system (PADSS) measures the discharge readiness of ambulatory surgical patients. Five items are assessed (see Table 21-4):
         (1) Vital signs.
         (2) Activity and mental status.
         (3) Pain.
         (4) Nausea and/or vomiting.
         (5) Surgical bleeding.
         (6) Intake and output.
      d. The modified post-anesthesia discharge scoring system (MPADSS) does not require voiding and drinking for discharge (Odom, 1997).
      e. The modified circulation Alderete score may be used for children 12 years of

Table 21-4.

Post-Anesthesia Discharge Scoring System

1. Vital Signs
   - 2 = within 20% of preoperative value
   - 1 = 20%-40% of preoperative value
   - 0 = 40% of preoperative value

2. Ambulation and mental status
   - 2 = oriented ˇ 3 and has a steady gait
   - 1 = oriented ˇ 3 or has a steady gait
   - 0 = neither

3. Pain or nausea/vomiting
   - 2 = minimal
   - 1 = moderate
   - 0 = severe

4. Surgical bleeding
   - 2 = minimal
   - 1 = moderate
   - 0 = severe

5. Intake and output
   - 2 = has had PO fluids and voided
   - 1 = has had PO fluids or voided
   - 0 = neither

Source: Chung, 1995.

age or less. A minimum Alderete score of 8 is generally required for discharge.

J. Outcome management.
   1. Disease-specific – Physiologic signs and symptoms (such as headaches, asthma attacks).
   2. General health – Functional or general well being (such as mobility, return to work/activities, productivity, self-image).
   3. Patient performance – Understanding and compliance with medical treatment plan (such as taking medications correctly, wound self-care).

K. Protocol development/usage.
   1. Moderate sedation training programs are standardized, competency-based, have established baseline educational requirements, and ensure comparable training throughout an institution. Key components of a moderate sedation education program include:
      a. Current basic cardiac life support certifi-
      cation (BCLS) and advanced cardiac life support certification (ACLS).
      b. Review of anatomy and physiology.
      c. Pre-procedural sedation assessment, ASA physical status classifications, and patient selection criteria.
      d. Moderate sedation vs. deep sedation, general anesthesia, and local anesthesia.
      e. Medications, dosages, administration rates, onset/duration/peak, adverse effects, contraindications, and reversal agents.
      f. Management and monitoring of patients before, during, and after moderate sedation.
      g. Management of emergency situations.
      h. Competency in operating and troubleshooting essential equipment.
      i. Patient education.
      j. Discharge criteria.
      k. Documentation and medico-legal issues.
      l. Pre- and post-testing, preceptorship to practice newly acquired skills, and regularly scheduled recertification (Janikowski & Rockefeller, 1998).
   2. Protocol for management of patients with latex sensitivity.
      a. Obtain thorough medical history: Food allergies, childhood or adult eczema, and asthma. Gender: 75% of latex-sensitive individuals are women.
         (1) Surgical history: Multiple surgeries, intra-operative events consistent with anaphylaxis, hypotension, reactions during dental or radiological procedures.
         (2) Occupational history: History of exposure, work-related symptoms, upper and lower respiratory symptoms.
         (3) Other symptoms: Itchy hands, localized angioedema, urticaria after touching poinsettia plants.
         (4) Pharmacy to prepare latex-free injectable medications when applicable.
      b. Provide latex-free environment (no direct patient contact with latex products).
         (1) List of safe alternative products.

(2) Set up a latex-free cart.

(3) Provide patient warning signs and alert bracelets (Williams, 1997).

Tuberculosis (TB) Skin Test Conversion

Patient Population: Adult and Pediatric

Tuberculosis infection is a communicable disease spreading from person to person by droplet nuclei. Once exposed, the bacteria, *Mycobacterium tuberculosis*, implants in lung tissue. Once implanted, the body is able to encapsulate the bacteria. The bacteria can then reside in the lungs for the lifetime of the individual and not develop into active TB. This condition is known as latent TB infection (LTBI). Once exposed, the screening tuberculin Purified Protein Derivative (PPD) test will become positive, although the individual is not infectious. Current focus within the U.S. is to find and treat LTBI with oral antibiotics. The first line of choice is Isoniazid (INH). The individual with LTBI is at risk for active TB disease if the body's immune defenses are no longer able to support shielding the bacterium from replication (Centers for Disease Control and Prevention [CDC], 2005). Health care workers must be knowledgeable and mindful of active TB disease and take appropriate steps to protect themselves and those around them from exposure.

A. Assess/screen/triage.

1. PPD screening (see Chapter 17, *Application of the Nursing Process in Ambulatory Care*, for PPD administration information).

   a. 5mm induration for immunocompromized clients.

   b. 10mm induration for people in high risk of exposure.

      (1) Health care workers.

      (2) Those with diabetes.

      (3) Those with chronic renal failure.

   c. 15mm induration for clients with no risk factors.

2. Assess for signs or symptoms of active TB disease.

   a. Hemoptysis.

   b. Fatigue.

   c. Weight loss.

d. Night sweats.

e. Chronic cough.

f. Fever.

3. If signs or symptoms of active disease exist, place client in respiratory isolation.

   a. Negative pressure room with door closed. If a negative pressure room is not available, place the patient in a single occupancy room and keep the door closed.

   b. All staff involved in direct patient care should don –95 or greater respirator.

   c. Place respiratory signage on door of client room.

   d. The patient should don a surgical mask when leaving the room.

4. If signs or symptoms of active disease do not exist, document history of exposure to TB.

B. Primary/secondary/tertiary prevention.

1. Primary prevention of active TB.

   a. Annual TB screening for health care workers and residents of long-term care facilities.

   b. Education regarding prevention of disease transmission.

   c. INH for 9 months for PPD conversions for patients without contraindications.

      (1) Education regarding signs of hepatotoxicity due to INH.

         (a) Anorexia.

         (b) Nausea.

         (c) Aches.

         (d) Upper abdominal pain.

         (e) Increased ALT levels (3 to 5 times higher than normal).

      (2) Risks of INH hepatotoxicity increased by:

         (a) Over 50 years of age – Increased risk.

         (b) Alcoholism or other active liver disease.

         (c) Postpartum 3 months post-delivery or less.

      (3) Risk of peripheral neuropathy due to INH increased by:

         (i) Individuals with diet deficient in B6.

         (ii) History of alcohol abuse.

(iii) History of diabetes.
(4) Possible fever or rash from INH.
2. Secondary prevention.
   a. Detection of active TB exposure.
   b. Completion of treatment course. Treatment is at risk due to extended treatment time frame. Education on importance of completion is imperative.
C. Clinical procedures.
  1. X-ray.
  2. Baseline labs.
  3. Screening PPDs for family members to rule out exposure source.
D. Care management.
  1. Health department.
  2. Infectious disease.
  3. Infection control services.
  4. Therapeutic communication.
E. Patient education.
  1. Process of tuberculosis infection and infection control measures.
  2. Medication management and length of treatment.
  3. Signs and symptoms of treatment complications (as stated in section B, "Primary/secondary/tertiary" above).
F. Advocacy.
  1. Centers for Disease Control and Prevention (www.cdc.gov).
  2. National Institutes of Health (www.nih.gov).
G. Telehealth practice.
  1. Recognition of signs and symptoms for active TB disease.
  2. Recognition of signs and symptoms for hepatotoxicity.
H. Communication/documentation.
  1. Patient record.
  2. Coordinate with the community health department reporting structure.
I. Outcome management.
  1. The patient understands disease process.
  2. The patient understands importance of completion of treatment.
  3. The patient is followed by health department to ensure completion of treatment.
  4. The patient is accepting of condition.

Depression and Suicide

Patient Population: Adult and Adolescent

A. Definitions.
  1. *Major depression* – Five or more symptoms of depression (see "Assess/screen/triage" section below).
  2. *Dysthymia* – Depression that is chronic in nature. Milder than major depression, lasting up to two years.
  3. *Atypical depression* – Depression that is accompanied by unusual symptoms, such as hallucinations or delusions.
  4. *Postpartum depression* – Feeling of sadness or "blue mood" after delivery. Usually induced by hormonal changes. True major depression after delivery is rare.
  5. *Premenstrual dysphoric disorder* – Feeling of depression with onset one week prior to menses. After onset of menstruation, symptoms resolve.
  6. *Seasonal affective disorder* – Feeling of depression that ensues during the autumn and winter months due to decreased length of sunlight.

One percent of all deaths that occur each year are due to suicide; 90% of those deaths are a result of a mood disorder or psychiatric illness (National Institutes of Health [NIH], 2000). For those attempting suicide but not succeeding, one-third will attempt again within 1 year; 10% of those will eventually succeed. Usually the attempt at suicide is staged for the possibility for rescue and is seen as a desperate cry for help. The health care provider needs to take the threat of suicide seriously and coordinate care to provide for the mental health services necessary to achieve emotional stability.

B. Assess/screen/triage.
  1. Common complaints of depression.
    a. Insomnia.
    b. Excessive sleeping.
    c. Change in appetite leading to weight gain or loss.
    d. Fatigue.
    e. Feelings of hopelessness, helplessness, worthlessness, self hate, and inappropriate guilt.
    f. Inability to concentrate.
    g. Withdrawal from social or usual activities.

h. Recurring thoughts of death or suicide.
i Lack of pleasure.
j. Low self-esteem.
k. Sudden bursts of anger.
2. Subjective assessment.
   a. Psychological review/history.
   b. Description of moods.
   c. Stressors.
   d. Thoughts of suicide or self-harm.
   e. If there are thoughts of suicide, is there a plan?
   f. Means to implement plan (such as poison, gun).
   g. Recreational drug or alcohol use.
   h. Medications.
C. Primary/secondary/tertiary prevention.
   1. Primary prevention.
      a. Always take threats of suicide seriously.
      b. Mental health evaluation is necessary.
      c. Utilize effective communication skills, especially empathetic listening. Many people who attempt suicide will talk about it first. Talking may be enough to prevent action.
      d. Sudden changes in behavior from anxiety to calmness in one who has history of suicide threat can be a sign that a decision to commit suicide has been made.
   2. Secondary prevention.
      a. Education on self care.
         (1) Get enough sleep.
         (2) Eat a healthy diet.
         (3) Exercise regularly.
         (4) Avoid alcohol or recreational drugs.
         (5) Participate in social events that bring joy.
         (6) Seek out faith-based and/or secular support.
   3. Tertiary prevention.
      a. Adding supplements to daily nutritional intake may be helpful.
         (1) Omega-3 fatty acids.
         (2) Folate (B9) in MVI: 400 to 800 micrograms.
         (3) The herbal supplement, St. John's Wort, has been shown to help some; however, this herb reacts with other medications such as antidepressants, birth control pills, pro-

tease inhibitors, theophylline, warfarin, and digoxin. The patient should counsel with a health care provider before adding St. John's Wort or any herbal remedy to daily regimen.
D. Clinical procedures (Institute for Clinical Systems Improvement [ICSI], 2004).
   1. Assessment for suicide risk.
   2. Antidepressant therapy.
      a. Selective Serotonin Reuptake Inhibitors (SSRIs).
      b. Secondary amine tricyclics.
      c. Monoamine oxidase inhibitors (MAOIs).
   3. Psychotherapy.
E. Collaboration/resource identification, and referral.
   1. For depression and suicidal ideation, mental health providers will need to be involved.
   2. For major depression and suicide attempt, hospitalization is necessary.
   3. Family members often feel responsible and will require mental health support.
F. Care management.
   1. Depression support groups provided by community services.
   2. Collaboration with mental health services.
   3. Ongoing medication management.
   4. Family/significant other support system.
G. Patient education.
   1. Signs and symptoms of worsening depression.
   2. Importance of medication compliance.
   3. Dangers of alcohol consumption while taking anti-depressants.
H. Advocacy.
   1. National Institute of Mental Health (www.nimh.nih.com).
   2. American Academy of Child and Adolescent Psychiatry (www.aacap.org).
I. Telehealth practice.
   1. Recognize signs and symptoms, and refer to a crisis center, police, and/or EMS (such as by calling 9-1-1) if necessary for management of suicide threat or attempt.
   2. Information resource.
   3. Therapeutic communication.
   4. Referral to community support.
J. Communication/documentation.
   1. Patient record.
   2. Maintain confidentiality.

3. Collaborate with tertiary care, if necessary.
K. Outcome management.
    1. The patient remains free from harm.
    2. The patient and family are involved in coordinated mental health care.
    3. The patient verbalizes self-help measures.
    4. The patient verbalizes information on community resources.

Acutely Ill Children and Adolescents

Fever

Patient Population: Acute, Pediatric

Fever is the most common cause for pediatric visits in ambulatory care. Fever, alone, is not an illness but the body's defense against infection. Most bacteria and viruses thrive in a 98.6°F temperature. The body's ability to increase temperature is a component of defense against organism growth. Young children will develop fevers with minor viral infections. In the past, fevers were thought to be dangerous, and antibiotic use to fight infections causing fevers was the treatment of choice, regardless of underlying sequellae. That practice, however, has led to microorganism mutation and inability for the antibiotic to be effective when the medication is truly needed. Untreated fevers caused by infection will seldom go over 105°F unless the child is overdressed or trapped in a hot place. The brain's thermostat will stop the fever from climbing above 106°F. Brain damage from a fever generally will not occur unless the fever is over 107.6°F (42°C) (Greene, 2004). The brain center will not allow the body to increase its temperature to fatal levels. Proper education on how to treat fevers is an important part of the ambulatory care nurse function.
A. Assess/screen/triage.
    1. History of fever.
        a. How long has the fever been present?
        b. Did the fever suddenly go up?
        c. Did the fever occur 4 to 6 hours after exposure to antigen?
        d. Pattern of fever and response to antipyretics.
    2. Emergent situations.
        a. Less than 90 days old with rectal temperature 100.2°F or greater.
        b. Three to 6 months old with temperature

of 101°F or greater.
        c. Six to 12 months old with temperature of 103°F or greater.
        d. Less than 2 years old with a fever lasting longer than 24 to 48 hours.
        e. Fever in older children lasting longer than 48 to 72 hours.
        f. Greater than 105°F unless the fever responds to antipyretics.
    3. Emergent symptomology needing immediate transport to an emergency department, such as by EMS (Schmitt, 2004).
        a. Confusion.
        b. Limp, weak, or not moving.
        c. Unresponsive.
        d. Bulging fontanel.
        e. Difficulty breathing.
        f. Stiff neck.
    4. Need to see a provider urgently.
        a. Irritability.
        b. Unable to move a limb.
        c. Accompanying earache, throat pain, or cough.
        d. Newborn.
        e. Signs of dehydration (such as dry mouth, no urine output for >12 hours).
        f. Immunosuppressed due to chronic condition or immunosuppressive therapy.
        g. Burning or painful urination.
B. Primary/secondary/tertiary prevention.
    1. Parent/patient education.
        a. Do not overdress.
        b. Keep room temperature comfortably cool.
        c. Lukewarm bath. Do not use cold bath or alcohol rub. Doing so will cool the skin, causing shivering and raising core temperature.
        d. Have the child drink cool liquids in unlimited amounts, as tolerated.
    2. Use of antipyretics.
        a. Use over-the-counter antipyretics, such as acetaminophen or ibuprofen, for fever over 102°F. Do not use ibuprofen for children under the age of 6 months.
        b. Alternate acetaminophen and ibuprofen, if needed.
        c. Do not give aspirin to children for treatment in fever because of the risk of Reye's Syndrome.

3. Infection control measures.
   a. Hand hygiene, with soap and water, or alcohol hand rub.
   b. Wash toys to prevent spread of germs.
   c. If the child is in daycare, choose an establishment that has 6 children or fewer in an area.
   d. "Cover your cough" education (CDC, 2006).
C. Clinical procedures.
   1. Blood samples.
   2. Urinalysis.
   3. Sputum culture.
   4. Lumbar puncture.
   5. X-rays as indicated.
D. Care management.
   1. Personal physician.
   2. Health clinics
   3. Telehealth triage.
   4. Therapeutic communication techniques utilized.
E. Patient education.
   1. Teach parents techniques for managing fever at home.
   2. Teach parents signs and symptoms of emergent situations.
   3. Teach parents infection control measures.
   4. Reassure parents that a fever is a normal response to help a child's body fight infection, usually caused by a virus.
   5. Inform that most fevers last 2 to 3 days.
H. Telehealth practice.
   1. Information resource for parents for fever control.
   2. Recognize emergent situations and refer for appointment, as necessary.
   3. Referral as necessary.
   4. Call back for fever lasting >3 days or if the child becomes worse.
I. Communication/documentation.
   1. Patient record.
   2. Telephone advice documentation.
J. Outcome management.
   1. Fever controlled.
   2. Antibiotic use for bacterial infections and not for viral infections.
   3. Parent verbalizes understanding of home treatment for fever.
   4. Parent understanding and supportive of treatment plan.

Ear Pain

Patient Population: Pediatric

Otitis media is the second most common diagnosis for sick child visits to pediatricians. Approximately 30% to 60% of children have at least one episode or acute otitis media by age one, and approximately 80% have had at least one episode by age 3. However, there is great variability in diagnostic criteria and approaches to therapy. Ear pain may also be due to inflammation of the auditory canal, most commonly caused by microorganism growth from water trapped after swimming.

A. Definitions.
   1. *Otitis Media* – Infection occurring just behind the eardrum. Presents as collection of fluid, bloody, or purulent, and is visible by otoscope.
   2. *Otitis Externa* – Infection of the ear canal. Canal will look reddened or infected.
B. Assess/screen/triage.
   1. Child's affect.
      a. Irritability or inconsolable crying.
      b. Malaise.
   2. Vital signs.
   3. Vomiting and/or diarrhea.
   4. Hearing screening: Child may experience temporary hearing loss due to fluid accumulation behind the ear.
   5. Severe pain followed by sudden relief may indicate a ruptured tympanic membrane. There may be cloudy fluid or pus drainage in the ear canal.
   6. Itchy and somewhat painful ear canal; discomfort when ear is moved up and down (signs of otitis externa).
C. Primary/secondary/tertiary prevention.
   1. Primary prevention of otitis media.
      a. For chronic otitis media, a myringotomy or tympanostomy may be performed to relieve fluid accumulation.
      b. Pneumoccocal conjugate vaccine administration.
      c. Annual influenza vaccine administration for children with recurrent infections.
      d. In children, Eustachian tubes become blocked easily. Educate parent on home prevention.
         (1) Wash hands and toys frequently.
         (2) For the child that is not breast fed,

hold the child upright while bottle feeding.

    (3) Place child in daycare that has 6 children or fewer in the area.

    (4) Avoid pacifier use.

    (5) Do not use antibiotics leftover from an unused prescription.

    (6) Keep child away from second-hand smoke.

    (7) The use of xylitol syrup (a natural sweetener) or chewing gum may reduce the incidents of ear infections.

2. Secondary prevention – Parent education regarding common causes of ear infections.
   a. Colds.
   b. Allergies.
   c. Second-hand smoke.
   d. Infected or overgrown adenoids.
   e. Excess mucous and saliva during teething.
   f. Drinking from a sippy cup or bottle while lying down.

3. Prevention of otitis externa (Schmitt, 2004).
   a. Limit number of hours the child spends in water.
   b. Do not insert cotton swabs into the ear canal.
   c. Dry the opening of the canal carefully after bathing or swimming.
   d. For recurrences, may prevent (but not treat acutely) by rinsing the ear canal with rubbing alcohol or 50% white vinegar solution after swimming.

D. Clinical procedures.
   1. Otoscope examination to visualize tympanic membrane.
   2. Pneumatic otoscopy to assess movement under slight pressure.
   3. Tympanogram and acoustic reflectometry.
   4. Antibiotics, if necessary.
      a. Children under 2 years old.
      b. Unresolved fever.
      c. Unimproved after 24 to 48 hours.
   5. Cerumen removal, if indicated.
   6. Acetaminophen or ibuprofen for pain and fever, as needed.
   7. Tympanocentesis – Invasive and painful technique using spinal needle attached to a vac-

uum trap for removal of fluid from behind tympanic membrane for assessment. Limited to research applications at present, but may become more common with increasing antibiotic-resistant organisms.

E. Care management.
   1. Otolaryngologist for possible myringotomy and tubes.
   2. Telehealth triage.
   3. Therapeutic communication techniques utilized.

F. Patient education.
   1. Home treatment and risk factors.
   2. Most ear infections resolve without use of antibiotics.
   3. May apply warm compresses to outer ear.
   4. Use over the counter pain preparations.
      a. Acetaminophen.
      b. Ibuprofen; do not use ibuprofen in children 6 months old or less.
      c. Do not use aspirin to treat pain in children.
      d. Complete entire course of antibiotics as prescribed.
      e. Return for ear check, if ordered.
      f. How to administer ear drops, if prescribed.
      g. White vinegar 50% solution rinses for mild otitis externa.

G. Advocacy.
   1. Provide referrals as necessary.
   2. Education.

H. Telehealth practice.
   1. Information resource.
   2. Triage/assessment.
   3. Referral as necessary.

I. Communication/documentation.
   1. Patient record.
   2. Telehealth advice documentation.

J. Outcome management.
   1. Fever controlled.
   2. Ear pain resolved.
   3. Antibiotic use for bacterial infections.
   4. Parent education.

Upper Respiratory Infection

Patient Population: Pediatric

Bacterial and viral upper respiratory infections affect the nasal passages, throat, bronchioles, and lungs. The most common upper respiratory infection is the common cold. There are over one-billion colds each year in the general population. For children under the age of 3 years, viral infections are the greatest cause of upper respiratory illness. Viruses, like the common cold, migrate from nasal and sinus passages to bronchioles and lungs. School-age children are at a higher risk of bacterial infection, caused by the bacterium *Mycoplasma pneumoniae*. The severity of illness may be mild to fatal. Infection hinders the lungs from ventilation and can lead to respiratory arrest and death.

A. Assess/screen/triage.
   1. Onset of symptoms.
   2. Vital signs.
   3. Auscultate lung sounds.
      a. Clear.
      b. Wheezing.
      c. Rales.
      d. Crackles.
      e. Diminished.
   4. Chest pain.
   5. Pulse oximetry.
   6. Work of breathing: Signs of distress.
      a. Inspiratory and expiratory motion.
      b. Lower chest retractions.
      c. Xiphoid retractions.
      d. Nasal flaring.
      e. Expiratory grunting.
B. Primary/secondary/tertiary prevention (Schmitt, 2004).
   1. Patient/parent education on respiratory etiquette, "Cover Your Cough" program (CDC, 2006).
      a. Infected individuals should sneeze or cough by covering their mouths with tissues or the sleeve of a garment.
      b. Throw the tissue away and wash hands with soap and water or hand sanitizer.
   2. Emphasize a healthy lifestyle.
   3. Pneumococcal vaccine administration.
   4. Influenza vaccine administration.
   5. Haemophilus Influenzae B vaccine administration.

   6. Wash hands and toys frequently.
   7. Avoid overusing antibiotics.
   8. Humidifier if air in the home is dry.
   9. Minimizing risk factors.
      a. Pollution.
      b. Second-hand smoke.
C. Clinical procedures.
   1. Pulse oximetry.
   2. Peak flow meter, if asthmatic.
   3. Nebulizer, if necessary.
   4. Blood samples for signs of bacterial infection and/or dehydration.
   5. X-ray, if indicated.
   6. Antibiotics, if necessary.
D. Care management.
   1. Providers.
   2. Telehealth triage.
   3. Utilization of home care, if necessary.
E. Patient/parent education (Schmitt, 2004).
   1. Course of infection: Within 2 to 7 days after exposure, the contaminated host has "caught a cold." At onset of symptoms, an infected child is contagious for the first 2 to 3 days of the viral infection.
   2. Signs and symptoms of ineffective airway.
   3. Signs and symptoms of ineffective breathing patterns.
   4. Over-the-counter medications.
      a. Antipyretics, such as acetaminophen and ibuprofen. Do not use aspirin.
      b. Decongestants.
   5. Nasal suctioning with a bulb syringe as needed for younger children.
   6. Nasal washes with worm water or saline nose drops as needed.
   7. Viral infections resolve without antibiotics. Antibiotic for bacterial infections.
   8. Home treatments to ease symptoms:
      a. Increased intake of fluids.
      b. Bedside steam.
      c. Increased rest.
   9. Monitoring fever, secretion changes, or other signs of worsening or secondary infection.
F. Advocacy.
   1. Provide referrals as necessary.
   2. Education.
G. Telehealth practice.
   1. Return call or appointment if symptoms

worsen.

2. Triage/assessment.
3. Referral as necessary.

H. Communication/documentation.
   1. Patient record.
   2. Telehealth advice documentation.

I. Outcome management.
   1. Infection resolved.
   2. Parent verbalizes understanding of home treatment and risk factors.
   3. Parent understanding and supportive of treatment plan.
   4. Complete entire course of antibiotics, as prescribed.

Nausea, Vomiting, and Diarrhea

Patient Population: Pediatric

Just as sneezing is the body's defense against allergens and pathogens, nausea, vomiting, and diarrhea is the body's way of eliminating the gastrointestinal tract of irritants. The most common diagnosis is viral gastroenteritis. At some time during their development, most children will have gastroenteritis, which is typically self-limiting. Pyloric stenosis, a congenital anomaly affecting 2 to 3 per 1,000 infants aged 0 to 6 months per year (NIH, 2004), is a less common but serious case of vomiting and diarrhea. Symptoms indicative of serious underlying disease process in all age groups include blood in emesis or stool, severe pain, uncontrolled fever, and absent or hyperactive bowel sounds. In all cases of nausea, vomiting, and diarrhea, there is a risk of dehydration due to fluid and electrolyte loss.

A. Assess/screen/triage (King, Glass, Bresee, & Duggan, 2003).
   1. Onset of symptoms.
   2. Color, frequency, amount, consistency of stool.
   3. Extent of emesis.
   4. Location, nature, and pattern of pain.
   5. Urinary output.
   6. Recent oral intake.
   7. Recent travel outside the U.S. (evaluation for parasites).
   8. Chronic conditions that may exacerbate risks from dehydration, such as immunosuppressive illnesses or therapies.
   9. Vital signs, including orthostatic vital signs.
   10. Weight.
   11. Skin turgor.
   12. Bowel sounds.
   13. Gastric distention.
   14. Child's affect.

B. Primary/secondary/tertiary prevention.
   1. Handle food properly.
   2. Wash hands thoroughly after using the toilet.

C. Clinical procedures.
   1. Blood specimen to assess hydration.
   2. Fluid replacement, including IV hydration, if indicated.
   3. Urine specimen.
   4. Stool cultures, if necessary.

D. Care management.
   1. Providers.
   2. Telehealth triage.

E. Patient education.
   1. Fluid/electrolyte replacement (Schmitt, 2004).
      a. Infants/toddlers:
         (1) Oral rehydrating solutions (ORS) for frequent, watery diarrhea. Avoid water, fruit juice, or soda.
         (2) For breast-fed infants, continue feeding at frequent intervals and supplement with ORS according to provider instructions.
         (3) For formula-fed infants, return to formula from ORS as soon as possible and supplement with ORS and solids according to provider instructions.
      b. School-age children: Sports drinks and other fluids, as tolerated. Avoid fruit juice and soda.
      c. Popsicles at any age.
      d. Once diarrhea has subsided, introduce starchy foods.
      e. Yogurt with active cultures for children >12 months will help restore GI flora.
   2. Parental instruction on signs and symptoms of dehydration.
      a. Dry mucous membranes.
      b. Low urinary output.
      c. Concentrated urine.
      d. Sunken eyes, fontanelles.
   3. Wash hands and toys frequently.
   4. Introduce new foods slowly.

F. Advocacy.

1. Provide referrals as necessary.
2. Education.

G. Telehealth practice.
   1. Information resource.
   2. Triage/assessment.
   3. Referral as necessary.
   4. Call back if signs of dehydration, if diarrhea persists >2 weeks, or the child becomes worse.

H. Communication/documentation.
   1. Patient record.
   2. Telehealth advice documentation.

I. Outcome management.
   1. Illness resolved.
   2. Electrolyte and fluid balance intact.
   3. Parent verbalizes understanding of home treatment.
   4. Parent understanding and supportive of treatment plan.

Acutely Ill Adult

Headache

Patient Population: Adult and Adolescent

Headache is one of the most common health complaints worldwide. Although population-based studies of chronic headache syndromes are limited, it appears that tension headaches are more prevalent than migraines, and that both affect women slightly more often than men (Rasmussen, 1991). Chronic headache syndromes affect the quality of life, but also cause millions of lost workdays and schooldays (Stang & Osterhaus, 1993)

A. Definitions.
   1. *Tension headache* – Headache typically starting in the back of the head radiating forward. Caused by tight, contracted muscles in shoulders, neck, scalp, and jaw. Brought on by stress, depression, anxiety, overwork, lack of sleep, not eating properly, and alcohol or drug use.
   2. *Migraine headache* – Severe, recurrent headache with other symptoms, including visual changes, nausea and vomiting, and photophobia. Starts on one side of the head and may spread to both sides. Some may have an aura before onset. Pain described as throbbing, pounding, or pulsating.
   3. *Cluster headaches* – Sharp, extremely painful headaches that tend to occur several times a day for months, then go away for a similar period of time. Occur more often in men. Can occur after the patient has fallen asleep, are located near or above the eye, and are associated with nasal congestion. More prevalent in men than in women.
   4. *Rebound headache* – Headache that occurs after taking medication for pain relief of headaches has been taken away. Reintroducing the pain reliever does not decrease pain. Usually treated with antidepressants.

B. Assess/screen/triage.
   1. Subjective data.
      a. History of headaches.
         (1) Age of onset.
         (2) Frequency and duration.
      b. Accompanying symptoms.
      c. Pain level on pain scale, such as 0 to 10 point scale (see Chapter 17, *Application of the Nursing Process in Ambulatory Care*).
      d. History of onset (sudden vs. gradual), association with activity, trauma, change in method of birth control or other hormonal changes.
      e. Location of onset.
      f. Visual changes.
      g. Precipitating, aggravating, and alleviating factors.
   2. Objective data.
      a. Neurological assessment.
      b. Vital signs.
   3. Emergent situations with presentation of headache.
      a. Sudden, severe onset with neurological symptoms including mental status.
      b. Headache with accompanying fever and neck stiffness may indicate meningitis.
      c. "Worst headache in my life" may indicate a medical emergency (for example, cerebral aneurysm).
      d. Headache with accompanying loss of memory.
      e. Headache that gets progressively worse over 24 hours.
      f. First time the patient has ever had a severe headache.

C. Primary/secondary/tertiary prevention.
    1. Adequate sleep.
    2. Nutritious eating habits.
    3. Routine exercise.
    4. Relaxation techniques.
    5. Stretching at least once an hour if the patient spends the day working at a desk/computer.
    6. Correct posture.
    7. Abstaining from smoke.
    8. Avoiding known personal triggers (such as chocolate).
D. Clinical procedures.
    1. Medications.
    2. Radiography including CT, MRI, X-ray.
    3. Lumbar puncture.
    4. Close monitoring of pain management.
    5. Place the patient in a darkened, quiet room, reclining with head supported and eyes closed. May apply warm or cool compresses to face/neck, depending upon facility protocol.
    6. Close monitoring of vital signs and neurological status in emergent situations.
E. Care management.
    1. Transfer to tertiary care in emergent situations.
    2. Medication management.
        a. Prophylactic: To prevent migraine or tension headaches.
            (1) Calcium channel blockers.
            (2) Tricyclic and SSRI antidepressants.
            (3) Monoamine oxidase inhibitors.
            (4) Beta blockers.
            (5) Serotonin antagonists.
            (6) Anticonvulsants.
            (7) Ergot derivatives.
        b. Acute treatment. For migraine headaches, prompt treatment is important to a good response.
            (1) Simple analgesics: Acetaminophen, ibuprofen, NSAIDs, aspirin.
            (2) Ergot alkaloids.
            (3) Triptans (such as sumitriptan).
            (4) Combination analgesics (such as caffeine and analgesics).
            (5) Narcotic analgesics.
            (6) Nasal spray: Dihydrogotomine (DHE-45), butorphanol, or sumatriptan.
            (7) Parenteral medication: Dihydro-

gotomine (DHE-45) or sumatriptan.
    3. Provider may refer for physical therapy, manipulation, or acupuncture.
F. Patient education.
    1. Identification of triggers. Client should keep a headache diary to help determine cause.
    2. Measures to ease discomfort.
        a. Relaxation techniques and other behavioral therapies.
        b. Medication management, if necessary.
    3. Prevention of headache.
G. Advocacy.
    1. National Migraine Association (www.migraines.org).
    2. National Institutes of Health (www.nih.org).
H. Telehealth practice.
    1. Triage for severity of illness.
    2. Information resource on pain management.
    3. Referral, if necessary.
I. Communication/documentation.
    1. Patient record.
    2. Telephone advice documentation.
J. Outcome management.
    1. Pain diminished on pain scale.
    2. Client verbalizes understanding of etiology.
    3. Client verbalizes preventive and treatment self-care interventions.
    4. Number of chronic or rebound headaches reduced or eliminated.

Low Back Pain

Patient Population: Adult

Low back pain can range from mild to severe and can last from 1 day to years. The pain can be caused by trauma or strain, or the pain can be referred pain and an indication of an underlying disease process. Pain that increases while lying down or resting could be an indication of organ pain. Pain that increases with movement typically involves muscle strain. Nerve pain signals the involvement of the spinal column (Hu, Tribus, Tay, & Carlson, 2003).
A. Definitions.
    1. *Acute back pain* – Sudden onset of pain which is temporary.
    2. *Chronic back pain* – Pain that is persistent and disabling, >3 months.

B. Assess/screen/triage.
1. Onset of pain.
2. Pain description (sharp, dull, aching, stabbing).
3. Level of pain on 0 to 10 scale.
4. Associated symptoms.
   a. Numbness.
   b. Urinary retention or incontinence.
   c. Constipation or loss of bowel control.
   d. Hematuria.
   e. Associated fever.
   f. Difficulty walking.
   g. Foot drop.
   h. Headache.
5. Medical history.
   a. Weight loss.
   b. Fever.
   c. Injuries.
   d. Osteoporosis.
   e. Steroid use.
   f. Cancer.
6. Medications.
C. Primary/secondary/tertiary prevention.
   a. Relaxation techniques.
   b. Weight loss, if necessary.
   c. Education on proper body mechanics.
   d. Education on back strengthening exercises.
   e. Healthy lifestyle.
   f. Women: Do not wear high heels.
D. Clinical procedures.
1. Radiography.
2. Intravenous Pyelography (IVP) if necessary for suspected kidney pathology.
3. Ultrasound, CT Scan or MRI, and Electromyelogram (EMG) for radicular pain.
4. Muscle relaxants.
5. Analgesia.
E. Care management.
1. Pain management to keep the patient comfortable enough to remain as active as possible.
2. Physical therapy.
F. Patient education.
1. Proper body mechanics.
2. Medication usage.
3. Maintain activities of daily living as pain allows. Bed rest is not recommended.
4. Alternate heat and ice on the affected area every 20 minutes.

G. Advocacy.
1. American Chronic Pain Association (www.theacpa.org).
2. National Institutes of Health (www.nih.gov).
3. National Chronic Pain Outreach Association (www.chronicpain.org).
H. Telehealth practice.
1. Triage for severity of illness.
2. Information resource.
3. Referral as necessary.
I. Communication/documentation.
1. Patient record.
2. Telehealth advice documentation.
J. Outcome management.
1. Resolution of acute pain.
2. Motor function intact.
3. Sensory function intact.
4. Patient accepting of treatment plan.

Acute Rhinosinusitis

Patient Population: Adult

Sinusitis in an infection or inflammation of the sinus cavities. Sinuses are air-filled chambers located around the nasal passages, the eyes, and head. There are 4 sets of sinus cavities in the human body: ethmoid, sphenoid, frontal, and maxillary. Mucous membranes in the sinuses are connected to nasal passages. Bacteria or allergens causing nasal irritation can travel along mucous membranes and settle in the sinus cavities. When mucous becomes thick and plugs the passageways to the sinus, pressure causes pain that is palpable over the sinus area. Millions of people suffer each year from allergy-induced irritation or infection of the sinuses, and millions of dollars are spent to relieve symptoms (NIAID, 2005).

A. Assess/screen/triage.
1. Objective data.
   a. Palpate sinuses for tenderness.
   b. Vital signs.
2. Subjective data.
   a. Drainage color and amount.
   b. Date of onset.
   c. History of sinus infections.
   d. Lack of improvement on decongestants.
   e. Other accompanying symptoms such as sore throat, fever, post nasal drip, ear

pain, dental pain, nasal speech, cough.
B. Primary/secondary/tertiary prevention.
  1. Cause of sinusitis: Ostia from sinus to nose become blocked.
    a. Excessive mucous production.
    b. Cilia not able to clear sinus cavity.
  2. Risk factors for sinusitis.
    a. Asthma.
    b. Recent upper respiratory infection.
    c. Overusing nasal decongestants.
    d. Deviated nasal septum.
    e. Frequent swimming and diving.
    f. Dental work.
    g. Air pollution or smoke.
    h. Gastroespophogeal reflux disease (GERD).
    i. Allergic rhinitis.
C. Clinical procedures.
  1. Radiography of sinus (X-ray, CT, or MRI) for persistent, recurring, or chronic sinusitis.
  2. Nasal smear.
  3. Sinus irrigation.
  4. Antibiotics for bacterial infection initially for 10 to 14 days, except azithromycin, which is prescribed for 3 days.
  5. Referral for surgical course for fungal infection.
D. Care management.
  1. Referral to otolaryngologist for unresolved or chronically recurring infection.
  2. Surgical procedure for fungal infection or threatened intraorbital or intracranial complications.
  3. Surgical procedure for polyps or deviated septum with accompanying infections.
E. Patient education.
  1. Humidifier.
  2. Nasal saline.
  3. Increase fluid intake.
  4. Warm compresses to face.
  5. Avoid temperature extremes.
  6. Avoid flying during upper respiratory infection.
  7. Over-the-counter decongestants (for example, pseudoephedrine) and anitcholinergics (for example, chlorpheniramine and diphenhydramine).
F. Advocacy.
  1. National Institute for Allergy and Infectious Diseases (www.niaid.nih.gov).
  2. National Institutes of Health (www.nih.gov).
G. Telehealth practice.
  1. Triage for severity of illness.
  2. Information resource on comfort measures.
  3. Referral as necessary.
H. Communication/documentation.
  1. Patient record.
  2. Telehealth advice documentation.
I. Outcome management.
  1. Resolution of acute infection.
  2. Decreased incident of infection.

Sexually Transmitted Diseases

Patient Population: Adult and Adolescent

Sexually transmitted diseases (STDs) are very common, affecting 1 in 4 adults in the U.S. STDs affect people of all social and income levels. Women are at greater risk of being infected than men, and younger women are at greater risk than those who are older. Women may develop health problems associated with STDs, such as infections spreading to the uterus and fallopian tubes leading to pelvic inflammatory disease (PID), a major cause of female infertility and ectopic pregnancy. Human papilloma virus (HPV) infections increase the risk of cervical cancer. HIV can be sexually transmitted, and upon progression to AIDS, may cause numerous debilitating symptoms and death (CDC, 1998). Prevention of STDs is a major nursing focus when caring for any sexually active female. Communication between sexual partners about sexual history and STDs is of primary importance. Counseling about testing for HIV and other STDs is one way that a professional nurse can make a difference in the long-term health status of patients. Providing reassurance about the confidential nature of the patient's treatment/testing is critical in gaining the trust of the patient and allowing him or her to share information necessary to develop a plan of care.
A. Assess/screen/triage.
  1. Determine factors.
    a. Number of sexual partners.
    b. Partner history of STDs.
    c. Personal history of STDs.
    d. History of abnormal Pap smears.
    e. Condom use.

2. Determine presence of partner violence.
3. Signs and symptoms of STDs.
    a. Many STDs have no symptoms.
    b. Vaginal burning, itching.
    c. Urethral burning, itching, discharge.
    d. Unusual vaginal discharge.
    e. Chancre or vaginal, perianal, or penile lesions.
    f. Rash.
    g. Acute discomfort/pain.
    h. Foul-smelling discharge.
    i. Pain during intercourse.
    j. Irritation or pain around the anus.
    k. Infection also possible in the oropharynx, conjunctiva, or disseminated gonococcal meningitis and endocarditis.
    l. Neonatal infection of eyes, scalp, or other areas.
4. Diagnosis.
    a. Vaginal/pelvic exam.
    b. Intraurethral swab.
    c. Culture.
    d. Slide prep for wet mount or gram stain.
    e. Pap smear.
    f. Colposcopy.
    g. Biopsy.
    h. Blood tests.
5. Treatment depends on the causative agent. Bacterial infections, such as gonorrhea, chlamydia, and syphilis, can be cured with antibiotics. Viral infections, such as HPV, herpes, and HIV, cannot be cured. Medications can be taken to control the symptoms, but there is no way to completely remove the virus from the body.
    a. Appropriate antibiotic(s).
    b. Antivirals.
    c. Antifungals.
    d. Ensure partner treatment of all partners.
B. Primary/secondary/tertiary prevention.
    1. Primary prevention.
        a. Annual health checks.
            (1) Pelvic exam.
            (2) Pap smear.
            (3) Screening of pregnant women.
            (4) Other tests, as indicated.
        b. Patient education.
            (1) Communication with sexual partner(s).
            (2) Abstinence.

               (3) Barrier protection using condoms, female condoms.
               (4) Signs and symptoms (and prevalence of infections with no symptoms).
    2. Secondary prevention.
        a. Education.
        b. Detection of asymptomatically infected persons.
        c. Identification of symptomatic persons unlikely to seek diagnosis and treatment.
        d. Effective diagnosis and treatment, counseling to complete treatment.
        e. Evaluation, testing, treatment, and counseling of sex partners.
        f. Pre-exposure vaccination if at risk for:
            (1) Hepatitis B.
            (2) Hepatitis A.
        g. Reporting requirements.
            (1) According to state law.
            (2) Reports are maintained in strictest confidentiality.
            (3) Most states require public health officials to verify diagnosis and treatment, and to notify contacts for screening and treatment.
    3. Tertiary prevention.
        a. Assisted lifestyle changes.
        b. Reinfection prevention education.
        c. Long-term effects.
            (1) Infertility or ectopic pregnancy.
            (2) Fetal risk.
            (3) Death.
        d. Support groups for people with herpes, HIV.
C. Clinical procedures.
    1. Pelvic/penile exam for patient and partner.
    2. Blood tests.
    3. Biopsy.
    4. Microscopy, including gram stain and wet prep for Trichomonas, yeast, and WBCs.
D. Care management.
    1. Providers.
    2. Health clinics, including public health clinics that offer free testing and treatment.
    3. Insurance/payer source.
    4. Telephone triage.
    5. Support groups.

E. Patient education.
1. Individualized teaching tailored to the patient.
2. Include specific actions the patient can take.
3. Use effective communication skills.
4. Use all opportunities for proactive interviewing.
F. Collaboration/referral.
1. Provide resources and referrals when appropriate.
a. Personal provider.
(1) Physician.
(2) Nurse practitioner.
(3) Certified nurse midwife.
(4) Staff nurse.
b. Planned Parenthood clinics and public health clinics.
c. Family/social services/community services.
d. Specialty groups.
e. Library and Internet information resources.
2. Provide education.
3. Support patient decision making.
G. Telehealth practice.
1. Information resource.
2. Triage/referrals.
3. Provide reassurance when indicated.
4. Maintain confidentiality.
H. Communication/documentation.
1. Patient record.
2. Telephone advice documentation.
3. Number system (for confidentiality purposes) vs. names, often used for STD/HIV testing.
I. Outcome measurement.
1. Early detection and treatment rate.
2. Risk-reducing behavior changes.
3. Improvement in health status.
4. Patient satisfaction.
J. Protocol development.
1. The CDC is a resource for protocol development (www.cdc.gov).
2. Areas for protocol development include:
a. Contact mechanisms for informing patients of test results.
b. Reporting of positive STD test protocols (usually based on government requirements). Partner identification may also be required.
c. Diagnosis/treatment protocols for patients and partners.
d. Domestic violence, substance abuse screening.

References

American Heart Association (AHA). (2005). CPR priorities for the healthcare provider. *Currents in Emergency Cardiovascular Care, 16*(4), 12-15.

American Society of Anesthesiologists (ASA). (1996). Practice guidelines for sedation and analgesia by non-anesthesiologists: A report by the American Society of Anesthesiologists Task Force on sedation and analgesia by non-anesthesiologists. *Anesthesiology, 84*(2), 459-471.

Association of Operating Room Nurses (AORN). (1996). *Recommended practices for monitoring the patient receiving intravenous conscious sedation. 1996 standards and recommended practices.* Denver, CO: Author.

Centers for Disease Control and Prevention (CDC). (2006). *Cover your cough.* Retrieved April 12, 2006, from http://www.cdc.gov/flu/protect/covercough.htm

Centers for Disease Control and Prevention (CDC). (1998). Guidelines for treatment of sexually transmitted diseases. *MMWR, 47*(RR-1), 1-118.

Chung, F. (1995). Recovery patterns and home-readiness after ambulatory surgery. *Anesthesia and Analgesia, 80*(5), 896-902.

Greene, A. (2004). *Fever.* Retreived February 25, 2006, from http://www.nlm.nih.gov/medlineplus/ency/article/003090.htm.

Hu, S.S, Tribus, C.B., Tay, B.K-B., & Carlson, G. (2003). *Disorders, diseases, and injuries of the spine. Current diagnosis and treatment in orthopedics* (3rd ed.). New York: Lange Medical Books/McGraw Hill.

Institute for Clinical Systems Improvement (ICSI). (2004). *Major depression in adults in primary care.* Bloomington, MN: Author.

Janikowski D., & Rockefeller, C. (1998). Awake and talking: Ambulatory surgery and conscious sedation. *Nursing Economic$, 16*(1), 37-43.

Joint Commission on Accreditation of Healthcare Organizations (JCAHO). (2005a). *Comprehensive accreditation manual for ambulatory care.* Oakbrook Terrace, IL: Author.

Joint Commission on Accreditation of Healthcare Organizations (JCAHO). (2005b). *2005 comprehensive accreditation manual for hospitals.* Oakbrook Terrace, IL: Author.

Joint Council of Allergy, Asthma and Immunology (JCAAI). (2005). The diagnosis and management of anaphylaxis: An updated practice parameter. *Journal of Allergy and Clinical Immunology, 115*(3 Suppl), S483-523.

King, C.K., Glass, R., Bresee, J.S., & Duggan, C. (2003). Managing acute gastroenteritis among children: Oral rehydration, maintenance, and nutritional therapy. *MMWR Recommendations and Reports, 52*(RR-16), 1-16.

Krause, R.S. (2005). *Anaphylaxis.* eMedicine by WebMD. Retrieved February 25, 2006, from http://www.emedicine.com/emerg/topic25.htm

National Institute for Allergy and Infectious Diseases (NIAID). (2005). *Allergy statistics.* Retrieved February 25, 2006, from http://www.niaid.nih.gov/factsheets/allergystat.htm

National Institutes of Health (NIH). (2000). *Let's talk about depression.* Publication 00-3561. 2000. National Institutes of Health.

National Institutes of Health (NIH). (2004). *Medical encyclopedia: Pyloric Stenosis.* Retrieved June 25, 2006, from http://www.nlm.nih.gov/medlineplus/ency/article/000970.htm

Odom, J. (1997). Conscious sedation in the ambulatory setting. *Critical Care Nursing Clinics of North America, 9*(3), 361-370.

Rasmussen, B.K. (1991) Epidemiology of headache in general population: A prevalence study. *Journal of Clinical Epidemiology, 44,* 1147.

Schmitt, B. (2004). *Pediatric telephone protocols, office version* (10th ed.). Elk Grove Village, IL: American Academy of Pediatrics.

Somerson, S.J., Husted, C.W., & Sicilia, M.R. (1995). Insights into conscious sedation. *American Journal of Nursing, 95*(6), 26-33.

Stang, P.E., & Osterhaus, J.T. (1993). Impact of migraine in the United States: Data from the National Health Interview Survey. *Headache, 33,* 29.

Williams, G.D. (1997). Preoperative assessment and health history interview. *The Nursing Clinics of North America, 32*(2), 395-416.

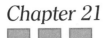
Care of the Acutely Ill Patient

This test may be copied for use by others.

COMPLETE THE FOLLOWING:

Name: _____

Address: _____

City: _____ State: _____ Zip: _____

Preferred telephone: (Home)_____ (Work)_____

E-mail_____

AAACN Member Expiration Date: _____

Registration fee: AAACN Member: $12.00
                   Nonmember: $20.00

Objectives

This educational activity is designed for nurses and other health care professionals who practice in ambulatory care. For those wishing to obtain CE credit, an evaluation follows. After studying the information presented in this offering, you will be able to:

1. Describe the assessment and care for life-threatening situations in ambulatory care.
2. Identify critical factors and care implications in the provision of ambulatory moderate sedation.
3. Identify the assessment and care for patients with acute illnesses commonly seen in ambulatory care settings.
4. Discuss patient and family education for acutely ill patients.

Answer Form:

1. If you applied what you have learned from this activity into your practice, what would be different?

_____

_____

_____

Evaluation

	Strongly disagree				Strongly agree
2. By completing this activity, I was able to meet the following objectives:					
a. Describe the assessment and care for life-threatening situations in ambulatory care.	1	2	3	4	5
b. Identify critical factors and care implications in the provision of ambulatory moderate sedation.	1	2	3	4	5
c. Identify the assessment and care for patients with acute illnesses commonly seen in ambulatory care settings.	1	2	3	4	5
d. Discuss patient and family education for acutely ill patients.					
3. The content was current and relevant.	1	2	3	4	5
4. The objectives could be achieved using the content provided.	1	2	3	4	5
5. This was an effective method to learn this content.	1	2	3	4	5
6. I am more confident in my abilities since completing this material.	1	2	3	4	5

7. The material was (check one) ___new ___review for me.

8. Time required to read this chapter: _____minutes

I verify that I have completed this activity: _____
                                                              Signature

Comments: _____

_____

_____

Posttest Instructions

1. To receive continuing education credit for individual study after reading the article, complete the answer/evaluation form to the left.

2. Detach and send the answer/evaluation form along with a check or money order payable to the *American Academy of Ambulatory Care Nursing (AAACN)*, East Holly Avenue Box 56, Pitman, NJ 08071–0056.

3. Test returns must be postmarked by August 1, 2011. Upon completion of the answer/evaluation form, a certificate for **1.7** contact hour(s) will be awarded and sent to you. Should the material contained in this chapter become outdated prior to the above expiration date, AAACN reserves the right to withdraw this CE test.

This activity is co-provided by the *American Academy of Ambulatory Care Nursing (AAACN)* and Anthony J. Jannetti, Inc. (AJJ). AJJ is accredited as a provider of continuing nursing education by the American Nurses' Credentialing Center's Commission on Accreditation (ANCC-COA). AAACN is a provider approved by the California Board of Registered Nurses, provider number CEP 05336.

This article was reviewed and formatted for contact hour credit by Sally S. Russell, MN, CMSRN, AAACN Education Director; and Candia Baker Laughlin MS, RN, C, Editor.

Chapter 22

Care of the Chronically Ill Patient

Jo Ann Appleyard, PhD, RN

Nancy M. Albert, PhD, CCNS, CCRN, CNA • Chronic Heart Failure

Candia Baker Laughlin, MS, RN, C • Chronic Obstructive Pulmonary Disease

Linda L. Edwards, RN, MHS, CDE • Diabetes Mellitus

Christine Schaefer, MSN, RN, CDE, BC-ADM • Diabetes Mellitus

Pamela Del Monte, MS, RN, C • Hypertension

Margaret Ross Kraft, PhD, RN • Osteoarthritis

Linda L. Gehring, PhD, APNP, RN, BC • Asthma

Stephanie G. Metzger, MS, RN, CPNP • Attention Deficit Hyperactivity Disorder

Renée Y. Cecil, BSN, RN • Sickle Cell Disease

Patient Prototypes

Adults
Chronic Heart Failure • Chronic Obstructive Pulmonary Disease • Diabetes Mellitus • Hypertension • Osteoarthritis
Children and Adolescents
Asthma • Attention Deficit Hyperactivity Disorder • Sickle Cell Disease

Objectives

Study of the information presented in this chapter will enable the learner to:
1. Discuss the role of ambulatory care nurses in caring for chronically ill patients in all age ranges.
2. Describe how ambulatory care nurses support chronically ill patients, develop effective self-management behaviors, adhere to complex medication regimens, and manage the effects of polypharmacy.
3. Identify the risk factors for common chronic conditions among children and adults.
4. Identify the essential elements of the nursing process for patients with common chronic illnesses.
5. Describe the treatment strategies for common chronic conditions for children and adults.

Key Points

1. Ambulatory care nurses have a great deal of contact with patients with chronic diseases, and besides assisting physicians in disease diagnosis and treatment, nursing responsibilities include assessment and management of disease progress, client education, and care management.
2. The ambulatory care nurse's most important role in working with chronically ill patients is to support and enhance the patient's self-management skills, including treatment adherence and medication management.
3. Patients with common chronic illnesses may present at almost any ambulatory care setting or telehealth encounter, requiring timely and knowledgeable assessment and care.

Modern medicine has been of immense benefit to humankind, bringing about cures to many deadly conditions, as well as the means to prevent multiple diseases. Conversely, millions of people currently suffer from chronic illnesses as a result of the miracles of modern medicine. Especially in developed nations, people are now living longer with diseases that cannot yet be cured, and the growing population of chronically ill people is causing great strain upon the health care resources of all countries. On the community and individual levels, chronic illness is also a significant burden. Many chronically ill people endure daily symptoms of their illness, including pain, limited mobility, weakness, and fatigue. They may be unable to engage in their normal daily activities, and they struggle with the financial burden of paying large medical bills. Communities must develop resources for assisting their chronically ill citizens, resulting in a constant need for leaders to make painful choices about funding both public and private programs designed to support the general good of the community.

This chapter addresses the ambulatory nurse's role in caring for the chronically ill patient, including information on self-management, as well as treatment adherence and content on selected chronic medical conditions. These include sickle cell disease, attention deficit hyperactivity disorder (ADHD), asthma, chronic heart failure (CHF), chronic obstructive pulmonary disease (COPD), diabetes, hypertension, and osteoarthritis.

Chronic Illness Self-Management

All people with chronic diseases need varying degrees of help from health care providers and the health care system; however, it is the individual who must manage the illness. Providers administer preventive measures, diagnoses, treatment interventions, and treatment plans, but it is the patient who must deal with illness and its consequences routinely. Furthermore, it is the patient who chooses how, or even whether, to engage in the medical process to be diagnosed and treated. In this country, most people with chronic disease receive a diagnosis during the trajectory of their disease, and people engage in treatment activities along a large continuum, ranging from no engagement to daily actions, to manage the illness.

Since most care of chronically ill patients takes place outside of acute or long-term care settings, ambulatory care nurses have a great deal of contact with chronic disease. This includes nurses in both primary and specialty care settings. Besides assisting physicians in disease diagnosis and treatment, nursing responsibilities include assessment and management of disease progress, patient education, and care management. In all facets of working with chronically ill patients, the ambulatory care nurse must be aware of the patient's abilities to manage that illness on his or her own. The nurse's most important role in working with a chronically ill patient is to support and enhance the patient's self-management skills, and this element of chronic disease management should be addressed at every patient visit.

Treatment adherence and medication management are two essential components of disease self-management in the care of patients with both acute and chronic illnesses. Patient adherence to medical treatment regimens has been studied for decades, and although the phenomenon is better understood, the causes of non-adherence are so complex that health care providers must spend a great deal of time assessing individual patient circumstances to ensure adequate adherence to chronic disease treatment regimens. This assessment and subsequent interventions to assist patients with adherence most often falls to professional nurses in ambulatory care settings because the medical visit providers do not have the time, and at times the skills, necessary to perform this aspect of care.

Similarly, medication management assistance is crucial to successful patient self-management of chronic disease. In particular, older patients with multiple conditions may experience polypharmacy, and they often struggle with the sheer logistics of taking all prescribed medicines as directed. Again, professional nurses have the time, knowledge, and skills to identify polypharmacy and to assist patients in the management of complex medication therapy. Increasingly, clinical pharmacists are available to help polypharmacy, but nurses often recognize the signs and symptoms of this medical treatment problem.

A. Dynamics of patient self-management in chronic illness.
1. Assumptions and operational definition.
    a. All health behaviors involve self-management.
    b. Effective self-management is essential for chronically ill patients to achieve optimal outcomes.
    c. Self-management in chronic illness is an enduring process, and patients experience a range of success in developing and carrying out self-management activities.
    d. Patients self-manage chronic diseases by actively self-monitoring their symptoms and relevant physiologic processes, making decisions about their behaviors related to their conditions, and actually engaging in those behaviors.

2. Theories contributing to understanding of patient self-management behaviors (Newman, Steed, & Mulligan, 2004).
    a. Social cognitive theory.
        (1) Behavior shaped by expectations of individuals.
        (2) Confidence, or expectations of succeeding or failing (self-efficacy), is key to patient success in disease self-management.
    b. Stress coping model – Developing successful coping strategies for stress caused by chronic disease is essential for effective self-management.
    c. Trans-theoretical model of social theory.
        (1) Readiness to change is an essential feature of effective self-management.
        (2) Interventions focus on patient motivations related to health behavior change.
    d. Cognitive behavioral therapy – Patients learn how their thoughts feed into their behavior, and they are assisted to modify how they think about themselves and their disease.
3. Tasks in chronic disease self-management (Lorig & Holman, 2003).
    a. Patients' perspectives about their diseases will change over time depending on many factors, including the severity of current symptoms.
    b. All chronically ill patients face three sets of tasks throughout their lives.
        (1) Learning and acting upon the knowledge and skills essential to effectively manage their conditions.
        (2) Managing their lives to change, maintain, and/or create new behaviors and life roles that are essentially satisfying.
        (3) Dealing with emotions resulting from the realities of having a chronic illness, including fear, anger, frustration, sadness, and depression.
4. Decision making in chronic disease self-management (Thorne, Paterson, & Russell, 2003).
    a. Patient decision making in self-management is a conscious process to gain control in the management of their disease.
        b. Initially, the challenges in self-management decision making are often overwhelming.
        c. Patients must learn to "listen to their bodies" as they experience various symptoms and pathophysiology of their disease.
        d. During decision making, patients are managing their lifestyle, treatment, and often the health care system itself.
        e. Although health care professionals can be instrumental in supporting patient decision making, the patient must want to be in control in order to make the most effective decisions regarding self-management.

B. Chronic disease self-management programs.
    1. Many programs are organized around disease entities, including chronic heart failure (CHF), chronic obstructive pulmonary disease (COPD), diabetes mellitus (DM), hypertension, and osteoarthritis.
        a. Recent meta-analysis of studies regarding the effectiveness of programs for diabetes, hypertension, and osteoarthritis showed that some programs, especially those for diabetes and hypertension, may have beneficial effects upon clinical measures of those diseases, specifically hemoglobin A1c and blood pressure levels.
        b. This same study also concludes it is currently not possible to determine which program interventions are the ones responsible for the beneficial effects (Chodosh et al., 2005).
    2. The Chronic Disease Self-Management Program (CDSMP), developed by Kate Lorig, David Sobel, and others, assists patients with one or more chronic illnesses to manage their conditions.
        a. Patients with different chronic conditions are educated together, often by a trained layperson who is also chronically ill, in developing self-management skills focusing on problem-solving, decision making, and confidence building (Linnell, 2005).
        b. The CDSMP implemented by Kaiser Permanente has been shown to be

effective in increasing self-efficacy in dealing with health problems, improving health status, and reducing health care utilization (Lorig, Sobel, Ritter, Laurent, & Hobbs, 2001).

3. The chronic care model (CCM), developed at Group Health Cooperative of Puget Sound, is a comprehensive model encompassing elements of the community, the health care system, and the health care provider organization (Bodenheimer, Wagner, & Grumbach, 2002a; 2002b).

   a. Six essential elements of CCM.

      (1) Community resources – Linkages with a broad array of community support services, including senior centers, transportation, nutrition support, and medication payment assistance programs.

      (2) Health care organization – Organization goals and leadership must put a priority on chronic care activities and provide the resources to support them; health care payers must also provide resources to support chronic care programs.

      (3) Self-management support – Involves collaborative relationships between patients and providers along with specific programs to assist patients to develop and improve essential self-management skills.

      (4) Delivery system design – Must reflect essential components of chronic disease care, including multidisciplinary teams and structures to support planned visits and appropriate followup care.

      (5) Decision support – Availability of evidence-based clinical practice guidelines, preferably in a format to constantly remind providers about appropriate care measures.

      (6) Clinical information systems – Systems must perform the functions of reminding providers about practice guidelines and patients about the need for periodic followup visits, providing feedback to providers about the status of patient chronic illness measures over time, and creating registries of patients with specific disease entities to conduct true population-based care.

   b. Chronic care model components all result in improved chronic disease outcomes according to a recent meta-analysis study; however, the study could not identify whether the whole model is essential or whether certain components are more effective than others (Tsai, Morton, Mangione, & Keeler, 2005).

C. Nursing practice elements that promote successful patient self-management in chronic disease.

  1. Skills and knowledge needed by the nurse:

   a. Critical thinking skills.

   b. Organization and planning skills.

   c. Demonstrated teaching skills.

   d. Negotiation skills.

   e. Assertiveness skills.

   f. Team management skills.

   g. Knowledge of determinants of patient self-management behavior.

   h. Knowledge of pathophysiology and management of appropriate chronic diseases, including the latest evidence-based medical and nursing practice guidelines.

   i. Knowledge regarding medical and community resources available to support patients with specific chronic diseases, including Internet resources.

  2. Nursing roles in chronic disease self-management.

   a. Teacher.

      (1) Teaching may occur individually or with groups of patients.

      (2) Content should be tailored to individual learning needs; patients who receive group education may also need individual teaching.

      (3) Disease-focused content should be accompanied with content to assist patients with specific knowledge and skills related to self-management.

   b. Advisor.

      (1) It is important to assume an advisor role (as opposed to "expert direc-

tor") to promote independent self-management skills with patients.

(2) Successful advising includes assisting patients to develop self-management strategies based on patient needs as well as disease-related consequences of alternative actions.

c. Partner.

(1) Holistic focus of nurses fosters their ability to serve as partners with patients in chronic disease self-management.

(2) A primary partnership strategy is assisting patients with achieving realistic, everyday, small changes in health behaviors to improve self-management (Linnell, 2005).

d. Multidisciplinary team leader and member.

(1) Patients working on chronic disease self-management are often best assisted by multidisciplinary health teams.

(2) Nurses frequently recognize the need for team support for patients and must do the work of mobilizing and leading the team efforts on the patient's behalf.

(3) In many settings, chronic disease support for patients is organized as a team effort, and nurses serve as both members and leaders of these teams.

D. Treatment adherence with chronically ill patients.

1. Brief review of the literature.

a. Patient adherence or compliance with treatment regimens has been the subject of many studies over the past 30 years; it is estimated only 50% of chronically ill patients adhere to their treatment or preventive care regimens (Sawyer & Aroni, 2003).

b. Although "adherence" and "compliance" are terms often used interchangeably, the term "adherence" is preferred because it connotes the patient's willing and active participation in the complex process of disease self-management (McDonald, Garg, & Haynes, 2002; Sawyer & Aroni, 2003).

c. Most of the studies related to adherence focus on medication management, and several of these document the cost-effectiveness achieved when patients do adhere to their medication plans (Wahl et al., 2005).

d. Recent studies demonstrate that chronically ill patients frequently struggle with medication adherence because of the high cost of drugs and limited insurance coverage for pharmaceuticals (Goldman et al., 2004; Mojtabai & Olfson, 2003).

e. A recent meta-analysis showed that effective interventions designed to help chronically ill patients with medication adherence tended to be complex and expensive; these interventions led to small, rather than large, improvements in adherence and treatment outcomes (McDonald et al., 2002).

f. A qualitative study performed in Scotland found that chronically ill patients disliked being dependent upon medications, but they recognized their dependence upon them. Most patients developed highly individual behaviors related to their medications, perhaps taking some quite regularly as prescribed and others irregularly, based on how they felt at the time (Townsend, Hunt, & Wyke, 2003).

2. Nursing interventions in promoting medication adherence.

a. With older adults, especially those with multiple medications for more than one chronic disease, using the principles of geragogy (art and science of helping older adults learn) is useful (Hayes, 2005).

(1) Verbal instructions must be accompanied by written instructions. Effective verbal and written instructions must follow certain guidelines.

(a) Verbal instructions should occur in a quiet place with the door shut to permit the instructor to speak louder and to minimize distractions.

(b) Verbal instructions should be delivered with slow, clear, and concise speech patterns.

(c) Use at least 14-point font for written materials.

(d) Use buff colored paper rather than bright white.

(e) Written instructions should be based on a 5th or 6th grade reading level.

b. Considerations when developing programs that promote medication adherence for older adults.

(1) Continuous, comprehensive patient assessment is a cornerstone of any adherence program, including identifying polypharmacy issues, as well as facilitating factors and barriers to taking prescribed medications.

(2) Self-medication practices that contribute to non-adherence to medication regimens include (Curry, Walker, Hogstel, & Burns, 2005):

(a) Discontinuing medications because of lack of funds or fears of side effects or dependency.

(b) Failing to follow food or alcohol-related recommendations when taking certain medications.

(c) Failing to keep track of medications as they are taken, resulting in missed doses or added doses.

(d) Taking over-the-counter (OTC) medications and/or herbal products as well as prescribed drugs for the same problem.

(e) Adding doses when symptoms are not relieved or skipping doses when symptoms are not present.

(f) Taking the wrong doses or using the wrong technique with inhalers, eye drops, suppositories, or injections.

(3) Adherence programs should emphasize effective self-medication practices, including (Curry et al., 2005):

(a) Patient knowledge of basic facts about their medications, such as name, desired action, dosage and timing, method of administration, adverse effects, and side effects.

(b) Specific knowledge about how to take medications and how and where they should be stored, including administration techniques, managing hard-to-swallow medications, the dangers of sharing medications or splitting doses to save money, and how to talk with providers when there are problems with medications.

(c) Where to obtain medications, the importance of selecting one pharmacy for all their medication needs, and how to find a pharmacy where adequate pharmacist support is assured.

(4) Evaluation of programs to promote medication adherence should be based on concrete evidence, such as (Curry et al., 2005):

(a) Patients do recognize and report medication adverse effects and side effects, as well as symptoms that may be related to medication interactions.

(b) Patients take their medications as prescribed and readily report medications that do not relieve their symptoms; conversely, they report when they perceive improvements in their conditions and ask about dosage adjustment or discontinuance of a medication.

(c) Patients are wary of direct-to-consumer marketing of drugs and are willing to engage their providers in meaningful discussions about whether newer or additional medications are warranted for their conditions.

(5) Medication management assistive

devices are available, and the technology in this area is constantly improving. Examples of current products include:

(a) Alarm watches, clocks, timers, and pagers to remind patients to take their medications at the appropriate times.

(b) Pill dispensers that organize medications according to time and day, by day, week, or month.

(c) Information may be obtained about medication assistive devices at www.epill.com/epill/ind.html (ePill.com, n.d.).

(6) Medicare recipients now have pharmacy benefit programs available to them. In addition, there are multiple drug payment assistance programs available through pharmaceutical manufacturers and other sources. Nurses working with chronically ill patients must have access to updated information to assist patients who cannot afford their prescribed medication regimens.

(a) Information regarding the Medicare benefit may be accessed through the Medicare Web site at www.medicare.gov (Centers for Medicare and Medicaid Services, n.d.).

(b) Information regarding other drug discount programs may be obtained through AARP's Web site at www.aarp.org/health/affordable_drugs (AARP, n.d.).

E. Issues with polypharmacy.

1. *Polypharmacy* has various definitions in the literature, but the most commonly offered definition in the U.S. literature involves patients with one or more conditions who are using multiple medications, some of which are not clinically indicated (Fulton & Allen, 2005). Polypharmacy issues exist along a continuum, ranging from increased health care expenses caused by the prescription of unnecessary medications to additional patient illness burden or death, resulting from the serious physiologic consequences of medication adverse reactions or interactions among multiple medications. Factors that may contribute to polypharmacy include:

a. Patient self medication with OTC products, vitamins, and herbal and other complementary remedies.

b. The patient seeks care from various health care providers, and there is no coordination among these providers in terms of their treatment plans.

c. Direct-to-consumer drug marketing.

d. Increased pressure on provider visit time; it is often easier for providers to write a prescription rather than take the time to fully assess the patient's situation and provide the education necessary to have the patient try a different mode of treatment.

2. Recommended methods to decrease the incidence of polypharmacy that should be used by ambulatory nurses (Fulton & Allen, 2005).

a. "Brown bag" approach to medication assessment – Ask the patient to put all medications, including vitamins, OTC products, and herbal remedies in a bag and bring them to the next visit.

(1) Use when the patient is new to the practice or clinic, or when the patient cannot provide a coherent account of what medicines and other products are used.

(2) Determine and document which medications and other products the patient is actually using.

(3) Consult with the prescribing provider and possibly a clinical pharmacist, if available, to determine which medications and other products the patient should be taking.

(4) Ask the patient for permission to discard the medications that are expired or are not currently prescribed; repeat this for vitamins and other products the patient uses.

(5) Set up and implement a medication education and adherence plan for

the patient, including the use of a medication assistive device.

b. Support the use of electronic medication records at the worksite.

   (1) If a computerized medication record system is already in use, become involved in quality management efforts to evaluate and improve the system.

   (2) If such a system is not in use, learn about how one could be developed or purchased, and become a champion for the implementation of electronic medication records.

   (3) Investigate how you can obtain hospital medical records for your patients when they are hospitalized.

c. Develop a self-education program regarding the interactions and adverse effects of medications commonly used in the ambulatory care setting; find resources to learn about OTC drugs and herbal products used by patients; search the literature for articles describing appropriate prescribing practices for the patient populations served.

Chronic Heart Failure

Patient Population: Adult
Nancy M. Albert PhD, CCNS, CCRN, CNA

Heart failure (HF) is a complex clinical syndrome in which the cardiac myocytes or contractile apparatus of the heart does not pump enough blood to meet the needs of the tissues (Hunt et al., 2005). Peripheral perfusion is altered, leading to subsequent mechanical, neuro-endocrine, and inflammatory responses in an attempt to improve systemic organ flow. Compensatory mechanisms fail to improve contractility over time and lead to a maladaptive state characterized by "ventricular remodeling" (myocyte hypertrophy, cardiac dilatation, and reshaping of the left ventricle from an elliptical to a spherical or globular shape), neurohormonal activation, and hemodynamic alterations (systemic and venous vasoconstriction, increased afterload and preload, and low cardiac output). Chronic myocyte dysfunction may be due to systolic left ventricular

dysfunction (ejection fraction below 40%) and/or preserved left ventricular function (HF with normal ejection fraction, known as diastolic dysfunction) due to changes in regional myocyte workload and/or passive tension, respectively (Albert, Eastwood, & Edwards, 2004; Hunt et al., 2005).

Patients with heart failure are evaluated based on the New York Heart Association (NYHA) functional status assessment or classification (Hunt et al., 2005). Class I reflects the ability to carry out ordinary exercise *without physical activity limitation* due to symptoms of fatigue, dyspnea, chest pain, or palpitations. Class II is designated when the patient is comfortable at rest but has symptoms with ordinary exercise, which causes a *slight limitation of physical activity*. In class III HF, less than ordinary activity results in symptoms; therefore, the patient has a *marked limitation of physical activity*. When the patient develops *discomfort with any physical activity or has symptoms at rest*, functional class IV is designated.

Stages of HF reflect a system of identifying overall status and treatment expectations for patients with suspected or known systolic dysfunction. Stage A represents people *at high risk for developing heart failure*. Medical conditions that place patients at high risk for HF are hypertension, diabetes mellitus, coronary artery disease, and family history of cardiomyopathy. In this stage, people are pre-HF. Stage B represents *asymptomatic left ventricular dysfunction*. In this stage, people have structural heart disease but have not experienced symptoms associated with HF; thus, this stage also reflects pre-HF. Many conditions and diseases can lead to Stage B, and most notable are asymptomatic valve dysfunction, previous myocardial infarction, and left ventricular remodeling including left ventricular hypertrophy and low ejection fraction. Stage C represents *symptomatic HF*. People may have signs and symptoms or have a history of symptoms, even though they are currently asymptomatic. In Stage C, NYHA functional class can span from I-IV. In addition to treatments that revise or attenuate left aventricular remodeling and neurohormonal activation; in this stage, treatment is escalated to include symptom management as well. Stage D represents *end-stage HF*. At this stage, management strategies no longer relieve symptoms. Myocyte, neurohormonal, and other changes escalate or are associated with disabling symptoms and poor quality of life. The ultimate goal of therapy at any stage of HF is to prevent or reverse progression of left ventricular remodeling (Hunt et al., 2005; Misra, Diwan, Mann, & Deswal, 2002).

A. Assessment, screening, and triage (Hunt et al., 2005; Jessup, 2003).
    1. History.
        a. History of chronic coronary artery disease, myocardial infarction, hypertension, diabetes, valve or thyroid disease, or anemia.
        b. Age (prevalence increases with age).
        c. Type of cardiac dysfunction (systolic versus preserved left ventricular function, right versus left HF), stage of syndrome severity (stages A through D), and functional limitations (NYHA functional classes I through IV).
        d. Proper intervention when managing or correcting precipitating disease processes can lead to reversal of HF (for example, surgical or interventional cardiac revascularization or valve repair; treatments that control diabetes, prevent anemia, lower blood pressure, maintain optimal renal function, prevent or limit atrial fibrillation, alter coronary artery plaque progression, and optimize thyroid function).
        e. Lifestyle issues.
            (1) Alcohol use/substance abuse.
            (2) Tobacco use.
            (3) Fluid indiscretion.
            (4) Diet (sodium and fat content).
            (5) Activity/exercise level.
            (6) Stress management.
            (7) Medication noncompliance.
            (8) Social isolation.
            (9) Economic constraints related to purchase of food and medications.
        f. Potentially detrimental medications:
            (1) Chronic non-steroidal anti-inflammatory drugs (NSAIDs) (sodium and water retaining effects).
            (2) High dose (> 325 mg/day) chronic aspirin (sodium and water retaining effects).
            (3) Decongestants (vasoconstriction).
            (4) Calcium channel blockers, except

amlodipine or felodipine (cardio-depressant effects).
            (5) First generation beta-blockers: Propranolol or timolol (cardio-depressant effects).
            (6) Class 1a and 1c anti-arrhythmic agents (cardiodepressant and proarrhythmia effects).
            (7) Sodium-based antacids.
            (8) Thiazolidinediones (sodium and water retaining effects).
            (9) Minoxidil (sodium retaining effects).
    2. Assess medication drug and dose history (including therapy adherence) related to "core" pharmacologic therapies for heart failure.
        a. Angiotensin converting enzyme (ACE) inhibitor with efficacy in heart failure.
            (1) Asymptomatic post myocardial infarction left ventricular systolic dysfunction: Captopril, lisinopril, ramipril, trandopril.
            (2) Ischemic or dilated cardiomyopathy: Captopril, enalapril, lisinopril, quinipril, fosinopril.
        b. Beta-adrenergic blocker with efficacy in heart failure.
            (1) Asymptomatic post myocardial infarction left ventricular systolic dysfunction: Carvedilol, atenolol, metoprolol tartrate, propranolol, timolol.
            (2) Ischemic or dilated cardiomyopathy: Carvedilol, metoprolol, succinate, and bisoprolol.
        c. Aldosterone antagonist.
            (1) Post-myocardial infarction left ventricular systolic dysfunction: Eplerenone.
            (2) Ischemic or dilated cardiomyopathy: Spironolactone.
        d. Loop diuretic (such as furseminde) if signs of volume overload.
        e. Digoxin in systolic heart failure, or heart failure with preserved left ventricular function due to hypertension or ischemic myocardial damage.
        f. Angiotensin II receptor blocker (ARB) when an ACE inhibitor is contraindicated or as adjunctive therapy.
            (1) Asymptomatic post-myocardial infarc-

tion left ventricular systolic dysfunction: Valsartan.

   (2) Ischemic or dilated cardiomyopathy: Candesartan, valsartan.

  g. Hydralazine/nitrate combination in self-
described African Americans who:

   (1) Remain symptomatic after treatment with an ACE inhibitor (or ARB)
and beta blocker, or

   (2) As an alternative to ACE inhibitor or
ARB when contraindicated due to
renal insufficiency/failure, hyper-
kalemia, angioedema, or bilateral
renal artery stenosis.

3. Assess signs and symptoms of volume overload. Note: Only 35% of patients have "congestive" signs (rales) or symptoms (edema);
therefore, the nurse must carefully assess
for sub-clinical volume overload (Albert,
Eastwood, & Edwards, 2004; Albert,
2005a).

  a. Dyspnea, orthopnea, paroxysmal noc-
turnal dyspnea.

  b. Edema, ascites, anasarca, acute pulmonary edema.

  c. Worsening cough or rales.

  d. Sudden, unexpected weight gain of two
pounds in one day or five pounds in one
week.

  e. New or worsening S_3 gallop, neck vein
distension, or elevated jugular venous
pressure (> 10 cm. H_2O pressure); positive hepatojugular reflux test.

4. Assess for signs and symptoms of resting
hypoperfusion that may occur with or without
volume overload (Albert, Eastwood, &
Edwards, 2004).

  a. Fatigue, decreased exercise tolerance.

  b. Mental obtundation, dizziness, lightheadedness.

  c. Nausea, anorexia, change in bowel
habits.

  d. Resting tachycardia (> 85 bpm),
decreased systolic blood pressure,
increased intra-cardiac pressures, and
pulsus alternans.

  e. Proportional pulse pressure < 25%. To
obtain proportional pulse pressure, sub-
tract diastolic blood pressure from sys-

tolic blood pressure, then divide results
by systolic blood pressure.

5. Assess for arrhythmias (palpitations, atrial
fibrillation, slow or rapid heart rate, dizziness, lightheadedness, syncope or near-syn-
cope, or irregular heart rate) and cardiac
device therapy functioning (Albert, 2004).

6. Assess serum lab work for electrolyte balance (basic metabolic panel, calcium magnesium), renal function (creatinine), thyroid
function, and ventricular function (B-type
natriuretic peptide [BNP] or N-terminal pro-
brain BNP [NT-proBNP]) (Silver et al., 2004).

7. Assess urinalyses results.

8. Assess electrocardiogram for QRS width,
intraventricular conduction delay, left ventricular hypertrophy, arrhythmias, myocardial
ischemia, injury or infarction, and proper
pacemaker function, when appropriate.

9. Assess for signs and symptoms of hypovolemia.

  a. Flat neck veins.

  b. Dry mucous membranes/mouth.

  c. Clear lung fields, absence of edema.

  d. Signs and symptoms of hypoperfusion
(refer to section 4 above, *Assess for
Signs and Symptoms of Resting
Hypoperfusion...*).

  e. Decreased frequency of urination or
urine volume, dark urine.

  f. Elevated blood urea nitrogen and creatinine.

  g. Dizziness/lightheadedness when changing from lying to standing/sitting that
lasts more than 15 minutes (sustained
orthostatic hypotension).

  h. Headache.

  i. Blurred vision.

10. Determine need for hospitalization (Albert,
Eastwood, & Edwards, 2004).

  a. Hypotension with organ hypoperfusion.

  b. Severe dyspnea.

  c. Profound volume overload, especially if
not relieved with intravenous loop diuretic agent administration in the outpatient
setting.

  d. Severe electrolyte imbalances.

  e. New onset of atrial fibrillation, non-sus-
tained ventricular tachycardia, or other

cardiac rhythm problem requiring immediate evaluation and treatment.

f. New onset of angina or refractory angina, clinical suspicion of myocardial infarction by signs and symptoms, laboratory values, or electrocardiograph reading.

g. Uncontrolled hypertension requiring immediate evaluation and treatment with intravenous agents.

h. Acute pneumonia concomitant with heart failure.

i. Advanced renal or hepatic disease with decompensated heart failure.

11. Determine need for critical care hospitalization due to complex decompensation (Albert, Eastwood, & Edwards, 2004).

a. Severe or refractory symptoms of volume overload and/or resting hypoperfusion (with metabolic sequellae) requiring intravenous preload and afterload reduction, intravenous inotropic therapies, and/or renal therapies (ultrafiltration).

b. Hemodynamic instability requiring right heart catheterization and continuous or intermittent hemodynamic monitoring to augment management of intravenous vasodilator and/or inotropic therapies.

c. Hypoxemia requiring respiratory support via ventilator.

d. Recent respiratory or cardiac arrest.

e. Shock.

f. Complex cardiac arrhythmias requiring close electrocardiographic monitoring and medication and/or technical therapies.

B. Primary, secondary, and tertiary prevention (Albert, Paul, & McCauley, 2003; Hunt et al., 2005).

1. Major modifiable primary and secondary prevention strategies:

a. Hypertension control.

b. Hyperlipidemia control.

c. Cigarette smoking cessation.

d. Promotion of aerobic exercise and regular activity.

e. Weight reduction, if overweight.

f. Prevention of glucose intolerance.

g. Alcohol cessation; limiting caffeine intake; habitual drug withdrawal.

h. Low sodium diet of 2,000 to 3,000 mg/day in Stage CHF.

2. Other secondary prevention strategies:

a. Self-management education related to fluid management (weight monitoring, fluid intake limitation, and managing thirst).

b. Compliance with pharmacologic therapies.

c. Yearly influenza vaccine; pneumococcal vaccine once, repeat after age 65 if first dose received before age 65 and it has been at least 5 years.

d. Regular physical examinations.

e. Social (family) support of life-style changes.

f. Treat depression, anxiety, anemia, renal dysfunction, and other medical conditions that can lead to worsening left ventricular dysfunction.

3. Tertiary prevention (Richards, Troughton, Lainchbury, Doughty, & Wright, 2005; Silver et al., 2004):

a. Prompt recognition and treatment of signs and symptoms of a worsening condition.

(1) Obtaining lab work of ventricular function (B-type natriuretic peptide); renal function (blood urea nitrogen, creatinine, glomerular filtration rate); basic electrolytes; calcium and magnesium; thyroid function; and complete blood count.

(2) Chest film to detect the presence of cardiac enlargement, pulmonary congestion, or other pulmonary disease and electrocardiogram to detect evidence of prior myocardial infarction, left ventricular hypertrophy, cardiac arrhythmia, cardiac dyssynchrony (conduction delays), or diffuse myocardial disease, as necessary.

(3) Pulmonary function test and 24 to 48-hour holter monitor, as necessary for pulmonary dysfunction and cardiac electrophysiology issues, respectively.

b. Identification and treatment of exacer-

bating factors:
  (1) See primary and secondary prevention.
  (2) New or worsening stress.
  (3) Atrial arrhythmias, especially tachyarrhythmias.
  (4) Infection.
  (5) Anemia.
  (6) Chronic obstructive pulmonary disease or asthma.
  (7) Pulmonary emboli.
  (8) Thyroid disease.
  (9) Environmental conditions.
  (10) Pregnancy.
  (11) Clinical depression.
  (12) Cardiac valve dysfunction (regurgitation and stenosis), cardiac congenital conditions.
C. Clinical procedures (Hunt et al., 2005; Jessup, 2003).
  1. Two-dimensional echocardiogram (coupled with Doppler flow study when possible) or radionuclide ventriculography: to evaluate the presence and severity of left ventricular systolic dysfunction (ejection fraction). These tests can reveal segmental wall motion abnormalities.
    a. Echocardiogram: Can assess chamber size, valve abnormalities, pericardial effusion, ventricular thrombus, presence of cardiac hypertrophy, and degree of cardiac dyssynchrony.
      (1) Echocardiogram is the single, most useful diagnostic tool in the evaluation of HF.
      (2) Echocardiogram is less expensive and more generally available than radionuclide ventriculography; it does not require preparation.
    b. Radionuclide ventriculogram requires venipuncture and radiation exposure; it does not require preparation.
  2. Special studies.
    a. Diagnostic right heart catheterization/hemodynamics: Catheter inserted into a vein and guided to the right side of the heart to determine low cardiac output and elevated right ventricular filling pressures. Uses local anesthetics; it does

not require preparation.
    b. Electrophysiologic testing: Heart catheterization that records electrical activity in the heart and can reveal serious rhythm disturbances after electrical stimulation.
    c. Maximal cardiopulmonary exercise testing: Graded treadmill or bicycle exercise protocol to measure total duration of exercise and peak oxygen consumption. Does not require preparation except to hold medications as necessary.
  3. Routine assessment, metabolic status assessment (diabetes, lipids, weight).
D. Collaboration/resource identification and referral (Grady et al., 2000).
  1. Ancillary services: Nutrition, social work, pharmacy, cardiac or physical rehabilitation, case manager.
  2. Preventive cardiologist, HF specialist cardiologist, palliative care medicine, endocrinologist, pulmonologist, nephrologist.
  3. Group therapy programs (smoking cessation, stress management, relaxation, regular group office visits), HF education/social support group.
  4. Cardiothoracic surgeon for hibernating myocardium, congenital conditions requiring surgical treatment, cardiac valve disorders, dyskinesis (with or without aneurysm) or local akinesis of left ventricle after transmural myocardial infarction (Leier, 2005).
E. Care management (Hunt et al., 2005).
  1. Medical therapies.
    a. Determine need for changes based on patient signs and symptoms or other objective measures (laboratory results, device or testing results).
    b. Routine medication up-titration (to target doses based on dosages used in large, randomized clinical trials) as tolerated for ACE inhibitors and beta-blocker therapies.
    c. Addition of medications if HF is worsening: Loop diuretic and digoxin therapies; aldosterone inhibitor, ARB or hydralazine/isosorbide dinitrate.
    d. Implantable cardioverter defibrillator and/or cardiac resynchronization therapy (CRT of bi-ventricular pacemaker), if

criteria for use are met (Brennan & Haas, 2005; Wickliffe & Leon, 2005).

2. Regular evaluation of self-care practices, education needs, and symptoms.

3. Regular surveillance monitoring via telephone or other means following an emergency department visit, inpatient hospitalization, or if history of therapy noncompliance.

4. Assess psychosocial issues: Anxiety, depression, social isolation.

5. If implantable cardiac device is in place (hemodynamic monitor, cardiac resynchronization therapy [CRT] and/or implantable cardioverter defibrillator with or without cardiac function parameters), regular surveillance of data after patient transmission to a secure computer server; regular consultation with electrophysiologist cardiologist team to ensure device is operating properly.

F. Patient education (Albert, Paul, & McCauley, 2003; Koelling, Johnson, Cody, & Aaronson, 2005).

1. Knowledge of heart failure, including prognosis; Signs and symptoms of worsening condition; when to access health care.

2. Medication management; adherence to prescriptions, side effects; polypharmacy issues.

3. Recommend a 2,000 to 3,000 mg sodium diet; low animal fat diet; limit alcohol intake; limit caffeine intake.

4. Fluid management; daily weight monitoring, fluid restriction/monitoring, tips to quench thirst.

5. Activity and exercise; increasing activity level safely including performing warm-up and cool-down exercises when exercising aerobically; prevention of overexertion.

6. Health promotion strategies.

   a. Self management of symptoms (dyspnea, weight gain, dizziness/lightheadedness).

   b. Risk factor modification (smoking, stress, alcohol, obesity, over-the-counter medications that may worsen HF).

   c. Followup management (flu shot, regular check-ups with HF team and other care providers to control other chronic conditions).

d. Self-monitoring of blood pressure and heart rate, including when to notify provider of changes.

e. If cardiac device (CRT-implantable cardioverter defibrillator) that has an internal alarm, takes steps recommended by provider when alarm sounds.

7. Prognosis counseling.

G. Advocacy: There is a great need for patient advocacy in HF. Current HF research literature has led to an alteration in patient management recommendations, and past assumptions regarding care no longer apply in today's health care environment. In the past, rest was promoted; currently, exercise and activity are promoted. In the past, beta-blocker therapy was contraindicated because it has a negative inotropic effect (worsens contractility); now, selective beta-blocker therapy is recommended because it favorably alters neurohormone levels and leads to regression on cardiac remodeling. Internal cardiac devices are becoming more sophisticated. For example, internal impedance cardiography is available through a CRT-implantable cardioverter defibrillator device. Nurses must understand newer technology and be able to interface with data provided to optimize care delivery. Nurses are a key link to physician ordering practices, especially when the nurse initiates communication with the physician regarding patient complaints, symptoms, and needs. Nurses must be proactive in clearly communicating the patient's situation and offering ideas based on current consensus recommendations so that patient quality of life is optimized and survival is prolonged. Nurses are stakeholders in outpatient disease management programs that transition patients from an acute hospitalization to the outpatient environment. Programs designed for primary care are successful in improving outcomes (Hershberger et al., 2005).

1. Nurse knowledge of advanced pathophysiology concepts (ventricular remodeling, neuroendocrine changes, effects on the vascular and end-organ systems).

2. Nurse knowledge of the hemodynamic goals of therapy (Albert, Eastwood, & Edwards, 2004):

   a. Optimized systolic blood pressure.

      (1) Lowest systolic blood pressure that

maintains mentation and urine output, and does not cause long suffering orthostasis (dizziness and light-headedness).

    (2) 80 mm Hg; 90 mm Hg in the frail elderly.

  b. Optimized afterload values and definitions if using non-invasive hemodynamic monitoring to guide therapy.

    (1) 800 to 1,200 dynes/sec/cm^{-5} or uses systolic blood pressure value.

    (2) Lowest value that leads to an increase/maintenance of cardiac index and does *not* cause systolic blood pressure and/or renal perfusion to fall, even if cardiac index is increased.

  c. Optimized preload values and definitions if using noninvasive hemodynamic monitoring to guide therapy.

    (1) Right atrial pressure of 5 to 8 mm Hg or 6 to 11 cm H_2O; right internal jugular venous pressure of <6 to 9 cm H_2O; pulmonary artery wedge pressure of 8 to 15 mm Hg.

    (2) The lowest preload value that can be maintained without a decrease in systolic blood pressure and/or cardiac index.

3. Nurse knowledge of the pharmacologic goals of therapy; steps to reach goals, and measures to minimize and/or alleviate side effects and complications.

4. Nurse understanding and communication of HF non-pharmacologic principles related to cardiac device management and self-care.

5. Common errors in patient management that can be overcome through advocacy (Albert, Paul, & McCauley, 2003):

  a. Nonaggressive treatment in managing concomitant hypertension.

  b. Inadequate patient, family, and caregiver education.

  c. Inappropriate treatment when HF is not due to systolic dysfunction.

  d. Close weight monitoring is not specifically stated and/or the patient does not understand what to do (self-management) with slight weight changes to decrease risk of worsening symptoms.

  e. Causes of patient noncompliance are not recognized and/or acted on appropriately.

  f. In patients with chronic coronary artery disease (three vessel disease) and systolic dysfunction, myocardial metabolic function must be assessed and revascularization must be considered.

  g. In patients with severe mitral regurgitation and systolic dysfunction, mitral valve repair is often not considered.

  h. In patients with cardiac devices (pacemakers, defibrillator, or hemodynamic monitor), care coordination with electrophysiology cardiologist is lacking.

  i. Heart transplantation referral is often delayed and severe decompensation or secondary multi-system organ failure develops.

  j. Cardiac rehabilitation program or an exercise prescription is underused.

  k. Home health care specialty program in HF is underused in home-bound patients.

  l. Suboptimal dosing (too low or too high) of ACE inhibitor, aldosterone inhibitor, digoxin, and/or beta-blocker may be based on concerns of possible side or adverse effects rather than on actual issues.

  m. Underdosing of diuretics when overt or sub-clinical signs and symptoms of volume overload persist.

  n. Failure to remove medications from the patient's pharmacologic profile that have been clearly shown to cause deleterious effects.

  o. Failure to offer self-management instructions to offset the development of symptoms of worsening condition. Assuming that telling the patient to "call your doctor" is adequate instruction when symptoms develop or worsen in severity.

  p. Not providing prompt response and early intervention to patients when they phone the office with complaints or new symptoms.

  q. Failure to communicate to the patient whom to call when symptoms occur.

Patients have multiple care providers and because symptoms of HF are often non-specific, patients do not know who to notify for problems.

H. Telehealth practice.
1. Rapid response telephone practice:
   a. Priority evaluation protocols that direct the patient to an immediate emergency department visit, when necessary.
   b. Assessment of past medical history and HF history.
   c. Cardiac medication assessment including recent changes or additions/deletions.
   d. Current symptom(s) assessment including onset and severity.
   e. Treatment plans for fluid overload, hypoperfusion, and for symptoms that reflect worsening HF with or without obvious volume overload. These plans need to offer specific treatment options (for example, additional dose of diuretic, hold ACE inhibitor) rather than just referring the patient to the emergency department or an office visit the following day.
2. Surveillance or vigilance monitoring programs:
   a. Physical and psychosocial status; current symptoms.
   b. Compliance with the pharmacologic and nonpharmacologic plan of care.
3. Patient education and counseling programs.
4. Care coordination programs.
I. Communication/documentation.
1. Subjective and objective assessment and plan of care.
2. Patient understands education taught and adherence with the plan of care.
3. Patient and/or nurse initiated followup telephone calls or results from another surveillance system, including cardiac device data.
4. Ancillary program results: Home health care or cardiac rehabilitation programs.
J. Outcomes management.
1. Determine standards of chronic HF care utilizing one or more of the following resources:
   a. American Heart Association/American College of Cardiology consensus rec-

ommendations for the management of chronic HF (Hunt et al., 2005).
   b. Heart Failure Society of America recommendations for the management of chronic HF (Heart Failure Society of America, 1999).
2. Identify outcomes and benchmarks.
   a. Based on national consensus performance measures/recommendations from the American Heart Association/ American College of Cardiology and the Joint Commission on Accreditation of Healthcare Organizations (JCAHO) (American College of Cardiology/American Heart Association Task Force on Performance, 2005b; JCAHO, 2005).
   b. Based on local or regional issues of concern (patient knowledge, co-morbid conditions, quality of life, self-care ability, coordination of care, promotion and/or adherence to standards, hospitalization intervals, mortality, etc.).
3. Develop interventions to meet outcomes.
   a. Multidisciplinary team.
   b. Physician champion who understands the complexity of HF and is an expert in this field of care.
K. Protocol development/usage (Albert & Young, 2001):
1. Pharmacologic therapy algorithms for ACE inhibitors, beta-blockers, diuretics, digoxin, hydralazine, nitrates, ARBs, and aldosterone antagonists.
   a. Initiation and up-titration schedules.
   b. Serum electrolyte, vital signs, and other monitoring.
2. Decision tree based on clinical severity of symptoms (mild, moderate, or severe).
3. Device therapy algorithms for CRT, implantable cardioverter defibrillator, and implantable hemodynamic monitor.
4. How to treat persistent:
   a. Volume overload.
   b. Dyspnea.
   c. Hypertension.
   d. Concomitant angina.
   e. Concomitant atrial fibrillation.
   f. Hypotension.

5. Education.
    a. Heart failure cause, signs and symptoms, chronicity, prognosis, and ways it can be controlled.
    b. Self-care actions.
    c. Who to call for symptoms and issues.
6. Surveillance/compliance monitoring questionnaire or system.
7. Patient-initiated communication (rapid-response program) algorithm regarding treatment options based on current symptom or signs.
8. Multidisciplinary consultation and support group expectations (such as an aggressive home care HF program).
9. When to consult a HF specialist.
10. When should a patient be directly hospitalized; routine floor versus intermediate care versus critical care environment.
11. End-of-life issues and guidelines (Albert, 2005b).

Chronic Obstructive Pulmonary Disease

Patient Population: Adult
Candia Baker Laughlin, MS, RN, C

Chronic obstructive pulmonary disease (COPD) is a major cause of morbidity and mortality, and like other chronic, virtually irreversible conditions, may require frequent office visits for ongoing management as well as for acute exacerbations. In countries from which data are available, the prevalence of COPD is estimated to range between 4 and 10% of the population, and is highest in countries in which cigarette smoking is most common (Ferguson & Make, 2005). It is currently the fourth leading cause of death in the U.S. and in the world, and further increases in the prevalence and the mortality are anticipated in the coming decades (Murray & Lopez, 1997a; 1997b). The costs of this disease are not only those associated with health care (physician office and emergency department visits and hospitalizations) and premature death, but also indirect costs due to lost work days.

The Global Initiative for Chronic Obstructive Lung Disease (GOLD) is a report from an expert panel convened in 1998 by the National Heart, Lung and Blood Institute (NHLBI) and the World Health Organization (WHO). The goals for the panel were to raise awareness of COPD and to promote control of this major public health concern. The consensus report was a first step, and many of the recommendation continue to be studied and refined as they are implemented (NHLBI/WHO Workshop, 2005).

The GOLD report defined Chronic Obstructive Pulmonary Disease (COPD) as, "A disease state characterized by airflow limitation that is not fully reversible. Airflow limitation is usually progressive and associated with an abnormal inflammatory response of the lungs to noxious particles or gases" (NHLBI/WHO, 2005, p.11). Emphysema is the abnormal enlargement of airspaces distal to the terminal bronchioles with destruction of their walls without obvious fibrosis (Ferguson & Make, 2005). Chronic bronchitis is the presence of a productive cough for 3 months in each of 2 successive years in those whom other causes of chronic cough have been excluded. Patients with unremitting asthma are also classified as having COPD. There are overlaps of these three disorders (for example, some patients have both asthma and chronic bronchitis), but there are also individuals with these diseases considered NOT to have COPD, while others do. The reversibility of the airflow limitation is the key diagnostic criteria. Alpha-1 antitrypsin (AAT) deficiency is a genetic abnormality that predisposes one to lung disease, such that those with this finding may develop COPD in their 30s or 40s, especially if they smoke.

A. Assess/screen/triage.
    1. History.
        a. Smoking history.
            (1) Age at initiation.
            (2) Average amount smokes since initiation in packs.
            (3) Date stopped, if patient stopped.
            (4) Occupational exposure to dusts or chemicals.
            (5) Symptomatic COPD typically found with 20 cigarettes/day for 20 or more years.
        b. Age: COPD usually presents in the 5th decade with a productive cough or acute illness. Dyspnea on exertion usually occurs in mid-60s to early 70s.
        c. Chronic cough with sputum production.
            (1) Initially occurs in morning.

(2) Daily volume rarely exceeds 60 cc.

(3) Mucoid, but becomes purulent with exacerbations.

   d. Wheezing may or may not be associated with cough or exertional dyspnea.

   e. Acute chest illness occurs intermittently and with increased frequency.

    (1) Increased cough.

    (2) Purulent sputum.

    (3) Wheezing.

    (4) Dyspnea.

    (5) Fever.

   f. Late stages of COPD.

    (1) Hypoxia with cyanosis.

    (2) Morning headaches suggest hypercapnia.

    (3) Hypercapnia with severe hypoxemia (end stage).

    (4) Cor pulmonale with right heart failure and edema.

    (5) Hemopytsis.

2. Physical examination.

   a. Chest auscultation.

    (1) Slowed expiration becomes more prolonged as disease progresses.

    (2) Wheezing.

    (3) Decreased breath sounds.

    (4) Heart sounds distant as anterior-posterior (A-P) diameter increases.

    (5) Coarse bi-basilar crackles.

   b. Positioning in end-stage disease – To relieve dyspnea; may lean forward with arms outstretched and weight supported on palms.

   c. Use of accessory muscles of neck and shoulders.

   d. Paradoxical in-drawing of lower interspaces (Hoover's sign).

   e. Expiration through pursed lips.

   f. Cyanosis.

   g. Enlarged, tender liver with right heart failure.

   h. Asterixis ("flapping tremor") with acute hypercapnia.

   i. Neck vein distention, especially during expiration.

3. Laboratory/radiology.

   a. Chest radiography.

    (1) Low, flat diaphragm.

    (2) Increased retrosternal airspace.

    (3) Long, narrow heart shadow.

    (4) Hyper-trans-radiance and bullae.

   b. Computed tomography (CT).

    (1) Not indicated for routine care since information rarely alters therapy.

    (2) Indicated for consideration of pulmonary resection or diagnosis of bronchiectasis.

   c. Pulmonary function tests (PFTs) – Necessary for diagnosing and assessing severity of obstruction.

    (1) Forced expiratory volume at 1 second (FEV1).

    (2) Forced vital capacity (FVC).

    (3) FEV1/FVC ratio.

    (4) Carbon monoxide diffusing capacity.

    (5) Spirometry with bronchodilators.

    (6) Arterial blood gases.

   d. Sputum culture for suspected infections.

4. Functional status.

   a. Impact on activities of daily living (for example, able to participate in activities outside the home, climbing stairs).

   b. Level of dependence on others (for example, ability to manage medications and prepare own meals).

   c. Nutritional status (for example, weight loss, protein intake, balanced intake).

   d. Rest and comfort (for example, ability to recline for sleep).

   e. Emotional status (for example, anxiety secondary to air hunger, depression).

5. Staging of COPD.

   a. Classification of severity of COPD (NHLBI/WHO, 2005).

    (1) Scores 0 ("at risk") to IV ("very severe COPD").

    (2) Uses symptoms, FEV1 and FEV1/FVC ratios.

    (3) Classification of Severity not yet validated (Vestbo & Lange, 2002).

   b. BODE.

    (1) Scores include:

     (a) **B**ody mass index (BMI).

     (b) **O**bstruction of airflow as indicated by FEV1.

     (c) **D**yspnea on Modified Medical Research Council dyspnea scale

(MMRC).
- (d) **E**xercise capability – 6-minute walk test.
- (2) Used to indicate risk of death.
- (3) Not fully adopted, in part because 6-minute walk test is difficult to administer in most office settings (Celli et al, 2004).

B. Primary, secondary, tertiary prevention.
1. Primary prevention.
   a. Risk factor identification.
      (1) Tobacco smoke.
      (2) Air pollution.
      (3) Hyper-responsive airways.
      (4) Second-hand smoke.
      (5) Occupational exposure to industrial pollutants.
      (6) Alpha 1-antitrypsin deficiency.
   b. Education programs.
      (1) National Lung Health Education Program.
      (2) American Lung Association.
      (3) Alpha 1 Association/Alpha One Foundation.
2. Secondary prevention.
   a. Smoking cessation.
      (1) Group therapy.
      (2) Pharmacologic therapy.
      (3) Hypnosis.
   b. Pharmacologic therapy.
      (1) Bronchodilators – Beta$_2$-agonists, anticholinergic agents, theophylline.
      (2) Corticosteroids.
      (3) Mucolytic agents.
      (4) Antibiotics, when indicated.
      (5) Psychoactive agents
      (6) Cardiovascular agents, as needed.
      (7) Immunizations (influenza annually and pneumococcal pneumonia once; repeat after age 65 at least 5 years after the first).
   c. Surgical treatments.
      (1) Bullectomy.
      (2) Lung volume reduction.
      (3) Lung transplantation.
3. Tertiary prevention.
   a. Pulmonary rehabilitation.
      (1) Exercise training that improves large muscle groups and relates to activities of daily living.
      (2) Education about the disease and behavioral changes.
      (3) Psychosocial support.
      (4) Breathing retraining.
      (5) Nutrition and weight control, including use of supplements, as indicated.
      (6) Mobilization of secretions.
      (7) Antioxidant vitamins (beta-carotene, vitamins C and E) supplements (recommendations not definitive).
   b. Long-term oxygen therapy.
      (1) Determination of need.
      (2) Oxygen systems.
      (3) Oxygen delivery methods.
      (4) Reimbursement criteria.

C. Clinical procedures.
1. Assisting with initiation of supplemental oxygen therapy.
2. Measuring pulse oximetry.
3. Drawing of arterial blood gases.
4. Spirometry.
5. Nebulizer mist treatment.
6. Pulmonary hygiene, such as percussion and postural drainage, suctioning.

D. Collaboration/resource identification and referral.
1. Primary care physician/nurse practitioner.
2. Pulmonologist.
3. Cardiologist.
4. Thoracic surgeon.
5. Respiratory therapist.
6. Home care nurse.
7. Nutrition counselor.
8. Home equipment and oxygen supplier.

E. Care management/telephone practice.
1. Frequency of followup calls based on severity of disease.
2. Assess for need of a followup visit/hospitalization.
   a. Response of symptoms to outpatient management.
   b. Ability to eat and sleep.
   c. Ability to walk between rooms (patient previously mobile).
   d. Family opinion of patient's ability to manage at home.
   e. High-risk co-morbid conditions.
   f. Prolonged, progressive symptoms.
   g. Altered mental capacity

　　　h.　Level of dyspnea
　　　i.　Sputum production.
　3.　Assess patient's understanding of current therapeutic regimen.
　4.　Assess psychosocial issues and home supports.
　5.　Maintain contact with home care providers.
　6.　Assess functioning of equipment.
　7.　Documentation of discussion and changes in care management.
F.　Patient education.
　1.　Smoking cessation (see Chapter 19, *Patient Education and Counseling*).
　2.　Oxygen therapy.
　3.　Medication management (Ferguson & Make, 2005).
　　　a.　Sympathomimetic agents – Have been the mainstay of COPD treatment.
　　　　　(1)　Selective beta-2 agonists (such as albuterol) provide rapid onset of bronchodilation.
　　　　　(2)　Role of long-acting beta-2 agonists (such as salmeterol and formoterol) still being determined.
　　　b.　Anticholinergic bronchodilators (such as ipratropium and triotropium) now considered integral part of treatment. May be used in combination with beta adrenergic agonists with additive effect compared to either agent alone.
　　　c.　Methylxanthines (aminophylline and theophylline). Use is controversial.
　　　d.　Corticosteroids, bursts and tapers and long-term therapy. Chronic administration may have severe adverse effects, but approximately 20% of stable COPD patients have improvement of airflow with oral corticosteroid therapy.
　　　e.　Mucokinetic agents. Little evidence supporting their effectiveness in COPD.
　　　f.　Antibiotics for acute exacerbation with purulent secretions. Culture and gram stain not required for initial management. Generally recommend prescription of amoxicillin, doxycycline, or trimethaprim-sulfamethoxazole for 10-day course.
　4.　Methods of mediation administration.
　　　a.　Oral.
　　　b.　Inhaled – Inhaled route preferred for

some bronchodilators because it may provide more direct effect on lungs with fewer systemic side effects.
　　　　　(1)　Metered dose inhalers.
　　　　　(2)　Spacers.
　　　　　(3)　Nebulizer mist treatments.
　5.　Nutrition.
　6.　Breathing techniques.
　7.　Exercising and pacing of activity.
　8.　Mobilization of secretions.
　9.　Prevention and treatment of infections.
　10.　Early recognition and seeking care for an exacerbation.
　11.　Travel guidelines (in-flight oxygen requirements).
　12.　Advance directives.
G.　Advocacy.
　1.　Interact with caregivers in other areas.
　2.　Meet with outpatient management team on a regular basis.
　3.　Patient support/education organizations, such as the American Lung Association Network (http://lungaction.com).
H.　Outcome management.
　1.　Improved exercise tolerance.
　2.　Decreased dyspnea.
　3.　Decreased anxiety/depression.
　4.　Improved quality of life and functional status.
　5.　Decreased healthcare utilization.
　6.　Improved survival rate.
I.　Protocol development/usage.
　1.　Cessation of smoking.
　2.　Pharmacologic therapy for the COPD patient.
　3.　Indications for long-term oxygen therapy.
　4.　Indications for emergency room evaluation and/or hospitalization of COPD patients with acute exacerbation.
　5.　Management of the preoperative patient with COPD.
　6.　Criteria for lung volume reduction surgery or lung transplantation, and assisted pre- and post-surgical care.

Table 22-1.

Diagnostic Criteria for Diabetes

	Fasting Gucose	Random	Comments
Not Diabetes	70-99 mg/dl		Screen after age 45 if no risk factors or symptoms.
Pre-Diabetes	100-125 mg/dl		Screen adults under age 45, including children if risk factors.
Diabetes	126 mg/dl or higher on 2 separate occasions or	200 mg/dl or higher with symptoms	

Diabetes Mellitus

Patient Population: Adult
Linda L. Edwards, RN, MHS, CDE
Christine Schaefer, MSN, RN, CDE, BC-ADM

Diabetes mellitus, a serious chronic disease, affects more than 20.8 million people in the U.S., consuming $132 billion health care dollars in 2002. Diabetes is the seventh leading cause of death in the U.S. People with diabetes are at increased risk for heart disease, strokes, blindness, kidney disease, and amputations (Centers for Disease Control and Prevention [CDC], 2005).

Approximately 75% of all people with diabetes receive their medical care in the primary care setting (Herbst, 2002). The nurse who works in an ambulatory setting, especially in primary care, can significantly and positively impact quality of care for people with diabetes by coordinating a multidisciplinary team utilizing the Chronic Care Model. In most successful interventions, the nurse acts as a central case manager, educating and coordinating care among multiple disciplines, including the primary care team, certified diabetes educators (CDEs), nurses and dietitians, endocrinologists, and other specialists, as needed (Wagner, 2000).

Diabetes care and management knowledge, tools, and strategies change frequently with the integration of new research evidence into practice. It may be difficult for the ambulatory care nurse to remain current in diabetes management issues in addition to other areas of practice. Many organizations are implementing basic competencies for nurs-

es in those areas of practice that include high-volume and high-risk patient groups. The ambulatory care nurse does not need to demonstrate *expert* knowledge and skill in *all* areas of diabetes care and education; however, it is recommended that the nurse demonstrate *basic* diabetes competencies.

A. Assess, screen, triage.
  1. Risk factors.
     a. Obesity.
     b. First degree relative with diabetes.
     c. High-risk population: African American, Hispanic, Native American, and Asian.
     d. Previous gestational diabetes, baby over 9 lbs, history of glucose intolerance.
     e. History of insulin-resistant syndrome or polycystic ovarian syndrome (PCOS).
  2. Diagnosis.
     a. Criteria (see Table 22-1).
     b. Type 1 diabetes.
        (1) Onset: Usually acute with pronounced symptoms.
        (2) Etiology: Autoimmune disease characterized by loss of pancreatic beta cell function.
        (3) Treatment: Insulin required in a regimen designed for the individual in a way that imitates non-diabetes insulin production (for example, 3 to 4 injections/day for optimal control).
     c. Type 2 diabetes.
        (1) Onset usually gradual, with or without symptoms in those with a fami-

ly history of type 2 diabetes, and other risk factors.

    (2) Insulin production at onset may be normal or elevated, but insulin resistance, elevated liver production of glucose, and other factors may prevent insulin from functioning normally.

    (3) Treatment includes healthy eating, exercise, oral medications, and/or insulin to control blood glucose levels.

3. Diabetes history.

  a. Diabetes: Date of diagnosis, success of previous treatment(s).

  b. Current status: Blood glucose (BG) patterns, acute complications, presenting problem(s), symptoms.

  c. Hypertension, other diagnoses, co-morbidities.

  d. Presence of diabetes complications, foot infections.

4. Life style.

  a. Current weight, weight changes.

  b. Eating patterns: Usual foods, meal/snack times, portion sizes.

  c. Exercise/activity patterns.

  d. Smoking and alcohol usage.

  e. Stress levels, coping skills, and stress management patterns.

  f. Social/family support systems.

5. Laboratory parameters.

  a. Blood glucose control: Fasting glucose, Hemoglobin A1c.

  b. Fasting lipid panel.

  c. Kidney function: Urine microalbumin and serum creatinine.

B. Primary, secondary, tertiary prevention.

1. Primary prevention: There is no known primary prevention strategy to prevent type 1 diabetes. The Diabetes Prevention Program Trials showed that people with pre-diabetes could significantly delay or even prevent the onset of type 2 diabetes by lifestyle modification (weight loss of 7% of body weight and moderate exercise 30 minutes per day, 5 days per week).

2. Secondary prevention: Preventing/delaying the onset of diabetes-related long-term complications through the achievement of appropriate blood glucose control, BP and lipid

management, through time.

3. Tertiary prevention: Management of the complications of diabetes, retinopathy, neuropathy, nephropathy, and cardiovascular complications to reduce to morbidity and mortality associated with these problems.

C. Clinical procedures *American Diabetes Association [ADA] Clinical Practice Recommendations* (ADA, 2005).

1. Blood glucose monitoring.

  a. Observe the patient perform BG test with own meter.

  b. Evaluate patient BG patterns on the patient's record.

2. Foot examination.

  a. Annual comprehensive foot examination, including evaluation of skin integrity, circulation status, sensitivity (using monofilament), and deformities.

  b. Visual inspection of feet at each visit for signs of infection.

3. Treatment plan.

  a. Medical nutrition therapy (MNT): Individualized meal plan, facilitated by an RD, CDE when possible, which addresses BG goals, patient goals, family/work schedule, cultural traditions, and timing according to medications/insulin being used.

  b. Medication.

    (1) Oral diabetes medications (see Table 22-2).

      (a) Sulfonylureas increase insulin production (may cause hypoglycemia).

      (b) Biguanides, thiazolidinediones improve effectiveness of insulin.

      (c) Alpha-glucosidase inhibitor, delay glucose absorption.

    (2) Insulin or insulin mixtures (see Table 22-3): very fast-acting, fast-acting, intermediate-acting, and long-acting.

    (3) Many new medications are in clinical trials, while others have been approved recently by the FDA (see Table 22-4).

  c. Physical activity: Negotiated level of activity, including type of exercise, inten-

Table 22-2.

Oral Diabetes Medications

Generic Name	Brand Name	Dosage Range	Comments
Sulfonylureas			
Glipizide	Glucatrol® Glucatrol XL®	2.5-40 mg 5-20 mg (once daily)	Once or twice daily dosing. Stimulates increased insulin production. May be used alone or in combination with Metformin®, Acarbose®, or insulin.
Glyburide	Diabeta Micronase®	1.25-20 mg	
Glimeperide	Glynase PresTab® Amaryl®	0.75-12 mg 1-8 mg once/day	**All in this class can cause hypoglycemia.**
Biguanides			**Contraindicated: Elevated creatinine.**
Metformin	Glucophage®	500-2550 mg twice daily dosing	**Caution: History of CHF.** May be used alone or in combination with sulfonylurea and/or insulin. May cause flatulence, diarrhea. Does not cause hypoglycemia when used alone.
Miglitinides			
Repaglinide	Prandin®	0.5-2 mg with meals	Short-acting, meal coverage, and may cause hypoglycemia.
Nateglinide	Starlix®	60-120 mg with meals	
Alpha-Glucosidase Inhibitors			
Acarbose	Precose®	75-300 mg	Taken 3 times/day with meals. Delays carbohydrate digestion and glucose absorption. Used alone or in combination with other orals/insulin.
Miglitol	Glyset®	25 mg tid	Take with first bite of food.
Thiozolodine Dione			**Contraindicated in those with impaired liver function, CHF.**
Pioglitizone	Actos®	15-45 mg daily	This class of drugs improves insulin sensitivity at cellular level; may cause edema, headache, weight gain.
Rosiglitizone	Avandia®	4-8 mg daily	
Combination drugs			
Glucovance	Glyburide® and Metformin®		All in this class have varying dose combinations.
Avandamet	Avandia® and Metformin®		
Metaglip	Glipizide® and, Metformin®		

Table 22-3.

Commonly Used Insulin Preparations

Insulin	Starts	Peaks	Ends	Check BG Effect
Rapid-acting Humulog® (Lispro) Novolog® (Aspart)	10 minutes	1.5 hours	3 hours	2-4 hours after injection
Fast-acting Humulin® Novolin® (Regular)	30 minutes	3-4 hours	3-7 hours	Before next meal
Intermediate-acting Humulin® N Novolin® N (NPH)	2 hours	4-12 hours	6-12 hours	AM dose: Before dinner PM dose: Before breakfast
Long-acting Lantus® (Glargine)	2-4 hours	Peakless	20-24 hours	Basal insulin, cannot mix with other insulins

Note: There are several pre-mixed insulin combinations (Humulin® 70/30 and Novolin® 70/30) also pre-mixed combinations of the newer insulin analogues (Humulog® Mix 75/25 and Novolog® Mix 70/30). Many insulin preparations and pre-mixed combinations are available in a variety of injection delivery devices, such as disposable and refillable pens.

Table 22-4.

Incretin Mimetics

Name	Action	Dose	Comments
Exenatide injection (Byetta®)	Stimulates post-meal insulin secretion, restores 1st phase insulin production	5 mcg bid for 1 month, then 10 mcg bid	For patients with type 2 diabetes on 2 or more oral meds w/o adequate control. Can cause nausea, fullness, weight loss.
Pramlintide injection (Simlin®)	Synthetic analogue of human amylin from beta cells. Helps to control post-meal glucose levels	Titrated doses injected before each meal	For patients with type 1 diabetes or those with type 2 diabetes treated with insulin. Insulin doses should be reduced. Can cause nausea.

Note: This is a new class of medications approved in 2005.
Source: Amylin Pharmaceuticals, Inc., 2006

sity, frequency, and timing in relation to meals and medications.

  d. Blood glucose monitoring: Frequency of routine testing, additional testing to determine causes of BG problems, such as hypoglycemia.

    (1) Hemoglobin A1c (A1c): A lab test that reflects a 3-month BG average and risk for microvascular disease.

    (2) A1c target: In general, less than 7.0%, ideal less than 6.0%.

    (3) Targets individualized to minimize risk of hypoglycemia.

  e. Followup plan: Includes expectations for both routine followup and when to contact physician when BG pattern changes or problems occur.

    (1) Next contact for routine review of BG patterns.

    (2) Next physician visit.

    (3) When lab tests are due.

    (4) When next eye exam and foot exam are due.

4. Blood pressure management.

  a. Target: <130/80.

  b. ACE inhibitors drug of choice for managing hypertension in people with diabetes, has additional renal-protective benefit.

  c. Additional agents may be needed to reach blood pressure target.

5. Lipid management.

  a. Nutrition management.

  b. Lipid-lowering drugs, if needed, to achieve LDL cholesterol level <100.

6. Management of hypoglycemia (in patients taking sulfonylureas and/or insulin).

  a. Assess for signs and symptoms each visit/encounter.

  b. Evaluate BG patterns for wide fluctuations which include BG below normal.

  c. Determine causes, whether clinical management or patient behavior, and implement intervention to reduce possibility of future episodes.

  d. Establish followup plan to be followed until BG stable.

7. Management of acute hyperglycemia, "sick days": Blood glucose over 240 mg/dl or presence of infection, gastroenteritis, other acute illness including fever, nausea, diarrhea.

  a. High-risk for severe hyperglycemia, dehydration, ketoacidosis; requires hospitalization if treatment delayed or inadequate.

  b. Requires immediate intervention: Guidance for the patient to maintain hydration and short-term, frequent advice about insulin adjustments, and blood glucose and urine ketone monitoring.

  c. Ambulatory IV fluid administration if patient unable to maintain hydration.

D. Collaboration, resource identification, and referral.

1. Endocrinology.

  a. Recommended for all patients with type 1 diabetes, those with multiple endocrinopathies, and those with other complex management issues.

  b. Provide ongoing support, education to primary care providers.

2. Certified diabetes educators: RNs, RDs, and other professionals with diabetes education experience who have passed the CDE examination (Franz, 2003).

  a. Provide patient education, individually or in groups, to support patient progress toward self-management.

  b. Provide education and support to the primary care team and other professionals regarding standards of care, management of complex issues, and changes in current knowledge base and state-of-the-art care.

3. Resources supporting appropriate routine care:

  a. Pharmacy.

  b. Ophthalmology.

  c. Podiatry.

  d. Exercise specialist, physical therapist.

  e. Mental health professionals.

4. Resources to manage diabetes complications/special needs.

  a. Nephrology.

  b. Cardiology.

  c. Neurology.

  d. Other as needed: Gastroenterology,

obstetrics and gynecology, urology and home care.

E. Care management (Ward & Rieve, 2001).

   1. Primary care.

      a. Blood glucose management and medication management in uncomplicated cases: Newly diagnosed and stable type 2 diabetes.

      b. Facilitate patient achievement of diabetes control goals and manage episodes of blood glucose variations to regain stability.

      c. Facilitate appropriate ongoing care and access to appropriate resources according to patient needs.

   2. Diabetes care management.

      a. The nurse should be trained in diabetes management/education, care management, and diabetes risk reduction strategies.

      b. Targets population segments that have dropped out of routine care, are at known risk for diabetes complications (elevated HbA1c levels), and/or those who frequently utilize health care resources inappropriately (frequent ED, hospital admissions).

      c. Provide diabetes management, education, access to appropriate resources, and followup for a pre-determined period of time or until the patient has engaged in the process of active participation in the care and management of his or her own diabetes.

      d. Goals: Improved clinical outcomes, risk reduction, reduced cost, appropriate resource utilization.

F. Patient education.

   1. Basic skills: Provided/coordinated by primary care team; immediate knowledge and skills the patient needs to perform the treatment plan safely without supervision (Edwards, 1999).

      a. Type of diabetes, treatment plan elements, BG targets.

      b. Eats reasonably appropriate meals at consistently spaced times (does not skip meals).

      c. BG monitoring.

      d. Takes medication(s)/insulin correctly.

      e. Recognizes signs/symptoms of hypoglycemia and treats promptly.

      f. Followup plan: When to call for BG extremes, routine followup, next steps.

   2. Intermediate: Referral to Diabetes Education Program, preferably ADA recognized as meeting the Standards of Care for Diabetes Self-Management Education Programs.

      a. *ADA Clinical Practice Recommendations*, 2005.

         (1) Usually group education programs provided by CDEs, which include expanded diabetes management education information and behavior change strategies.

         (2) The patient is able to make appropriate decisions about daily BG management issues and effectively manage BG fluctuations.

         (3) The patient actively participates in his or her own care and uses health care resources appropriately.

   3. Advanced: The patient has knowledge, skill, and motivation to design his or her own treatment plan to meet individual needs.

      a. Example: Type 1 patient who proactively anticipates insulin needs based upon variations in food intake and exercise.

      b. Provided by expert diabetes team, experienced in insulin intensification.

   4. Community support groups.

      a. Frequently provided by ADA local chapters (www.diabetes.org).

      b. May be facilitated by organizations providing care for patients with unique or similar needs (such as Spanish-speaking communities, etc.).

   5. Special needs: Additional education may be needed for individuals experiencing unique problems (such as visual impairment, renal dialysis, stroke rehabilitation, etc.).

G. Advocacy.

   1. Facilitate appropriate communication between patient and physician.

   2. Facilitate access to appropriate resources.

   3. Provide patient-focused, flexible support and interventions.

   4. Promote positive, pro-active expectations

with the patient, physician, and other providers.

H. Telehealth practice.
   1. Support day-to-day blood glucose management.
   2. Patient access for acute situations.
   3. Reminders: Annual lab tests, and eye and foot examinations.
I. Communication/documentation.
   1. Baseline.
      a. General health status.
      b. Current diabetes control.
      c. Patient competencies.
   2. Patient goals.
      a. Blood glucose and HbA1c targets.
      b. Lipid and blood pressure targets.
      c. Weight.
      d. Life style changes.
      e. Management of co-morbidities.
   3. Progress.
      a. Clinical targets.
      b. Accomplishment/readjustment of patient goals through time.
J. Outcome management.
   1. Individual outcomes.
      a. Demonstrated competencies.
      b. Quality of life.
   2. Clinical.
      a. Process criteria.
         (1) Documented performance of recommended annual lab tests.
         (2) Documented performance of annual eye, foot examinations.
      b. Outcome criteria.
         (1) Lab values in target ranges.
         (2) Eye, foot examinations with normal results.
         (3) BP managed within target range.
      c. Resource utilization/cost outcomes.
         (1) ED visits and hospitalizations.
         (2) PCP visits for recommended routine care.
K. Protocol development/usage.
   1. ADA Standards: Criteria by which regulatory bodies (such as CMS and JCAHO) evaluate quality of care provided by health care organizations and by managed care organizations.
   2. Diabetes treatment algorithms or guidelines.

      a. Promote consistent level of care throughout an organization.
      b. Guide provider through steps to advance therapy to help patients achieve diabetes control goals in an efficient and appropriate manner.
   3. Nursing care pathways: Useful to promote consistent level of care, timely patient access to appropriate care and education, and continuity of care throughout an organization (Zander, 1997).
      a. Newly diagnosed Type 1 or Type 2 diabetes.
      b. Diabetes "out-of-control," "sick day" management.

Hypertension

Patient Population: Adult
Pamela Del Monte, MS, RN, C

Hypertension is the most common primary diagnosis in the U.S., with 35 million office visits per year. Hypertension is present in approximately 50 million Americans, with prehypertension present in 59 million. Healthy People 2010 set a goal of hypertension control at 50% of the population, and control rates are still far below that goal (CDC/NIH, 2000). Fewer than 60% of adults with a diagnosis of hypertension receive treatment, and fewer than 40% are controlled to levels of 140/90 or below (NHLBI, 2003). Persons with conditions such as diabetes or chronic kidney disease and hypertension should be treated to achieve blood pressure levels of 130/80 or below (NHLBI, 2003). Adults 55 years of age and older have a 90% lifetime chance of developing hypertension. It is a significant risk factor for kidney disease, adverse cardiac events, and stroke, and the higher the blood pressure, the greater the risk. Complications of hypertension can be prevented or delayed with screening, early detection, and early and adequate blood pressure control. Lifestyle modifications are paramount in the management of hypertension and prehypertension. The ambulatory care nurse is well positioned to increase awareness and to serve as a potent motivator for these patients, especially given that they often feel well without obvious symptoms (see Table 22-5).

A. Assessment/screening/triage.

Table 22-5.

Classification of Blood Pressure for Adults Aged 18 and Older

BP Classification	SBP mm Hg	DBP mm Hg
Normal	<120	and <80
Prehypertension	120-139	or 80-89
Stage 1 hypertension	140-159	or 90-99
Stage 2 hypertension	≥160	or >100

Note: Based on the average of 2 or more properly measured, seated BP readings on 2 or more office visits.

Source: NHLBI, 2004a.

1. Evaluation.
   a. Assess lifestyle; identify other cardiovascular risk factors and associated disorders.
   b. Assess for identifiable causes of high blood pressure.
   c. Assess for presence/absence of target organ damage and cardiovascular disease.
2. Risk factors.
   a. Family history of hypertension, cardiovascular disease, coronary artery disease.
   b. Patient history of diabetes, elevated lipid levels, or renal disease.
   c. Medication history: To include prescription medications, over-the-counter drugs, and herbal supplements.
   d. Patient lifestyle history: To include physical inactivity, smoking, sodium intake, inadequate intake of fruits, vegetables and potassium, alcohol intake.
   e. Patient demographics: Age; race; gender.
   f. Weight and height; body mass index (BMI).
3. Physical assessment.
   a. Blood pressure measurement.
      (1) Auscultate blood pressure readings with patient seated for at least 5 minutes in a chair, feet on floor, and arm supported at heart level.
      (2) Use an appropriately sized cuff and cuff bladder.
      (3) No caffeine, smoking, or exercise for 30 minutes prior to reading.
      (4) Take 2 measurements and average the readings.
      (5) Verify blood pressure readings in contra-lateral arm.
      (6) Assess standing blood pressure readings, especially with risk of postural hypertension, before starting medications and when changing dosing.
   b. Examine optic fundi.
   c. Calculate BMI and measure waist circumference.
   d. Palpate thyroid.
   e. Make thorough exam of heart and lungs, including heart sounds.
   f. Auscultate for carotid, abdomen, and femoral bruits.
   g. Examine abdomen – Palpate for enlarged kidneys, masses, distended urinary bladder, abnormal aortic pulsations.
   h. Palpate lower extremities for edema and pulses.
   i. Neurological assessment.
4. Lifestyle assessment.
   a. Excess body weight.
   b. Excess dietary sodium intake.
   c. Inadequate physical activity.
   d. Inadequate intake of fruits, vegetables, and potassium.
   e. Excess alcohol intake.
B. Primary, secondary, tertiary prevention.
   1. Primary prevention.
      a. Identify those at risk and educate to risk factors and lifestyle modifications.
      b. Self blood pressure monitoring.
         (1) Calibrate equipment.
         (2) Have patient demonstrate technique.
         (3) Review patient log of blood pressure readings.
         (4) Validate self blood pressure measurements.
      c. Ambulatory blood pressure monitoring.
         (1) Provides blood pressure information during activities of daily living and sleep.
         (2) Levels correlate with target organ injury.

d. Weight appropriate to height.
e. Physical activity (aerobic) of 30 minutes most days of the week.
f. Dietary modifications; Dietary Approaches to Stop Hypertension (DASH) eating plan (NHLBI, 2003).
  (1) DASH diet is an evidence-based eating plan that is low in saturated fat, cholesterol and total fat, reduced consumption of red meats, sweets, and sugar-containing beverages. There is concomitant emphasis on fruits, vegetables, and low-fat dairy products. The eating plan is rich in magnesium, calcium, protein, and fiber. Sodium consumption is limited from 1,500 to 2,400 mg/day.

2. Secondary prevention.
a. Identify patients where lifestyle modifications have not achieved blood pressure control.
b. Adequate antihypertensive medication and dose.

3. Tertiary prevention.
a. Minimize target organ damage (heart, brain, eyes, kidneys).
b. Additional laboratory and diagnostic tests/procedures to monitor therapy and target organ function.

C. Clinical procedures.
1. Pharmacological management.
a. Diuretics.
b. Beta blockers.
c. ACE Inhibitors.
d. Angiotensin II antagonists.
e. Calcium channel blockers.
f. Alpha-blockers.
g. Central alpha-2 agonists.
h. Direct vasodilators.

2. Followup monitoring – Scheduled visits, monthly or less, until blood pressure goal is reached. Include blood pressure monitoring, discussion, and re-emphasis on lifestyle modifications.

3. Hypertensive emergencies.
a. Hypertensive emergency.
  (1) Severe elevation of BP (>180/120 mm Hg) complicated by evidence of impending or progressive target organ dysfunction.
  (2) Goals of therapy include:
    (a) Continuous monitoring of blood pressure and administration of appropriate parenteral antihypertensive agents.
    (b) Immediate mean arterial blood pressure reduction of no more than 25% within minutes to 1 hour. Further decrease, if stable, to 160/100 to 110 mm Hg within 2 to 6 hours. Further gradual decrease of blood pressure over the next 24 to 48 hours.
    (c) Minimization and prevention of target organ damage for either maintained elevations or from too rapid and vast a decrease in blood pressure.
    (d) Determine organic and treatable cause(s) of elevated blood pressure.
b. Hypertensive urgencies.
  (1) Severe elevation of BP without progressive target organ dysfunction.
  (2) Goal of therapy includes:
    (a) Pharmacological intervention with short-acting oral agents.
    (b) Blood pressure reduction within a few hours, followed by several hours of observation.
    (c) Confirmed followup appointment, within 1 to a few days, prior to discharge from emergency department.

D. Collaboration.
1. Utilize services, including but not limited to pharmacy, nurse case managers, registered dieticians, licensed nutritionists, and health education.
2. Reinforce patient education with patient and significant other(s).
3. Manage co-morbidities.
a. Co-morbidities, such as diabetes, require lower blood pressure targets.
b. Co-morbidities may benefit or be adversely affected. May require medication adjustments for blood pressure control.
4. Utilize specialty services, as needed.

E. Care management.
    1. Reinforce lifestyle modification instruction/education.
    2. Regular evaluation of blood pressure control.
    3. Barriers to prevention.
        a. Cultural norms.
        b. Inadequate attention to health education by clinicians.
        c. Cost for services, clinical and education.
        d. Integrating physical activity into daily lifestyle.
        e. Lack of healthy food choices in workplace, schools, restaurants, and at home.
        f. Cost of healthier food products.
        g. Amounts of sodium in packaged/prepared/restaurant foods.
    4. Referrals as necessary.
        a. Cardiology.
        b. Nephrology.
        c. Ophthalmology.
        d. Neurology.
        e. Nutrition counseling.
F. Patient education.
    1. Goal setting.
    2. Lifestyle modifications.
        a. Dietary modifications.
            (1) DASH eating plan.
            (2) Limit alcohol intake.
        b. Activity modifications.
            (1) Increasing activity safely.
            (2) Integrating activity into daily activities.
    3. Risk factor modification.
        a. Weight appropriate to height.
        b. Smoking cessation.
    4. Adherence to regimen.
        a. Medication administration.
            (1) Compliance with prescription.
            (2) Side effects.
            (3) Nonprescription medications.
            (4) Herbal supplements.
    5. Typical lack of overt symptoms.
    6. Followup and access to health care.
        a. Routine followup for monitoring of blood pressure control.
        b. Emergency access for signs and symptoms of untoward event. These can include:
            (1) Onset of severe headaches.
            (2) New onset of mental status changes.
            (3) New onset of vision changes.
            (4) Numbness and weakness.
            (5) Chest pain.
            (6) Palpitations.
            (7) Shortness of breath.
    7. Self-monitoring of blood pressure.
G. Advocacy.
    1. Health care resources.
    2. Access to health care.
    3. Health education.
H. Telehealth practice.
    1. Assessment and triage.
        a. Onset of symptoms.
        b. Pertinent history, including medications and how they are being taken.
        c. Current blood pressure readings.
        d. Associated symptoms: Severe headache, visual changes, weakness, numbness, and chest pain.
        e. Nurse recommended changes or follow up care.
I. Communication/documentation.
    1. Documentation/log of self-measured blood pressure readings. Bring log to all appointments.
    2. Documentation of all patient encounters.
    3. Documentation and evaluation of teaching plan.
J. Outcome management.
    1. Lifestyle modification adherence.
    2. Medication adherence.
    3. Blood pressure readings to target optimal/normal.
    4. Lower blood pressure targets if diabetes, chronic kidney disease.
    5. Minimize target organ damage.
K. Protocol development/usage.
    1. Teaching plans.
    2. Lifestyle modifications.
        a. Diet.
        b. Physical activity.
        c. Alcohol intake.
        d. Smoking cessation.
    3. Medication dosage and side effects.

Osteoarthritis

Patient Population: Adult
Margaret Ross Kraft, PhD, RN

Arthritis is the most prevalent chronic condition and leading cause of disability in the U.S., with 1 out of every 3 adults affected (American Arthritis Foundation, 2005). Osteoarthritis, also known as degenerative joint disease (DJD), is the most common type of arthritis and is generally a disease of older adults, especially older women. After the age of 75, some degree of osteoarthritis is found in almost all persons. It occurs as the result of normal "wear and tear" on joints, but its presence can be hastened through repetitious joint strain, injury, and/or obesity. This disease is manifested by progressive degeneration of cartilage in joints, usually weight-bearing joints, although any joint could be affected. As cartilage becomes thin, bone ends come closer together, bone spurs develop at tendon and ligament attachment sites, synovial fluid may leak, and cysts may develop on the bone (Gulanick, Klopp, Galanes, Gradishar, & Puzas, 1998). The result is impaired joint functioning. Early treatment is essential to prevent limitation in daily activities.

A. Assess/screen/triage.
  1. History.
     a. Risk factor screening.
        (1) Repetitive joint motion, including occupational activities.
        (2) Familial tendency.
        (3) Obesity.
     b. Symptom assessment.
        (1) Pain.
        (2) Changes in mobility: Maintenance of mobility in older adults can mean the difference between living independently in the community and institutionalization.
        (3) Body image changes.
  2. Physical assessment/joint assessment: Check for tenderness on palpation, bony enlargement, crepitus on motion, and/or limitation of joint motion.
     a. Spine.
     b. Knees.
     c. Fingers.
     d. Hips.

B. Primary, secondary, tertiary prevention.
  1. Primary prevention: Maintain ideal body weight.
  2. Secondary prevention.
     a. Treatment to reduce pain.
     b. Therapy and exercise for maintenance of joint mobility.
  3. Tertiary prevention.
     a. Referral to dietitian for weight reduction.
     b. Rehabilitation after joint surgery to promote mobility.

C. Clinical procedures.
  1. Surgical interventions.
     a. To correct deformities.
     b. To improve function.
     c. To relieve pain.
     d. To prevent deformity (Harkness & Dincher, 1996).
  2. Common surgical interventions.
     a. Tendon transplants.
     b. Synovectomy.
     c. Total joint replacement.

D. Care management.
  1. Treatment is aimed at relieving pain, which tends to be worse in the morning or after any extended period of inactivity, and at keeping the joint working by reducing strain and relieving stiffness and swelling (Ebersole & Hess, 2001).
     a. Maintenance of optimal joint function.
     b. Position changes.
     c. Joint support.
     d. Medication for control of pain and inflammation.
     e. Hot or cold packs.
        (1) Moist heat (such as pads, soaks, paraffin baths).
        (2) Ice packs for duration of no more than 20 minutes.
     f. Adequate regular and intermittent rest periods.
     g. Use of adaptive equipment, as necessary.
     h. Elimination of stressors.
  2. Prevention of progressive disability.

E. Patient education.
  1. Medication management.
     a. Acetaminophen: First choice of medication, this medication belongs to a class

of drugs called analgesics (pain relievers) and antipyretics (fever reducers). Acetaminophen relieves pain in mild arthritis but has no effect on the underlying inflammation, redness, and swelling of the joint. Side effects are rare.

b. Salicylates: Used to relieve pain, reduce fever, and relieve some symptoms caused by arthritis, such as swelling, stiffness, and joint pain.
   (1) Teach side effects (for example, GI upset, bruising).
   (2) Toxicity of sustained use of large doses (for example, ototoxicity).
   (3) Teach precautions/contraindications.

c. Non-steroidal anti-inflammatory drugs (NSAIDs) and COX2 inhibitors (such as celecoxib [Celebrex®]):
   (1) Evaluate for GI upset, which is a major risk for older adults.
   (2) Monitor for increased bruising.
   (3) All sponsors of marketed prescription NSAIDs, including celecoxib (Celebrex®), a COX-2 selective NSAID, have been asked to revise the labeling for their products to include a warning that highlights the potential for increased risk of cardiovascular (CV) events and serious, potential life-threatening gastrointestinal (GI) bleeding associated with their use.

d. Corticosteroids: Preferred for short-term therapy for acute exacerbations. Corticosteroids are not used systemically for osteoarthritis, although they are sometimes used as a local injection into an affected joint.

e. Muscle relaxants:
   (1) May be used for painful muscle spasms.
   (2) Caution about drowsiness and driving.

f. Topical application of anti-inflammatory or deep heat creams for short-term pain relief.
   (1) Wear cotton gloves, if applied to hands.
      (2) Wash hands thoroughly to avoid irritation to non-medicated body areas.

2. Weight control: Excess weight stresses involved joints.

3. Exercise program: Stressing the importance of gentle exercise to maintain joint mobility. Exercise in warm swimming pools may be very helpful in improving joint function.
   a. Maintain range of motion (ROM) of all joints.
   b. Encourage rest between activities.
   c. Evaluate pain during exercise.
   d. Discuss environmental barriers to mobility.
   e. OT/PT/RT/KT consult(s) as indicated.

4. Teach relaxation and stress reduction techniques.

5. Teach ADL adaptations.

6. Orthopedic consultation regarding possible joint replacement.

F. Telehealth practice.
   1. Evaluate for exacerbation of symptoms.
   2. Assess compliance with medication and diet regimen.

G. Documentation – Subjective and objective data are documented along with the nursing assessment and treatment plan.

H. Outcomes management.
   1. Pain reduction.
   2. Increased mobility and functional status.
   3. Improved quality of life.

Asthma

Patient Population: Pediatric
Linda L. Gehring, PhD, APNP, RN, BC

Asthma is the most common chronic disease of childhood, and it is found in all age groups. Over 9 million children under the age of 18 have been diagnosed with asthma. This is over 12% of the children under 18 years of age, and of those diagnosed, 75% of the diagnoses are made in children under 5 years of age. Asthma is diagnosed with increasing frequency in children, although it is often overlooked because asthma is frequently confused with allergies, upper respiratory infections, bronchitis, and pneumonia. Both chronic and acute asthma are primarily managed in outpatient and other ambulatory care settings.

It is important to understand exactly what asthma is. Asthma is defined as chronic inflammatory disorder of the airways. Chronically inflamed airways are hyper-responsive to triggers, which can lead to acute asthma exacerbation. Exposure to triggers contributes to an increased level of airway inflammation with edema, acute bronchoconstriction, and mucus plug production. The airway inflammation process occurs on a cellular level through mast cell activation and inflammatory cell infiltration, including activation of eosinophils, airway macrophages, neutrophils, and lymphocytes. These cellular changes lead to edema, denudation, and disruption of the bronchial epithelium, collagen disposition beneath the basement membrane, goblet cell hyperplasia (leading to mucus hyper-secretion), and smooth muscle thickening. Recent research shows that the these cellular conditions are often, but not always, features of mild to moderate asthma (National Asthma Education and Prevention Program [NAEPP], 2002).

A. Respiratory system – Anatomy and physiology.
   1. The lungs receive oxygen-rich fresh air through the trachea when one inhales.
   2. The lungs remove poor air (carbon dioxide) from the system when one exhales.
   3. Exchange gas through air sacs (alveoli).
      a. Oxygen passes into the blood for transport to all cells of the body.
      b. Carbon dioxide passes from blood into the lungs.
B. Nursing assessment and monitoring.
   1. Nursing history: Perform at each visit for acute or chronic management.
      a. Obtain patient symptom history, including the frequency of the symptoms.
      b. Inquire when the symptoms started, whether they are worse night or day, possible triggers, illness (fever, vomiting, diarrhea, etc.).
         (1) What were the symptoms?
         (2) When did the symptoms start?
         (3) When are the symptoms worse day or night?
         (4) What were the possible triggers?
         (5) What action did the parent/caretaker take to relieve the symptoms, and did it help?
      c. Assess the parent/caretaker's ability to recognize their child's signs and symp-

toms of an impending exacerbation, administer medications properly, and adhere to asthma action plan.
      d. Review peak flow diary.
      e. Assess impact of asthma on quality of life of children and family.
         (1) Does play/activity/excitement trigger symptoms: Coughing wheezing, shortness of breath, chest discomfort, and fatigue?
         (2) Is the child unable to keep up with peers or has to stop to rest?
         (3) Does the parent/caretaker restrict the child's participation in gym or sports?
         (4) Is the child's or the parent/caretaker's sleep interrupted by the child's symptoms or the need for extra treatments during the night?
         (5) Are family plans altered or cancelled due to the child's asthma?
         (6) Is the child absent from school excessively or is school performance affected?
         (7) Is the parent/caretaker missing a lot of work in order to care for the child and take him or her to appointments?
      f. Is the child growing and developing appropriately? Any problems with growth and development, such as obesity, can complicate asthma.
      g. Is the child tolerating his or her medications or treatments?
      h. Does the parent have a prescription plan to cover the cost of medications and insurance coverage for equipment?
   2. Physical assessment: Perform at each visit for acute or chronic management.
      a. Respiratory assessment:
         (1) Check vital signs and respiratory rate.
         (2) Observe symptoms.
         (3) Observe the child's behavior and activity level. The child with uncontrolled asthma may be restless, apprehensive, or sit upright in three point/orthopedic position.
         (4) Assess use of accessory muscles, retractions, and nasal flaring as the

Table 22-6.

Classification of Severity of Asthma

	Clinical Features Before Treatment			
Classification	**Days with Symptoms**	**Nights with Symptoms**	**FEV$_1$ or PEF (% predicted normal)**	**PEF Variable**
Severe persistent	Continual	Frequent	$\leq$60% predicted	> 30%
Moderate persistent	Daily	>1time a week	>60% <80% predicted	> 30%
Mild persistent	>2 times a week	>2 times a month	$\geq$80% predicted	20-30%
Mild intermittent	$\leq$2 times a week	$\leq$2 times a month	>80% predicted	< 20%

Source: National Asthma Education and Prevention Program, 2002; NHLBI, 2002.

child struggles to breath.
  (5) Assess children who experience repeated exacerbations and/or have poorly controlled asthma for barrel chest, elevated shoulders, and increased accessory muscle use because of air trapping.
  (6) Auscultate the lungs for adventitious breath sounds and air movement. It is important that the stethoscope be placed directly on the skin. It is inappropriate to listen through the child's clothing. Expiratory phase may be prolonged (wheezing may or may not be heard depending on the intensity of bronchospasm and obstruction of air movement as a result of increased airway inflammation).
  (7) Check oxygen saturation by pulse oximetry.
  b. Assess height and weight, and plot on growth chart to assess growth and development.
3. Diagnostic studies – Determine the reversibility of the breathing problem (asthma is reversible).
  a. Spirometry (may not be feasible in children under 4 years of age).
  b. Pulmonary function tests (may be used in children under 4 years of age).
  c. Determine the level of asthma severity (see Table 22-6) to prioritize educational goals.
    (1) Define individualized asthma manage-

ment plan.
    (2) Determine appropriate level of nursing intervention.
C. Clinical manifestations and therapeutic interventions.
  1. Airway smooth muscle contraction, bronchoconstriction, and mucus plugs lead to symptoms.
    a. Coughing (which may occur in spasms).
    b. Wheezing.
    c. Shortness of breath.
    d. Chest discomfort.
    e. If this continues, the chest may tighten and pain may be felt.
    f. It is important to understand that some children may only have occasional coughing while others have daily coughs.
  2. Common therapeutic modalities.
    a. Nursing interventions – Background knowledge.
      (1) The aim of asthma care is to:
        (a) Maintain asthma control.
        (b) Prevent exacerbation of symptoms.
        (c) Use the least amount of medication to maintain normal peak flow measures and normal activity while maintaining minimal risk of side effects.
      (2) The onset of asthma symptoms can be related to family history of asthma or allergy, present allergies,

Table 22-7.

Common Asthma Triggers/Irritants and Avoidance Strategies

Trigger	To Avoid
Dust mite allergens (not visible to the naked eye)	Focus on bedroom Wash bed linens and blankets once a week in hot water Encase pillows and mattresses in airtight covers Remove carpets, especially in sleeping rooms Use vinyl, leather, or plain wooden furniture instead of fabric-upholstered furniture Damp dust the area
Cockroaches	Minimal use of pesticides Eliminate food, water, and entry points Use baits, keep away from children
Allergens from animals with fur	Remove animals from the home, or at least from the sleeping area Use HEPA air filtering system Remove carpet and other reservoirs for allergies in the bedroom Wash pets weekly
Outdoor pollens	Close windows and doors Use air conditioner, not fans Visit an air conditioned mall or movie theater
Outdoor and indoor mold	Remain indoors when pollen and mold counts are highest (midday) Contained in damp soil or leaves, plastic toys and equipment Increase kitchen and bathroom ventilation Repair leaky faucets Clean mold with mild bleach solution
Indoor mold	Reduce dampness in the home; clean any damp areas frequently
Tobacco smoke	Avoid it (smoking or secondary smoke) Ask others to take it outside Odor of smoke residue is also a trigger
Air pollution	Stay indoors on Ozone Action Days
Cold and infection	Wash hands frequently Encourage yearly flu shots
Exercise	Plan warm up activates Allow time for pre-medication
Strong odors	Avoid the use of fragranced self care product, cleaning products, candles, and room fresheners
Weather	Watch at times of sudden weather changes Cover mouth and nose in cold weather

Source: Fight Asthma Milwaukee, 2005.

Table 22-8.

Stepwise Approach for Managing Infants and Young Children (5 Years of Age and Younger)

STEP 1 Mild Intermittent	STEP 2 Mild Persistent	STEP 3 Moderate Persistent	STEP 4 Severe Persistent
No daily medications needed	Low-dose inhaled corticosteroid, *Or* cromolyn, *Or* leukotriene receptor agonist	Preferred Low to Medium dose inhaled corticosteroid and long-acting inhaled beta$_2$ agonist, *Or* Medium-dose inhaled corticosteroid alone, *Or* Low-dose inhaled corticosteroid and either leukotriene receptor antagonist or theophylline.	Preferred High-dose inhaled corticosteroid with long acting bronchodilator If needed, add systemic corticosteroids 2mg/kg/day.

Source: National Asthma Education and Prevention Program, 2002. NHLBI, 2002.

prenatal exposure to secondary smoke, viral infection, male gender, and low birth weight.

(3) Triggers that can cause asthma episodes include upper respiratory tract infections, animals, dust, mold, cockroaches, smoke pollution, exercise, cold air, and other conditions like gastroesophageal reflux, sinusisis, and rhinitis (see Table 22-7).

b. Nursing intervention – Asthma treatment is divided into two classifications:

(1) The long-term control or preventive maintenance medications consist of the anti-inflammatory agents (administered daily whether or not symptoms are present).

(2) Quick relief therapy is used to provide symptom relief and treat acute exacerbations (administered daily whether or not symptoms are present).

(3) It is crucial that the nurse understand these concepts for control of inflammation (long-term control therapy) and bronchospasm (quick-relief therapy).

c. Nursing intervention – Assessing and teaching.

(1) Keep it simple.

(2) Encourage the caregiver to decide which asthma topic he or she would like to cover first.

(3) Patient education: Five key messages included in patient education.

(a) Basic facts about asthma.

(b) Role of medication.

(c) Skills: Inhaler and spacer use; nebulizer use, cleaning, disinfecting, and maintenance; self-monitoring (peak flow meter).

(d) Environmental (triggers) control measures.

Table 22-9.

Stepwise Approach for Managing Children (over 5 Years of Age)

			STEP 4 **Severe Persistent**
		STEP 3 **Moderate** **Persistent**	Preferred High-dose inhaled corticosteroid with long-acting inhaled beta$_2$ agonist If needed, add systemic corticosteroids 2 mg/kg/day
	STEP 2 **Mild Persistent**	Preferred – Low-to-medium dose inhaled corticosteroid and long-acting beta$_2$ agonist, *Or* Low to medium- dose inhaled	
STEP 1 **Mild Intermittent**	Preferred Low-dose inhaled, *Or* cromolyn, leukotriene modifier or nedocromil, *Or* Sustained-release theophylline		
No daily medications needed			

Note: The stepwise approach presents guidelines to assist clinical decision making. Asthma is highly variable; clinicians should tailor specific medication plans to the needs and circumstances of individual patients. Gain control as quickly as possible; then decrease treatment to the least medication necessary to maintain control. A rescue course of systemic corticosteroid (prednisolone) may be needed at any time and step. In general, use of short-acting beta$_2$ agonist on a daily basis indicates the need for additional long-term control therapy; consultation with an asthma specialist is *recommended* for patients with moderate or severe persistent asthma in this age group. Consultation should be considered for all patients with mild persistent asthma.

Source: National Asthma Education and Prevention Program, 2002. NHLBI, 2002.

(e) When and how to take rescue actions (including written individualized asthma action management/action plan).

(4) Include interventions to meet the goals of education and promote optimal self and parent/caretaker management.

   (a) Explain the concept of chronic airway inflammation and bronchospasm.

   (b) Define the roles of medication: Long-term control agents (anti-inflammatory agents) and quick relief agents (bronchodilators) (see Tables 22-8 and 22-9 for a stepwise approach to asthma control and treatment recommendations for each level of severity).

   (c) Identify the patient's long-term control medicines by name and emphasize that medications must be taken whether or not symptoms are present.

   (d) Identify the patient's quick-relief medications (brand and generic), which are used only on an as-needed basis to relieve breakthrough symptoms. Caution the patient and the parent/caregiver against the use of over-the-counter cough or cold medicine.

(e) Individualize the administration of each medication with the child and caregiver. Which is best based on developmental level of the child, level of asthma severity, medication formulation, availability, cost, and convenience?

    (i) Inhaler (spacer).

    (ii) Oral.

    (iii) Dry powdered device.

    (iv) Nebulizer.

(f) Demonstrate proper medication technique, including use of a chamber and proper seal on mouthpiece or of facemask, and have the child/caregiver complete a return demonstration (evaluate regularly). Many erroneously administer nebulizer treatments to infants and toddlers by "blow-by," rather than by a properly fitted and firmly-sealed mask.

(g) Teach symptom monitoring and peak flow monitoring, if applicable.

(h) Teach environmental/trigger control measures. Help caretaker prioritize control measures.

(i) Agree upon an "Asthma Action Plan" for daily care and for exacerbations.

3. Asthma action plan.

  a. Provide every child with a written individualized asthma management/action plan to include:

    (1) Routine treatment.

    (2) Pre-exercise treatment.

    (3) Plan for emergency exacerbation.

  b. Establish that parents/caretakers know how and when to implement their child's action plan. The written asthma management plan includes:

    (1) Medications: Name, dose, and how and when to administer.

    (2) Peak flow monitoring instructions/parameters (if appropriate).

    (3) How and when to take rescue action and call the doctor or go to the emergency room.

    (4) Clarify that the parent/caretaker will make a plan to educate others involved in the child's care, such as school nurse, teacher, coach, babysitter, daycare personnel, and other back-up family members.

  c. Supply the parent/caretaker with resource materials and written instructions as part of the child's asthma management plan.

    (1) How to recognize the signs and symptoms of worsening asthma.

    (2) How to treat worsening asthma, as well as how and when to seek medical attention or take rescue action (for example, call the primary care provider, go to the emergency room or call Emergency Management Services, such as 9-1-1).

    (3) Routine treatment, pre-exercise treatment, and an action plan for exacerbations.

  d. Principles of maintenance therapy.

    (1) Start medications at a high dose to correct the symptoms quickly, which assists with adherence.

    (2) Step down once control is achieved.

    (3) Maintain the lowest dose of medicine that controls asthma.

    (4) Step up and down as indicated by the child's action plan (see Tables 22-8 and 22-9).

4. Clinical procedures while at the ambulatory care facility.

  a. Medication administration for acute asthma exacerbation.

    (1) Administer *short-acting bronchodilators*, usually albuterol diluted in normal saline via nebulizer or metered dose inhaler (MDI) via spacer, as prescribed.

    (a) Relaxes the muscles that tighten around the airways.

    (b) Helps to stop exacerbations when they happen.

    (c) Helps with the asthma symptoms that accompany exercise.

(2) Administer *oral corticosteroids*, as prescribed (1 to 2 mg/kg/day in two divided doses for 3 to 10 days, with maximum dose 60 mg/day).

    (a) Used for flare-ups or severe asthma episodes.

    (b) Taken in addition to controller and quick relief.

    (c) Helps decrease swelling and mucus production in the airways.

(3) Perform and document respiratory assessment and peak flow rate (children 5 years of age) before and after administering treatments.

(4) Prepare to send child home if improved.

(5) Specify a plan for followup.

(6) Give specific instructions outlining steps the parent/caretaker is to do if the child worsens.

(7) If the child worsens or does not respond to treatment (no improvement in breath sounds or symptoms, hypoxia/oxygen requirement, or other complicating condition) send the child to the emergency room.

  b. Review and update, as indicated, the child's immunizations. Children with asthma should receive an annual influenza immunization.

5. Care management.

  a. Coordination of care: Work with the parent/caretaker to meet the goals of treatment within the context of the child's development, environment, home routine, school/daycare, activities, and insurance coverage.

    (1) The goals of care management are:

      (a) Prevent chronic and bothersome symptoms (such as nocturnal cough).

      (b) Maintain normal pulmonary function (80% or better of the personal best peak flow rate).

      (c) Maintain normal participation in activities/exercise/sports.

      (d) Prevent breakthrough symptoms, exacerbations, emergency room visits, and hospitalizations.

      (e) Provide optimal pharmacotherapy with the least amount of side effects and expense.

      (f) Assist the patient/family's prioritize and organize/plan care to meet their needs and expectations with asthma management.

    (2) Teach peak flow monitoring, as appropriate.

      (a) It can be a reliable tool for children 5 years of age or older.

      (b) Establish each child's personal best expiratory flow rate; it is the highest number (or maximum rate of exhalation expressed as liters per minute) that the patient can achieve when they are well.

    (3) Define the patient's green, yellow, and red zones.

      (a) The green zone is 80% to 100% of the personal best.

      (b) The yellow zone is 50% to 80% of the personal best.

      (c) The red zone is 50% or below of the personal best.

    (4) Peak flow monitoring facilitates identification of an impending exacerbation before the onset of signs or symptoms because the peak flow rate may drop into the yellow zone, and the action plan can be initiated even before other signs are manifest.

  b. Teach medication use and administration.

    (1) Include the following interventions to meet the goals of education and promote optimal self-parent/caretaker management.

      (a) Concept of chronic airway inflammation and bronchospasm.

      (b) Define the roles of medication: Long-term control agents and

Table 22-10.

Medication Adverse Effects

Medication	Adverse Effects
Short and long-acting bronchodilators	Increased heart rate, tremors, headache (short duration)
Leukotriene modifiers	Gastrointestinal upset
Inhaled corticosteroids	Thrush, dysphonia, high doses may have systemic effects
Systemic corticosteroids	Many – Increased appetite, stomach aches, mood changes, fluid retention, diabetes, osteoporosis

Source: Fight Asthma Milwaukee, 2005.

quick relief agents (see Tables 22-8 and 22-9, which outline the stepwise approach to therapy and treatment recommendations for each level of severity).

(c) Identify the patient's long-term control medication(s) by name (brand and generic) and emphasize that they must be taken whether or not symptoms are present (see Table 22-10).

6. Nurse as advocate: Actions/implications for nurses as per the National Asthma Education and Prevention Program (NAEPP) (2002).

a. Be familiar with the real costs (both financial and psychosocial) of asthma care to patients in the community.

b. Identify available community resources (social services, government-sponsored programs, and voluntary organizations) to help meet the financial needs of patients. Some communities have summer camps for children with asthma where they receive education and medical supervision.

c. Assess whether prescribed medications, treatments, equipment, and/or diagnostic procedures are covered by the patient's insurance.

d. If necessary, contact the payer and be prepared to provide documentation explaining why the medication, treatment, equipment, or diagnostic procedure is medically necessary.

7. Telehealth practice.

a. For asthma sick calls.

(1) Identify the main symptom(s).

(2) Identify onset and duration of the symptom(s).

(3) Assess level of respiratory distress: Ask about respiratory rate, retractions, accessory muscle use, work of breathing, activity level/tolerance, any change in level of alertness, and ability to talk and carry on a conversation. If possible, talk to the child or have the child sing a song to determine presence of dyspnea or increased work of breathing.

(4) Ask the caller what action has been taken to treat the symptom(s) and be specific.

(a) For example, if the parent reports that the child is being given nebulizer treatments, ask questions and document precisely (for example, "The child is given albuterol 0.25 ml in NaCl via nebulizer every 6 hours for the last 48 hours").

(b) Assess the child's response to

        treatments.

    (c) Also, ask if the child is taking any other medications or if over-the-counter medications have been tried.

    (d) If the patient monitors peak flow, inquire about peak flow rate before and after treatment.

    (e) Compare to baseline and determine zone: Green, yellow, or red.

  (5) Assess for symptom(s) indicating other conditions that also need evaluation: Fever, vomiting, diarrhea, rash, pain, injury, or change in mental status.

  b. Collaborate with the physician to plan treatment and determine level of care: Increase treatments, keep child inside in air conditioning during hot weather, change medication/prescribe medication (for example, burst of oral prednisone), arrange to see the patient in the office, or instruct the parent/caretaker to take the child to the emergency room.

  c. Advise the parent/caretaker to call back as needed with any questions or concerns if the child doesn't improve or if condition worsens.

8. Communication.

  a. Assess for common fears and misconceptions that can lead to poor adherence and increased symptoms. Contrary to the beliefs of some:

  (1) Asthma is NOT caused by an emotional problem.

  (2) Asthma involves chronic inflammation, and the child needs ongoing treatment, even when there are no symptoms.

  (3) Asthma medications are NOT addictive and CANNOT lose their effectiveness over time. One of the most common mistakes made in asthma management is delaying the start of treatment to wait and see if it will get better or go away on its own. Another common problem is not

replacing MDIs frequently enough and using an empty inhaler. If the medication is taken daily at recommended doses, then most MDIs last a month.

  (4) Activities/exercise should NOT be restricted.

  (5) Inhaled or oral corticosteroids are NOT the same as anabolic steroids, and not all steroids are dangerous.

  (6) Asthma exacerbations DO NOT occur suddenly without warning.

  (7) Medication administration via nebulizer is NOT superior to MDI/spacer.

9. Outcome management.

  a. Document specify/quantify breakthrough symptoms.

  b. Document number of courses of oral corticosteroids.

  c. Record number of emergency room visits and hospitalizations.

  d. Document number of school days missed by the patient and workdays lost by the parent/caretaker because of asthma.

  e. Consider referral to an asthma specialist for patients with a history of:

  (1) A life-threatening exacerbation.

  (2) Child not meeting the goals of asthma therapy after 3 to 6 months of treatment.

  (3) Signs, symptoms, or response to treatment are atypical.

  (4) Presence of other complicating conditions. Other/additional diagnostic testing is indicated.

  (5) Adherence problems.

  (6) Child has severe persistent asthma or has been treated with two or more bursts of oral corticosteroids in 1 year or requires daily oral corticosteroids.

10. Resources for protocol development (see Table 22-11).

Table 22-11.

Resources for Protocol Development

National Heart, Lung and Blood Institute
National Institutes of Health
P.O. Box 30105
Bethesda, MD 20824-0105
301-251-1222
www.nhlbi.nih.gov/nhlbi/nhlbi.htm

The American Lung Association
1740 Broadway
New York, NY 10010
800-LUNG USA
http://www.lungusa.org

Allergy and Asthma Network/Mothers of Asthmatics
3554 Chain Bridge Road
Suite 200
Fairfax, VA 22030-2709
800-878-4403
www.podi.com/health/aanma

Asthma and Allergy Foundation of America
1125 15th Street NW
Suite 502
Washington, DC 20005
800-7 ASTHMA
www.aafa.org

Association of Asthma Educators
1215 Anthony Avenue
Columbia, SC 29201
888-988-7747
www.asthmaeducators.org

National Asthma Educator Certification Board (NAECB)
1150 18th Street NW
Suite 900
Washington, DC 20036
202-785-3355
www.naecb.org

Attention Deficit Hyperactivity Disorder

Patient Population: Pediatric and Adolescent
Stephanie G. Metzger, MS, RN, CPNP

Attention deficit hyperactivity disorder (ADHD) is the most common neurobehavioral disorder of childhood (American Academy of Pediatrics, 2001).

ADHD begins in childhood, but it is important not to lose sight of the fact that inattention, hyperactivity, and impulsivity are present in varying degrees in all children. However, when these behaviors become clinical features with associated impairments in academic and social functioning, the diagnosis of ADHD is considered. The American Psychiatric Association (2000) definition of ADHD is "...a persistent pattern of inattention and/or hyperactivity-impulsivity that is more frequently displayed and more severe than is typically observed in individuals at a comparable level of development..." (p.85).

In 1998, the National Institutes of Health recognized ADHD as a severe public health issue, which served to mitigate the dispute regarding this often controversial diagnosis. In the U.S., ADHD affects 3% to 5% of children, or as many as 2 million children. Symptom onset of ADHD may present in children as young as 3 years of age, with the mean age of diagnosis being between 8 and 9 years of age (National Institutes of Health, 2000). ADHD is a disorder of childhood that often continues into adolescence and adulthood, and may lead to considerable impairments, including decreased achievement and legal system difficulties. It is estimated that ADHD is present in 6% of the adult population, and that two-thirds of individuals with childhood ADHD retain the symptoms into adulthood. ADHD may be overlooked as an adult diagnosis because symptoms may be more subtle and be associated with adaptive symptoms without impairment (Wender, Wolf, & Wasserstein, 2001). There are several suspected etiologies of ADHD, including genetic origins, environmental factors, insults to the central nervous system, and neuroanatomic or neurochemical factors.

A. Assess/screen/triage.
   1. Classic symptoms of ADHD (Dreyer, 2006).
      a. Impulsivity, inattention, and hyperactivity are uniquely manifested according to developmental stages.
      b. In preschool children aged 3 to 5 years, clinical presentation includes:
         (1) Inattention.
         (2) Aggression, primarily hitting others.
         (3) Restlessness.
         (4) Fearlessness.
         (5) High activity level .
         (6) Arguing and demanding behaviors.
         (7) Frequent accidental traumas.

(8) Spilling and breaking things.

(9) Frequent temper tantrums.

(10) Noisiness and interrupting behaviors.

c. In school-aged children, aged 6 to 12 years, clinical presentation includes (Evans, Allen, Moore, & Strauss, 2006; Scahill & Schwab-Stone, 2000):

(1) Poor peer relationships (the hallmark presentation).

(2) Work is poorly organized, careless, and incomplete.

(3) Behavior is intrusive and interrupting (for example, blurted out answers).

(4) Inability to wait his or her turn in activities and games.

d. In adolescents aged 13 to 18 years, clinical presentation includes (Barkley, 2004; Wolraich et al., 2005):

(1) Restlessness more than hyperactivity.

(2) Lack of follow-through on tasks.

(3) Lack of organization in life.

(4) Independent academic assignments incomplete.

(5) Risk-taking behaviors often employed.

2. ADHD is a behavioral diagnosis because no medical test exists to confirm or exclude the diagnosis. Brain imaging, electroencephalograms, and thyroid hormone level testing are not recommended. There are various ADHD assessment tools and rating scales that may be helpful in diagnosis (see Table 22-12). Diagnosis of ADHD is based on the criteria outlined in the Diagnostic and Statistical Manual of Mental Disorders DSM-IV-TR (American Psychiatric Association, 2000).

a. Based on criteria, ADHD sub-types are determined by the level of cognitive functioning, inattentive behavioral functioning, and hyperactive-impulsive behavior.

(1) Attention deficit hyperactivity disorder, combined type.

(2) Attention deficit hyperactivity disorder, predominately inattentive type.

(3) Attention deficit hyperactivity disorder, predominantly hyperactive-impulsive type.

(4) Attention deficit hyperactivity disorder, not otherwise specified (does not meet the full criteria for diagnosis, but impairment is present).

b. Additional requirements include:

(1) Symptoms must be present prior to the age of 7.

(2) Must be present for 6 months or more.

(3) Must present in at least 2 settings: School, home, and community.

(4) Must cause significant impairment in social, academic, or occupational function.

3. It is imperative that these criteria be stringently followed to ensure that ADHD is the correct diagnosis. The controversy surrounding ADHD and treatment stems from rapid diagnosis that may not follow these criteria. The clinical assessment used for diagnosis includes the following (American Academy of Pediatrics, 2000; Bauchner, 2000; Dulcan, 1997):

a. Child/adolescent interview.

b. Parent interview and reports.

Table 22-12

ADHD Assessment Tools

AD/HD Rating Scale IV – http://adhdwarehouse.com

ANSER system – http://www.epsbooks.com/dyanmic/catalog/series

BASC: Behavior Assessment System for Children – http://agsnet.com/ags

Brown Attention Deficit Disorder Scales – http://www.drthomasebrown.com

Child Behavior Checklist – http://www.pubol.duke.edu/centers/child/fasttrack

Conners Rating Scales Revised – short and long forms – www.pearsonassessments.com

Early Childhood Inventory – http://www.checkmateplus.com/product

McCarney Attention Deficit Disorder Scales (ADDES) – www.hes-inc.com

Pediatric Symptom Checklist – www.brightfutures.com

SNAP-IV – http://www.adhd.net/

Vanderbilt Scales – http://peds.mc.vanderbilt.edu/VCHWEB

---

c. School-based assessment to include as many past and present teachers as possible.
d. Review of academic achievement to include grades and standardized test scores.
e. Reports from others involved with child, such as:
    (1) Counselors.
    (2) Social workers.
    (3) School personnel and daycare/childcare personnel.
    (4) Family members such as grandparents, siblings, etc.
    (5) Community-based activity personnel, such as coaches and clergy.
f. Use of a standardized rating scale, of which many are available.
g. Complete health history and physical examination.
h. Clinical observations.

B. Primary, secondary, tertiary prevention.
1. Common co-morbid conditions present in individuals with ADHD (Adesman, 2003; American Academy of Pediatrics, 2000; Bauchner, 2000; Brown, 2000; Costello, Foley, & Angold, 2006).
    a. Disruptive behavior disorders – Prevalence 10% to 44% overall.
        (1) Conduct disorder (10% to 40 %): A repetitive and persistent behavior pattern where individual rights and societal norms and rules are violated (American Psychiatric Association 2000; Scahill & Schwab-Stone, 2000).
            (a) Aggressiveness.
            (b) Deceitfulness/theft.
            (c) Damage of property.
            (d) Serious violation of rules.
        (2) Oppositional defiant disorder (19% to 44%): A recurrent pattern of negativistic, defiant, disobedient, and hostile behavior towards authority (American Psychiatric Association 2000; Scahill & Schwab-Stone, 2000).
            (a) Present 6 months or longer.
            (b) Clinically significant in social and academic functioning.

            (c) Does NOT meet criteria for conduct disorder.
            (d) Not present only during a psychotic or mood disorder.
    b. Psychiatric disorders.
        (1) Bipolar disorder.
        (2) Depressive disorder.
        (3) Anxiety disorder.
        (4) Obsessive compulsive disorder.
    c. Tic/movement disorders.
    d. Learning disorders.
        (1) Auditory (central auditory processing disorder).
        (2) Visual.
        (3) Reading.
        (4) Mathematics.
        (5) Written language.
        (6) Spatial.
    e. Developmental language disorders.
    f. Pervasive developmental disorder.
    g. Mental retardation.
    h. Sensory integration disorder.
2. Secondary co-morbidities (American Academy of Pediatrics, 2000). These psychological sequellae are often preventable with proactive interventions. The presence of primary or secondary co-morbidities worsens the prognosis and may indicate the need for pharmacologic and non-pharmacologic intervention.
    a. Low self-esteem.
    b. Lack of social skills.
    c. Lack of positive peer interactions.
    d. Impaired judgment.
    e. Psychosomatic complaints.
    f. Family conflict.
    g. Anxiety.
    h. Substance abuse.

C. Clinical procedures.
1. Treatment goals – ADHD is a chronic condition. The goal of treatment is to reduce the major symptoms of ADHD and to advance functioning in each area of impaired functioning. For some individuals, impaired functioning is present only in an academic environment, while for others, activities within the home and community cause an equal amount of impairment as the academic environment. For these latter individuals, a 7-day-

per-week treatment plan is needed to maximize outcomes. In the treatment plan, the clinician and the family incorporate the evaluation of baseline functioning inside and outside of the school arena, identify target outcomes based on precise symptoms and impairments, and review outcomes.

2. Pharmacological treatment of ADHD – Use of psychostimulants has long been the cornerstone of treatment (MTA Cooperative Group, 1999a, 1999b). Each of the psychostimulant categories is potentially effective in treating ADHD, including both methylphenidates and amphetamines (see Table 22-13). At least 80% of children will respond to stimulant medication if trialed in a systematic fashion. If one psychostimulant is not effective, another may be tried (American Academy of Pediatrics, 2001). All initiation trials should be done 7 days per week to allow for comprehensive evaluation of efficacy and side-effects, including parental observations and evaluation of medication in all arenas (Zamerkin & Ernst, 1999). Individual response may differ depending on side effect profile and comorbid conditions. No parameter predicts optimal stimulant dose or schedule, and titration is individualized for optimal effects with minimal side effects (American Academy of Pediatrics 2001).

   a. Psychostimulant categories available for treatment vary by onset of action and duration of positive behavioral effects.

     (1) Longer-acting preparations have greatly reduced or eliminated issues of frequent dose administration, privacy and security problems, and rebound effects.

     (2) Psychostimulant titration is based on the discriminating between inadequate dosing, wear-off effects, and medication effects. Dosing is initiated at a low level with titration upward using a consistent titration system with incremental increases (American Academy of Child and Adolescent Psychiatry, 2002).

     (3) Due to the variations in the duration of action, dosing schedules may be

very flexible, and careful monitoring may provide valuable information to determine an individualized dosing plan combining forms of drugs (Kratochvil,2003).

     (4) All of these psychostimulant medications are Schedule II Controlled Substances, controlled by federal regulation due to the high potential for abuse. Prescriptive authority for scheduled substances varies by state.

   b. Alternatives to stimulants.

     (1) Atomoxetine (Strattera®).

       (a) Recently approved by FDA for use in children with ADHD.

       (b) Presynaptic norepinephirine reuptake inhibitor.

       (c) Not a scheduled substance and renewable.

       (d) Low abuse potential and useful for children living in environments where stimulant medications may not be secure.

       (e) Expensive as compared to stimulants.

       (f) Used as an alternative to stimulant if stimulant worsens tic disorder.

       (g) Maximal response may be delayed for 2 to 4 weeks, requiring concurrent stimulant use, initially.

       (h) Duration of action – 24 hours.

       (i) Few published studies despite increasing popularity.

       (j) New toxicity alerts.

         (i) Black box warning: Increased risk of suicidal ideation in children/adolescents but not in adults. Close monitoring during initiation and titration, increase or decrease.

         (ii) Warning section labeling: Liver toxicity. Monitor for dark urine, itchy skin, jaundice, RUQ pain.

     (2) Antidepressants – If necessary, use these pharmacologic interventions;

Table 22-13.

ADHD Psychostimulant Medications

Brand/Generic Name	Daily Dose	Onset of Action	Duration of Action	Special Considerations
Methylphenidate Preparations				
Ritalin®/ Methylphenidate	2.5-60 mg/day	20-30 minutes	3-4 hours	
Ritalin SR®/ Methylphenidate SR	20-60 mg/day	60-90 minutes	6 hours	Must be swallowed intact
Ritalin LA®/ Methylphenidate ER	20-60 mg/day	30 minutes-2 hours	7-9 hours	
Focalin™/ d-methylphenidate	2.5-20 mg/day 20 mg maximum	60-90 minutes	4 hours	May be crushed
Focalin XR™/ d-methylphenidate	5-20 mg/day	Within 60 minutes	12 hours	Sprinkle capsules
Metadate CD™/ Methylphenidate controlled delivery	20-60 mg/day	30-120 minutes	7-9 hours	Sprinkle capsules
Amphetamine Preparations				
Concerta®/OROS Methylphenidate	18-72 mg/day	30-120 minutes	12 hours	Must be swallowed
Adderall®/ Amphetamine Salts	20-60 mg/day	30-60 minutes	6-7 hours	May be crushed
Adderall XR®/ d,-l-amphetamine	5-30 mg/day	1-2 hours	12 hours	Sprinkle on apple-sauce without absorption delay
Dexedrine®/ dextroamphetamine	2.5-40 mg/day	20-60 minutes	3-4 hours	
Dexedrine Spansule®/ Dextroamphetamine - SR	4-40 mg/day	60-90 minutes	6-7 hours	Must be swallowed

beyond the first line drugs (stated above), co-morbidities must be considered. Use of the following pharmacologic interventions requires psychiatric specialization (Waxmonsky, 2005).

(a) Tricyclics:

(i) Imipramine (Tofranil®); desipramine (Norpramin®); nortripyline (Aventil®, Pamelor®).

(ii) FDA preliminary analysis of data shows that taking antidepressants may increase suicidal thoughts and actions in about 1 out of 50 people 18 years or younger. At the time of this publication deadline, no final conclusion had been made regarding labeling requirements.

(iii) Consider for use if tics or insomnia are triggered by stimulant treatment.

(iv) Perform electrocardiogram (EKG) and blood pressure monitoring baseline and when therapeutic dose is reached due to potential cardiac effects.

(v) Assess family history of arrhythmias.

(vi) Educate the individual and family regarding possible cardiotoxicity symptoms (such as chest pain, especially with exercise, shortness of breath).

(b) Aminoketones.

(i) Bupropion (Wellbutrin®, Wellbutrin SR® & XL®)

(ii) Selective serotonin reuptake.

(iii) Studies are few, but research shows that the same dosing parameters used for depression are necessary for ADHD treatment.

(iv) FDA preliminary analysis of data shows that taking antidepressants may increase suicidal thoughts and actions in about 1 out of 50 people 18 years or younger. No final conclusion regarding labeling requirements at the time of publication.

(v) No cardiac conduction delays; EKG monitoring not required.

(vi) Lowers seizure threshold – Contraindicated with seizure disorder diagnosis.

Do not use concurrently with other drugs that reduce seizure threshold.

(vii) Do not use with current or prior diagnosis of anorexia nervosa or bulimia due to higher incidence of seizures.

(c) Antihypertensive medications (Posey, Puntney, Sasher, Kem, & McDougle, 2004).

(i) Although used for treatment of ADHD, clonidine (Catapres®) and guanfacine (Tenex®) are approved only for the treatment of hypertension; clonidine is approved only for adolescent and adult hypertension, while guanfacine is approved for adults only. There is some debate as to their use with stimulants (Wilens & Spencer, 1999; 2000). Psychiatric use is off label and considered under various circumstances, including:

(A) Children who are very hyperactive, impulsive, aggressive.

(B) Children who are able to attend to schoolwork or when engaged in activity, but are otherwise very active.

(C) Children whose parents object to the use of stimulant medications.

(D) Children living in environments where stimulant medications may not be secure.

(ii) Blood pressure monitoring required. Concern regarding cardiac effects: Hypotension/rebound hypertension especially 2 to 4 days after abrupt withdrawal.

(iii) Guanfacine is less sedating than clonidine.

3. Behavioral treatment of ADHD – Behavioral treatment is the other main treatment mode for ADHD. In many instances, these interventions are a valuable adjunct in treatment. However, behavioral treatment ranks second to pharmacologic intervention in the management of ADHD (Barkley, 2004; Bauchner, 2000; MTA Cooperative Group, 1999a, 1999b).
   a. Behavioral treatments range from direct behavior modification through cognitive-behavioral strategies, to behavioral interventions based on the principles and application of social learning theory.
   b. Implementations vary from a simple star chart to a sophisticated establishment of a token economy for home and school, integrated by structured communication, such a daily report card.
   c. The exploration of the many different types of behavioral treatment is outside the scope of this chapter, but it is important to recognize the role of such treatment and the availability for use in the time constraints of daily practice.
4. If medication and behavioral treatments are being used and the child is unresponsive, then the diagnosis must be reconsidered and co-morbidities must be ruled out.
5. Alternative and complementary therapies for ADHD (Arnold, 2001; Cala, Crismon, & Baumgartner, 2003). Alternative and complementary therapies are available and may be beneficial. Trials must include full disclosure between the clinician and the family regarding potential costliness and lack of scientific data. As with any therapy, if it is not decreasing the target behaviors, the parents must be encouraged and supported in the decision to abandon. Examples include but are not limited to:
   a. Dietary changes.
   b. Vitamin supplementation.
   c. Relaxation/ biofeedback/hypnotherapy.
   d. Massage.
   e. Herbal healing.
   f. Vision/oculovestibular therapy.
   g. Magnet therapy.
D. Care management (Lopez, Toprac, Crismon, Boemer, & Baumgartner, 2005; Power, 2002;

Rushton, Fant, & Clark, 2004).
1. Multi-modal treatment is important to achieve optimal outcomes.
2. Key psychosocial interventions include assuring the patient and parent that:
   a. No medical test available to confirm diagnosis.
   b. ADHD does not result from poor parenting.
   c. ADHD symptoms are beyond the control of the child.
3. Emotional responses are fluid and inconsistent.
   a. Guilt.
   b. Anger.
   c. Stress.
   d. Chronic sorrow as grief response.
4. Chronicity model: Long-term management for greatest impact on outcome.
E. Patient education.
1. Therapeutic adherence.
   a. Proactivity is key.
   b. Assess for ADHD in other family members, especially those responsible for the care of the child.
      (1) Keep medication regime simple.
      (2) Written instructions and reminders.
      (3) Technology aides, if accessible within family.
2. Types of adherence.
   a. Adherent – Overly.
      (1) ADHD lives in home.
      (2) Child is lost in environment.
   b. Adherent – Appropriate.
   c. Non-adherent – Accidental.
      (1) Forgotten dose.
      (2) Sudden financial crisis.
   d. Non-adherent – Unknown etiology.
      (1) Thoroughly reassess the patient.
      (2) Use team approach in reassessment, if possible.
3. Everyone involved and aware of the treatment plan and outcomes.
   a. Obtain written permission to communicate with school, outside agencies, and all persons providing care.
   b. Provide ongoing appropriate education and resources.
4. Planning transitions.
   a. Set developmentally appropriate goals.
   b. Start early – Resources may be limited,

Table 22-14.

ADHD Internet Resources

A to Z Disorder Guide – NYU Child Study Center – http://www.aboutourkids.org
ADHD Support Company – http://www.adhdsupportcompany.com
American Academy of Child & Adolescent Psychiatry – http://www.aacap.org (Facts for Families)
American Academy of Pediatrics (AAP) – http://www.aap.org
Attention-Deficit Disorder Association (ADDA) – http://www.add.org
Children and Adults with Attention Deficit Hyperactivity Disorder – http://www.chadd.org
Center for Complementary and Alternative Pharmacotherapy – http://www.mcphs.edu/altmed
Council for Learning Disabilities – http://cldinternational.org
Comprehensive Treatment for Attention-Deficit Disorder – http://www.ctadd.com
Education Resources Information Center (ERIC) – http://ericir.syr.edu
Food and Drug Administration – http://www.fda.gov/cder/pediatric
Guide to Popular Natural Products – Facts and Comparisons – www.drugfacts.com
Holistic Kids Integrative Pediatric Medical Education Report – www.holistickids.org
Internet Resource for Special Children – http://www.irsc.org
Learning Disabilities Association of America (LDA) – http://www.ldanatl.org
Learning Disorders http://pbs.org/wgbh/misunderstoodminds
National Attention Deficit Disorder Association – http://www.add.org
National Information Center for Children and Youth with Disabilities http://www.nichy.org
National Institute on Drug Abuse – http://nida.nih.gov
National Institute of Mental Health (NIMH) – http://www.nimh.nih.gv
National Mental Health Association – http://www.nmha.org
NIH: National Center for Complementary and Alternative Medicine – http://www.nccam.nih.gov
NIH Office of Dietary Supplements – http://ods.od.nih.gov
Parent Advocacy Coalition for Educational Rights (PACER) Center – http://www.pacer.org
Pediatric Development and Behavior – http://www.dbpeds.org

creativity is essential.

   c. Go slowly – Build upon each success.

F. Advocacy.

   1. Support the parent as ultimate child advocate.

   2. Special services at schools protected by federal laws.

     a. *Individuals with Disabilities Education Act of 1990* (IDEA) (PL 101-476).

       (1) Established the principle of free, appropriate education in the least restrictive environment for all children with disabilities, the right to due process, appropriate assessment, and that each child with a disability has an individualized education plan.

       (2) Children with ADHD are eligible for special services if they meet the criteria of "other health impaired" (defined as any acute or chronic condition that results in limited alertness and thereby impairs educational performance), "learning disabled," or "emotionally disturbed." The child is eligible for special services if the ADHD has a significant impact on the child's education.

     b. Section 504 of the *Rehabilitation Act of*

1973 (PL 93-112).

(1) Provides that individuals with disabilities cannot be discriminated against in any program or activity receiving federal funds.

(2) Allows for classroom accommodations for children whose disability is causing problems that are not specifically academic.

(3) Children with ADHD may have accommodations, such as repeating instructions, modified tests or homework, daily school-home notes, extra time to complete assignments, typed rather then handwritten assignments, or teacher-checked assignment books.

3. Resources available to parents, providers, and the public are shown in Table 22-14.

G. Telehealth practice.

1. May utilize telehealth practice when a therapeutic plan is established and the patient is stable.

2. Especially useful for evaluation of confounding factors.

   a. Substitute teacher, difficult academic work, peer conflicts.

   b. Change in home routine, change in sleep habits, recent illness.

3. Useful for recommendations for discussion with counselor.

H. Communication/documentation.

1. Document subjective and objective on the medical record, along with the nursing assessment and treatment plan.

2. Document involvement in counseling/behavioral interventions.

3. Communicate with other members of the team, including physician, social worker, psychologist, etc., as appropriate.

I. Outcomes management.

1. Parent and child report of progress.

2. Report cards and comments on behavior.

3. Rating scales scored and compared to establish progress.

4. Teacher feedback during parent conferences.

Table 22-15.

Nomenclature of the Four Major Variants

Full Name	Abbreviation
Sickle cell disease-SS	SCD-SS
Sickle cell disease-SC	SCD-SC
Sickle cell disease-Sβ° thalassemia	SCD- Sβ° thal
Sickle cell disease-Sβ+ thalassemia	SCD- Sβ+ thal

Source: NHLBI, 2004b.

Sickle Cell Disease

Patient Population: Pediatric
Renée Y. Cecil, BSN, RN

Sickle cell disease is an autosomal recessive disorder characterized by the production of abnormal hemoglobin causing a decrease in red blood cell survival and polymerization of red blood cell (sickling). In the U.S., 1 in 10 African Americans has sickle cell trait, and 1 in 325 has sickle cell disease. Sickle cell trait is not a disease. It is the carrier state and does not cause symptoms except under extreme circumstance (NHLBI, 2004b). The complications in sickle cell disease are due to vaso-occlusion (blockage of blood vessels) and chronic anemia. There are four major variants of the disease (see Table 22-15). Newborn screening has played a significant role in decreasing mortality and morbidity by providing early identification of affected babies. This early identification provides the opportunity for early intervention. Currently 49 states and the District of Columbia have newborn screening programs which identify sickle cell disease (CDC, 2006). The complications of sickle cell disease are episodic and severity can be different for each individual, as well as being different for one individual throughout their lifetime (Aliyu, Tumblin, & Kato, 2006). Individuals with sickle cell diseases are now frequently surviving beyond 50 years of age (Aliyu et al., 2006).

Sickle Cell Disease:
General Health Maintenance

Individuals with sickle cell disease should receive the same general health care as individuals without the disease. However, whenever possible, they should also be followed in an organized sickle cell program or in a place where providers have knowledge of the disease and experience with its management (NHLBI, 2004b).

A. Physical examination.
   1. Frequent visits.
      a. Every 2 to 3 months during the first 2 years of life.
      b. After the age of 2 years depending upon patient/family needs; at minimum, every 6 months.
   2. Immunizations.
      a. Should receive all routine immunizations.
      b. Additional immunizations include:
         (1) Pneumococcal polysaccharide vaccine (PPV23) at age 2 years and 5 years.
         (2) Influenza vaccine yearly.
   3. Penicillin prophylaxis for prevention of pneumococcal infection.
      a. Penicillin VK 125 mg orally BID (2 months to 3 years of age).
      b. Penicillin 250 mg orally BID (over 3 years of age).
      c. Erythromycin if there is a penicillin allergy.
   4. Nutrition.
      a. Encourage breastfeeding for infants.
      b. No need for iron supplements unless proven to be iron-deficient. May lead to iron overload in individuals with sickle cell disease.
      c. Folic acid 1 mg orally daily to reduce the risk of bone marrow aplasia.
B. Laboratory evaluation to establish baseline.
   1. Complete blood count with reticulocyte count at each visit.
   2. Hemoglobin F percent every 6 months until age 2 years, then yearly.
   3. Renal function yearly after 12 months of age.
   4. Liver function yearly after 12 months of age.
   5. Routine urinalysis yearly after 12 months of age.
C. Special studies.
   1. Transcranial Doppler Ultrasound (TCD).
      a. Abnormally high flow velocity in the middle cerebral or internal carotid arteries is associated with an increased risk of stroke.
      b. Recommended starting at 2 years of age; done yearly if normal.

2. MR studies.
   a. Done to detect the presence of "silent" cerebral infarcts. Individuals with "silent" infarcts are at a higher risk for having overt stroke.
   b. Should be done yearly until age 5 years and then every other year.
3. Neuropsychological testing, as indicated.
   a. Abnormal TCD and/or MR studies.
   b. Deterioration in school performance.
4. Pulmonary function tests.
   a. Done for those with history of recurrent acute chest syndrome and low baseline oxygen saturation.
   b. Oxygen saturation assessed at each office visit.
D. Patient/family education – Age appropriate.
   1. Fever.
      a. Indication of potentially life-threatening bacterial infection.
      b. Seek medical care immediately for temperature greater than or equal to 101°F and/or signs of infection.
      c. Do not give antipyretics at home.
      d. Importance of penicillin prophylaxis.
   2. Growth and development.
      a. Tend to be smaller than their peers.
      b. Delayed development of secondary sexual characteristics.
   3. Chronic anemia.
      a. Jaundice due to hemolysis. Not significant unless accompanied by other symptoms.
      b. Parents should be taught to palpate and measure spleen.
      c. Parents should be reassured that heart murmur due to chronic anemia does not require further evaluation.
   4. Dental.
      a. Subacute bacterial endocarditis (SBE) prophylaxis is required for patients with a history of rheumatic heart disease, mitral valve prolapse, heart murmurs, those with implanted venous access catheters, and orthopedic prosthesis (NHLBI, 2004b).
      b. Hospitalization and red blood cell transfusion prior to any procedure requiring general anesthesia.

5. Eye.
   a. Eye examination by ophthalmologist yearly beginning at age 5 years.
   b. Ophthalmologist should be a retinal specialist.
E. Painful episodes.
   1. Potential site.
      a. Limbs.
      b. Abdominal viscera.
      c. Ribs.
      d. Sternum.
      e. Vertebrae.
      f. Skull bones.
   2. Precipitating factors.
      a. Most have no precipitating factor.
      b. Extreme changes in temperature.
      c. Physical and psychological stress.
      d. Infection.
      e. Dehydration.
   3. Severity.
      a. Range from mild (able to treat at home) to excruciating (requiring hospitalization).
      b. Duration can be hours to weeks.
      c. Most are not life-threatening.
   4. Recording pain (Platt & Sacerdote, 2002).
      a. Location of pain.
      b. Other symptoms such as fever, nausea, cough.
      c. Character of the pain – Deep, burning, throbbing.
      d. Aggravating and alleviating things – What makes it worse and what makes it better.
      e. Timing – When did it start, does it come and go.
      f. Environment and effect – Activity and location when pain began, does pain affect daily routine.
      g. Severity – Do not over estimate, this could lead to being over medicated.
   5. Treatment.
      a. Increase fluids, especially water.
      b. Rest and relaxation.
      c. Distraction.
      d. Massage.
      e. Warm compress.
      f. Medications.
         (1) Acetaminophen – Do not use if there is a fever. Always take tem-
perature first.
         (2) Ibuprofen and ketorolac – Do not use if there is a fever. Always take temperature first.
         (3) Acetaminophen with codeine – Mild opiate; do not use if there is a fever.
         (4) Stronger opiates, as needed.
      g. If home management is unsuccessful or if there is a fever, the patient/parent should call the health care provider and go to the emergency room for evaluation and IV pain management.

Sickle Cell Disease: Complications and Management

A. Fever and infection: Alteration in thermodynamics.
   1. Overview.
      a. Temperature greater than or equal to 101°F may be indicative of life-threatening bacterial infection.
      b. Increased susceptibility to bacterial infection due to decreased splenic function. The infection often has no focus.
      c. Leading cause of death in sickle cell disease-afflicted children under the age of 5 years.
      d. Most common causative agents: *Streptococcus pneumoniae, Haemophilus influenzae, Salmonella.*
      e. Considered a medical emergency because the risk of death from overwhelming sepsis is high.
   2. Assessment.
      a. Signs and symptoms of infection.
      b. Possible bone infection (osteomyelitis): pain and swelling over an extremity, elevated white blood cell count, fever (Wethers, 2000a).
      c. Refer for acute care management.
   3. Medical management.
      a. History and physical examination.
      b. Complete blood count with differential, reticulocyte count, and blood cultures.
      c. Chest X-ray if indicated for children, strongly recommended for those under 3 years of age.
      d. The following tests as indicated: Urinalysis, urine culture, throat culture,

stool culture, virology evaluation, lumbar puncture.

  e. IV hydration, IV antibiotics, antipyretics.

  f. Consult hematology team.

4. Nursing intervention/patient/family education.

  a. Emphasize that a fever in a child with sickle cell disease can be indicative of a life-threatening bacterial infection. Promote adequate hydration.

  b. Immediate medical attention is needed for temperature greater than or equal to 101°F.

  c. Do not give antipyretics before calling the health care provider.

  d. Penicillin prophylaxis should be given as directed. It is very important that the child does not miss a dose. Call for refills before medication runs out.

  e. Caregiver should demonstrate the ability to take a temperature.

  f. Instruct caregiver to call if child has diarrhea, vomiting, productive cough, irritability, or if the child "just doesn't seem right."

  g. Encourage good primary care followup and keeping immunizations up-to-date. Immunizations should include pneumococcal vaccine and influenza vaccine.

B. Vaso-occlusive painful episode: Alteration in comfort.

  1. Overview.

    a. Most common type of vaso-occlusive episode.

    b. Due to the blockage of small blood vessels by sickle cells leading to decreased oxygen perfusion, ischemia, infarction, and pain. May be precipitated by extreme changes in temperature, stress, infection, dehydration, and hypoxia.

    c. Most are not life-threatening.

    d. Account for most hospitalizations.

    e. Onset is sudden, unpredictable, recurrent, and variable. Can be in any and all parts of the body.

    f. Dactylitis or hand-foot syndrome.

      (1) Usually occurs in children between 6 months and 2 years.

      (2) Acute painful swelling of one or more extremities.

      (3) Duration is approximately 1 week. Can reoccur.

      (4) Can be predicative of severe disease.

  2. Assessment.

    a. Location, onset, and severity of pain. Is it typical or atypical of vaso-occlusive pain. Use appropriate pain scales to classify severity of pain as mild, moderate, or severe.

    b. Medications taken, dose taken, time of last dose, and response to medication.

    c. Pain medications that have worked in the past.

    d. Effective non-pharmacologic therapies used.

    e. Rule out possibility of trauma.

    f. Refer for acute care management if home management unsuccessful.

  3. Medical management.

    a. Requires prompt evaluation and treatment.

    b. Past medical history.

      (1) Baseline hemoglobin, hematocrit, O_2 saturation.

      (2) Allergies.

    c. Physical examination including appropriate laboratory studies and X-rays, as indicated.

    d. IV hydration.

    e. Combination drug therapy – Opioids with NSAIDs and/or acetaminophen.

  4. Nursing intervention.

    a. Response to medication.

    b. Respiratory status. Encourage ambulation and use of incentive spirometer.

    c. Possible side effects to medication such as puritis, over sedation, and GI complaints. Administer stool softener, diphenhydramine, and Mylanta®, as indicated.

    d. Patient/family education.

      (1) FARMS (Platt & Sacerdote, 2002).

        F – Fluids and Fever – Drink plenty of fluids and seek immediate medical care for fever.

        A – Air – Maintain adequate oxygen.

        R – Rest – Get plenty of sleep, rest when needed, no over-exertion.

M – Medication – Take medication as directed.
S – Situations – Avoid getting too hot or too cold, smoking, alcohol, and illegal drugs.

(2) Side effects of medication, correct dosing of medication, types of non-pharmacologic treatments.

(3) Parents should be aware that opioids can lead to severe constipation.

(4) Clinical parameters for seeking medical attention – pain unrelieved or of increasing severity despite home management, fever greater than or equal to 101°F.

(5) Incentive spirometer when managing pain at home.

C. Acute exacerbation of anemia: Alteration if fluid volume; alteration in tissue perfusion.

1. Transient red cell aplasia.
   a. Overview.
      (1) Bone marrow viral suppression of red blood cell production.
      (2) Usual cause – Parvovirus B19. There is no recurrence of parvovirus infections (Sarjeant & Sarjeant, 2001).
      (3) May require hospitalization and red cell transfusion if decreasing hemoglobin results in symptoms of cardiac compromise.
      (4) Recovery usually in 7 to 10 days (Serjeant & Serjeant, 2001).
   b. Assessment.
      (1) Assess for fever, cough, rash.
      (2) Determine if child has tachypnea, tachycardia, listlessness, or pallor. Is spleen palpable?
      (3) Refer for acute care management.
   c. Medical management.
      (1) Complete blood count with reticulocyte count, parvovirus titers (should do parvovirus polymerase chain reaction (PCR) test, and repeat in one week if negative), type and cross for possible red blood cell transfusion, blood culture if febrile.
      (2) IV hydration, IV antibiotics, if indicated.
      (3) Red blood cell transfusion, if indicated.

d. Nursing intervention.
   (1) Monitor hemoglobin/hematocrit, reticulocyte count.
   (2) Monitor for signs of cardiovascular compromise due to decreased hemoglobin.
   (3) Isolate from others at increased risk for infection, such as pregnant women, those who are immuno-compromised, and others with hemolytic anemias.
   (4) Patient/family education.
      (a) Usual cause – Parvovirus B19. Does not recur; self-limiting.
      (b) Seek medical attention if the child has a fever greater than or equal to 101°F, is pale, more tired, has rapid heart beat, or rapid breathing.
      (c) May require hospitalization and red cell transfusion if decreasing hemoglobin results in symptoms of cardiac compromise.
      (d) Siblings and other at-risk family members should be tested.

2. Acute splenic sequestration: Alteration in fluid volume.
   a. Overview.
      (1) Intrasplenic trapping of red blood cells which cause a precipitous fall in hemoglobin level and the potential for hypoxic shock (NHLBI, 2004b). Spleen becomes large and tender.
      (2) Potentially life-threatening.
      (3) Usually requires hospitalization and possibly red blood cell transfusion if decreasing hemoglobin results in symptoms of cardiac compromise.
      (4) Usually occurs between the ages of 3 months and 5 years of age in those with SCD-SS. May occur later in other variants. Recurrence is common (NHLBI, 2004b).
   b. Assessment.
      (1) Onset of symptoms: Fever, irritability, tachypnea, tachycardia, listlessness, pallor, left-sided abdominal pain.
      (2) Spleen size and mark location.

(3) Baseline hemoglobin/hematocrit and spleen size.

(4) Refer for acute care management.

c. Medical management.

(1) Complete blood count with reticulocyte count, type and cross for possible red blood cell transfusion, and blood culture if febrile.

(2) IV hydration and IV antibiotics, if indicated.

d. Nursing intervention.

(1) Monitor hemoglobin/hematocrit, reticulocyte count.

(2) Monitor for signs of cardiovascular compromise due to decreased hemoglobin.

(3) Assess spleen size hourly and mark location.

(4) Mark level of spleen at discharge.

(5) Patient/family education.

(a) Seek medical attention if the child has a fever greater than or equal to 101°F, is pale, more tired than usual, or has rapid hear beat, rapid breathing, complaint of left side abdominal pain.

(b) Teach family how to palpate spleen.

(c) Explain that splenic sequestration often recurs and child may need to be started on a chronic transfusion program. Splenectomy may be indicated, particularly if recurrence occurs while on a transfusion program.

(d) Maintain adequate fluid intake.

D. Acute chest syndrome: Alteration in gas exchange.

1. Overview.

a. Defined as an acute illness characterized by fever and respiratory symptoms, accompanied by a new pulmonary infiltrate on a chest X-ray (NHLBI, 2004b).

b. Frequent cause of death in both children and adults.

c. The second most common cause of hospitalizations in patients with sickle cell disease (NHLBI, 2004b).

d. Most common complication of surgery and anesthesia (NHLBI, 2004b).

e. When caused by infection the most common organisms are *Streptococcus pneumoniae* and *Haemophilus influenzae* (Serjeant & Serjeant, 2001).

2. Assessment.

a. Assess for fever, cough, chest pain, shortness of breath, and oxygen saturation.

b. Assess for history of painful episode, medications taken, and decreased activity.

c. Refer for acute care management.

3. Medical management.

a. Complete blood count, reticulocyte count, blood cultures, type and cross, chest X-ray, and monitor oxygen saturation.

b. Carefully monitor IV hydration.

c. Supplemental oxygen as needed.

d. IV antibiotics. Pain medication, antipyretics, and bronchodilators, as indicated.

e. Red blood cell transfusion, as indicated.

4. Nursing intervention.

a. Monitor hydration; Very important to avoid over hydration. Carefully monitor intake and output.

b. Encourage use of incentive spirometer and encourage ambulation.

c. Monitor vital signs and laboratory values carefully.

d. Patient/family education.

(1) Instruct patient to complete course of antibiotics.

(2) Use of incentive spirometer.

(3) Importance of ambulation.

(4) Seek medical attention if child has fever greater than or equal to 101°F, chest pain, difficulty breathing.

E. Priapism: Alteration in comfort.

1. Overview.

a. Sustained, unwanted, and painful penile erection usually unrelated to sexual activity (Mantadakis, Ewalt, Cavender, Rogers, & Buchanan, 2000).

b. Due to vaso-occlusion causing obstruction of the venous drainage of the penis (NHLBI, 2004b).

c. Can occur as early as 4 years old (Serjeant & Serjeant , 2000).

d. Types.
   (1) Prolonged priapism last for more than 3 hours. (NHLBI, 2004b) Considered a urologic emergency (Mantadakis et al., 2000).
   (2) Stuttering priapism lasts for less than 3 hours, but more than a few minutes. Resolves spontaneously (NHLBI, 2004b).
   (3) Associated with an increased incidence of impotence.
2. Assessment.
   a. Assess time of onset, presence of trauma, infection, or drug use.
   b. Assess for fever, dysuria and dehydration.
   c. Assess type of home management.
   d. History of prior episodes and effective treatments.
   e. Refer for acute care management.
3. Medical management.
   a. Complete blood count with reticulocyte count.
   b. IV hydration and IV morphine.
   c. Encourage patient to empty bladder.
   d. Consult urology for possible penile aspiration if above management unsuccessful after 2 hours.
   e. Red blood cell transfusion, if indicated.
4. Nursing intervention/patient/family education.
   a. Explain to the patient that it is very important to let someone know right away when an episode begins.
   b. What to do at home: Drink plenty of fluids, attempt to empty bladder, take analgesics, and take a warm shower or bath.
   c. Seek medical care if unresolved after 2 hours.

F. Cerebrovascular accident (stroke): Alteration in neurological status.
   1. Overview.
      a. About 10% of children with SCD-SS are at risk for stroke (Wethers, 2000b).
      b. Usually infarctive in young children (Stuart & Nagel, 2004).
      c. The peak incidence is between 2 and 5 years (Stuart & Nagel, 2004).
      d. Risk factors include history of tran-

sient ischemic attack, low steady state hemoglobin level, high leukocyte count, raised systolic blood pressure, history of acute chest syndrome, abnormal TCD and hypoxemia (Stuart & Nagel, 2004).
   2. Assessment.
      a. Onset of symptoms.
      b. Assess for fever, headaches, syncope, altered mental status, weakness, visual changes, seizures.
      c. History of previous neurological events.
      d. Refer for emergency care.
   3. Medical management.
      a. Complete physical with neurological examination.
      b. Immediate CT scan, exchange transfusion, ICU admission and MR studies.
      c. Chronic transfusion program.
      d. Consult neurologist.
   4. Nursing intervention/patient/family education.
      a. Seek medical attention immediately for any symptoms of stroke.
         (1) Sudden weakness or tingling of an arm, leg, or the whole body, and facial changes.
         (2) Loss of vision or speech.
         (3) Sudden strong headache described as the "worst headache ever had."
         (4) Fainting, dizziness.
      b. Encourage compliance with transfusion, medications, and rehabilitation.

G. Gallbladder disease (gallstones): Alteration in comfort.
   1. Overview.
      a. Chronic hemolysis and increased bilirubin turnover leads to a high incidence of pigment gallstones (NHLBI, 2004b).
      b. Biliary sludge (viscous material) may be a precursor to the development of gallstones (NHLBI, 2004b).
      c. Gallstones can be detected in children as young as 2 years of age.
      d. Risk factors include high bilirubin levels, low hemoglobin F, and increasing mean red cell volume (Serjeant & Serjeant, 2001).
      e. May cause blockage of common bile duct.
   2. Assessment.

a. Onset of symptoms, may be precipitated by eating fatty or fried foods.
b. History of previous episodes.
c. Assess for fever, increased scleral icterus, nausea, vomiting, and right upper quadrant abdominal pain.
d. Refer for acute management if febrile or in severe pain.

3. Medical management.
   a. Abdominal ultrasound.
   b. Liver function test and bilirubin profile.
   c. If recurrent episodes, cholecystectomy with pre-operative transfusion.

4. Nursing intervention/patient/family education.
   a. Seek medical attention if child has fever, right upper quadrant abdominal pain, nausea, vomiting, or increased jaundice.
   b. Dietary – Avoid fatty and fried foods.
   c. Explain need for pre-operative transfusion if surgery, is indicated.

H. Renal complications: Alteration in tissue perfusion; Alteration in elimination.
   1. Overview.
      a. There are many abnormalities in renal function and structure due to chronic anemia and vaso-occlusion. (Serjeant & Serjeant, 2001).
      b. Inability to concentrate urine leading to a high incidence of enuresis, nocturia, and polyuria.
      c. Problems noted to occur involving the kidneys:
         (1) Proteinuria, may be indicative of glomerular sclerosis
         (2) Hematuria, secondary to papillar necrosis.
         (3) Urinary tract infections.
         (4) Renal failure.
   2. Assessment.
      a. Yearly routine urinalysis.
      b. Assess for worsening anemia.
   3. Medical management.
      a. Dependent on symptoms.
      b. Consult urology and nephrology, as indicated.
      c. Red cell transfusion as indicated.
   4. Nursing intervention/patient/family education.
      a. Encourage adequate fluid intake.
      b. Should have easy access to bathroom

particularly during school hours. School should be provided with written information on the needs of the child.
c. Enuresis is not a cause for disciplinary action.
d. Use of bed-wetting alarm when indicated.
e. Instruct on signs and symptoms of urinary tract infection.

I. Avascular necrosis: Alteration in comfort and mobility.
   1. Overview (NHLBI, 2004b).
      a. Most prevalent in patients with SCD-SS.
      b. Most often involves the femoral and humeral heads.
   2. Assessment.
      a. Assess for pain in hip or shoulder.
      b. Assess for impaired mobility.
   3. Medical management.
      a. Physical examination.
      b. X-ray and MRI of affected joints.
      c. Consult orthopedic surgery.
      d. Treatment may include chronic transfusion to promote healing, crutches, and braces.
      e. Surgery may be indicated if palliative treatment is unsuccessful.
   4. Nursing intervention/patient education.
      a. Seek medical attention for pain, particularly when bearing weight or attempting to use arms.
      b. Instruct the patient to maintain followup with orthopedics.
      c. Encourage patient to avoid weight bearing and to use crutches as indicated.
      d. Explain necessity of pre-operative transfusion, if surgery is indicated.

J. Retinopathy: Alteration in vision.
   1. Overview (NHLBI, 2004b).
      a. Non-proliferative disease includes conjunctival vascular occlusions, iris atrophy, retinal hemorrhages, retinal pigmentary changes, and other abnormalities. High rate of spontaneous regression and lack of progression.
      b. Proliferative disease involves the growth of abnormal vascular fronds that predispose the patient to vitreous hemorrhage and retinal detachment. Increased risk of visual loss from hemorrhage and reti-

nal detachment.

   c. Individuals with SCD-SC are at higher risk.

2. Assessment.
   a. Complaints of visual disturbances.
   b. When was patient's last ophthalmology appointment?
   c. History of previous retinopathy.
   d. History of trauma to the eye.

3. Medical management.
   a. Yearly examination by ophthalmologist who specializes in diseases of the retina.
   b. Treatment reserved for disease that has progressed to the proliferative stage.
   c. Methods of treatments include laser photocoagulation and vitrectomy if retinal detachment or vitreous hemorrhage is present.

4. Nursing intervention/patient education.
   a. Seek medical attention in the event of eye trauma, changes in vision, bleeding in the eye.
   b. Stress importance of yearly eye examination by ophthalmologist.

K. Leg ulcers: Alteration in skin integrity.
1. Overview.
   a. Causes chronic disability in 10% to 15% of older SCD-afflicted children and adults. Result of localized tissue death (Platt & Sacerdote, 2002).
   b. Usually occurs in areas with less subcutaneous fat, thin skin, and decreased blood flow (Trent & Kirsner, 2004).
   c. Heals much slower than venous ulcers and tends to recur. Patients may experience significant disfigurement (Trent & Kirsner, 2004).

2. Assessment.
   a. Vascular history and current medications.
   b. Level of pain and signs of infection.
   c. Examine leg for skin integrity, discoloration, edema, and temperature.
   d. Vital signs including pedal pulses.
   e. Assess for other causes, such as diabetes mellitus, varicose veins, and collagen vascular disease (NHLBI, 2004b).
   f. Refer for acute care management, particularly if signs of cellulitis.

3. Medical management.

   a. History and physical examination.
   b. Diagnostic tests: X-ray, MRI, Doppler ultrasound.
   c. Treatment options include topical treatments, dressings, surgical interventions, and systemic medications (Trent & Kirsner, 2004).
   d. Pain management.
   e. Red blood cell transfusion therapy.

4. Nursing intervention/patient education.
   a. Instruct patient to avoid trauma, wear properly fitting shoes, use insect repellent, maintain good personal hygiene, and use lotions to prevent dry skin.
   b. Instruct the patient to keep the wound clean, change dressing as directed, drink plenty of fluids, maintain nutritious diet, and take medications as directed.
   c. Encourage bed rest and leg elevation to promote healing.
   d. Explain reason for transfusion therapy.

L. Triage.
1. Fever: Fever greater than or equal to 101°F is a medical emergency, refer for acute care management.
2. Vaso-occlusive pain: Assist with home management. If home management is unsuccessful or if the patient has a fever, refer for acute care management.
3. Transient red cell aplasia: If afebrile, monitor lab values to assess increasing anemia. If febrile and signs of cardiac compromise, refer for acute care management.
4. Splenic sequestration: Medical emergency. Assess symptoms and level of spleen.
5. Acute chest syndrome: Attempt to differentiate between vaso-occlusive painful episode and acute chest syndrome. Refer for acute care management if febrile, difficulty breathing, cough.
6. Priapism: Assist with home management. If not resolved within 2 hours, refer for acute care management.
7. Cerebrovascular accident: Medical emergency. Refer to emergency room.
8. Gallbladder disease: Jaundice only, encourage increased fluids. Jaundice accompanied by nausea, vomiting, abdominal pain and fever, refer for acute care management.

9. Renal: Consult urology and nephrology as needed.
10. Avascular necrosis: Assist with home management. If fever, severe pain, and impaired mobility, refer for acute care management.

M. Care management, communication, and documentation.
   1. If care is not provided by a sickle cell program, it should be coordinated with a hematologist experienced in the care of individuals with sickle cell disease.
   2. Assist the patient/family in keeping a diary regarding care.
   3. Followup telephone calls as indicated to discuss current condition, lab values, diagnostic tests, need for followup.
   4. Document complete history and recommendation.
   5. Develop protocols for each complication.

Sickle Cell Disease: Current Therapies

A. Red blood cell transfusions.
   1. Indications.
      a. Episodic transfusions for acute severe anemia, pre-operative, hypoxia/acute chest syndrome.
      b. Chronic transfusions for stroke, abnormal TCD, debilitating pain, recurrent splenic sequestration, recurrent and severe acute chest syndrome.
   2. Goals of therapy.
      a. Episodic transfusions – Correction of anemia and increase oxygen carrying capacity.
      b. Chronic transfusion – To reduce hemoglobin S percent to less than 30%.
   3. Complications.
      a. Volume overload.
      b. Iron overload.
      c. Alloimmunization and delayed transfusion reaction.
      d. Infection.
   4. Education.
      a. Explain the need for need for transfusion.
      b. Inform patient/family about the importance of maintaining the transfusion regimen.
      c. Risk of transfusion reaction.

d. Eventual need for chelation therapy due to iron overload.

B. Hydroxyurea.
   1. Chemotherapeutic agents that increase the percent of fetal hemoglobin in the red blood cell. In high percents, fetal hemoglobin can prevent the formation of sickle cells.
   2. Decreases the rate of bone marrow production of red blood cells, white blood cells, and platelets.
   3. Goals of therapy.
      a. Reduce the occurrence of acute chest syndrome, severe pain, and the need for transfusions.
      b. Increase the production of fetal hemoglobin, which reduces sickling, vaso-occlusion, and hemolysis.
      c. Raises hemoglobin level.
   4. Education.
      a. How medication should be taken.
      b. Side effects of medication.
      c. Need for frequent laboratory evaluations.

C. Bone marrow transplantation.
   1. Only cure for sickle cell disease.
   2. Very risky.
   3. Requires matched, related donor, such as an unaffected sibling.
   4. Candidates usually have severe disease that makes taking the risk of transplant worthwhile.

Sickle Cell Disease: Psychosocial Management

A. Multidisciplinary team approach.
   1. Patient and family.
   2. Physician, nurse, and social worker.
   3. Psychologist.
   4. Community organization

B. School/work.
   1. Frequent absences from work or school.
   2. Families should have documentation that school or work may be interrupted due to complications of the disease.
   3. Schools should have printed materials regarding care of the child with sickle cell disease in school. Need for fluids, bathroom breaks, who to call if child should become ill.
   4. Assess need for episodic homebound education.

Sickle Cell Disease: Resources

A. Local comprehensive sickle cell center.

B. Sickle Disease Association of American (National) (www.sicklecelldisease.org). Several cities have local chapters.

C. Local social service agencies.

D. General sickle cell disease information - Emory site (www.scinfo.org).

E. National Institute of Health, National Heart Lung and Blood Institute, Division of Blood Disorders and Resources.

F. Mid-Atlantic Sickle Cell Disease Consortium (MASCC) Practice Guidelines (www.pitt.edu/~marhgn/guide.pdf).

References

AARP. (n.d.). *Affordable prescription drugs for men and women over 50, cost of medicines.* Retrieved December 7, 2005, from http://www.aarp.org/health/affordable_drugs

Adesman, A. (2003). A diagnosis of ADHD? Don't overlook the probability of comorbidity! *Contemporary Pediatrics, 20*(12), 91-106.

Albert, N.M. (2004). Ventricular dysrhythmias in heart failure. *Journal of Cardiovascular Nursing, 19*(Suppl), S11-S26.

Albert, N.M. (2005a). Maximizing acute care opportunities for improving outcomes. In N.M. Albert & R.J. Trupp (Eds.), *Novel approaches in the diagnosis and treatment of heart failure.* AACN news supplement. Thorofare, NJ: Slack, Inc.

Albert N.M. (2005b). Cardiovascular. In K.K. Kuebler, M.P. Davis, & C.D. Moore (Eds.), *Palliative practices: An interdisciplinary approach* (pp. 121-156). Mosby: St. Louis, MO.

Albert, N.M., Eastwood, C.A., & Edwards, M.L. (2004). Evidence-based practice for acute decompensated heart failure. *Critical Care Nurse, 24*(6), 14-24, 26.

Albert, N.M., Paul, S., & McCauley, K.M. (2003). Living with heart failure: Promoting adherence, managing symptoms and optimizing function. In M. Jessup & K.M. McCauley (Eds.), *Heart failure: Providing optimal care* (pp. 145-164). Elmsford, NY: Blackwell Publishing.

Albert, N., & Young J. (2001). Heart failure disease management: A team approach. *Cleveland Clinic Journal of Medicine, 16*(1), 53-62.

Aliyu, Z.Y., Tumblin, A.R., & Kato, G.J. (2006). Current therapy of sickle cell disease. *Haematologica/The Hematology Journal, 91*(10), 7-10.

American Academy of Child and Adolescent Psychiatry. (2002). Practice parameter for the use of stimulant medications in the treatment of children, adolescents, and adults. *Journal of American Academy of Child and Adolescent Psychiatry, 41*(2 Suppl), 26S-49S.

American Academy of Pediatrics. (2000). Clinical practice guideline: Diagnosis and evaluation of the child with attention-deficit/hyperactivity disorder. *Pediatrics, 105,* 1158-1170.

American Academy of Pediatrics. (2001). Clinical practice guideline: Treatment of the school-aged child with attention-deficit/hyperactivity disorder. *Pediatrics, 108,* 1033-1044.

American College of Cardiology/American Heart Association Task Force. (2005a). *ACC/AHA 2005 guideline update for the diagnosis and management of chronic heart failure in the adult: A report of the American College of Cardiology/American Heart Association Task Force on practical guidelines.* Retrieved August 17, 2005, from http://www.acc.org/clinical/guidelines/failure/index.pdf

American College of Cardiology/American Heart Association Task Force. (2005b). ACC/AHA clinical performance measures for adults with chronic heart failure. *Journal of the American College of Cardiology, 46,* 1144-1178.

American Diabetes Association (ADA). (2005). Clinical practice recommendations. *Diabetes Care, 28*(Suppl.1), S3.

American Psychiatric Association. (2000). *Diagnostic and statistical manual of mental disorders* (4th ed.). Washington, DC: Author.

Amylin Pharmaceuticals, Inc. (2006). *Byetta and Symlin.* Retrieved March 22, 2005, from http://www.amylin.com

Arnold, L. (2001). Alternative treatments for adults with attention-deficit hyperactivity disorder (ADHD). *Annuals New York Academy of Science, 931,* 310-341.

Arthritis Foundation. (n.d.). *The facts about arthritis.* Retrieved October 24, 2005, from http://www.arthritis.org/resources/gettingstarted/default.asp

Barkley, R. (2004). Adolescents with attention-deficit/hyperactivity disorder: An overview of empirically based treatments. *Journal of Psychiatric Practice, 10*(1), 39-56.

Bauchner, H. (2000). ADHD: A new practice guideline from the American Academy of Pediatrics. *Archives of Diseases in Childhood, 83,* 63.

Bodenheimer, T., Wagner, E.H., & Grumbach, K. (2002a). Improving primary care for patients with chronic illness. *Journal of the American Medical Association, 288*(14), 1775-1779.

Bodenheimer, T., Wagner, E.H., & Grumbach, K. (2002b). Improving primary care for patients with chronic illness: The chronic care model, Part 2. *Journal of the American Medical Association, 288*(15), 1909-1914.

Brennan, T.D., & Haas, G.D. (2005). The role of prophylactic implantable cardioverter defibrillators in heart failure: Recent trials usher in a new era of device therapy. *Current Heart Failure Reports, 2*(1), 40-45.

Brown, T. (Ed.) (2000). *Attention-deficit disorders and comorbidities in children, adolescents, and adults.* Washington DC: American Psychiatric Press, Inc.

Cala, S., Crismon, A., & Baumgartner, J. (2003). A survey of herbal use in children with attention-deficit-hyperactivity disorder or depression. *Pharmacotherapy, 23*(2), 222-230.

Celli, B.R., Cote, C.G., Marin, J.M., Casanova, C., Montes de Oca, M., Mendez, R.A., et al. (2004). The body- mass index, airflow obstruction, dyspnea, and exercise capacity index in chronic obstructive pulmonary disease. *New England Journal of Medicine, 350,* 1005.

Centers for Disease Control and Prevention (CDC). (2005). *National diabetes fact sheet.* Retrieved May 25, 2006, from http://www.cdc.gov/diabetes/pubs/factsheet.htm

Centers for Disease Control and Prevention (CDC). (2006). *Newborn screening quality assurance program: 2005 annual summary report.* Retrieved April 22, 2006, from http://www.cdc.gov/labstandards/nsqap.htm.

Centers for Disease Control and Prevention (CDC), & National Institutes for Health (NIH). (2000). *Healthy people 2010: Heart disease and stroke.* Retrieved April 22, 2006, from

http://www.healthypeople.gov/Document/HTML/Volume1/
12Heart.htm#_Toc490544222

Centers for Medicare and Medicaid Services (CMS). (n.d.). *The official U.S. government site for people with Medicare.* Retrieved December 7, 2005, from http://www.medicare.gov

Chodosh, J., Morton, S.C., Mojica, W., Maglione, M., Suttorp, M.J., Hilton, L., et al. (2005). Meta-analysis: Chronic disease self-management programs for older adults. *Annals of Internal Medicine, 143*(6), 427-438.

Costello, E., Foley, D., & Angold, A. (2006). 10-year research update review: The epidemiology of child and adolescent psychiatric disorders: II. Developmental epidemiology. *Journal of the American Academy of Child and Adolescent Psychiatry, 45*(1), 8-25.

Curry, L.C., Walker, C., Hogstel, M.O., & Burns, P. (2005). Teaching older adults to self-manage medications: Preventing adverse drug reactions. *Journal of Gerontological Nursing, 31*(4), 32-42.

Dreyer, B. (2006). The diagnosis and management of attention-deficit/hyperactivity disorder in pre-school children: The state of our knowledge and practice. *Current Problems in Pediatric and Adolescent Health Care, 36*, 6-30.

Dulcan, M. (1997). Practice parameters for the assessment and treatment of children, adolescents, and adults with attention-deficit/hyperactivity disorder. *Journal of American Academy of Child and Adolescent Psychiatry, 36*(10 Suppl.), 85S-121S.

Ebersole, P., & Hess, P. (2001). *Geriatric nursing and healthy aging.* St. Louis: Mosby.

Edwards, L.L. (1999). Phased competency: A new model to prepare nurses for enhanced roles in diabetes disease management. *Disease Management and Health Outcomes, 5*(5), 253-261.

Epill.com. (n.d.). *Medication reminders.* Retrieved December 7, 2005, from http://www.epill.com/epill/ind.html

Evans, S., Allen, J., Moore, S., & Strauss, V. (2006). Measuring symptoms and functioning of youth with ADHD in middle schools. *Journal of Abnormal Child Psychology, 33*(6), 695-706.

Ferguson, G.T., & Make, B. (2005). Overview of management of stable chronic obstructive pulmonary disease. *UpToDate® OnLine 14.1.* August, 2005.

Fight Asthma Milwaukee (FAM) Allies. (2004). *Asthma tool kit.* Milwaukee, WI: Lead Agency Children's Hospital and Health Systems.

Franz, M. (Ed.) (2003), *A core curriculum for diabetes education* (5th ed.). Chicago: American Association of Diabetes Educators.

Fulton, M.M., & Allen, E.R. (2005). Polypharmacy in the elderly: A literature review. *Journal of the American Academy of Nurse Practitioners, 17*(4), 123-132.

Goldman, D.P., Joyce, G.F., Escarce, J.J., Pace, J.E., Solomon, M.D., Laouri, M., et al. (2004). Pharmacy benefits and the use of drugs by the chronically ill. *Journal of the American Medical Association, 291*(19), 2344-2350.

Grady, K.L., Dracup, K., Kennedy, G., Moser, D.K., Piano, M., Stevenson, L.W., et al. (2000). Team management of patients with heart failure. A statement for healthcare professionals from the cardiovascular nursing council of the American Heart Association. *Circulation, 102*, 2443-2456.

Gulanick, M., Klopp, A., Galanes, S., Gradishar, D., & Puzas, M.K. (1998). *Nursing care plans: Nursing diagnosis and intervention* (4th ed.). St. Louis: Mosby.

Harkness, G., & Dincher, J. (1996). *Medical-surgical nursing: Total patient care* (9th ed.). St. Louis: Mosby.

Hayes, K. (2005). Designing written medication instructions: Effective ways to help older adults self-medicate. *Journal of Gerontological Nursing, 31*(5), 5-10.

Heart Failure Society of America (HFSA). (1999). HFSA guidelines for management of patients with heart failure caused by left ventricular systolic dysfunction – Pharmacological approaches. *Journal of Cardiac Failure, 5*(4), 357-82.

Herbst, K.L. (2002). Insulin strategies for primary care providers. *Clinical Diabetes, 20*, 11-17.

Hershberger, R.E., Nauman, D.J., Byrkit, J., Gillespie, G., Lackides, G., Toy, W., et al. (2005). Prospective evaluation of an outpatient heart failure disease management program designed for primary care: The Oregon model. *Journal of Cardiac Failure, 11*, 293-298.

Hunt, S.A., Abraham, W.T., Chin, M.H., et al. (2005). *ACC/AHA 2005 guideline update for the diagnosis and management of chronic heart failure in the adult: A report of the American College of Cardiology/American Heart Association Task Force on Practical Guidelines.* Retrieved August 17, 2005, from http://www.acc.org/guidelines/failure/index.pdf

Jessup, M. (2003). Defining heart failure: Systolic versus diastolic dysfunction, differential diagnosis, initial testing. In M. Jessup & K.M. McCauley (Eds.), *Heart failure: Providing optimal care* (pp. 51-70). Elmsford, NY: Blackwell Publishing.

Joint Commission on Accreditation of Healthcare Organizations (JCAHO). (2005). *Disease specific care. Request for public comment on disease-specific care standardized heart failure measure set.* Retrieved September 23, 2005, from http://jcaho.org/dscc/dsc/performance+measures/heart+failure+measure+set.htm

Koelling, T.M., Johnson, M.L., Cody, R.J., & Aaronson, K.D. (2005). Discharge education improves clinical outcomes in patients with chronic heart failure. *Circulation 111*, 179-185.

Kratochvil, C. (2003). Newer agents and formulations for the treatment of ADHD. *Advanced Studies in Medicine, 3*(5C), S452-S457, S464-S465.

Leier, C.V. (2005). A heart failure specialist's perspective on cardiac surgery for heart failure. *Current Heart Failure Reports, 2*(1), 46-53.

Linnell, K. (2005). Chronic disease self-management: One successful program. *Nursing Economic$, 23*(4), 189-191, 196-188.

Lopez, M., Toprac, M., Crismon, M., Boemer, C., & Baumgartner, J. (2005). A psychoeducational program for children with ADHD or depression and their families: Results from the CMAP feasibility study. *Community Mental Health Journal, 41*(1),51-67.

Lorig, K.R., & Holman, H. (2003). Self-management education: History, definition, outcomes, and mechanisms. *Annals of Behavioral Medicine, 26*(1), 1-7.

Lorig, K.R., Sobel, D.S., Ritter, P.L., Laurent, D., & Hobbs, M. (2001). Effect of a self-management program on patients with chronic disease. *Effective Clinical Practice, 4*(6), 256-262.

Manatadakis, E., Ewalt, D.H., Cavender, J.D., Rogers, Z.R. & Buchanan, G.R. (2000). Outpatient penile aspiration and epinephrine irrigation for young patients with sickle cell anemia and prolonged priapism. *Blood, 95*(1), 78-82.

McDonald, H.P., Garg, A.X., & Haynes, R.B. (2002). Interventions to enhance patient adherence to medication prescriptions:

Scientific review. *Journal of the American Medical Association, 288*(22), 2868-2879.

Misra, A., Diwan, A., Mann, D.L., & Deswal, A. (2002). Asymptomatic left ventricular dysfunction: An overlooked part of the continuum of heart failure. *Heart Failure Monitor, 3*(2), 42-48.

Mojtabai, R., & Olfson, M. (2003). Medication costs, adherence, and health outcomes among Medicare beneficiaries. *Health Affairs (Millwood), 22*(4), 220-229.

MTA Cooperative Group. (1999a). A 14-month randomized clinical trial of treatment strategies for attention- deficit/hyperactivity disorder. *Archives of General Psychiatry, 56*, 1073-1986.

MTA Cooperative Group. (1999b). Moderators and mediators of treatment response for children with attention- deficit/hyperactivity disorder. *Archives of General Psychiatry, 56*, 1088-1096.

Murray, C.J., & Lopez, A.D. (1997a). Global mortality , disability, and contribution of risk factors: Global Burden of Disease Study. *Lancet, 349,*1436.

Murray, C.J., & Lopez, A.D. (1997b). Alternative projections of mortality and disability by cause 1990-2020: Global Burden of Disease Study. *Lancet, 349,* 1498.

National Asthma Education and Prevention Program. (2002). *Update expert panel report 2: Guidelines for the diagnosis and management of asthma.* (NIH Publication No. 97-4051). Bethesda, MD: Author.

National Heart, Lung and Blood Institute (NHLBI). (2003) *The DASH eating plan.* (NIH Publication No. 03- 4082). Bethesda, MD: Author.

National Heart, Lung and Blood Institute (NHLBI). (2004a). *Seventh report of the Joint National Committee on Prevention, Detection, Evaluation, and Treatment of High Blood Pressure (JNC7).* (NIH Publication No. 04-5230). Bethesda, MD: Author.

National Heart, Lung and Blood Institute (NHLBI). (2004b). *The management of sickle cell disease* (4th ed.). (NIH Publication No. 04-2117). Bethesda, MD: Author.

National Heart, Lung and Blood Institute, & World Health Organization Workshop (NHLBI/WHO). (2005). *Global strategy for the diagnosis, management, and prevention of chronic obstructive lung disease: Executive summary 2005. Global Initiative for Chronic Obstructive Lung Disease (GOLD).* Retrieved February 27, 2006, from http://www.goldcopd.com

National Institutes of Health (NIH). (2000). Consensus Development Conference Statement: Diagnosis and treatment of attention-deficit/hyperactivity disorder (ADHD). *Journal of American Academy of Child and Adolescent Psychiatry, 39,*182-193.

Newman, S., Steed, L., & Mulligan, K. (2004). Self-management interventions for chronic illness. *Lancet, 364*(9444), 1523-1537.

Platt, A.F., & Sacerdote, A. (2002). *Hope and destiny.* Roscoe, IL: Hilton Publishing Company.

Posey, D., Puntney, J.,Sasher, T., Kem, D., & McDougle, C. (2004).Guanfacine treatment of hyperactivity and inattention in pervasive developmental disorders: A retrospective analysis of 80 cases. *Journal of Child and Adolescent Psychopharmacology, 14*(2), 233-241.

Power, T. (2002). Role of parent training in the effective management of attention-deficit/hyperactivity disorder. *Disease Management in Health Outcomes, 10*(2), 117-26.

Richards, A.M., Troughton, R., Lainchbury, J., Doughty, R., & Wright, S. (2005). Guiding and monitoring of heart failure therapy with NT-proBNP: Concepts and clinical studies. *Journal of Cardiac Failure, 11*(5 Suppl), S34-S37.

Rushton, J., Fant, K., & Clark, S. (2004). Guidelines in the primary care of children with attention- deficit/hyperactivity disorder. *Pediatrics, 114*(1), 23-28.

Sawyer, S.M., & Aroni, R.A. (2003). Sticky issue of adherence. *Journal of Paediatrics and Child Health, 39*(1), 2-5.

Scahill, L., & Schwab-Stone, M. (2000). Epidemiology of ADHD in school-aged children. *Child and Adolescent Psychiatric Clinics of North America, 9*, 541-55.

Serjeant, G.R., & Serjeant, B.E. (2001). *Sickle cell disease.* New York: Oxford University Press.

Silver, M.A., Maisel, A., Yancy, C.W., McCullough, P.A., Burnett, J.C., Francis, G.S., et al. (2004). BNP consensus panel 2004: A clinical approach for the diagnostic, prognostic, screening, treatment monitoring, and therapeutic role of natriuretic peptides in cardiovascular diseases. *Congestive Heart Failure, 10*(5 Suppl 3), 1-30.

Stuart, M.J., & Nagel, R.L. (2004). Sickle-cell disease. *Lancet, 364*, 1343-60.

Thorne, S., Paterson, B., & Russell, C. (2003). The structure of everyday self-care decision making in chronic illness. *Quality Health Research, 13*(10), 1337-1352.

Townsend, A., Hunt, K., & Wyke, S. (2003). Managing multiple morbidity in mid-life: A qualitative study of attitudes to drug use. *British Medical Journal, 327*(7419), 837.

Trent, J.T., & Kirsner, R.S. (2004). Leg ulcers in sickle cell disease. *Advances in Skin & Wound Care, 17*(8), 410-416.

Tsai, A.C., Morton, S.C., Mangione, C.M., & Keeler, E.B. (2005). A meta-analysis of interventions to improve care for chronic illnesses. *American Journal of Managed Care, 11*(8), 478-488.

Vestbo, J., & Lange, P. (2002). Can GOLD stage 0 provide information of prognostic value in chronic obstructive pulmonary disease? *American Journal of Respiratory and Critical Care Medicine, 166*, 329.

Wagner, E. (2000). The role of patient care teams in chronic disease management. *British Medical Journal, 320*, 569-572.

Wahl, C., Gregoire, J.P., Teo, K., Beaulieu, M., Labelle, S., Leduc, B., et al. (2005). Concordance, compliance and adherence in healthcare: Closing gaps and improving outcomes. *Healthcare Quarterly, 8*(1), 65-70.

Ward, M.D., & Rieve, J.A. (2001). The role of case management in disease management. In W.E. Todd & D. Nach (Eds.), *Disease management: A systems approach to improving patient outcomes.* Chicago: American Hospital Publishing, Inc.

Waxmonsky, J. (2005). Nonstimulant therapies for attention-deficit hyperactivity disorder (ADHD) in children and adults. *Essential Psychopharmacology, 6*(5), 262-76.

Wender P., Wolf, L., & Wasserstein J. (2001). Adults with ADHD: An overview. *Annals of New York Academy of Science, 931,* 1-16.

Wethers, D.L. (2000a). Sickle cell disease in childhood: Part I. Laboratory diagnosis, pathophysiology, and health maintenance. *American Family Physician, 62*(5), 1013-1020.

Wethers, D.L. (2000b). Sickle cell disease in childhood: Part II. Diagnosis and treatment of major complications and recent advances in treatment. *American Family Physician, 62*(6), 1309-1314.

Wickliffe, A.C., & Leon, A.R. (2005). Pacing and heart failure: Should all patients receive a biventricular device? *Current Heart Failure Reports, 2*(1), 35-39.

Wilens, T., & Spencer, T. (1999). Combining methylphenidate and clonidine: A clinically sound medication option/and affirmative rebuttal (debate forum). *Journal of American Academy of Child and Adolescent Psychiatry, 38,* 614-622.

Wilens, T., & Spencer, T. (2000). The stimulants revisited. *Child and Adolescent Psychiatric Clinics of North America, 9,* 573-603.

Wolraich, M., Wibbelsman, C., Brown, T., Evans, S., Gotlieb, E., Knight, J., et al. (2005). Attention-deficit/hyperactivity disorder among adolescents: A review of the diagnosis, treatment and clinical implications. *Pediatrics, 115,* 1734-1746.

Zametkin, A.J., & Ernst, M. (1999). Problems in the management of attention-deficit-hyperactivity disorder. *New England Journal of Medicine, 340,* 1766-1767.

Zander, K. (1997). Classic nursing management skills and disease management: Something old, something new. *Seminars for Nurse Managers, 5*(2), 85-90.

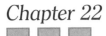
Care of the Chronically Ill Patient

This test may be copied for use by others.

COMPLETE THE FOLLOWING:

Name: _____

Address: _____

City: _____ State: _____ Zip: _____

Preferred telephone: (Home)_____ (Work)_____

E-mail_____

AAACN Member Expiration Date: _____

Registration fee: AAACN Member: $12.00
                              Nonmember: $20.00

Answer Form:

1. If you applied what you have learned from this activity into your practice, what would be different?

_____

_____

_____

Evaluation	Strongly disagree				Strongly agree
2. By completing this activity, I was able to meet the following objectives:					
a. Discuss the role of ambulatory care nurses in caring for chronically ill patients in all age ranges.	1	2	3	4	5
b. Describe how ambulatory care nurses support chronically ill patients, develop effective self-management behaviors, adhere to complex medication regimens, and manage the effects of polypharmacy.	1	2	3	4	5
c. Identify the risk factors for common chronic conditions among children and adults.	1	2	3	4	5
d. Identify the essential elements of the nursing process for patients with common chronic illness.	1	2	3	4	5
e. Describe the treatment strategies for common chronic conditions for children and adults.	1	2	3	4	5
3. The content was current and relevant.	1	2	3	4	5
4. The objectives could be achieved using the content provided.	1	2	3	4	5
5. This was an effective method to learn this content.	1	2	3	4	5
6. I am more confident in my abilities since completing this material.	1	2	3	4	5

7. The material was (check one) ___new ___review for me.

8. Time required to read this chapter: _____minutes

I verify that I have completed this activity: _____
                                                                              Signature

Comments: _____

_____

_____

Objectives

This educational activity is designed for nurses and other health care professionals who practice in ambulatory care. For those wishing to obtain CE credit, an evaluation follows. After studying the information presented in this offering, you will be able to:

1. Discuss the role of ambulatory care nurses in caring for chronically ill patients in all age ranges.
2. Describe how ambulatory care nurses support chronically ill patients, develop effective self-management behaviors, adhere to complex medication regimens, and manage the effects of polypharmacy.
3. Identify the risk factors for common chronic conditions among children and adults.
4. Identify the essential elements of the nursing process for patients with common chronic illnesses.
5. Describe the treatment strategies for common chronic conditions for children and adults.

Posttest Instructions

1. To receive continuing education credit for individual study after reading the article, complete the answer/evaluation form to the left.

2. Detach and send the answer/evaluation form along with a check or money order payable to the *American Academy of Ambulatory Care Nursing (AAACN)*, East Holly Avenue Box 56, Pitman, NJ 08071–0056.

3. Test returns must be postmarked by August 1, 2011. Upon completion of the answer/evaluation form, a certificate for **2.0** contact hour(s) will be awarded and sent to you. Should the material contained in this chapter become outdated prior to the above expiration date, AAACN reserves the right to withdraw this CE test.

This activity is co-provided by the *American Academy of Ambulatory Care Nursing (AAACN)* and Anthony J. Jannetti, Inc. (AJJ). AJJ is accredited as a provider of continuing nursing education by the American Nurses' Credentialing Center's Commission on Accreditation (ANCC-COA). AAACN is a provider approved by the California Board of Registered Nurses, provider number CEP 05336.

This article was reviewed and formatted for contact hour credit by Sally S. Russell, MN, CMSRN, AAACN Education Director; and Candia Baker Laughlin MS, RN, C, Editor.

Chapter 23

Care of the Terminally Ill Patient

Rebecca Elliott Bryan, MS, RN, C

Objectives

Study of the information presented in this chapter will enable the reader to:

1. Recognize the issues that are affecting End-of-Life (EOL) care in our country.
2. Identify appropriate pain interventions for terminal patients.
3. Identify appropriate symptom management measures which cross many terminal diseases.
4. Identify the ethical and legal issues patients, families, and caregivers must face.
5. Recognize the impact of a culturally diverse population in caring for the terminally ill.
6. Apply communication principles important to EOL care.
7. Identify key issues for care of the patient at the time of death.
8. Recognize the role of the nurse in advocating for quality of care at EOL.

Key Points

1. Quality end-of-life care is an important but challenging goal for nurses in ambulatory care.
2. Pain management is complex, but nurses are key in performing good pain assessment and maintaining open dialogue with the patient, family, and physicians.
3. Nurses must work to coordinate optimal pharmacologic and non-drug treatments for end-of-life symptoms, such as dyspnea, cough, anorexia, constipation, diarrhea, nausea/vomiting, depression, anxiety, fatigue, and weakness.
4. Issues of ethical decision making, legal rights of patients and families, and cultural considerations are particularly important in care of the terminally ill patient.
5. Nurses facilitate the grief process by assessing grief and assisting survivors to complete the tasks of the grief process.
6. The nurse is often the one to facilitate a dignified, comfortable death that honors patient and family choices.

Joanne Lynne, MD, with the Americans for Better Care of the Dying, and Dame Cicely Saunders, founder of the Hospice movement, share a common concern and desire for refocusing the medical community on the dying process. There are several issues that have influenced this need to refocus. Since the early 1900s, institutions have replaced the home as the most common place where death occurs. Because of this institutional approach, care is more likely to be given by strangers/health care professionals than family members (Field & Cassel, 1997). Sadly, almost half of conscious hospitalized patients have serious pain in the days before death (Lynne, 2000). One-third of Medicare recipients are in nursing homes during their last year, and of these residents with serious pain, only one-third receive any treatment (Lynne, 2000). More than 4 of every 5

Americans die after they have started receiving Medicare benefits, and 9 of every 10 Medicare patients who died had a chronic illness (heart disease, stroke, chronic lung, dementia, or cancer) in their last year of life (Lynne, 2000).

Chronic illness is a relatively new experience in American society, since most of the above mentioned diseases, with the exception of dementia, have had monumental breakthroughs in treatment over the last 50 years that have changed them from acute to chronic processes. Serious chronic disease at the end of life has become a common cause of bankruptcy and the source of most family caregiving burdens.

Nursing has, over the last 10 years, become aware of the need to include end-of-life care in educational programs. The Robert Wood Johnson

Table 23-1.

Comparison of Deaths in America 1900 vs. 2000

Health Care Issue	1900	2000
Age at death	46 years	78 years
Top causes of death	Infection	Cancer
	Accident	Organ system failure
	Childbirth	Stroke/dementia
Disability leading up to death	Not much	2 to 4 years before death
Financing of care of the dying	Private and modest	Public and substantial
		83% on Medicare
		Approximately 50% of women die on Medicaid

Source: Lynne, 2000.

Foundation supported a project by the American Association of Colleges of Nursing and the City of Hope National Medical Center to provide an extremely comprehensive curriculum for training nurses through their End-of-Life Nursing Education Curriculum. This curriculum is the primary source for information in this chapter.

Death and Dying in America: Current Issues

A. Health care delivery system issues at end of life (EOL).
  1. Some misperceptions include:
      a. Doctors see death as a failure.
      b. Laws make adequate treatment of pain care difficult.
      c. Health care systems aim to make money on false hope.
  2. Reality of the situation is that nurses have built a health care system around the epidemiology of a past era – Resuscitation, surgeries, and hospitals are now readily available (see Table 23-1).
      a. Americans are living longer.
      b. Period of time of living with progressive and eventually fatal illness is generally prolonged and marked with functional dependency on others.
      c. Technological advances have led to the medicalization of care at the end of life.
      d. The focus toward cure has lead to therapeutic optimism.

e. Health professionals are uncomfortable in discussing end-of-life concerns with patients and families.
  3. Barriers to quality end-of-life care.
      a. Patients and families state that their two greatest fears associated with death are being a burden to family and being in pain (National Hospice and Palliative Care Organization [NHPCO], 2005).
      b. Patients worry that they will be abandoned by the health care provider when "nothing more can be done."
      c. Families may be uncertain about how to provide physical care and adjust to role changes (Egan & Labyak, 2001).
      d. Inappropriate use of aggressive curative treatments can prolong the dying process and contribute to physical and emotional distress.
      e. Health care professionals receive little training regarding the safe and effective means of controlling pain and other symptoms.
      f. Hospice and palliative services are not well understood; rules and regulations often impede admittance to the programs, and there is a reluctance to take away "hope."
B. Hospice care.
  1. Hospice definition: Comprehensive services are provided by an interdisciplinary team wherever the patient is; includes physicians,

nurses, social workers, chaplains, counselors, certified nursing assistants, therapists, and volunteers (NHPCO, 2005).

2. Eligibility criteria:
   a. The patient's doctor and the hospice medical director use their best clinical judgment to certify that the patient is terminally ill with a life expectancy of 6 months or less (if the disease runs its normal course).
   b. The patient chooses to receive hospice care rather than curative treatments for his or her illness.
3. Payment for care:
   a. Medicare pays the hospice a per diem rate that is intended to cover virtually all expenses related to addressing the patient's terminal illness.
   b. There may be differing intensities of care during the course of the disease. The Medicare Benefit affords four levels of care:
      (1) Routine home care.
      (2) Continuous home care.
      (3) Inpatient respite care.
      (4) General inpatient care.
   c. Hospices that are Medicare certified must offer all services required to palliate the terminal illness, even if the patient is not covered by Medicare and does not have the ability to pay.

C. Palliative care.
   1. Definition: Palliative care is both a philosophy of care and an organized, highly structured system for delivery of care.
      a. The goal is to prevent and relieve suffering and to support the best possible quality of life for patients and their families, regardless of the stage of the disease or the need for other therapies.
      b. Palliative care expands traditional disease-model medical treatments to include the goals of enhancing quality of life, optimizing function, helping with decision making, and providing opportunities for personal growth.
      c. It can be delivered concurrently with life-prolonging care or as the main focus of care (NHPCO, 2005).

2. Offered by health providers such as hospices, hospitals, home health agencies, or nursing facilities, often through collaboration by two or more such entities.
3. Licensed physicians and advanced practice nurses can bill Medicare, Medicaid, and other third party payers.
4. Most common approaches:
   a. Inpatient care with a multi-disciplinary consultation service.
   b. Community-based, out-patient settings that provide consultation services and/or case management services that help patients and their families access resources in their community. These programs may provide volunteer assistance.
5. Funding of palliative care programs is a major issue.

D. Common principles of hospice and palliative care:
   1. The patient and family are the unit of care; quality can only be viewed subjectively.
   2. Attention is given to physical, psychological, social, and spiritual needs.
   3. The interdisciplinary team is the key to providing holistic, comprehensive care and works with the patient and family to develop goals.
   4. Education about the dying process is vital, as well as management of care, medications, and emotional needs.
   5. Bereavement support and interventions begin at admission to the program with attention to anticipatory needs and continue well beyond a year following the patient's death.

E. Assessment of quality of life (QOL).
   1. QOL encompasses all dimensions of a person and can only be defined by the patient based on his or her own life experience. As the disease progresses and there is physical decline, the psychological, spiritual, and social dimensions take on added meaning and purpose (Egan & Labyak, 2001).
   2. Physical well-being is a concern as the disease progresses and debility, organic, and metabolic changes affect the physical well-being of the patient. Pain is an important concern, as well as dyspnea, GI disturbances,

delirium, agitation, fatigue, and loss of appetite.

3. Family members can develop or have existing physical needs that impact their ability to care for the patient and themselves.

4. Psychological well-being is important because patients experience a wide range of emotional responses to illness including anxiety, sadness, fear, depression, denial, loneliness, hope/hopelessness, and guilt/anger.

   a. Communication and support for working through unresolved issues may affect suffering.

   b. The meaning of illness, along with physical and social attributes, greatly impacts emotional responses.

   c. Coping strategies that have been helpful in the past should be explored, along with possible strategies.

5. Social well being is at risk because the social structure and integrity of the family is threatened.

   a. Becoming a burden is often a concern.

   b. Children manifest their emotional concerns in ways that may not be easily discerned.

   c. Financial concerns may arise due to lost income as well as health care expenses.

6. Spiritual well being is often the key to transcending losses and finding meaning in life.

   a. Religion and spirituality are complementary concepts (Highland, 2000).

      (1) Religion gives expression to a person's beliefs, values, and practices.

      (2) Spirituality involves the human capacity to transcend self and connect with others, surrounding and powers outside of self, and exists independent of affiliation with an organized religion.

   b. The dying process can challenge a person's religious and/or spiritual sense of hope.

   c. Religious and/or cultural rituals are important means of support for both patients and their families.

F. Opportunities for growth at the EOL.

1. Personal growth is challenged in the midst of struggles to overcome physical, emotional,

and spiritual distress.

2. The meaning of hope shifts from that of cure to one in which individuals strive to reach personal end-of-life closure goals.

3. Many who die from a more progressive illness are able to overcome immeasurable suffering and emerge with a sense of wellness even as they are dying. Patients who die from sudden or traumatic deaths and their families may miss similar opportunities for growth (Byock, 1996).

4. Professionals find that acceptance of the dying process as a natural part of the life cycle is one of the first steps in learning how to view death as an achievement instead of a failure.

G. The role of the nurse in expanding EOL principles across all settings.

1. The importance of PRESENCE: Some things cannot be fixed (Rando, 1984).

   a. No one can change the inevitability of death.

   b. No one can erase the anguish felt when someone he or she loves dies.

   c. Everyone must face the fact that he or she, too, will die.

   d. No matter how hard one tries, the perfect words or gestures to relieve patient and family distress rarely, if ever, exist.

   e. It is often enough to just be with the person.

2. The use of "presence" with the dying patient and family is to allow oneself to enter into another's world and to respond with compassion (O'Connor, 2001).

3. Nurses are a constant across all settings and can impact quality EOL closure by identifying persons with any life-threatening illness or condition. A very useful technique is to ask, "Is the patient now sick enough that it would not be a surprise if he or she died in the next 3 to 12 months?" This may identify patients who would otherwise not be recognized in need of palliative care (Lynne, 2000, p. 86).

4. Nurses play an important role in expanding the concept of healing.

   a. At EOL, nursing care shifts from a focus of recovery to an understanding of "healing" (Coyle, 2001).

b. A "good death" is defined by the perspective of the individual, but criteria generally include being free from pain or other distressing symptoms, and the patient and family having adequate time to address concerns and bring closure.

Pain Management: Challenges of the Multiple Dimensions

A. Pain is defined by the International Association for the Study of Pain (IASP) as "an unpleasant sensory and emotional experience associated with actual or potential tissue damage, or described in terms of such damage" (IASP, 1994, p. 1). It is a multidimensional experience that involves sensory, affective, cognitive, behavioral, and socio-cultural components (Byock, 1997).

1. McCaffery and Pasero (1999) state that pain is "whatever the person says it is, experienced whenever they say they are experiencing it" (p. 15). This definition describes the subjectivity of pain.

2. Patients may not be able to report their level of pain at the very end of life, so nurses and caregivers must be able to recognize signs that the patient may be in pain and assume that there may be pain by observing potential physical manifestations.

B. Statistics from the last decade have shown how poorly pain was being treated and how pain management has improved.

1. Multiple studies have shown that no matter what the disease process, the patient may have inadequate pain relief, which hastens death by:
   a. Increasing physiological stress.
   b. Suppressing immunity.
   c. Decreasing mobility, which increases strain on other physiological functions.

2. Pain relief not only enhances the individual's quality of life, but may allow the patient to "let go" at the end of life.

C. There are multiple barriers to adequate pain relief.

1. Health care professionals' barriers.
   a. Inadequately informed of good method-

ology for pain control.
   b. Concern about regulation of controlled substances.
   c. Fears of patient addiction.

2. Patients' barriers.
   a. Reluctant to report that they are in pain out of fear of addiction.
   b. Concern that their physician may not treat the underlying disease if they report they are in pain.
   c. Anxiety about paying for the medications the physicians have ordered.

3. Nurses are the key to reducing barriers to adequate pain relief. Performing a good pain assessment will help physicians understand what factors to consider in providing good pain relief. An opportunity for open dialogue concerning patient/caregiver's fears and concerns is critical to providing adequate pain relief.

D. Pain assessment (American Pain Society [APS], 1999; Levy, 1996; McCaffery & Pasero, 1999).

1. Pain history involves the family/caregiver as well as the patient's self-report.

2. People are often unable to use the word "pain," so words such as "ache" and "hurt" may need to be interchanged. Listen carefully to the words the patient may use to describe his or her pain to evaluate his or her level of stoicism.

3. Location of the pain is important. Should the patient report "pain all over," it may be a sign of existential distress. Existential distress occurs at time when a person questions the meaning of his or her life. This response encompasses the physical, psychosocial, and spiritual angst that may occur at EOL (Ferrel & Coyle, 2001).

4. Intensity is a way to quantify pain and is usually measured with a scale from 1 to 10. If patients cannot use numbers, try categories (no pain, mild, moderate, strong) or faces to describe how they feel.

5. Quality of pain is generally divided into nociceptive or neuropathic.
   a. Nociceptive is related to damage to bones, tissues, or organs and is usually described as aching, throbbing, squeezing, cramping pain.

b. Neuropathic is due to damage to the nervous system and is usually described as burning, tingling, electrical, or shooting (for example, diabetic neuropathy or shingles).

6. Pattern of pain may be constant or intermittent (referred to as "breakthrough").

7. Aggravating/alleviating factors need to be reviewed. What makes the pain better or worse?

8. Pharmacologic interventions need to be assessed, including:
   a. Drugs the patient has already tried.
   b. Whether they have been effective.
   c. What adverse effects resulted?
   d. What has been ordered and what they are actually taking and how.
   e. Over-the-counter, recreational, and herbal products.

9. The meaning of pain to the patient is important for understanding how one may be able to help relieve the pain. Cultural and religious beliefs may influence the meaning of pain.

E. Physical examination contributes to determining the underlying cause of the pain.

1. Observe for non-verbal cues of pain, especially if the patient is unable to report pain; cues include signs of fatigue, grimaces, moans, irritability, holding, or bracing.

2. Examine sites for trauma, skin breakdown, changes in bony structures.

3. Palpate areas for tenderness, auscultate lungs and bowels for abnormal sounds, and percuss abdomen for gas or fluid accumulation.

4. Conduct a neurological examination to evaluate sensory and/or motor loss, as well as changes in reflexes.

F. Reassessment of the pain is critical to determine if changes are needed in the analgesic regimen.

1. Timing of reassessment is determined by the degree to which the patient's condition and pain state is changing.

2. Reassessment should always be done within 24 hours of change of medication.

3. A pain diary kept by the patient or caregiver can be a very helpful tool:
   a. Times of dose of medicine with time of relief.

b. Intensity of pain prior to and after medication.

G. Pain versus suffering at the EOL.

1. Existential distress, fear of dying, and grief may alter expressions of pain.

2. Management of pain must be an interdisciplinary approach, with any and/or all modalities of pain relief allowed.

H. Pharmacological therapies are optimal when there is close collaboration with physicians, pharmacists, nurses, and caregivers to evaluate all factors that affect the patient's pain control.

1. Acetaminophen.
   a. Analgesic, antipyretic.
   b. Can cause liver dysfunction in doses higher than 4,000mg/day.

2. Non-steroidal anti-inflammatory drugs (NSAIDs), such as aspirin, ibuprofen, and naproxen. These should not be used with people with GI distress or bleeding disorders (McCaffery & Pasero, 1999).
   a. Inhibit prostaglandins. Useful in relieving bone pain and dysmenorrhea.
   b. COX-2 NSAIDs (such as Celecoxib®) provide the same action but appear to have less risk of GI bleeding, renal dysfunction, and generalized bleeding. However, many have been voluntarily removed from the U.S. market because of the risk of cardio- and cerebrovascular events.
   c. The FDA has requested that all marketed prescription NSAIDs (COX-2 selective and non-selective) be labeled with a boxed warning regarding increased risk of serious cardiovascular thrombotic events, myocardial infarction, and stroke.
   d. NSAIDs have a ceiling effect. Increasing the dose beyond the ceiling does not help analgesia.
   e. Concurrent use of corticosteroids increase adverse effects of NSAIDs.

3. Opioids are narcotic analgesics (for example, codeine, morphine, hydrocodone, hydromorphone, fentanyl, methadone, and tramadol). Note: Merperidine (Demerol®) and Darvon® or Darvocet® are NOT indicated in end-of-life care because they may cause seizures (APS, 1999).

a. Allergic reactions are rare. If a patient says they are allergic, further questioning may reveal that they may have developed nausea and vomiting (adverse effect). Contraindicated only when the patient reports hypersensitivity reaction such as wheezing or edema.

b. Respiratory depression is rare but greatly feared. It is usually preceded by sedation, and the greatest prevalence of this is after the first dose of a narcotic-naive patient. Morphine has been found to help patients in respiratory distress due to COPD/emphysema because it relaxes the muscles around the lungs and allows lungs to expand.

c. Constipation is a significant adverse effect of opioid therapy, which results from a reduction in peristalsis and increased reabsorption of water. After initiating opioids, a stool softener and laxative should always be available at the first signs of constipation, and then should be administered regularly.

d. Sedation can occur, yet tolerance generally develops to this effect.

e. Urinary retention is common in opioid-naive patients when delivered intrathecally or epidurally.

f. Nausea and vomiting may occur and are best treated with antiemetics.

I. Routes of administration for pharmacologic therapies (APS, 1999; McCaffery & Pasero, 1999) are determined by the patient's ability to self medicate and ability to swallow, and the family's comfort level in administration.

1. Oral route includes use of immediate-release tablets, long-acting tablets, and liquids, which may be given to be swallowed or absorbed sublingually.

a. Oral delivery can provide equivalent analgesia when compared to IM, IV of SQ routes.

b. Prior to death, approximately 80% of patients need alternative routes.

2. Rectal route is useful for long-acting opioid tablets when the patient is no longer able to swallow. Plasma concentration of morphine after rectal placement is approximately 90% of concentrations achieved when the drug is given orally. Delivery via this route may be difficult for family members.

3. Transdermal administrations are accomplished through placement of a patch placed over non-hairy skin with good capillary flow. One drug commonly administered by this method is fentanyl (Duragesic®).

a. There is a delay in peak onset (8 to 12 hours), so other routes must be continued until peak is reached.

b. Fever and cachexia may accelerate drug distribution.

4. Topical anesthetics can be used for isolated, brief pain conditions but are not found to be appropriate for chronic, long-term pain.

5. Parenteral routes:

a. Intravenous may be useful when the patient cannot swallow or when the GI tract is altered. Home administration is complicated, unless PICC line, port-a-cath, or other implanted device is available.

b. Subcutaneous boluses have a slower onset and lower peak effect. This is a good option for use in home with a continuous pump.

c. Intramuscular is not recommended for outpatients due to wide variability in absorption, and it requires that a family member be comfortable or available to deliver.

6. Spinal route allows delivery of drugs in combinations, but it is complex, requires special knowledge for health care professionals, and may be a burden for the caregiver.

J. Principles regarding the use of analgesics.

1. The World Health Organization (WHO) (1998) provides a guide to selecting the initial analgesic choice and dosing, with continued reassessment necessary to modify the treatment plan based on the patient's response.

a. Mild pain (1 to 3 on the 0 to 10 scale), a non-opioid should be prescribed.

b. Moderate pain (4 to 6) calls for the addition of opioids in low doses.

c. Severe pain (7 to 10) indicates the need for higher doses of opioids, starting at the appropriate level for pain and titrate as needed to achieve pain relief.

d. Weak opioids (codeine) may not be the drug of choice in moderate pain; smaller doses of opioids, such as morphine, are just as effective and can be easily titrated for relief.

2. Use of long-acting and breakthrough medications.

a. Begin with immediate-release formulations as needed to relieve pain. Once the patient has achieved pain relief for 24 to 48 hours, calculate the 24-hour dose of opioid and convert to long acting formulation. For example, the patient who has been taking 60mg of liquid morphine in a 24-hour period may be converted to MS Contin® 30mg every 12 hours or fentanyl (Duragesic® 25) mcg every 72 hours.

b. Sustained-release formulation and around-the-clock dosing should be used for continuous pain syndromes.

c. Immediate-release formulations should be made available for breakthrough pain. The dose of immediate-release is usually 10% to 20% of the total 24-hour dose of the routine opioid every 1 to 2 hours prn. Therefore, if the 24-hour dose of MS Contin® is 200mg, the breakthrough dose should be 20 to 40 mg starting with the lower dose and titrating, as needed. Immediate-release medication can be repeated as often as every hour, since the peak effect of oral opioids is 1 hour.

d. Breakthrough pain can be incident-related (movement), idiopathic, or end-of-dose failure.

e. Titration should be based upon patient goals, requirements for supplemental analgesics, pain intensity, severity of undesirable or adverse drug effects, measures of functionality, sleep, emotional state, and patients'/care givers' reports of the impact of pain on quality of life.

3. Switch to a different opioid when the current one becomes ineffective after an adequate upward titration of the dose or if it produces adverse effects.

K. Special populations (APS, 1999; McCaffery & Pasero, 1999).

1. Children are often under-treated due to misguided fears of addiction or the belief that children do not feel pain due to underdeveloped nervous systems.

2. Elderly patients are often under-dosed. Even though treatments may start at slightly lower doses, they should be titrated aggressively.

3. The number of persons with a history of substance abuse are increasing. A thorough assessment of the pain and their addiction risk is critical.

a. An interdisciplinary team approach is important.

b. Realistic goals must be established.

c. Provide a structured and safe environment for patients and their support persons.

d. Co-morbid psychiatric disorders are common, particularly depression, personality disorders, and anxiety disorders. Treatment of these underlying problems may reduce aberrant behaviors and make pain control more effective.

e. Consistency is essential.

f. Tolerance must be considered, thus opioid doses may require more rapid titration and may be higher than patients without a history of substance abuse.

g. At the end of life, rehabilitation is not a goal, but prevention of withdrawal from opioids, benzodiazepines, and alcohol should be monitored.

4. Uninsured and poor persons are at risk for inadequate pain control at the end of life. Many analgesics, especially the newer and more sophisticated formulations, can be extremely expensive. Generic, immediate-release formulations are usually less expensive. Pharmaceutical companies often have patient assistance programs that provide analgesics at no cost. Hospice is mandated to provide analgesics in their per diem coverage.

L. Nonpharmacological techniques (McCaffery & Pasero, 1999).

1. Cognitive behavioral therapies, such as relaxation, guided imagery, distraction, support groups, and pastoral counseling, are

useful adjuncts to analgesic therapies. They may be used after administering a break-through dose of medication to help reduce pain.

2. Physical measures produce relaxation and relieve pain. Massage, heat/cold therapy, and repositioning/bracing are different techniques.

3. Complementary therapies (herbals, magnets, acupuncture) have little evidence to support their efficacy, but are being used with increasing frequency in conjunction with pharmacologic agents.

M. Pain management during the last hours of life.

1. Decreased consciousness may make assessment complicated. If the patient is unable to report pain, non verbal cues must be relied upon to measure pain levels.

2. If the patient did not previously have pain but now appears to be in pain, first rule out other potential causes of distress (such as constipation, anxiety). A therapeutic trial of opioids may be indicated to determine if the behaviors diminish.

3. The dosage of opioids given during the last hours of life should be based upon appropriate assessment and reassessment.

   a. The nurse should provide pain relief, and the fear of sedation or respiratory depression should not limit the use of opioids. The American Nurses Association (ANA) position statement, *Promotion of Comfort and Relief of Pain in Dying Patients* (1995), supports the nurse in the role of "increasing titration of medication to achieve adequate symptom control, even at the expense of maintaining life or hastening death secondarily, is ethically justified" (p. 1).

   b. Studies have shown that the opioid requirements during the last 24 hours of life remained low for the majority of patients; patients who did require significant increases do not have a different survival rate as compared to those who remained on stable dosing (Thorns & Sykes, 2000).

4. The dose of opioid needed to produce relief may be decreased during the final hours of

life. Decreased renal function is one contributing factor.

5. Metabolites of opioids, particularly morphine, may accumulate due to renal dysfunction. These metabolites can produce hallucinations, myoclonus, and a hyper-irritable state. Should this occur, a change to another opioid, such as hydromorphone, may be indicated.

N. Intractable pain at the end of life.

1. Pain may become intractable, even with aggressive titration of standard opioid and other therapies. Sedation may be the only alternative to provide comfort. Before sedation is initiated, several issues must be addressed.

   a. All possible etiologies and treatments have been considered and ruled out.

   b. The patient or surrogate should be instructed on the expected outcomes and goals of sedation, and informed consent must be obtained. Many members of the health care team who have been involved in the case should be called upon to provide support to the patient and family.

2. Aggressively increasing the existing opioid may be sufficient for most patients. However, benzodiazepines may be added to induce sedation and reduce the likelihood of myoclonus or other symptoms.

O. Suffering and existential distress are common at the end of life and add to the complications of determining the extent of physical pain. Although nurses may be able to provide relief of physical symptoms, they need to be constantly aware of the effects of psychological and spiritual distress, and the need for an interdisciplinary approach for comprehensive pain management.

Symptom Management

Multiple symptoms are common at the end of life. Nurses must work closely with all on the care team to coordinate optimum pharmacologic and non-drug treatments. Patients and families require extensive teaching and support for symptom management. The key nursing roles in symptom management include patient advocacy, assessment, pharmacologic treatments, non-pharmacologic treatments, and patient/family education about the symptoms, their role in the dying process, and interventions that will be most helpful.

A. Essential elements of symptom management.
1. Assessment and evaluation of interventions used so far.
2. Interdisciplinary teamwork ensures that optimal care is delivered. Close collaboration is important between nurses and physicians, as well as with all who provide care in the home/facility.
3. Insurance coverage and other financial concerns may be important factors for some families and should be considered in the overall care plan.
4. Criteria for ordering diagnostic test: If no change in management will result, tests should be questioned for appropriateness.

B. Symptoms and suffering: As with pain, other physical and psychological symptoms create suffering and distress. Psychosocial interventions are needed to complement pharmacologic strategies.

C. There are many physical and psychological symptoms common at the end of life. The following are important due to the distress they cause patients and families:
1. Respiratory: Dyspnea and cough.
2. GI: Anorexia, constipation, diarrhea, nausea/vomiting.
3. Psychological: Depression, anxiety.
4. General: Fatigue and weakness.

D. Dyspnea is defined as distressing shortness of breath.
1. Dyspnea is caused by pulmonary compromise (tumor, aspiration, effusions, emboli, bronchospasm, or ascites); cardiac-related issues (congestive heart failure [CHF], pulmonary edema, pulmonary hypertension or anemia); neuromuscular disorders (amyotrophic lateral sclerosis [ALS], myasthenia gravis, cerebrovascular disease, or trauma); anxiety, pneumothorax, or metabolic disorders; obesity; and psychological or physiological distress.
2. Assessment of dyspnea is like assessment of pain in that the subjective report of the patient is the only reliable indicator of this symptom. Assessment includes:
   a. Effect on functional status.
   b. Factors that improve or worsen this symptom.
   c. Assessment of breath sounds.
   d. Presence of chest pain or other pain that may compound the problem.
   e. Oxygenation status.
3. Clinical assessment determines any underlying pathophysiology.
   a. History should assess for:
      (1) Acute or chronic dyspnea.
      (2) History of smoking.
      (3) Heart or lung disease.
      (4) Concurrent medical conditions.
   b. Physical exam assesses:
      (1) Respiratory rate and depth.
      (2) Use of accessory muscles.
      (3) Presence of unilateral or bilateral crackles, rales, rhonchi.
      (4) Presence of pain with respiratory movement.
      (5) Functional status.
4. Treatment of dyspnea would involve treating the symptom while determining whether or not to treat the underlying cause (such as antibiotics for infection or management of tumor progression). Both pharmacologic and non-pharmacologic management should be initiated.
   a. Pharmacologic: Opioids, bronchodilators, diuretics, benzodiazpines, non-benzodiazepine anxiolytic, steroids, antibiotics, and anticoagulants. Note: Recent studies have shown morphine nebulizers to be helpful with severely compromised patients.
   b. Non-pharmacologic treatment techniques may include:
      (1) Oxygen.
      (2) Pursed-lip breathing.
      (3) Energy conservation.
      (4) Fans, air conditioners to circulate air.
      (5) Elevation of the head of the bed and support of the patient to sit in a forward and upright position.
      (6) Music.
      (7) Counseling in the use of cognitive

behavioral, interpersonal, and complementary therapies.

c. Other treatments may include: Blood transfusions, paracentesis to reduce ascites, radiation therapy to shrink tumor, stent tube placement to open occluded airway, or thoracentesis.

E. Cough, like dyspnea, can be debilitating for the patient, causing pain, fatigue, vomiting, and insomnia.

1. Possible causes include: Infection, bronchitis, aspiration, obstruction, medication, asthma, esophageal reflux, COPD, heart failure, sinusitis, environmental irritation, pulmonary fibrosis, pneumothorax, pulmonary embolism, or malignant involvement of lung or pleura.

2. Assessment is done via a history and physical, which include information about precipitating and relieving factors, presence of sputum production, and presence of blood.

3. Pharmacologic treatment includes bronchodilators, cough suppressants, opiates or local anesthetics, cough expectorants, antibiotics, steroids, anticholinergics, and nebulized saline.

4. Non-pharmacologic techniques include cool mist humidification, elevating the head of the bed, and caffeinated beverages.

F. Anorexia and cachexia can be the most distressing for patients and families.

1. Anorexia is defined as the loss of the desire to eat or a loss of appetite.

2. Cachexia is a general lack of nutrition and wasting occurring in the course of a chronic disease.

3. Weight loss is present in both, but cachexia is also a result of metabolic abnormalities. The etiology of cachexia is rarely reversible.

4. Aggressive nutritional treatment does not improve survival or quality of life and may actually create more discomfort for the patient. Artificial nutrition involves a medical procedure requiring serious consideration because it can cause serious morbidity and financial cost.

5. Causes of anorexia and cachexia may be:

a. Disease-related (infection, pain, nausea and vomiting, constipation, metabolic, delayed gastric emptying, malabsorption, bowel obstruction, intra-cranial pressure).

b. Psychological (depression, anxiety).

c. Treatment related following chemotherapy and radiation.

6. Treatment goal is eating for pleasure. Patients should be encouraged to eat small frequent meals with little odor.

7. Appetite stimulants (such as megacepam) may prove helpful in increasing intake.

8. Small amounts of alcohol, dronabinol (Marinol®), or corticosteroids may increase appetite.

9. Antiemetics may be helpful in increasing gastric emptying.

G. Constipation is defined as the infrequent passage of stool, associated with symptoms of rectal pressure, straining, cramps, distension, and/or sensation of bloating. Prevention is key.

1. Causes include: Obstruction (may be partial or complete, and may be due to tumor in or compression of the bowel), hypercalcemia, hypokalemia, spinal cord compression, concurrent disease such as diabetes, diverticulitis, adhesions, dehydration, inactivity, and pain. Medications can lead to constipation: Opiates suppress peristalsis, antidepressants slow motility, and antacids cause hardening of stool.

2. Assessment should include:

a. Bowel history, frequency, and use of medications; should also take into account the patient's definition of constipation, with the goal being to establish what is normal for that patient.

b. Abdominal assessment to rule out obstruction: Examine for bowel sounds, bloating, tenderness, percussion, and rectal assessment.

c. A rectal examination should not be done in the neutropenic patient without careful consideration.

d. Medications need to be reviewed with special interest in herbals.

3. Treatment – If the cause cannot be eliminated, then a bowel regime should be initiated. A minimum goal is for a bowel movement every 72 hours, regardless of intake. Bowel obstruction should be ruled out before any

treatment is initiated.

a. Medications include stool softeners and laxatives. Suppositories and/or enemas should be considered when the patient is no longer able to tolerate oral medications.

b. Dietary and fluid interventions include encouragement of fluid intake and high-fiber foods.

H. Diarrhea is the frequent passage of loose, non-formed stool. Diarrhea may dramatically impact a person's quality of life. It can cause fatigue, electrolyte abnormalities, and depression, and may lead to skin breakdown and dehydration. Psychologically, it may increase anxiety and fear of appearing in public.

1. Diarrhea may be disease-related.
   a. AIDS-related bacterial and parasitic infection.
   b. Partial bowel obstructions.
   c. Malabsorption.
   d. Excessive dietary fiber.
   e. Hyperthyroidism.
   f. Irritable bowel syndrome.

2. Diarrhea may be treatment-related.
   a. Mucositis secondary to chemotherapy and radiation.
   b. Infections secondary to immunosuppression.
   c. Dumping syndrome secondary to drugs, herbs, and over-the-counter medications.

3. Assessment requires a careful bowel history, medication history and assessment of the nature and frequency of the stools, as well as hydration.
   a. The onset/suddenness is important. A rapid onset may indicate fecal impaction with overflow.
   b. Watery stools in large amounts are consistent with colonic diarrhea.
   c. Foul-smelling, fatty, pale stools are associated with malabsorption.
   d. Laxative over-usage may include cramping, urgency, or fecal leakage.
   e. Lab tests to evaluate for infectious processes may be considered for blood, fat, mucous, and pus in stool.

4. Treatment is for the underlying cause, as appropriate.
   a. Initiate a clear liquid diet; advance to solids but avoid milk, proteins, fats, and high gas-forming foods.
   b. Promote hydration.
   c. Medications may be prescribed, such as opioids, bulk-forming agents, antibiotics, and steroids.

I. Nausea and vomiting have an extremely complex pathophysiology. They may be acute, anticipatory, or delayed.

1. Causes may be:
   a. Physiological: Gastric irritation and stasis, constipation, intestinal obstruction, pancreatitis, ascites, liver failure, intractable cough, and radiation effects. All cause stimulation of vagal and sympathetic pathways. Metabolic causes include hypercalcemia, uremia, infection, and drugs that stimulate the chemoreceptor zone. CNS causes are increased intracranial pressure and pain.
   b. Psychological: Emotional factors can be a result of stimulation of emetic receptors in the brain.
   c. Treatment-related: Chemotherapy, radiation therapy.
   d. Vestibular disturbances: Toxic action of drugs (such as ASA, opiates) and local tumors within the brain stimulate the vestibular apparatus.

2. Clinical assessment should include:
   a. Past history and effectiveness of treatment.
   b. Identification of those activities that may precipitate or alleviate nausea/vomiting.
   c. History of consistency, frequency, and volume of emesis; associations with position changes; and contributing factors such as pain, constipation, or anxiety.

3. Treatment is dictated by the presumed cause. Treat underlying cause and try any interventions that have worked in the past.
   a. Anticholinergics treat motion sickness, intractable vomiting or small bowel obstruction.
   b. Antihistamines are used for increased intracranial pressure, peritoneal irritation, or vestibular causes.

c. Prochlorparazine (Compazine®) is used for routine palliative care.

d. Steroids are appropriate for cytotoxic-induced emesis.

e. Metoclopramide (Reglan®) can treat gastric stasis or ileus.

f. Haloperidol (Haldol®) is used to treat opioid and chemically or mechanically induced nausea.

g. Lorazepam (Ativan®) is most effective in treating anxiety-induced nausea.

h. Non-pharmacologic techniques include distraction, relaxation, acupuncture, music therapy, and hypnosis.

i. Serving meals at room temperature and avoiding strong odors may be helpful.

J. Fatigue is "a subjective perception and/or experience related to disease, emotional state, and/or treatment. It is multidimensional, is not easily relieved by rest, and has a profound impact on the dimensions of quality of life... is influenced by the cultural context of the individual and is associated with a reduced capacity to carry out expected or required daily activities" (Ferrell, 2000, p. 42). Fatigue is often associated with anorexia; however, improving intake has not been shown to alleviate this symptom.

1. Causes include:

a. Disease-related anemia, electrolyte imbalances, malnutrition, infection, hyperglycemia, fever, pain, organ failure, or CNS injury.

b. Psychological influences include somatic symptoms associated with depression, inactivity/immobility, spiritual distress, and adverse environment.

c. Treatment-related, such as inadequate rest, unrelieved symptoms, medications, effects from chemotherapy, radiation, or surgery.

d. Unrelieved symptoms, such as diarrhea or vomiting, may cause or increase fatigue.

2. Assessment is primarily subjective with objective evaluation playing a lesser part.

a. Subjective data.
   (1) Feeling weak and/or tired.
   (2) Duration.
   (3) Pattern.

(4) Functional status, ability to perform ADLs.
(5) Anxiety.
(6) Difficulty concentrating.
(7) Nausea.

b. Objective data.
   (1) Presence of fever.
   (2) Pulse rate and strength.
   (3) Dyspnea on exertion.
   (4) Assessment of hydration (such as skin turgor).
   (5) Neuromuscular strength tests, symmetry and endurance of upper and lower extremities.

3. Treatment for fatigue may include both pharmacological and non-pharmacological interventions.

a. Pharmacologic treatments include corticosteroids, antidepressants, SSRIs, Tricyclic antidepressants, and stimulants (Kazanowksi, 2001).

b. Non-pharmacologic interventions include taking frequent rest periods, using energy-conserving techniques, and provision of assistance that helps the person maintain independence and functional abilities as long as possible.

K. Depression can be described as a broad spectrum of responses that range from "expected, transient, and non-clinical sadness to extremes of major clinical depressive disorder and suicidality" (Pasacreta, Minarik, & Nield-Anderson, 2001, p. 264). Depression and anxiety are frequent co-morbid factors in chronic medical illness. Persistent feelings of helplessness, hopelessness, inadequacy, depression, and suicidal ideation are not normal at the end of life and should be aggressively evaluated and treated.

1. Causes may be:

a. Disease-related: Pain, abnormal metabolic states, organic mental disorders, or drug reactions or withdrawal.

b. Psychological: Fear of death, loss of independence or control, changes in body image or social factors, such as financial and family issues, contributing to distress, and exacerbating depression.

c. Treatment-related: Numerous medications associated with depression include antihypertensives, analgesics, antiparkinsonism agents, steroids, chemotherapeutic agents, hormones, alcohol, amphetamines, and others.

2. Interdisciplinary team assessment.
   a. Somatic complaints, such as lack of appetite, insomnia, pervasive helplessness and hopelessness, psychomotor agitation, and diminished energy, may be a result of disease and treatment effects. More reliable symptoms, such as a depressed appearance, fearfulness, withdrawal, self-pity, and a sense of punishment, should be evaluated in the terminally ill (Matzo & Sherman, 2001).
   b. Previous psychiatric history treatment should be assessed.
   c. Presence of risk factors, such as living alone, lacking a support system, uncontrollable symptoms, presence of multiple deficits (such as inability to walk, loss of bowel and bladder control, sensory loss).
   d. Suicide lethality should be assessed by evaluating the presence of a suicidal plan, method to carry out the plan, availability of resources to carry out the plan, ability to communicate intent, and intended outcome (gesture or serious attempt to die). Patients with immediate, lethal, and precise suicide plans and resources to carry out the plan should be immediately evaluated by a psychiatric professional or placed in an appropriate close supervisory state (see *Ethical Issues in EOL Care* section, Assisted Suicide, I.6).

3. Treatment.
   a. Pharmacologic interventions include SSRI and tricyclic antidepressants, stimulants, non-benzodiazepines, and steroids.
   b. Non-pharmacologic interventions may include:
      (1) Promoting and facilitating as much autonomy and control as possible.
      (2) Increasing patient and family participation in care.

(3) Life review to assist the terminally ill patient to focus on accomplishments and promote closure and resolution of life events.
(4) Grief counseling to assist in dealing with past, present, and future loss.
(5) Maximizing symptom management to decrease physical stressors.
(6) Assisting the patient to draw on previous sources of strength, such as faith and belief systems.

L. Anxiety is a subjective feeling of apprehension, tension, insecurity, and uneasiness usually without a known specific cause.
   1. Causes may be medications or substances, such as stimulants, thyroid replacement hormones, neuroleptics, corticosteroids, digitalis, antihistamines, anticholinergics, and analgesics. Non-pharmacologic etiology may be such issues as facing uncertain futures; lifestyle changes; concerns over finances, dependency, and disability; and confrontation of family conflicts.
   2. Assessment should be frequent because patients with a terminal diagnosis may undergo rapid changes in lifestyle and physical well being. Symptoms may include chronic apprehension, inability to sleep or relax, difficulty in concentrating, and/or persistent thoughts, ideas, or impulses.
   3. Treatment:
      a. Pharmacological treatment includes antidepressants, benzodiazepines, neuroleptics, and non-benzodiazepines.
      b. Non-pharmacologic techniques include acknowledgment of the patient's fears, allowing the patient to articulate anger with appropriate reassurance and support, providing concrete information, encouraging the use of a stress diary, maximizing symptom management, and promoting the use of relaxation and guided imagery techniques.

M. Delirium/agitation/confusion: Delirium is an acute change in cognition or awareness. Agitation presents as a symptom accompanying delirium. Confusion refers to disorientation, inappropriate behavior or communication, and/or hallucinations.

1. Causes may be infection, medications, metabolic abnormalities, hypoxemia, renal or hepatic failure, constipation, bladder distension, or rapid withdrawal of medications. In older adults, bladder infection should be ruled out with any sudden change in mental status.
2. Assessment should include physical assessment, history of onset, and probability of any spiritual distress.
3. Treatment may include use of neuroleptics or benzodiazepines for acute agitation, evaluation of current medications to eliminate any nonessential drugs, and initiation of antibiotics for bladder infections. Family education is important because they may be very disturbed by changes in the patient. Relaxation, massage, and acupuncture therapies have been found to be beneficial.

Ethical Issues in EOL Care

A. Medical technology, changes in family and social systems, managed care, and multiple health care choices have added to the complexity of end-of-life care.
B. Key issues that affect nursing practice include:
   1. Lack of available family and community caregivers.
   2. Increased fear of litigation.
   3. An aging baby boomer population.
   4. Lack of knowledge about appropriate end-of-life treatment.
   5. Legalization of assisted suicide.
   6. Access to hospice services.
   7. Reimbursement for care.
C. End-of-life care raises questions about the meaning of life, dependency on others, the meaning of pain and suffering, and illness and death.
D. The nurse's role in addressing ethical issues is complex, understanding that each member of the care team comes with his or her own values, morals, and life experiences. The role of each member of the team is to work together so that the patient/family can make fully informed decisions with full knowledge of their options.
E. Shared decision making has taken on a new role because the nature of the professional-patient relationship has shifted from medical paternalism to patient self-determination. The elements of shared decision making are:
   1. Balance of objective and subjective data.
   2. Balance of participation and authority.
   3. Focus on understanding.
   4. Process-oriented.
   5. Robust interpretation of informed consent.
F. The fundamental principle of ethical decision-making is respect for the inherent worth, dignity, and human rights of each individual.
G. Issues of decision making and communication at EOL are complex and often provide challenges. Chapter 8, *Legal Aspects*, and Chapter 14, *Ethics*, provide information about ethical principles and legal regulation of patients' and families' rights that are particularly important to consider with a terminally ill patient.
H. Advance care planning is a process of decision making and communication of those decisions between the person and his or her family, friends, physicians, and other health care providers who ensure that the patient's choices are known, preferably long before a crisis situation, or when wishes can no longer be communicated.
   1. Advance care planning involves the patient deciding and designating whom they would like to make health care decisions for them in the event they cannot make them for themselves.
   2. Decision making is an ongoing, dynamic process; the patient and/or proxy have the right to change their decisions at any time.
   3. Decisions communicated ahead of time decrease the chances of conflict in future decision, decrease the potential for ethical dilemmas, and take the burden off the family and health care team.
   4. Several states now provide a shortened form of the living will that is signed by the physician, so it then becomes a physician's order for life-sustaining treatment. Patients with a terminal illness should keep these documents in plain sight in their homes so that emergency personnel and caregivers have information of the patient's wishes readily available.
I. Prolongation of life and quality of life are at the center of palliative care discussions.
   1. Life-sustaining treatment (LST).

    a. It may be appropriate to relieve symptoms, but in other cases, it may be seen as prolonging the suffering of a patient who is dying.

    b. It may allow time for the patient and family to become prepared and able to say their goodbyes.

    c. It may allow the patient and family to get affairs in order or to complete their emotional/spiritual tasks of dying.

    d. It may include resuscitation, hydration, nutrition, mechanical ventilation, or dialysis (Ferrell, 2000).

2. Palliative treatments (surgery, chemotherapy, radiation) may relieve symptoms to improve quality of life and decrease suffering.

3. Curative intent is aimed at ameliorating the disease process.

4. An ethical dilemma that may arise is whether or not a patient should be treated for a secondary problem, such as an infection, or if death is pending.

5. Withholding/withdrawing of treatment is usually done because of patient choice, undesirable quality of life, burdens outweighing benefits, or prolongation of the dying process. Common situations include withdrawal of medically provided hydration or nutrition, ventilation, CPR, and/or dialysis. The decision to withdraw or withhold is a decision that allows the disease to progress on its natural course. It is not a decision/action intended to cause death.

6. Do Not Resuscitate/No Code orders confirm that if a cardiopulmonary arrest occurs, no resuscitative measures are initiated. This requires a written physician order. It is not required by standard or law for admission to hospice.

7. Assisted suicide refers to a practice whereby a person other than the patient provides a means to a patient with the knowledge that a patient will use the means to commit suicide (Field & Cassel, 1997). Oregon voters approved physician-assisted suicide (PAS) in 1997 via the *Oregon Death with Dignity Act.* Data in Oregon has shown that although Oregonians have had the right to use PAS, very few patients actually go through the act after receiving the prescriptions. Patients report that they requested the medications primarily out of concern over uncontrollable pain or becoming a burden after loss of independence (Oregaon Hospice Association [OHA], 2004). Requests for PAS should alert the nurse that this is the first expression of unrelieved suffering of whether physical, psychological, social, or spiritual nature (Emanuel, von Guten, & Ferris, 1999).

    a. Nurses have the responsibility to respond to requests for a PAS in a way that supports the needs and expectations of the patient while offering care that is both ethical and legal.

    b. The ANA has based its position on PAS from the philosophical stance of respect for patients that is extensively explicated in the *Code of Ethics for Nurses with Interpretive Statements* (ANA, 2001). The position states that nursing may not deliberately act to terminate the life of any person, and that it has a social contract with society that is based on trust. While nursing practitioners are committed to the patient's right to self-determination, nurses are not obligated to comply with all requests.

    c. Nurses need to develop sensitivities and skills to preserve the integrity of clinical care and professional life.

    d. Nurses have the right to conscientiously object to participating in situations that they may find morally objectionable.

    e. Nurses strive to remain committed to the delivery of patient care and non-abandonment. There may be situations in which nurses need to remove themselves from the care of a particular patient based on an ethical objection. Nurses are obligated to provide for the patient's safety and seek alternative sources of care (Matzo & Sherman, 2001).

8. Situations in which conflicts regarding the belief of the beneficial nature of treatment occur are referred to as medical futility and are common reasons for ethics consults. These conflicts often involve failure in communication related to prognosis or benefits

versus burden of treatment options (Emanuel et al., 1999).

9. Issues of care and comfort are central to the patient-nurse relationship. The responsibility of the nurse to the patient is competence, compassion, support, and advocacy, with integrity being foremost in the relationship.

J. Palliative care begins from the time of diagnosis and is applied aggressively to assure comfort throughout the course of an illness. While some disease processes, such as cancer, allow for more definitive lines between curative and palliative approaches, those lines are vaguer with other diseases such as COPD and CHF.

K. The prevention and relief from suffering and provision of comfort to both the patient and his or her family are essential because they adapt to advancing illness and EOL issues. Symptom management supports a holistic approach of physical, psychological, social, and spiritual care.

L. Often nurses are concerned about how their actions will affect the timing and circumstances of a patient's death. They worry that they will "cause" the death if they administer adequate narcotics at the end of life. The increasing titration of medication to achieve adequate symptom control, even if hastening death secondarily, is ethically justified (ANA, 1995). Those who work with patients at the end of life often report that patients who are in pain often pass when their pain is under control, as the body is relaxed and suffering is assuaged.

M. Issues of justice impact EOL care.
1. Quality EOL care is not consistently available to all people.
2. Health care systems are beginning to identify and understand the need for the incorporation of quality palliative and hospice care. However, rural hospitals that are struggling to maintain financial solvency may be having a hard time justifying the expense of these programs and are likely to cut them from their budgets.
3. After the death of the patient, there is a responsibility to support the family through bereavement. This is mandated by Medicare in the hospice benefit; however, most hospices provide bereavement services in their community to families whether the patient

was on the hospice service or not.
4. Families shoulder the financial burden of caregiving in the home and/or need for placement of patients in nursing homes. Families are often drained of future financial stability.

N. Each state's *Nurse Practice Act* and other public health regulations provide essential information related to EOL care, such as the pronouncement of death, prescriptive practices, and laws governing controlled substances and disposition of opioids in the home after death.

O. When ethical dilemmas occur, the nurse's role is as advocate, with the responsibility to assure that the patient and family fully understand the options available so they can make informed decisions, and to facilitate that the patient and family wishes are clarified and communicated to the interdisciplinary team of caregivers.

Cultural Considerations at EOL

A. Cultural practices are defined as a system of shared symbols, serving as guides for interactions with others. It is more than race/ethnicity.
1. Cultural practices provide safety and security, integrity and belonging.
2. Culture is fluid, constantly evolving in response to historical and other factors (Koenig, 1997).
3. Every culture has a worldview or construct of reality that defines the individual within that reality. Therefore, a patient's cultural background is fundamental in defining his or her purpose in life (Matzo & Sherman, 2001).
4. One's culture provides a prescription for behaviors on how one is to conduct life and approach death.

B. Cultural communication issues at EOL include:
1. Interpreters may be needed. Family members should not be used as they may interject their own beliefs and values. The purpose of the meeting should be explained to the interpreter, and the family should meet him or her in advance, if possible, to develop a feeling of trust and to determine a level of understanding of the situation, as well as the family's beliefs and need for information.
2. Conversational style is also important;

patients should be asked how they should be greeted (first name, last name) and the nurse should determine whether the patient speaks for himself or if a family member will serve as a spokesman.

3. Personal space needs can be determined by observing the patient's reactions to posturing and space. This should also be observed with eye contact and touch. Patients should always be asked for permission before they are touched.

4. Evaluation of the patient/family view of health care professionals is also important.

5. Members of the health care team should assess and discuss the relationship of the patient and family, and determine who is the spokesperson. This becomes an issue in respect to confidentiality; family members and friends may request information. It may be best to ask the patient/family to select one person to serve as the key contact for information.

6. People of different cultural backgrounds have different views of full disclosure of diagnosis and prognosis to the patient.

C. Beliefs regarding death/dying, the afterlife, and bereavement vary within different cultural frameworks.

Effective Communication

One aspect of nursing care that has been neglected in the past is how to talk to patients/families about dying. Although this has been incorporated in most curricula for nurses and physicians, it is still given very little attention. Communication involves strong collaboration between members of the interdisciplinary team, including the patient/family.

A. Communication is both verbal and non-verbal (body language, eye contact, gestures, voice intonation). Meaning of the communication is interpreted as it is perceived by the receiver of the communication.

B. Nurses as educators always need to be aware that too much information can be overwhelming and that different people absorb information through a variety of communication forms.

C. The palliative care plan has individualized goals based upon needs and overall condition. The patient/family must be a vital part of this planning. Clear and dynamic communication between all members of the team is imperative to excellent care.

1. Expectations expressed by patients/families need to be addressed with respect, honesty, and guidance in exploration of realistic options.

2. The entire team needs to have a clear understanding of these expectations and a clear plan of how to help these expectations be met.

3. As issues of conflict arise, nurses should plan to initiate patient/family and relevant team member meetings.

D. Listening is being present physically, mentally, and emotionally. Presence (effective listening) occurs at 5 different levels (Ray, 1992).

1. Hearing.
2. Understanding.
3. Retaining information.
4. Analyzing and evaluating information.
5. Helping/active empathizing.

E. Guidelines for encouraging free conversation (Eagan & Labyak, 2001).

1. Set the right atmosphere.
2. Evaluate if the patient/family member wants to talk.
3. Practice principles of attentive listening. Allow for silence, acknowledge feelings, ask for clarification to avoid misunderstanding, take your time before giving advice, and encourage reminiscing.

F. There are several factors that may make effective communication difficult at EOL (Eagan & Labyak, 2001).

1. The family system may have little experience with death in the family, and coping skills may be minimal.

2. There may be inability to care for the patient within the family unit due to physical or emotional issues.

3. The crisis of impending death in a loved one affects family members' ability to comprehend information.

4. Family dynamics and security may be affected by financial concerns brought about by payment for medical expenses, lost time from work, and the cost of care giving.

5. The educational level and ability to read can influence the way in which information should be communicated to patients to ensure informed decision-making.

6. Communication and comprehension may be affected by physical limitations, such as medical interventions, disease processes, and pre-existing conditions.

7. Fear of the future, anger, anticipatory grieving of the loss of self or another, and spiritual concerns all need to be explored by the interdisciplinary team.

8. Changes in family dynamics/roles during illness will evolve.

9. Past coping experiences may help predict how individuals cope in new situations.

10. Family caregivers require extensive support for the stress and burden of care giving. Caregiver support groups can help coping with the feelings and stresses that arise.

11. Patients and families are often overwhelmed with a sense of helplessness. They may have a sense of loss of control.

12. Denial can be an effective coping strategy that allows the individual and family to integrate the impact of diagnosis/prognosis.

G. Health care professionals' behaviors greatly influence communication outcomes. Barriers to effective communication include:

1. Fear of one's own mortality.

2. Lack of personal experience with death and dying.

3. Fear of expressing emotion; showing tears may cause avoidance of difficult topics.

4. Fear of being blamed for causing a death when there are unrealistic expectations for cure.

5. Fear of not knowing the answer to a question or whether to be honest when answering a question.

6. Disagreement with patient/family decisions.

7. Lack of knowledge of the patient/family's culture, end-of-life goals, wishes, and/or needs.

8. Unresolved personal grief.

9. Ethical concerns.

10. Desire to keep physical and/or emotional distance from patients.

H. Breaking bad news or talking about death is a difficult task in our culture. While physicians generally break the bad news, nurses constantly are in a position of reinforcing that news and providing clarification. The nurse should approach such a situation in the following manner:

1. Plan what is to be said ahead of time and organize thoughts. Anticipate questions that may be asked.

2. Establish a rapport. One may want to ask a team member who has established rapport to attend.

3. Set aside appropriate amount of time and clear the area of distractions.

4. Find out what the patient/family may already know.

5. Find out how much the individual wants to know; avoid making assumptions about this.

6. Use language that they will understand.

7. Evaluate the body language, emotional status, educational level, and ability/manner of speaking.

8. Be sensitive to/respectful of cultural issues.

9. Continually assess the patient/family's understanding and adjust appropriately.

I. Should conflict amongst the team members occur (professional and patient/family), the nurse should take a step back, identify his or her own emotions, define the area of conflict, and obtain agreement on that area of difference, even if it cannot be resolved.

J. The role of the nurse in pediatric EOL care includes working with patient, siblings, and often a large family. Because of the sensitivity to the issues in dealing with dying children, nurses working in pediatric EOL care must rally a variety of team members to assist.

1. Children usually know they have a terminal illness even if they are not directly given this information. Children can usually detect subtle changes in the way staff and family members react to them, care for them, and talk to them.

2. It is the nurse's responsibility to respect patients' choices and decision making while assessing opportunities for open communication and education. The patient needs support and caring without being denied any realistic hope.

3. A child needs to be communicated with at his

or her level of understanding.

4. A child may let the nurse know he or she is finished talking by walking away, moving away to play, changing the subject, changing body posture, and/or other non-verbal cues that signify withdrawal.

5. Often presence is the most powerful intervention for both children and their families.

6. Parents and sibling(s) should be encouraged to care for the child. Life review is often very helpful.

7. Siblings should be assessed because they are often forgotten as parents focus on the dying child.
   a. Assess for acting out, and negative or the "perfect child" behavior.
   b. Allow the sibling to continue his or her extracurricular activities by finding resources and support people to take the sibling to these activities.
   c. Allow siblings to verbalize feelings in a safe place without feeling as though they are making their parents feel worse.

Grief, Loss, and Bereavement

As a death-denying society, Americans often deny the need to express grief and feel the pain that accompanies a loss, both which are beneficial to healing. The nurse's role includes facilitating the grief process by assessing grief and assisting the survivor to feel the loss, express the loss, and complete the tasks of the grief process. Grief affects survivors physically, psychologically, socially, and spiritually.

A. Grief is a process that begins before death for the patient and survivors as they anticipate and experience loss. It is the individualized feelings and responses that an individual makes to real, perceived, or anticipated loss (Doka, 1989).
   1. Grief process is not always orderly and predictable.
   2. There is a series of stages and/or tasks that the survivor moves through to help resolve grief (Lindemann, 1994).
   3. The survivor may never "get over" a loss, but may heal and learn to live with a loss and/or live without the deceased.

B. Mourning is the outward, social expression of loss and is often dictated by cultural norms, customs, practices (including rituals), and traditions. It is also influenced by the individual's personality and life experiences (Corless, 2001).

C. Bereavement includes grief and mourning – the inner feelings and outward reactions of the survivor.

D. It is the nurse's responsibility to be aware of the cultural characteristics of grief and mourning for patients and family members.

E. Bereavement interventions should be based on the type of grief being displayed.
   1. Anticipatory grief occurs before loss and is associated with diagnosis of an acute or chronic illness. Examples include grief reactions to actual or fear of potential loss of health, independence, body part, financial stability, choice, or mental function.
   2. Normal or uncomplicated grief reactions can be physical, emotional, cognitive, and/or behavioral.
   3. Risk factors of complicated grief include sudden or traumatic death, death of a child, multiple losses, unresolved grief from prior losses, concurrent stressors, and lack of support system or faith system. Reactions may include severe isolation, violent behavior, suicidal ideation, workaholic behavior, or replacing loss and relationship quickly. Complicated grief can be described as:
      a. Chronic – Characterized by normal grief reactions that do not subside and continue over long periods of time.
      b. Delayed – Characterized by normal grief reactions that are suppressed or postponed, and the survivor consciously or unconsciously avoids the pain of the loss.
      c. Exaggerated – Survivor resorts to self-destructive behaviors, such as suicide.
      d. Masked – Survivor is not aware that behaviors that interfere with normal functioning are the result of the loss.

F. Disenfranchised grief occurs when a loss is experienced and cannot be openly acknowledged, socially sanctioned, or publicly shared. This may occur with ex-spouses, lovers, co-workers, children experiencing the death of a step-parent, woman with a terminated pregnancy, or partners of HIV/AIDS patients.

G. Children's grief is based on developmental stages (Wolfelt, 1990). Children's grief is often not recognized by adults who are dealing with their own sense of grief and loss and have not realized the impact on the children involved. Adults often try to hide their own feelings of loss in order to protect children.

1. Symptoms of unresolved grief in younger children include nervousness, uncontrollable rages, frequent sickness, accident prone-ness, hyperactivity, nightmares, compulsive behavior, and dependency on remaining adults.

2. Symptoms of unresolved grief in older chil-dren include difficulty concentrating, forget-fulness, poor school work, insomnia or sleep-ing too much, reclusiveness, antisocial behav-ior, resentment of authority, over-dependence, talk of or attempted suicide, nightmares, fre-quent sickness, eating disorders, or experimen-tation with drugs, alcohol, or sex.

H. There are many theorists who have developed stages of grief and a series of tasks for survivors to successfully complete their grief work (Corless 2001; Kubler-Ross, 1969). Remember that although these tasks are focused on the survivor, it can be modified for the patient because grief work begins with the patient with the realization that they are on their end of their life journey. Stages include:

1. Stage of notification and shock.
   a. Task – Share acknowledgment of the reality of loss.
   b. Characteristics – Assist the survivor in coping with the initial impact of death; the survivor may have feelings of numb-ness, shock, poor daily functioning.

2. Experiencing the loss emotionally and cogni-tively.
   a. Task – Share in the process of working through the pain of the loss.
   b. Characteristics – The survivor may feel anger at the person who died; the sur-vivor was abandoned by them. Anger may be directed at the physician, nurse, family, or friends. There may be a lack of interest in daily life, apathy, or disor-ganization.

3. Reintegration.
   a. Task – Reorganize and restructure fami-ly systems and relationships.
   b. Characteristics – The survivor finds hope in the future, feels more energetic, participates in social events, and finally accepts the death.

I. Grief assessment includes the patient, family, and significant others. It is ongoing throughout the course of an illness and for the bereavement period after the death for the survivors. Nurses should assess:

1. Type of grief, reactions, stages and tasks, and factors that may affect the grief process:
   a. Personality of the individuals and their previous coping skills/experience of losses.
   b. History of substance abuse, mental ill-ness, or suicidal tendencies.
   c. Relationship to the deceased and age.
   d. Religious/spiritual belief system and cul-tural traditions.
   e. Type of death and preparation for the death.
   f. Concurrent stressors, support systems.

2. Many caregiver survivors do not care for themselves while caring for the patient. Nurses may want to suggest a thorough physical examination and psychosocial and spiritual evaluation.

J. Bereavement interventions may come from a variety of resources and should include an inter-disciplinary approach based upon the plan of care that has been developed after the assess-ment. Interventions may include:

1. Presence, active listening, touch, silence.
2. Identification of support systems.
3. Use of bereavement specialists, bereave-ment resources (hospice is a primary source to use).
4. Normalizing the grief process and individual differences.
5. Actualizing the loss and facilitating living with-out the deceased.
6. Public funerals, memorial services, rites, rit-uals, and traditions.
7. Spiritual care.

K. Bereavement interventions for children and parents are often available through community hospices and schools. Parents may be encouraged to attend support groups in the community.

L. No one can predict when the grief work will be complete, as there will always be times when a memory, object, anniversary, or feelings of loss will occur.

M. The nurse will, at one time or another, experience death anxiety and/or a sense of cumulative loss and grief.
   1. Working with dying patients can trigger the nurse's awareness of his or her personal losses or fears about death or mortality.
   2. Death anxiety occurs when the nurse is confronted with fears about death and has few resources or support systems to explore and express thoughts and emotions about dying/death.
   3. When overwhelmed by death anxieties, nurses may use defenses to allay fears including focusing only on physical care needs or evading emotionally sensitive conversations. This may result in emotional distancing at a time when patients and families need intensive interpersonal care.
   4. Personal death awareness allows the nurse to come to a sense of comfort to explore, experience and express his/her personal feelings regarding death (Vichon, 2001).
   5. Cumulative loss is a succession of losses experienced by nurses who work with patients with life-threatening illnesses often on a daily basis. When the nurse is exposed to death frequently, he or she may not have the time to resolve the grief issues.

N. Nurses new to working with dying patients may need to emotionally and spiritually adapt to caring for the terminally ill. The five stages of adaptation include intellectualization, emotional survival, depression, emotional arrival, and deep compassion (Matzo & Sherman, 2001). Working through these stages is crucial to assist the nurse in relieving his or her anxiety and to attain professional growth in adapting to caring for patients at the end of life.

O. Factors that influence the nurse's adaptation process include:
   1. Professional training and ability to verbalize feelings and emotions.
   2. Personal death history – Experiences on a personal and/or professional level.
   3. Life changes and how the nurse has coped with those changes.
   4. Support systems – Presence or absence of people who can provide emotional support.

P. Systems that are available for nurse support.
   1. Balance - the ability to provide compassionate, quality care to dying patients and their families and find personal satisfaction in work as a professional.
   2. The support system should be evaluated to determine if it inhibits or supports professional growth, adaptation, and development in caring for dying patients and families.
   3. Formal support systems can include preplanned gatherings where team members can express feelings in a safe environment, post-clinical debriefings, and ceremonies or programs to acknowledge and express grief (memorial services).
   4. Informal support is derived from co-workers, peers, or other team members.
   5. Spiritual support may be provided by pastoral care workers or the nurse's personal spiritual aid.

Q. Nursing care and responsibilities to the dying patient and family do not end with the death of the patient. Nurses, as all professionals, must recognize and respond to their own grief in order to provide quality palliative care.

Preparation and Nursing Care For the Time of Death

A. To be an effective caregiver to the dying patient and his or her significant others, the nurse must come to terms with his or her own mortality and view of dying and death. The death of a patient with a terminal illness forces the nurse to acknowledge that a cure cannot always be achieved. A nurse may be exposed to death during his or her entire career.
   1. The nurse has a more "real" exposure to death than other health care professionals.
   2. The final days to hours before a patient dies may be the most significant moments for a patient and his or her family while preparing

for death, saying goodbyes, and completing EOL closure tasks.

3. The nurse is often the one to facilitate a dignified, comfortable death that honors patient/family choices.

4. The nurse may take on many roles as advocate, companion on the journey, professional care giver, educator, and facilitator of resources.

5. The nurse's challenge is to gain knowledge and skills to promote competence and provide dignified EOL care in any practice setting.

B. Interpersonal competence includes empathy, unconditional positive regard, genuineness, and critical thinking skills (Berry & Griffie, 2001).

C. Professionals specializing in the care of the dying (nurses in hospice, spiritual counselors, social workers, volunteers, nursing aides) should be utilized as a resource. The team can help assess individual situations, identify problems, issues, and opportunities specific to the patient/family.

D. Dying is a unique experience. There is no typical death. Each person dies in his or her own way, own time, with his or her own culture, belief system, values, and unique relationships with others.

E. Patients who are aware that they are dying usually know where and with whom they want to die. Nurses need to advocate for these patient/family choices.

F. Dying is a physical, psychological, social, and spiritual event with the patient and family together as the unit of care.

G. The nurse works as an advocate for patient/family choice no matter what the setting (hospital, home, nursing facility, prison, hospice).

1. A part of this advocacy is to support the patient/family in the decision to die where he or she wants to and with whom he or she wishes.

2. Each setting should provide a supportive physical environment.

3. The nurse should avoid a change of setting in the final stages of life. The setting should be changed only if all options have failed and preferably only if the patient and family request the change.

4. Options in care, education about care, and/or increased support so the patient can

die where he or she chooses should be provided as early as possible so the patient and family are not making rash decisions.

H. The team must be open and honest to promote trust and informed decision making.

1. Information should be conveyed in simple, uncomplicated terms.

2. Avoid overloading, overwhelming the patient/family by providing simple answers to questions in accordance with the patient/family understanding and readiness for responses.

3. Family members may be tired, have difficulty concentrating, and focus on the present and not the future. The nurse may need to answer the same questions, provide the same information repeatedly as the family may be in crisis and the ability to retain information may be greatly diminished.

4. Patients often have a greater awareness that they are dying than those around them. If the patient asks if he or she is dying, be honest, then explore the patient's fears and concerns.

5. If the family is fearful of the patient knowing he or she is dying, address these concerns by educating the family that the patient may already know he or she is dying and encourage open, honest communication while respecting the patient/family requests.

a. The family may need education about the signs and symptoms of the dying process – what may happen, what they can expect regarding physical changes, and psychosocial and spiritual needs.

b. Care management is easier to educate if the patient is assessed earlier vs. later in the dying process. Generally, the more the family is involved in the care of the patient, the better they cope after the death (Matzo & Sherman, 2001).

6. Maintaining presence is the most important role nurses have; providing companionship, active listening, and reassurance that someone will be available during the dying process.

7. Hope is important to address. Knowing what the patient's hopes are, realistic or unrealistic, will help the team determine the course

of action and resources needed.

I. The imminently dying patient: Signs, symptoms, and nursing interventions.

    1. Prognosis is affected by the disease, the patient's will to live, and completion of life closure goals.

    2. Signs and symptoms of the dying process only serve as a guideline. Not all patients experience all symptoms, and the signs and symptoms do not necessarily occur in sequence.

    3. The dying process is a natural slowing down of physical and mental processes and may occur weeks, days, or only hours prior to death.

    4. Psychological and spiritual symptoms include fear of dying; abandonment or the unknown; withdrawal from family, friends, and caregivers; and/or increased focus on spiritual issues.

    5. Physical symptoms include confusion, disorientation, delirium, and restlessness. One may also see weakness and fatigue, decreased oral intake, increased drowsiness, sleeping and decreased responsiveness, decreased or lack of swallow reflex, surges of energy, fever, changes in bowel elimination (constipation or incontinence).

    6. Universal symptoms of imminent death are decreased urine output, cold and mottled extremities, vital sign changes, respiratory congestion (bubbling) and breathing pattern changes (Karnes, 1986).

    7. There are several booklets available through hospice that are good to share with family members that help explain these changes and guide them through the process of the body shutting down.

J. The death vigil occurs when death is imminent. Family will often want to be constantly at the bedside during the hours to days before death. In some situations, however, they may be uncomfortable due to their own fears. Education and support to the family is important at this time.

    1. Common fears include:

        a. Fear of being alone with the patient.

        b. Fear that the patient will have a painful death and/or they will have to watch the patient suffer.

        c. Fear of being alone with the patient when he or she dies and that they will not know what to do.

        d. Fear that they will not know if the patient has died.

        e. Fear of giving the last dose of pain medication and hastening death.

    2. Nursing interventions include:

        a. Calming family fears, reassuring the family that the patient will be kept as comfortable as possible.

        b. Educating the family about the signs and symptoms of the dying process, death, what they should do if they suspect the patient has died, and that they should call the nurse for any questions they may have at any time.

        c. Intensive physical comfort care including mouth care, turning and positioning, and pain and symptom management.

        d. Offering spiritual comfort through presence, prayer, rites, and rituals.

        e. Honor cultural beliefs, traditions, rites, and rituals.

K. Telling the family that the patient has died should be done with sensitivity. Provide small amounts of information at the family's level of understanding. Information about the death may need to be repeated due to the family feeling overwhelmed or shocked by the actual death.

L. Signs of death include absence of heart beat or respirations, release of stool and urine, eyes remain open with fixed pupils, pale body color, body temperature drops, and jaw may fall open.

M. In order to pronounce the death, the nurse should know practice setting guidelines and state procedures for reporting suspicious or existing circumstances of a death. If the patient is an organ donor, follow the procedure, as planned.

N. Preparing the body after death:

    1. Removal all tubes, IVs, and medical supplies to provide a personal closure experience for the family, leaving the family with memories of the deceased as a loved one rather than a patient.

    2. Bathe and dress the body, placing dressings on leaking wounds and diaper for incontinence.

        a. Position the body in proper alignment,

place dentures in the mouth.
  b. Ask the family to assist if they want and to provide clothing if they prefer.
3. Be aware of cultural practices with preparing the body.
O. Time with the body and removal of the body should be appropriate to the family's need to say goodbye.
  1. Rigor mortis occurs 2 to 4 hours after death. After the body is positioned, air may escape lungs and those present may hear a sighing sound, similar to breathing. Alert the family to this possibility.
  2. At the time of removal of the body, ask the family if they have preferences to covering or uncovering the face and whether or not they want to be in the room when the body is actually removed.
P. The nurse may want to assist the family with phone calls. The nurse should be the one to contact physicians, co-workers, or other health care agencies involved.
Q. In a home setting, refer to local/state laws regarding destruction of patient medications. If the family asks the nurse to leave medications for them, the nurse should assess reasons/issues for the request. Offer to call the physician, as indicated, for an assessment of the survivor's issue/problem and/or to obtain a prescription unique to their needs.
R. Funeral arrangements are best completed prior to death, but that option is not always available. If the family requests, provide options to promote family choice.
S. Following the death, the nurse should initiate bereavement support by providing compassion, active listening, presence. In addition, the nurse should assess grief reactions and assess risk factors. For survivors who may need continued bereavement support, refer to community resources, such as hospice and support groups.
T. When a child dies, encourage the parents to hold the child. Wrap babies snugly in a blanket. Allow siblings to participate in rituals, traditions, and encourage life review.
U. The nurse may experience feelings of anxiety when caring for a dying patient, caring for a dead body, or supporting the family. Nurses grieve the loss of their patients and should not work in iso-

lation while providing care for an imminently dying patient. Post-clinical debriefings can assist the nurse in exploration and expression of feelings of loss and grief.

Advocating for Quality Care at EOL

A. Costs of EOL care.
  1. Patients admitted to hospitals today are more critically ill, their length of stay has decreased, and there is a massive increase in ambulatory services. There is a trend towards increased utilization of home care services as patients are discharged to the home and long-term care facilities with serious illnesses and multiple needs (Ferrell, 2000).
  2. The health care system is straining under the effects of rapid change. Certain managed care plan restrictions particularly affect people with advanced illness, such as:
    a. Limiting the scope of benefits to reduce costs.
    b. Financial incentives for practitioners and providers to provide less care.
    c. Patient services that require pre-authorization.
    d. Coverage for services provided only by designated physicians and health care providers.
  3. Increased costs and health care spending for EOL care are influenced by such factors as population growth, general inflation in the economy, and medical inflation. Efforts to control costs and reduce spending are placing increased pressure on Medicare, Medicaid, and Social Security programs.
    a. Medicare covers 83% of those who die each year who are 65 years or older and younger persons with disabilities and certain illnesses.
    b. Medicaid pays for a smaller portion of health care costs and larger portion of long-term care.
    c. Other sources include private insurance, veterans' benefits, and an ever-increasing load on out-of-pocket payments by patient/family.

4. Restrictions that limit access to EOL care are:
   a. Rules regarding eligibility.
   b. Tendency to discourage new enrollment or to continue enrollment of sicker individuals to certain health plans.
   c. Poor access for populations at risk: Elderly, pediatric patients, the homeless, and the uninsured.
   d. Delayed referral to hospice and palliative care programs.
5. Nurses must be conscious of financial costs as well as the burden of treatments and therapies on the patient/family.
6. Interdisciplinary teamwork extends to community resources. Early access of needed resources can significantly decrease stressor and the perception of burden, especially for patients/families that do not have extended family to assist the primary care giver.
7. Caring for the dying patient can exhaust a family's financial resources because of missed work and out-of-pocket medical costs. An increasing amount of payment for care has shifted to the patient/family. The inability to access services that allow patients to remain at home and instead turn to institutional care actually increases costs of care covered by private and public sources.
8. The death of the patient has typically not been seen as a positive outcome of care. Improving care at the EOL can be determined by measuring outcomes that reflect the positive outcomes of quality EOL closure. Strategies to reduce cost at EOL include (Field & Cassel, 1997):
   a. Attention to realistic outcomes of care.
   b. Better understanding and utilization of advanced directives.
   c. Increased use of hospice and palliative care services are strategies that can reduce costs at the end of life (Field & Cassel, 1997).

B. The nurse's role in improving care systems.
1. Nurses need to take an active role leading reform because current services and reliability are woefully inadequate.
2. Specific skills, attitudes, and behaviors are helpful in this work, and they must be learned and taught.
3. When the care system has especially serious shortcomings in serving its community, professionals have similarly strong obligations to correct those shortcomings.
4. The history of reform in EOL care has been dominated by nursing.
5. The aim of reform should be to provide a care system that can make the following seven promises to a patient who is at the EOL (Lynne, 2000).
   a. Good medical treatment.
   b. Never overwhelmed by symptoms.
   c. Continuity, coordination, and comprehensiveness.
   d. Well-prepared, no surprises.
   e. Use of patient and family resources.
   f. Make the most of every day.
6. Nurses, individually and collectively as a profession, play a vital role in improving care at the end of life.
   a. Nurses can encourage, contribute to, and collaborate with efforts to make transfers less frequent and less disruptive.
   b. Nurses can develop and implement standardized protocols and measures of success for populations.
   c. Nurses should be familiar with the settings that their EOL patients utilize including their personnel, practices and potentials (for example, the ambulatory care nurse could sit in on a hospice team meeting, visit the hospital, talk to the discharge nurse, etc.).

References

American Association of Colleges of Nursing (AACN) & the City of Hope National Medical Center. (2000). *The end-of-life nursing education consortium curriculum.* Washington, DC: Author.

American Nurses Association (ANA). (1995). *Position statement on comfort and relief of pain in dying patients.* Kansas City, MO: Author.

American Nurses Association (ANA). (2001). *Code of ethics for nurses with interpretive statements.* Kansas City, MO: Author.

American Pain Society (APS). (1999). *Principles of analgesic use in the treatment of acute pain and cancer pain* (4th ed.). Glenview, IL: Author.

Berry, P., & Griffie, J. (2001). Planning for the actual death. In B.R. Ferrell & N. Coyle (Eds.), *Textbook of palliative nursing* (pp. 382-396). New York, NY: Oxford University Press.

Byock, I. (1996). The nature of suffering and the nature of opportunity at the end of life. *Clinics in Geriatric Medicine, 12*(2), 237-251.

Byock, I. (1997). *Dying well: The prospects for growth at the end of life.* New York: Riverhead Books.

Corless, I.B. (2001). Bereavement. In B.R. Ferrell & N. Coyle (Eds.). *Textbook of palliative nursing* (pp. 352- 362). New York: Oxford University Press.

Coyle, N. (2001). Introduction to palliative nursing care. In B.R. Ferrell & N. Coyle (Eds.). *Textbook of Palliative Nursing* (pp. 3-6). New York: Oxford University Press.

Doka, K. (1989). *Disenfranchised grief: Recognizing hidden sorrow.* New York: Lexington Books.

Egan, K.A., & Labyak, M.J. (2001). Hospice care: A model for quality end-of-life care. In B.R. Ferrell & N. Coyle (Eds.). *Textbook of palliative nursing* (pp. 7-26). New York: Oxford University Press.

Emanuel, L.L., von Gunten, C.F., & Ferris, F.D. (Eds.). (1999). *The EPEC curriculum: Education for physicians on end-of-life care.* Retrieved April 30, 2006, from http://www.epec.net/EPEC/Webpages/Ecommerce/itemDetail.cfm?productID=74

Ferrell, B.R. (2000). Analysis of palliative care. *Journal of Palliative Care, 16*(1), 39-47.

Ferrell, B.R., & Coyle, N. (Eds.). (2001). *Textbook of palliative nursing.* New York: Oxford University Press.

Field, M.J., & Cassel, C.K. (Eds.). (1997). *Approaching death: Improving care at the end of life (Report of the Institute of Medicine Task Force).* Washington, DC: National Academy Press.

Highland, M.E.F. (2000). Providing spiritual care to patients with cancer. *Clinical Journal of Oncology Nursing, 4*(30), 115-120.

International Association for the Study of Pain (IASP). (1994). *IASP pain terminology.* Retrieved March 6, 2006, from http://www.iasp-pain.org/terms-p.html

Karnes, B. (1986). *Gone from my sight: The dying experience.* Stillwell, KS: Author.

Kazanowski, M. (2001). Symptom management in palliative care. In M. Matzo & W. Sherman (Eds.), *Palliative care nursing: Quality care to the end-of-life* (pp. 327-361). New York: Springer Publishing Company.

Koenig, B.A. (1997). Cultural diversity in decision-making about care at the end of life. In M.J. Field & C.K. Cassel (Eds.), *Approaching death: Improving care at the end of life* (pp. 363-382). Washington, DC: National Academy Press.

Kubler-Ross, E. (1969). *On death and dying.* New York: MacMillan.

Levy, M.H. (1996). Pharmacologic treatment of cancer pain. *The New England Journal of Medicine, 335*(15), 1124-1132.

Lindemann, E. (1994). Symptomatology and management of acute grief. *American Journal of Psychiatry, 151*(6 Sesquicenntenial Suppl.), 155-160.

Lynne, J. (2000). Sick to death and not going to take it anymore. Accelerating change today for America's health. *Promises to keep: Changing the way we provide end of life care.* Washington, DC: The National Coalition on Health Care, The Institute for Health Care Improvement.

Matzo, M.L., & Sherman, D.W. (Eds.). (2001). *Palliative care nursing: Quality care to the end of life.* New York: Springer Publishing Company.

McCaffery, M., & Pasero, C. (1999). *Pain: Clinical manual* (2nd ed.). St. Louis, MO: Mosby.

National Hospice and Palliative Care Organization (NHPSO). (2005). *Hospice fact sheet.* Alexandria, VA: Author.

O'Connor, C.I. (2001). Characteristics of spirituality, assessment, and prayer in holistic nursing. *Nursing Clinics of North America, 36*(1), 33-46.

Oregon Hospice Association (OHA). (2004). *Death with Dignity Act revisited.* Portland, OR: Satelitte Publishing.

Pasacreta, J., Minarik, P., & Nield-Anderson, L. (2001). Anxiety and depression. In B.R. Ferrell & N. Coyle (Eds.), *Textbook of palliative nursing* (pp. 269-289). New York: Oxford University Press.

Rando, T.A. (1984). *Grief, dying and death: Clinical interventions for caregivers.* Champaign, IL: Research Press Co.

Ray, M.C. (1992). *I'm here to help (a hospice worker's guide to communicating with dying people and their loved ones).* New York: Bantam Books.

Thorns, A., & Sykes, N. (2000). Opioid use in last week of life and implications for end-of-life decision-making. *Lancet, 356*(9227), 398-399.

Vichon, M.L.S. (2001). The nurse's role: The world of palliative care nursing. In B.R. Ferrell & N. Coyle (Eds.), *Textbook of palliative nursing* (pp. 647-662). New York: Oxford University Press.

Wolfelt, A. (1990). Bereavement and children: Adolescent mourning, a naturally complicated experience. Part II. *Bereavement Magazine,* March/April, 34-37.

World Health Organization. (1998). *Cancer pain relief and palliative care in children.* Geneva, Switzerland: Author.

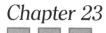
Care of the Terminally Ill Patient

This test may be copied for use by others.

COMPLETE THE FOLLOWING:

Name: _____

Address: _____

City: _____ State: _____ Zip: _____

Preferred telephone: (Home)_____ (Work)_____

E-mail_____

AAACN Member Expiration Date: _____

Registration fee: AAACN Member: $12.00
                   Nonmember: $20.00

Answer Form:

1. If you applied what you have learned from this activity into your practice, what would be different?

_____

_____

_____

Evaluation	Strongly disagree				Strongly agree
2. By completing this activity, I was able to meet the following objectives:					
a. Recognize the issues that are affecting End-of-Life (EOL) care in our country.	1	2	3	4	5
b. Identify appropriate pain interventions for terminal patients.	1	2	3	4	5
c. Identify appropriate symptom management measures which cross many terminal diseases.	1	2	3	4	5
d. Identify the ethical and legal issues patients, families, and caregivers must face.	1	2	3	4	5
e. Recognize the impact of a culturally diverse population in caring for the terminally ill.	1	2	3	4	5
f. Apply communication principles important to EOL care.	1	2	3	4	5
g. Identify key issues for care of the patient at the time of death.	1	2	3	4	5
h. Recognize the role of the nurse in advocating for quality of care at EOL.	1	2	3	4	5
3. The content was current and relevant.	1	2	3	4	5
4. The objectives could be achieved using the content provided.	1	2	3	4	5
5. This was an effective method to learn this content.	1	2	3	4	5
6. I am more confident in my abilities since completing this material.	1	2	3	4	5

7. The material was (check one) ___new ___review for me.

8. Time required to read this chapter: _____minutes

I verify that I have completed this activity: _____
                                              Signature

Comments: _____

_____

_____

Objectives

This educational activity is designed for nurses and other health care professionals who practice in ambulatory care. For those wishing to obtain CE credit, an evaluation follows. After studying the information presented in this offering, you will be able to:

1. Recognize the issues that are affecting End-of-Life (EOL) care in our country.
2. Identify appropriate pain interventions for terminal patients.
3. Identify appropriate symptom management measures which cross many terminal diseases.
4. Identify the ethical and legal issues patients, families, and caregivers must face.
5. Recognize the impact of a culturally diverse population in caring for the terminally ill.
6. Apply communication principles important to EOL care.
7. Identify key issues for care of the patient at the time of death.
8. Recognize the role of the nurse in advocating for quality of care at EOL.

Posttest Instructions

1. To receive continuing education credit for individual study after reading the article, complete the answer/evaluation form to the left.

2. Detach and send the answer/evaluation form along with a check or money order payable to the *American Academy of Ambulatory Care Nursing (AAACN)*, East Holly Avenue Box 56, Pitman, NJ 08071–0056.

3. Test returns must be postmarked by August 1, 2011. Upon completion of the answer/evaluation form, a certificate for **1.5** contact hour(s) will be awarded and sent to you. Should the material contained in this chapter become outdated prior to the above expiration date, AAACN reserves the right to withdraw this CE test.

This activity is co-provided by the *American Academy of Ambulatory Care Nursing (AAACN)* and Anthony J. Jannetti, Inc. (AJJ). AJJ is accredited as a provider of continuing nursing education by the American Nurses' Credentialing Center's Commission on Accreditation (ANCC-COA). AAACN is a provider approved by the California Board of Registered Nurses, provider number CEP 05336.

This article was reviewed and formatted for contact hour credit by Sally S. Russell, MN, CMSRN, AAACN Education Director; and Candia Baker Laughlin MS, RN, C, Editor.

Glossary

Absence Seizure – Resulting in brief loss of consciousness, usually 10 seconds or less, with the absence of hypertonicity or muscular contracture.

Accessibility of Care – Refers to the ease with which consumers can initiate interaction with a clinician about health problem/s; includes activities to eliminate barriers raised by geography, financing, culture, race, language, etc.

Accreditation Association for Ambulatory Health Care (AAAHC) – A private, non-profit agency that offers voluntary, peer-based review of the quality of health care services of ambulatory health organizations, including ambulatory and office-based surgery centers, managed care organizations, as well as Indian and student health centers, among others.

Advanced Cardiac Life Support (ACLS) – Protocols and algorithms created through the American Heart Association to provide guidelines for medical management of cardiac arrest and/or arrhythmia, respiratory arrest and/or respiratory support, and stroke.

Advance Directives – Allow competent adults to make certain kinds of health care decisions in advance of an acute (such as a car accident) or chronic (such as Alzheimer's or cancer) incapacity, thus ensuring that their wishes are respected even if they are unable to communicate them directly; three types are living wills, durable power of attorney for health care, and "DNR" ("Do Not Resuscitate" order).

Advocacy – Act or process of advocating or supporting (a cause or proposal) on behalf of another.

Ambulatory Care – Outpatient care in which patients stay less than 24 hours and are discharged to their normal residential situation after care.

Ambulatory Care Nursing – A specialty practice area that is characterized by nurses responding rapidly to high volumes of patients in a short span of time while dealing with issues that are not always predictable.

Americans with Disabilities Act (ADA) – Prohibits discrimination on the basis of disability in employment, state and local government, public accommodations, commercial facilities, transportation, and telecommunications.

Anaphylactoid Reaction – An allergic reaction induced by drug infusion: Anaphylactoid reactions are not caused by IgE.

Anaphylaxis – An allergic reaction caused by immune globulins "IgE" that affects whole body systems; can be fatal if not immediately treated.

APCs – Ambulatory Patient Classifications; used by the Center for Medicare and Medicaid Services for prospective payment in hospital outpatient departments and ambulatory surgery centers: based on procedures and adjusted for severity.

APGs – Ambulatory Patient Groups; patient classification system designed to explain amount and type of resource used in ambulatory care visit.

Assisted Suicide – A practice whereby a person other than the patient provides a means to a patient with the knowledge that a patient will use the means to commit suicide.

Asthma – Chronic inflammatory disorder of the airways; chronically inflamed airways are hyperresponsive to triggers, which can lead to acute asthma exacerbation; exposure to triggers contributes to an increased level of airway inflammation with edema, acute bronchoconstriction, and mucus plug production.

Asthma Action Plan – A written individualized asthma management/action plan that includes routine treatment, pre-exercise treatment, and a plan for emergency exacerbation.

Attention Deficit Hyperactivity Disorder (ADHD) – A persistent pattern of inattention and/or hyperactivity- impulsivity that is more frequently displayed and more severe than is typically observed in individuals at a comparable level of development.

Atypical Depression – Depression that is accompanied by unusual symptoms, such as hallucinations or delusions.

Aura – Subjective indication of oncoming seizure; patients may describe a change in vision, taste, or smell pursuant to the onset of seizure activity.

Automated External Defibrillator (AED) – Device delivering electrical joules in response to shockable cardiac arrhythmias utilizing ACLS protocol.

Autonomy – Self-determination; the freedom to choose one's course of action.

Balanced Scorecard – Graphic or pictorial display of the organization's indicators chosen to support the strategic plan and vision of the organization; allows for examination of relationships among the separate indicators (care, quality, financial, operational, etc.).

Basic Life Support (BLS) – Process of providing circulation and respiration through artificial means (for example, chest compressions and rescue breathing) in an organized, scientifically proven way in an effort to sustain life until advanced care can be provided.

Benchmarking – A continuous measurement of a process, product, or service in comparison to those of the toughest competitor, to those considered industry leaders, or to similar activities in the organization and using the information to change/improve practices, resulting in superior performance as determined by measured outcomes.

Beneficence – Doing good: requires defining what is meant by good in the situation.

Bereavement – Includes grief and mourning; the inner feelings and outward reactions of the survivor.

Body Mass Index (BMI) – Weight (kilograms) ÷ Height (meters)^2; or Weight (pounds) X 703 Height (inches)^2

Capitation – Method for funding expenses of enrollees in prepaid health plans; pays providers a fixed fee per member regardless of whether or not the service is provided; for example, a plan pays a per member per month (PMPM) amount to a physician group to provide primary care services for each enrollee in the plan.

Care Coordination – A process that seeks to achieve the optimal cost-effective use of scarce resources by helping individuals obtain health and appropriate social and life support services that meet the unique needs of individuals at a given point in time or across the life span.

Case Management – A collaborative process of assessment, planning, facilitation, and advocacy for option and services to meet an individual's health needs through communication and available resources to promote quality cost-effective outcomes; a method for managing the provision of health care to members/patients with catastrophic or high-cost medical conditions.

Centers for Medicare and Medicaid Services (CMS) – Formerly Health Care Financing Administration, or HCFA; division within the U.S. Department of Health and Human Services that determines the standard rules and reporting mechanisms for health care services.

Certification – Process that uses predetermined standards to validate and recognize an individual's knowledge, skills, and abilities in a defined functional and clinical area of specialty practice.

Certified Diabetes Educators – Registered nurse, registered dietitian, and other professionals with diabetes education experience who have passed the CDE examination.

Chronic Bronchitis – The presence of a productive cough for 3 months in each of 2 successive years in an individual whom other causes of chronic cough have been excluded.

Chronic Obstructive Pulmonary Disease (COPD) – Disease state characterized by airflow limitation that is not fully reversible: airflow limitation is usually progressive and associated with an abnormal inflammatory response of the lungs to noxious particles or gases.

Clinical Care Classification (CCC) – Formerly Home Health Care Classification (HHCC); Saba's Georgetown System for Patient Problems, Interventions, and Outcomes.

Clinical Practice Guidelines – Statements that have been systematically developed to assist practitioners and patients in making decisions about appropriate health care for specific clinical circumstances.

Cluster Headaches – Sharp, extremely painful headaches that tend to occur several times a day for months, then go away for a similar period of time; can occur after patient has fallen asleep, located near or above the eye, and associated with nasal congestion.

Collaboration – Working together toward a common goal; to pursue a common purpose and a sharing of knowledge to resolve problems, decide issues, and set goals within a structure of collegiality.

Commercial Indemnity Plans – A type of insurance contract in which the insurer pays for care received up to a fixed amount per encounter or episode of illness.

Competence – Having the ability to demonstrate the technical, critical thinking, and interpersonal skills necessary to perform one's job responsibilities.

Confidentiality – To protect the patient's and family's right to privacy regarding information that the nurse or institution holds about the patient.

Confusion – Disorientation, inappropriate behavior or communication, and/or hallucinations.

Copayment – Out-of-pocket expense paid by an individual for a specific service defined in the insurance plan.

Cost Benefit Analysis – A formal financial analysis completed by organizations to determine the cost of a program, projected revenues, and to identify and quantify program benefits; includes assumptions about specific expenses and potential revenue based on projected volumes.

CPT – *The Physicians' Current Procedural Terminology*, published by the American Medical Association; the internationally recognized coding system for reporting medical services and procedures.

Credentialing – Review and verification of credentials (education, training, licensure, certification, experience) of nurses. In some cases (such as most nursing homes and an increasing number of other health care facilities), this includes performing criminal background checks.

Cultural Competence – Requires developing cultural awareness (conscious learning process through which one becomes appreciative and sensitive to the cultures of other people), cultural knowledge (process of understanding the key aspects of a group's culture), cultural skill (ability to collect relevant data regarding health histories and perform culturally specific assessments), and cultural encounter (process that encourages one to engage directly in cross-cultural interactions with people from culturally-diverse backgrounds).

Decision Support Systems – Automated tool that enhances the nurse's ability to make decisions in semi-structured, uncertain situations by bringing necessary information, evidence, expertise, and resources to the point of care.

Deductible – Amount an insured individual is responsible to pay before insurance pays. For example, an individual may have a $200 deductible for hospitalization before the remainder of the hospital stay is covered.

Delegation – The transfer of responsibility for the performance of a task from one person to another.

Delirium – An acute change in cognition or awareness with agitation presenting as a symptom accompanying delirium.

Deontology – Also known as duty-based ethics; based on the belief that there are duties to which one must be faithful and which one is obligated to carry out because these duties are owed to all human beings and because of the expectations implied by one's professional role.

Depression (major) – Five or more symptoms of depression.

Diagnostic Related Groups (DRGs) – A system for classifying hospital inpatients into groups requiring similar quantities of resources according to characteristics such as diagnosis, age, procedure, complications, and comorbidities.

Dietary Approaches to Stop Hypertension (DASH) – Evidence-based eating plan that is low in saturated fat, cholesterol, and total fat; reduced consumption of red meats, sweets and sugar-containing beverages; concomitant emphasis on fruits, vegetables, and low-fat dairy products; rich in magnesium, calcium, protein, and fiber; sodium consumption is limited from 1,500 to 2,400 mg/day.

Distance Learning – Provides access to learning modalities initially designed to reach/include persons in rural/isolated areas, providing educational opportunities/resources.

Domain of Ambulatory Nursing Practice – The overall scope of nursing practice in the ambulatory arena; it includes attributes of the environment in which practice occurs, patient requirements for care, and specific nursing role dimensions.

Dyslipidemia – See *Hyperlipidemia*.

Dysthymia – Depression that is chronic in nature; milder than major depression, lasting up to two years.

Education Process – Systematic planned course of action consisting of two major interdependent operations: teaching and learning.

Emergency Medical Treatment and Active Labor Act (EMTALA) – Federal law passed in 1986 to ensure patient access to emergency services regardless of ability to pay.

Emotional Intelligence – Ability to accurately perceive one's own and others' emotions, to understand the signals that emotions send about the relationship, and to manage one's own and others' emotions.

Emphysema – The abnormal enlargement of airspaces distal to the terminal bronchioles with destruction of their walls without obvious fibrosis.

Environmental Management – The assurance of appropriate management plans to provide a safe, accessible, effective, and functional environment of care.

Epilepsy – Diagnosis for congenital or acquired brain disease resulting in seizure activity.

Equal Employment Opportunity Commission (EEOC) – A federal agency that enforces regulations concerning equal opportunity.

Ethics – A branch of philosophy dealing with the values related to human conduct, with respect to the rightness or wrongness of certain actions; and to the goodness and badness of the motives and ends of such actions; a set of moral principles or values, the principles of conduct governing an individual or a group.

Ethnopharmacology – Emerging field of research that is increasingly focusing on the effect of genetic and cultural factors on absorption, metabolism, distribution, and eliminations and the mechanism of action and effects of drugs.

Evidence-Based Practice – The conscientious, explicit, and judicious use of current best evidence in making decisions about the care of individual patients; combines research and clinical expertise.

Existential Distress – Occurs at a time when a person is questioning the meaning of his or her life. This response encompasses the physical, psychosocial, and spiritual angst that may occur at end of life.

Fee for Service – Reimbursement method in which payment is made for each service or item.

Fidelity – Faithfulness; involves duty owed to patients, families, and colleagues to do what one says.

Focal Seizure – Seizure activity initiating from one side of the brain; presentation of seizure activity is seen on the opposite side of the body; may or may not generalize to include both sides of the body.

Food Guide Pyramid (United States Department of Agriculture) – Provides a visual key to the proper dietary balance of the five food groups.

Grand mal seizure (Tonic-clonic seizure) – Increased neuronal activity in the brain with presenting loss of consciousness, muscle rigidity, involuntary muscular twitching, and incontinence.

Grief – The individualized feelings and responses that an individual makes to real, perceived, or anticipated loss.

Health Care Financing Administration (HCFA) – See *CMS*.

Health Care Financing Administration [HCFA] Common Procedure Coding System (HCPCS) – A uniform method for health care providers and medical suppliers to report professional services, procedures, and supplies to health care plans.

Health Care Team – Includes the patient, family, and other members of the health care system who are involved in the development and implementation of the care plan.

Health Insurance Privacy and Portability and Accountability Act (HIPAA) – Federal law establishes a "floor" for privacy protection and implementing privacy and security regulations; applies to all health plans, health care clearinghouses, and those health care providers (including nurses) who bill electronically for their services; basically provide that patients have a right to control their information and must "authorize" use or disclosure of their health information.

Health Maintenance Organization (HMO) – A health plan that uses physicians as gatekeepers. In this model the patient chooses a primary care provider (PCP) who is responsible for all aspects of care management and who must authorize (gatekeeper) or give permission for referral to other providers; another model of HMO places risk on the providers for medical expenses. In this instance, providers are encouraged to provide appropriate medical services but not medically unnecessary services in exchange for larger premiums.

Heart Failure – A complex clinical syndrome in which the cardiac myocytes or contractile apparatus of the heart does not pump enough blood to meet the needs of the tissues; peripheral perfusion is altered, leading to subsequent mechanical, neuro-endocrine, and inflammatory responses in an attempt to improve systemic organ flow; compensatory mechanisms fail to improve contractility over time and lead to a maladaptive state characterized by "ventricular remodeling."

HEDIS® – A set of standardized performance measures designed to assure that purchasers and consumers have the information they need to reliably compare the performance of health plans; sponsored and maintained by NCQA.

Hospice – Comprehensive services are provided by an interdisciplinary team wherever the patient is and include physicians, nurses, social workers, chaplains, counselors, certified nursing assistants, therapists, and volunteers.

Hyperlipidemia – An elevation of any lipid in blood plasma; increased levels of Low Density Lipoprotein (LDL) incorporate themselves into fatty plaque development on the intima wall of the blood vessel causing atherosclerotic changes, stiffening of the arteries and reducing blood flow to vital organs.

Hypertensive Emergency – Severe elevation of BP (>180/120 mm Hg) complicated by evidence of impending or progressive target organ dysfunction.

ICD 9-CM (*International Classification of Diseases,* 9th revision, Clinical Modification) – Published by the U.S. National Center for Health Statistics; the internationally recognized system for the purposes of international morbidity and mortality reporting; in the United States, used for coding and billing purposes.

Independent Practice Association (IPA) – A legal entity whose members are independent physicians who contract with the IPA for the purpose of having the IPA contract with one or more HMOs.

Informed Consent – Process by which a patient is provided relevant information about a proposed procedure, test, or course of treatment; given an opportunity to ask questions; and asked to voluntarily agree.

International Classification of Nursing (ICNP®) (International Council of Nursing [ICN]) – Combinatorial terminology for nursing practice that facilitates cross-mapping of local terms; represents nursing phenomena (diagnoses), nursing activities (interventions), and nursing outcomes that nurses use across the world in all settings of care.

Interstate Compacts – Allow that nurses may practice across state lines, physically or electronically, unless under discipline or a monitoring agreement that restricts interstate practice. Nurses are licensed where they live (the "home state").

Joint Commission on Accreditation of Healthcare Organizations (JCAHO) – An independent, not-for-profit organization, which evaluates and accredits more than 15,000 health care programs in the United States.

Justice – Fair, equitable distribution of resources.

Managed Care – A system that combines financing and care delivery through comprehensive benefits delivered by selected providers and financial incentives for enrolled members to use these providers: goals of managed care are quality, cost-effectiveness, and accessible health care. It is a coordinated system of health care, which achieves outcomes (reduced utilization and improved population health) through preventive care, case management, and the provision of medically necessary appropriate care.

Medicaid – A plan jointly funded by federal and state governments, introduced in 1966 to cover poor individuals; it is managed by each state.

Migraine Headache – Severe, recurrent headache with other symptoms, including visual changes, nausea and vomiting, and photophobia; starts on one side of the head and may spread to both sides; some may have an aura before onset; pain is described as throbbing, pounding, or pulsating.

Moderate Sedation – Use of medication resulting in amnesia and/or analgesia to sufficiently blunt but not remove a patient's protective reflexes in order to allow the performance of a procedure or test; patient should exhibit a state of reduced consciousness that allows the patient to tolerate unpleasant procedures while retaining the ability to independently and continuously maintain cardiorespiratory function and appropriately respond to physical stimulation and/or verbal commands.

Mourning – The outward, social expression of loss and is often dictated by cultural norms, customs, and practices including rituals and traditions; is also influenced by the individual's personality and life experiences.

NCQA – A not-for-profit, independent organization that assesses, evaluates, and publicly reports on the quality of health plans, health care provider groups, and individual physicians.

Nonmaleficence – Acting in such a way that avoids harm, either intentional harm or harm as an unintended outcome.

North American Nursing Diagnosis Association (NANDA) Nomenclature – Nursing diagnoses used by nurses to document nursing diagnoses in all settings where nursing care is delivered.

Nursing Informatics – A specialty that integrates nursing science, computer science, and information science to manage and communicate data, information, and knowledge in nursing practice.

Nursing Interventions Classification (NIC) – Taxonomy for classifying nursing interventions; used in all settings where care is delivered to document nursing interventions; developed by a team at University of Iowa lead by McCloskey and Bulechek.

Nursing Management Minimum Data Set (NMMDS) – Data set developed by Delaney and Hubner for use by managers in all nursing care settings; it contains 17 defined data elements that include environment, nurse resources, nursing care staff, and financial resources.

Nursing-Sensitive Outcomes – Changes in the actual or potential health status, behavior, or perceptions of individuals, families, or populations that can be attributed to nursing interventions provided.

Nursing Services – Organized services delivered to groups of patients by nursing staff; includes nursing care as well as services to support or facilitate direct care, such as referral and coordination of care.

Obesity – Body weight 120% of ideal; body mass index (BMI) equal to or greater than 27; or adipose deposition patterns.

Occupational Safety and Health Administration (OSHA) – Branch of U.S. Department of Labor responsible for enforcing laws and regulations on workplace safety.

Omaha VNA System– The Omaha VNA's system for problems, interventions, and outcomes; used by nurses to describe and document care in community settings; contains 40 nursing problems (diagnoses) and a number of associated nursing interventions and outcomes (composed of knowledge, behavior, and status subscales).

Orientation – A structured plan created by the organization to "on-board" new staff to provide smooth assimilation into a new position; key components include a general organizational overview, department specifics, and individualized job duties.

Osteoarthritis – Disease manifested by progressive degeneration of cartilage in joints; as cartilage becomes thin, bone ends come closer together, bone spurs develop at tendon and ligament attachment sites, synovial fluid may leak, and cysts may develop on the bone; also known as degenerative joint disease (DJD).

Otitis Externa – Infection of the ear canal.

Otitis Media – Infection occurring just behind the eardrum; presents as collection of fluid, bloody or purulent, visible by otoscope.

Out-of-Pocket Expense – Refers to the portion of health care cost for which the individual is responsible.

Ozbolt's Patient Care Data Set (PCDS) – Taxonomy used by nurses to document care in all settings, but primarily developed for the acute care setting comprises nursing diagnoses, patient care actions, and nursing outcomes.

Pain – An unpleasant sensory and emotional experience associated with actual or potential tissue damage, or described in terms of such damage.

Palliative Care – Both a philosophy of care and an organized, highly structured system for delivery of care whose goal is to prevent and relieve suffering and to support the best possible quality of life for patients and their families, regardless of the stage of the disease or the need for other therapies.

Patient Education – Process of assisting people to learn health-related behaviors (knowledge, skills, attitudes, and values) so they can incorporate them into their everyday lives.

Pediatric Advanced Life Support (PALS) – Protocols and algorithms created through the American Heart Association to provide guidelines for medical management of potentially fatal health conditions in the pediatric population, and to provide guidelines for medical management of cardiac arrest and/or arrhythmia and respiratory arrest and/or respiratory support.

Peer Review – Process of reviewing and assessing the clinical competence and conduct of health professionals on an ongoing basis; an integral part of quality assessment and improvement processes.

Performance Improvement – Systematic analysis of the structure, processes, and outcomes within systems for the purpose if improving the delivery of care.

Perfusion – Tissues in the body exchanging metabolic waste (carbon dioxide) and receiving oxygen through arterial/venous circulation.

Perioperative Nursing Data Set (PNDS) – Developed by the Association of Operating Room Nurses; used by perioperative registered nurses and surgical service managers in a variety of perioperative settings.

Physician Hospital Organization (PHO) – Legal organization often developed for purposes of contracting with managed care plans; links physicians to specific hospitals for hospitalization care.

Point of Service (POS) – A plan that defines service providers in the service area outside of the usual preferred provider network.

Polypharmacy – Involves clients with one or more conditions who are using multiple medications, some of which are not clinically indicated.

Post-ictal Period – Time after a seizure for which the client may present with confusion and lethargy.

Postpartum Depression – Feeling of sadness or "blue mood" after delivery; usually induced by hormonal changes.

Precertification – Process of obtaining authorization or certification from a health plan for routine hospital admissions, referrals, procedures, or tests.

Preferred Provider Organization (PPO) – Program in which contracts exist between the health plan and care providers at a discount for services; typically, the plan provides incentives for patients to use in-network providers as opposed to nonparticipating providers (independent/noncontracted) through decreased co-payments.

Premenstrual Dysphoric Disorder – Feeling of depression with onset one week prior to Menses; after onset of menstruation, symptoms resolve.

Presence – Effective listening; occurs at 5 different levels: hearing, understanding, retaining information, analyzing and evaluating information, and helping/active empathizing.

Priapism – Sustained, unwanted, and painful penile erection usually unrelated to sexual activity, due to vaso-occlusion causing obstruction of the venous drainage of the penis.

Primary Care – The provision of integrated, accessible health care services by clinicians who are accountable for addressing a large majority of *personal* health care needs, developing a sustained partnership with patients, and practicing in the context of family and community.

Primary Prevention – Includes health promotion (HP) interventions and specific protections (SP); may be directed at individuals, groups, or populations; targeted at well populations or those already ill (for example, HP = nutrition education; SP = use of seat belts, avoidance of allergans, or inoculations).

Productivity – Measure of the efficiency with which labor and materials are converted into service or care; volume of output related to amount of resources consumes/used to produce a specified output/services.

Rebound Headache – Occurs after taking medication for pain relief of headaches has been taken away; reintroducing the pain reliever does not decrease pain.

Relative Value Unit (RVU) – Established by HCFA/CMS to approximate the work, practice expense, and malpractice expense for delivery of physician services.

Report Cards – Identify performance measures that include quality indicators (immunization, Pap smear, and mammogram rates), utilization indicators (membership, access, finances, hospital, and ER admission), and satisfaction levels; consumers use report card data to compare the performance of different organizations against a predetermined standard/best practice.

Research Utilization – A process of using research findings as a basis for practice; typically based on a single study.

Resource-Based Relative Value System (RBRVS) – A classification system that attempts to assign within a defined setting the resource requirements based on weights according to relative cost of each service.

Respiratory Arrest – Lung tissue is not able to receive carbon dioxide or give oxygen to circulating blood.

Risk Management – An organization-wide program to identify risks, control occurrences, prevent damage, and control legal liability; a process whereby risks to an institution are evaluated and controlled.

Root Cause Analysis – A method to determine the fundamental reason that causes variation in performance.

Seasonal Affective Disorder – Feeling of depression that ensues during the autumn and winter months due to decreased length of sunlight.

Secondary Prevention – Involves early diagnosis and prompt treatment to avoid disability (for example, screening, biopsies, medication, surgery).

Seizure – Increased neuronal activity in the brain caused by disease process or trauma leading to hypertonicity and muscular contracture.

Sickle Cell Disease – An autosomal recessive disorder characterized by the production of abnormal hemoglobin causing a decrease in red blood cell survival and polymerization of red blood cell (sickling).

SNOMED-CT® – Systematic Nomenclature for Medicine-Reference Terminology (College American Pathology) comprehensive, multiaxial nomenclature classification system created for the indexing of the entire medical and health care vocabulary.

Splenic Sequestration – Intrasplenic trapping of red blood cells which cause a precipitous fall in hemoglobin level and the potential for hypoxic shock.

Standard – An authoritative statement developed and disseminated by a professional organization or governmental or regulatory agency by which the quality of practice, services, research, or education can be judged.

State Practice Acts – A combination of laws and regulations that define and regulate practice of medicine, nursing, and other health professions.

Status Epilepticus – Increased neuronal activity in the brain resulting in seizure activity that continues for more than 10 minutes; considered a medical emergency.

Strategic Planning – The continuous process of systematically evaluating the nature of the ambulatory care organization, defining its long-term objectives, identifying quantifiable goals, developing strategies to reach these objectives and goals, and allocating resources to carry out these strategies.

Supervision – The direction and oversight of the performance of others.

Telehealth – Delivery, management, and coordination of health services that integrate electronic information and telecommunications technologies to increase access, improve outcomes, and contain or reduce costs of health care.

Telehealth Nursing – Delivery, management, and coordination of care and services provided via telecommunications technology within the domain of nursing; encompassing practices that incorporate a vast array of telecommunications technologies (telephone, fax, electronic mail, Internet, video monitoring, and interactive video) to remove time and distance barriers for the delivery of nursing care.

Telephone Nursing – All care and services within the scope of nursing practice that are delivered over the telephone; component of telehealth nursing practice restricted to the telephone.

Telephone Triage – An interactive process between the nurse and patient that occurs over the telephone and involves identifying the nature and urgency of client health care needs and determining the appropriate disposition; a component of telephone nursing practice that focuses on assessment and prioritization and referral to the appropriate level of care.

Tension Headache – Caused by tight, contracted muscles in shoulders, neck, scalp, and jaw; brought on by stress, depression, anxiety, overwork, lack of sleep, not eating properly, and/or alcohol or drug use.

Tertiary Prevention – Involves rehabilitation to return to maximum use of remaining capacities (such as maximizing functional status of the COPD patient with pulmonary toilet and oxygen administration).

TriCare – A federal program providing coverage to families of active duty military personnel, military retirees, spouses, and dependents which replaced CHAMPUS (Civilian Health and Medical Program of the United States).

Type 1 Diabetes – Onset usually acute with pronounced symptoms: autoimmune disease characterized by loss of pancreatic beta cell function; insulin required in a regimen designed for the individual in a way that imitates non-diabetes insulin production.

Type 2 Diabetes – Onset usually gradual, with or without symptoms in those with family history of type 2 diabetes, and other risk factors; insulin production at onset may be normal or elevated, but insulin resistance, elevated liver production of glucose, and other factors may prevent insulin from functioning normally; treatment includes healthy eating, exercise, oral medications, and/or insulin to control blood glucose levels.

Usual, Customary, and Reasonable (UCR) – A method used to determine if a fee is usual, customary, and reasonable; customary based on a percentile of aggregated fees charged in the geographic area for the same service; usual refers to fees normally charged by a doctor or health care provider for a service.

Utilitarianism – Also known as consequence-based ethics; the theory that seeks to choose the thing that will offer the most good to the greatest number of people, increase pleasure, and avoid pain.

Utilization Management – The second process of care coordination across the continuum of care; the management and evaluation of the medical necessity, appropriateness, and efficiency of the use of health care services, procedures, and facilities under the auspices of the applicable health benefit plan.

Ventilation – Mechanism by which the blood gives off carbon dioxide and takes on oxygen in the lungs.

Ventricular Fibrillation – Fatal heart arrhythmia that results in pulselessness; ventricles contract in an unorganized manner resembling a quiver and produce no cardiac output.

Ventricular Tachycardia – Fatal heart arrhythmia with wide QRS complexes; not necessarily resulting in pulselessness initially; rapid rate of ventricular contraction inhibits adequate blood filling and decreased cardiac output.

Veracity – Truth telling.

* Definitions taken from text.

Index

C

AAACN Education Resources

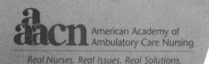

American Academy of Ambulatory Care Nursing

Real Nurses. Real Issues. Real Solutions.

Education Resources

Are you looking for great ideas for nurse staffing?

AAACN has developed an excellent springboard for you to find *the best staffing model for your ambulatory setting.*

Ambulatory Care Nurse Staffing: An Annotated Bibliography

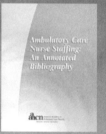

Product #P043
Member: $29
Non-Member: $34

The bibliography is just what you need to:
- Assess and plan your staffing needs
- Evaluate your staff's workload
- Adjust staffing mix
- Plan for new nursing positions
- Support staffing changes to management and prepare reports
- Design evidence-based research studies

Contents

Over 75 references:
A comprehensive summary of landmark articles, from classic to current, on nurse staffing.

Focus areas
- Scope and dimension of ambulatory care nursing practice
- Ambulatory care nursing workload, nursing intensity, and patient classification
- Ambulatory care nurse staffing

Orienting your staff has just become easier!

AAACN's guide helps you develop a customized orientation process for new employees based on specific competencies.

Guide to Ambulatory Care Nursing Orientation & Competency Assessment

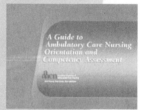

Product #P044
Member: $59
Non-Member: $69

- *No more guess work!* Select the competencies you need to match with a staff member's duties.
- *Better staff understanding!* Fundamental competencies are fully defined, so staff members know exactly what is expected regarding professional performance.
- *Improved outcomes!* Develop competencies based on ambulatory care practice standards to help enhance patient care.

The orientation and competency assessment guide incorporates the three roles of ambulatory care nursing practice:
- Organizational/Systems
- Clinical Nurse
- Professional Nurse

The competencies are designed for Registered Nurses, and can be easily adapted for Licensed Vocational/Practical nurses and other staff.

Do you need help starting or improving your telehealth services?

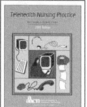

Product #P040V06
Member: $19
Non-Member $24

Telehealth Nursing Practice Resource Directory, *2006 Edition*

The 2006 edition of the Telehealth Nursing Practice Resource Directory contains a current and relevant listing of resource information for use by healthcare providers that will help improve the quality, efficiency and effectiveness of your telehealth practice. If you are looking for Professional Standards, Decision Support and Practice Support Tools, Textbooks, Articles, Standard Reference Works, Web sites, Newsletters, Continuing Education, Associations & Organization Consultants, or Outsourced Call Center Services, this guide can help you locate the resources you need.

P.O. Box 56, Pitman, NJ 08071-0056 • 800-AMB-NURS, Fax: 856-589-7463
Order on our Web site: www.aaacn.org • Email: aaacn@ajj.com • *Join AAACN when you order and receive member prices!*

* Prices as of this printing are subject to change without notice.

TELEHEALTH RESOURCES

Telehealth Nursing Practice Core Course CD-ROM

Earn 9.1 contact hours

The CD-ROM has been updated to reflect current practices and terminology. The CD also includes the course hand-outs. If you are a telehealth nurse or have staff who are providing patient care via the telephone in any setting, this course is a great way to orient nurses new to the role of telehealth practice, enhance knowledge of telehealth practice, provide staff education and training in telehealth.

Product #P041V05

Member: $119.00   Non-Member: $159.00

Telehealth Nursing Practice Core Course (TNPCC) Manual, 2nd Edition, 2003

Earn 20 contact hours

The TNPCC manual focuses on the essential competencies associated with delivering nursing care to patients via telecommunications technologies. This manual was developed by telehealth experts. Use this manual to orient nurses new to the role of telehealth practice, enhance knowledge of telehealth practice, and provide staff education and training in telehealth.

Product #P041V03

Member: $69.00   Non-Member: $79.00

Certification in Telephone Nursing Practice

Certification in telephone nursing practice is offered through the National Certification Corporation (NCC), 312-951-0207 or www.nccnet.org

---

Ambulatory nurses are everywhere caring for you PRODUCTS

Tote Bag
Green and white expandable tote with adjustable straps and outside pocket.
Product #P051
Price: $6.00

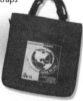

Logo Pin
Wear this pin proudly to show your commitment to excellence in ambulatory care through your membership in AAACN.
Product #P050
Price: $9.00

Twist Action Pen
Twist action pen is green with gold slogan.
Product #P052
Price: $4.00

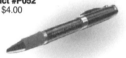

Stainless Steel Travel Mug
16 oz. Green Acrylic Travel Mug with slogan. Stainless steel interior keeps coffee extra hot. Gift box included.
Product #P054
Price: $6.00

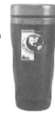

Post It Note Cube
Cube contains 285 – 2 3/4" x 2 3/4" sheets with green imprint on post its and sides of cube.
Product #P053
Price: $6.00

SUBSCRIPTION

Viewpoint Newsletter
(free with membership) Institutional subscription published bi-monthly. Each issue contains a CE article.
Product #NL - $80 per year

CD-ROMS

EARN 1.5 Contact Hours

Audio seminar CDs provide current information on hot topics. Each CD offers 1.5 contact hours and contains the slides/materials used during the live seminar.

Member: $109.00   Non-Member: $139.00

Visit our Web site: www.aaacn.org for the CD-ROM topics recorded monthly during each live audio seminar.

A complete 2005 **annual conference** CD-ROM or individual session audio CDs are available at www.netsymposium.com or call Digitell at 800-679-3646.

"Telephone Triage book for CEU is excellent."
Anna Doremus, RN, BSN, MSA, Jacobstown, NJ

3 Easy Ways to order from AAACN

ONLINE at:
www.aaacn.org

FAX with credit card information to: 856-218-0557

MAIL with payment to:
American Academy of Ambulatory Care Nursing
East Holly Avenue/Box 56
Pitman, NJ 08071-0056

Join below and receive member prices • Prepayment required • Sorry, no phone orders

QUANTITY	PRODUCT #	ITEM DESCRIPTION	PRICE	TOTAL

Name _____

Shipping Address ☐ home ☐ work

Facility Name

City _____ State _____ Zip _____

☐ home
Preferred Phone ☐ work _____

E-mail address _____

Method of Payment: ☐ Check ☐ Cash ☐ Credit Card

__ American Express __ Mastercard __ Visa Exp. Date _____

Account # __ __ __ __ - __ __ __ __ - __ __ __ __ - __ __ __ __

Name on card _____

Signature _____

Credit card billing address if different from shipping address _____

TAX ID: 51-023 1130
DUNs: 209739138

A credit coupon will be issued for overpayments under $15

P06I

	Subtotal	
	Shipping Total	
	Join AAACN Today	
	GRAND TOTAL	

Order Total	UPS Ground	UPS 2nd Day Air
Up to $24	$4	$12
$25 - $49	$6	$14
$50 - $99	$9	$16
$100 - $149	$11	$19
$150 - $199	$15	$24
$200 - $299	$20	$27
$300 - $500	$23	$30

Canadian orders
☐ Add 25% of subtotal for UPS Standard
☐ Add 25% of subtotal for Airmail Parcel Post
International Orders, except Canada
☐ Add 25% of subtotal for Airmail Parcel Post

AAACN Membership Application
Categories of Membership

☐ **Active (RN)** $130
Available to any registered nurse.

☐ **Affiliate** $105
Professional interested in ambulatory care nursing.

☐ **LPN/LVN** $105

☐ **Senior** $70
Active member for 3 years and reached age 62.

☐ **Student** $70
Course of study for initial licensure - enclose proof of enrollment.

Membership Fee Dues and contributions are not deductible as a charitable organization, but may qualify as a business expense. Membership year is January 1 – December 31. After you complete your first year of membership, you will be cycled into the group membership year. Your dues for the second year will be prorated accordingly.

Please circle one answer for each question.

1. Position
(1) Administrator/Director
(2) Manager/Supervisor
(3) Staff Nurse/Clinical Practitioner
(4) Educator
(5) Researcher
(6) Nurse Practitioner
(7) Consultant
(8) Other _____

2. Practice Setting
(1) University Hospital
(2) Group Practice/Health Center
(3) Community/Private Hospital
(4) Managed Care/HMO/PPO
(5) Military
(6) Free Standing Facility
(7) University/College/ Educational Institution
(8) Public Sector/Community Health Center/Public Health
(9) Other _____

3. Highest Level of Education Completed
(1) LPN/LVN
(2) Diploma—Nursing
(3) Associate Degree—Nursing
(4) Associate Degree—Other
(5) Bachelor's Degree—Nursing
(6) Bachelor's Degree—Other
(7) Master's Degree—Nursing
(8) Master's Degree—Other
(9) Doctorate Degree, Nursing
(A) Doctorate Degree, Other

4. If you are involved in clinical care, please circle the area that best describes your practice.
(1) Family Practice
(2) Internal Medicine
(3) Pediatrics
(4) Behavioral Health
(5) Obstetrics/Gynecology
(6) General Surgery
(7) Oncology
(8) Orthopaedics/Rehabilitation
(9) Ambulatory Surgery

(A) Telehealth
(B) Primary Care
(C) Medical Specialties
(D) Surgical Specialties
(E) Multispecialty Clinic
(F) Other _____

5. If you are in an administrative/ managerial position, please check ONE area that best describes your area of responsibility.
(1) Physician Group Office Practice/Primary Care
(2) Hospital-based Emergency Services
(3) Urgent/Immediate Care Center
(4) Ambulatory Surgery
(5) Community/Public Health
(6) Employee/Occupational Health
(7) Specialty/Sub-specialty Physician Practice
(8) Oncology Clinic
(9) Triage
(A) Rehabilitation Outpatient
(B) Nurse-Managed Center

(C) Patient Education
(D) Staff Education
(E) Information Management

6. Are you Certified?
(1) Ambulatory Nursing ANCC
(2) Telehealth NCC
(3) Both

7. Choose membership in one special interest group (SIG).
(1) Pediatrics
(2) Telehealth Nursing Practice
(3) Staff Development
(4) Veterans Affairs
(5) Tri-Service Military
(6) Leadership
(7) Patient Education

8. Salary (Confidential)
(1) Less than $25,000
(2) $25,000 - $44,999
(3) $45,000 - $64,999
(4) $65,000 - $84,999
(5) $85,000 - $105,000
(6) more than $105,000

9. Select the journal you would like to receive as part of your membership benefits.
☐ NEC - Nursing Economic$
☐ DNJ - Dermatology Nursing
☐ PED - Pediatric Nursing
☐ MSJ - MEDSURG Nursing

10. How did you hear about AAACN?
(1) A member
(2) Web site
(3) Viewpoint
(4) Colleague
(5) AAACN Conference
(6) Another Conference
(7) AAACN Enews
(8) Certification organization

Date of birth _____

Who referred you to AAACN? _____

☐ AAACN occasionally makes available its members' information to organizations and vendors that provide products and services of value to the ambulatory care nursing community. If you prefer not to be included in these lists, please check the box provided.

M06I   AJJ-0306-R-25C